ANNALS OF THE NEW YORK ACADEMY OF SCIENCES

Volume 725

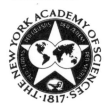

EDITORIAL STAFF

Executive Editor
BILL M. BOLAND

Managing Editor
JUSTINE CULLINAN

Associate Editor
TRUMBULL ROGERS

The New York Academy of Sciences
2 East 63rd Street
New York, New York 10021

CELLS AND CYTOKINES IN LUNG INFLAMMATION

ANNALS OF THE NEW YORK ACADEMY OF SCIENCES
Volume 725

CELLS AND CYTOKINES IN LUNG INFLAMMATION

Edited by Michel Chignard, Marina Pretolani, Patricia Renesto,
and B. Boris Vargaftig

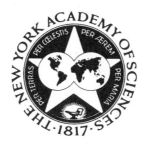

The New York Academy of Sciences
New York, New York
1994

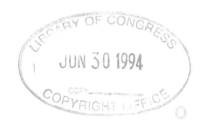
Cover: Photomicrograph showing in pink the staining of T-lymphocytes migrating to the bronchial submucosa and epithelium of an allergen-challenged guinea pig. Kindly provided by Dr. José Roberto Lapa e Silva, Universidade Federal do Rio de Janeiro, Brazil.

Library of Congress Cataloging-in-Publication Data

Cells and cytokines in lung inflammation / edited by Michel Chignard . . . [et al.].
        p.   cm. — (Annals of the New York Academy of Sciences, 0077-8923   ;   ISSN v. 725)
    Includes bibliographical references and index.
    ISBN 0-89766-855-3 (cloth : alk. paper). — ISBN 0-89766-856-1 (pbk. : alk. paper)
        1. Pneumonia—Pathophysiology—Congresses.   2. Cytokines—Pathophysiology—Congresses.   3. Inflammation—Mediators—Congresses.
    4. Respiratory epithelium—Congresses.   I. Chignard, Michel.   II. Series.
        [DNLM: 1. Respiratory System—immunology—congresses.   2. Lung—physiopathology—congresses.   3. Pneumonia—physiopathology—congresses.
    4. Pneumonia—immunology—congresses.   5. Imunity, Cellular—congresses.
    6. Cytokines—immunology—congresses.   W1 AN626YL v. 725 1994 / WF 140
    C393 1994]
    Q11.N5 vol. 725
    [RC771]
    616.2'407—dc20
    DNLM/DLC   94-18939
    for Library of Congress   CIP

BiComp/PCP
Printed in the United States of America
ISBN 0-89766-855-3 (cloth)
ISBN 0-89766-856-1 (paper)
ISSN 0077-8923

ANNALS OF THE NEW YORK ACADEMY OF SCIENCES
Volume 725
May 28, 1994

CELLS AND CYTOKINES IN LUNG INFLAMMATION[a]

Editors
MICHEL CHIGNARD, MARINA PRETOLANI, PATRICIA RENESTO,
AND B. BORIS VARGAFTIG

Conference Organizers
M. CHIGNARD, M. PRETOLANI, P. RENESTO, AND B. B. VARGAFTIG

Advisory Committee
M. K. CHURCH, PH. GODARD, P. M. HENSON, S. T. HOLGATE, L. G. LETTS,
R. MOQBEL, A. TONNEL, AND B. B. VARGAFTIG

CONTENTS

[a] The papers in this volume were presented at the 1993 Conference on Cells and Cytokines in Lung Inflammation, held in Paris, France, at the Institut Pasteur from June 24 to 25, 1993.

Part 6: Chronic Airway Inflammation and Lung Injury

Part 7: Perspectives and Pharmacological Approaches

Financial assistance was received from:

Major funder
- INSTITUT PASTEUR

Supporters
- INSTITUT DE RECHERCHES INTERNATIONALES SERVIER
- LABORATOIRES GLAXO
- LABORATOIRES SQUIBB
- PIERRE FABRE MÉDICAMENTS
- RHÔNE-POULENC RORER
- SCHERING-PLOUGH RESEARCH INSTITUTE

Contributors
- AMERSHAM FRANCE
- CIBA-GEIGY
- CLINISCIENCE
- DOMPÉ FARMACEUTICI
- EUROMEDEX
- ICI PHARMACEUTICALS GROUP
- IMMUNOTECH
- MERCK & CO., INC., U.S.A.—RESEARCH LABORATORIES
- MERCK FROSST CANADA—CENTRE FOR THERAPEUTIC RESEARCH, CANADA
- PFIZER
- SMITH KLINE BEECHAM LABORATORIES PHARMACEUTIQUES
- SMITH KLINE BEECHAM PHARMACEUTICALS
- THE WELLCOME FOUNDATION LTD.

Preface

B. BORIS VARGAFTIG

Unité de Pharmacologie Cellulaire
Unité Associée IP/INSERM 285
Institut Pasteur
25, Rue du Dr. Roux
75724 Paris cedex 15
France

Lungs are becoming fashionable. They not only ensure gas exchanges, their primary function, but are also recognized as a site of metabolism for mediators, hormones, and xenobiotics, as a source of other mediators and of cytokines, and as a target for circulating or locally generated hormones. They fully participate in homeostasis. Lungs are also becoming fashionable for medical and social reasons: they are involved directly or indirectly by new or revived diseases, including AIDS, new forms of infections (infections brought by the increased age pyramid in industrial countries, tuberculosis, pneumonia by *P. carinii*), diseases originating from or aggravated by the deterioration of the environment, including asthma, and diseases originating from smoking. Acute respiratory problems are initiated by trauma or sepsis, and seem to have maintained the same mortality for a long time. On the other hand, cytokines have also become fashionable, particularly because of the astonishing progress of molecular biology and because of the recognition of their involvement in diseases. The growing extension of interest in lungs and cytokines led to a situation that is reminiscent of that of Monsieur Jourdain, the bumptious character in the play *Le bourgeois gentilhomme,* written in 1670 by Molière (1622–1673). Indeed, Monsieur Jourdain wanted to become a poet and was very surprised when told that anyone can speak and write either "poetry" or "prose," and that he had spoken "prose" since he was a child. By analogy, many scientists are non-self-aware "pneumologists," since they work on themes involving the lungs, even though they may not recognize that they do.

This explains the interest raised by the meeting held at the Institut Pasteur in June 1993, under the title "Cytokines and Cells in Lung Inflammation," from which selected contributions were drawn for inclusion in the present volume. We hope that this will start a tradition of similar meetings, adapting the scientific programs to progress in the field, to the discovery of new cytokines and cell networks, and to the recognition of new pathologies involving those apparently dissimilar topics.

Role of T Cells and T-Cell-Derived Cytokines in the Pathogenesis of Allergic Diseases

E. MAGGI AND S. ROMAGNANI

Clinical Immunology Department
Institute of Clinica Medica III
University of Florence
50134 Florence, Italy

INTRODUCTION

The interaction between environmental allergens and the immune system is critical to the development of human allergy. This interaction is presumably initiated by uptake and presentation of allergens by MHC class II-positive accessory cells to helper T (Th) lymphocytes. Activated Th cells then induce B lymphocytes to produce allergen-specific antibodies, mainly belonging to the IgE class. However, the origin of the preferential IgE antibody production in individuals genetically determined to recognize allergen epitopes is still unclear. In the last few years a great deal of progress in the knowledge of the cellular and molecular signals responsible for IgE antibody synthesis and for the induction of allergic inflammation has been achieved. There is a general consensus that T-cell-derived interleukin-4 (IL-4) and interferon-γ (IFN-γ) are the main regulatory cytokines of IgE production, with opposite effects. Their pathophysiological role in atopy has clearly been established by both *in vitro* and *in vivo* studies. Convincing evidence is also accumulating to suggest that Th lymphocyte subsets producing IL-4 and IL-5, but not of limited amounts of IFN-γ, accumulate in the blood and/or target organs of patients with helminth infections or atopic disorders. These cells can account for the IgE antibody formation and eosinophilia observed in these patients. Both the presence of T cells at sites of allergic inflammation and the recruitment of T cells in disease models suggest that T cells are involved in the local expression of allergic inflammation.[1–5]

In this paper we describe the mechanisms involved in the regulation of human IgE synthesis; then we analyze the functional characteristics of Th1 and Th2 response and how allergens selectively expand T cells with Th2 profile. Finally, the cytokine profile of T cells infiltrating the target organs of allergic inflammation and the modulatory signals able to inhibit the Th2 response in allergic patients are examined.

MECHANISMS INVOLVED IN THE INDUCTION AND REGULATION OF HUMAN IgE SYNTHESIS

A reciprocal role of IL-4 and IFN-γ-producing CD4+ Th cell subsets in the regulation of human IgE synthesis was first provided in our laboratory by assessing the activity of large numbers of T-cell clones (TCC) derived from different lymphoid organs. When TCC or their supernatants were checked for their ability to induce the synthesis of IgE and to produce IL-2, IL-4, and IFN-γ, a significant positive correlation between helper function for IgE and production of IL-4 was found.[6] In contrast, there was a significant inverse correlation between the IgE helper activity of TCC and their ability to produce IFN-γ.[6] The opposite regulatory role of IL-4 and IFN-γ in the synthesis of human IgE was confirmed by the observations that recombinant IL-4, as well as IL-13, can induce the synthesis of IgE in peripheral blood mononuclear cell, and this effect is inhibited by addition of recombinant IFN-γ, IFN-α, IL-12, PGE2.[6-8]

The activity of IL-4 alone, however, is not sufficient for the induction of human IgE synthesis. Both recombinant IL-4 and IL-4-containing supernatants are consistently ineffective in inducing IgE synthesis by highly purified B cells.[9] Direct evidence that physical interaction between T and B cells is required for IL-4-dependent IgE synthesis was provided by double-chamber system experiments in which T and B cells were separated by a millipore membrane permeable to molecules but not to cells. In this system, IgE synthesis occurs only when T and B cells are cultured in the same chamber.[9] Several data have confirmed our first observations that IgE synthesis is dependent on two main signals delivered by CD4+ T cells to B cells: the first signal is due to soluble T-cell factors such as IL-4 and IL-13, acting on the same receptor and inducing on B cells a sterile ε-germ line transcript. The second signal (leading to a productive ε-transcript) is mediated by T–B cell-to-cell, MHC class II-unrestricted physical contact mainly due to the interaction between CD40L (on activated T cells) and CD40 molecules (on B cells).[10] Very recently it has been described that also mast cells or basophils, through CD40L molecule on their surface and IL-4 production, can directly support the two signals for IgE synthesis by B cells.[11] Other molecule(s), however, are certainly involved in such noncognate activation signal; membrane TNF-α (on T cells)–TNF-α receptor (on B cells) interaction, EBV infection of B cells, and corticosteroids can mimic the *in vitro* effect of CD40L–CD40 signal.[12-14] All these findings strongly suggest that Th cells and mainly those displaying peculiar cytokine pattern, play a central role in mechanisms of induction and regulation of human IgE synthesis and, more importantly, as we will see later, also in the pathogenesis of allergic disorders.

FUNCTIONAL PROPERTIES OF HUMAN Th1 AND Th2 CELLS

In recent years it has become clear that T helper (Th) lymphocytes, which are required for both cell-mediated and humoral immune responses, are composed by distinct subsets distinguished by different patterns of cytokine production. In the murine system, CD4+ T cells can be subdivided into at least two main groups coded as Th1 and Th2, differing in their cytokine profile. The initial observation by Mosman *et al.*[15] that repeated stimulation of murine CD4+ T helper (Th) lymphocytes *in vitro* with given antigens results in the development of a restricted and stereotyped pattern of cytokine production that frequently falls into Th1 or Th2 phenotype has been widely confirmed in both the murine and human systems.[16,17]

Since no highly specific surface marker is available to date in order to phenotypically identify the different CD4+ T cell subsets, both murine and human Th1 and Th2 cells are currently recognized on the basis of their cytokine secretion profile and effector functions. In murine systems Th1 cells produce interleukin-2 (IL-2), interferon-γ (IFN-γ), and lymphotoxin (TNF-β) and promote both macrophage activation that results in delayed-type hypersensitivity (DTH), antibody-dependent cell cytotoxicity, and production of opsonizing antibodies, particularly of the IgG2a class, required for clearance of infection caused by intracellular organisms; Th2 cells secrete IL-4, IL-5, IL-6, IL-10, and IL-13, provide optimal help for production of antibodies, mainly of IgE and IgG1 isotypes, and mucosal immunity, through production of growth and differentiation factors for mast cells and eosinophils and facilitation to IgA synthesis.[16]

Evidence for the existence of human Th1 and Th2 cells was first provided by establishing CD4+ TCC specific for peculiar antigens. The majority of TCC specific for purified protein derivative (PPD) of *Mycobacterium tuberculosis* derived from normal donors secreted IL-2 and IFN-γ, but not IL-4 and IL-5, following stimulation with either specific antigen or phorbol myristate acetate plus anti-CD3 monoclonal antibody, whereas under the same experimental conditions, most TCC specific for the *Toxocara canis* excretory/secretory antigen (TES) derived from the same health donors secreted IL-4 and IL-5, but not IL-2 or IFN-γ.[18] IL-6, IL-10, and IL-13 tend to segregate less clearly among human CD4+ subsets than in the mouse.[19] In the absence of clear polarizing conditions leading to stereotyped Th1 or Th2 patterns, murine and human CD4+ T-cell subsets with a less differentiated lymphokine profile than producing both Th1- and Th2-type cytokines, designed Th0, usually arise, which are responsible for intermediate effects depending on the ratio of cytokines produced and the nature of responding cells.[20,21]

Human Th1 and Th2 clones not only differ for different profiles of cytokine secretion but also for their responsiveness to cytokines. IL-4 potentiated the antigen-induced proliferation and cytokine production of Th2, but not of Th1, clones. In contrast, IFN-γ selectively inhibited the proliferative response and cytokine production by Th2 clones. Unlike in the murine system, IL-10 significantly inhibited the proliferation and the cytokine production of both Th1 and Th2 human T-cell clones in response to either the specific antigen or PHA.[19] Finally, human Th1 and Th2 clones also differ for their cytolytic potential and mode of providing help for B-cell antibody synthesis. Th2 clones that usually lack cytolytic potential induce IgM, IgG, IgA, and IgE synthesis by autologous B cells in the presence of the specific antigen, with an Ig response that is proportional to the number of Th2 cells added to B cells.[22] In contrast, Th1 clones (that usually are cytolytic) provide B-cell help for IgM, IgG, IgA (but not IgE) synthesis at low T-cell:B-cell ratios. At T-cell:B-cell ratios higher than 1:1, a decline in B-cell help could be observed, which was related to Th1 lytic activity against autologous antigen-presenting B cells.[22] This may represent a mechanism for the down-regulation of antibody responses *in vivo* as well. On the other hand, the failure of Th2 cells to express antigen-dependent cytolytic activity against autologous APC may account, at least in part, for the long-term ongoing IgE antibody responses seen in patients with atopy or helminth infections.

ALLERGENS SELECTIVELY EXPAND T CELLS SHOWING TH2-LIKE CYTOKINE SECRETION PROFILE

The findings just reported encouraged investigations into whether alterations in IgE-regulatory mechanisms are involved in the genesis of human diseases characterized by hyperproduction of IgE. An attractive hypothesis to explain the increased production of allergen-specific IgE is that it may result from modified regulation of cytokines derived from T cells. This view is supported by the analysis of cytokine production by allergen-specific T cells. In contrast to TCC specific for bacterial antigens derived from PB of atopic donors that showed a prevalent Th0/Th1 phenotype, the great majority of allergen-specific CD4 + TCC derived from the same donors expressed a Th2/Th0 phenotype, with high production of IL-4 and no (or low) production of IFN-γ.[23-25] The reason why allergens preferentially expand Th2-like CD4 + T cells is still unclear. One possibility is that it is due to their peculiar physicochemical structure. Polyphenol-rich compounds have been shown to activate preferentially Th2 cells.[26] Some determinants are coexpressed by major allergens and parasitic antigens: helminths, that usually induce Th2 responses, release proteolytic enzymes and some allergens are also proteases. The allergen structure *per se* does not, however, explain the induction of Th2-like responses. Allergen-specific TCC derived from nonatopic donors preferentially express a Th1/Th0 profile.[24] On the other hand, CD4 + T cells from atopic subjects are able to produce IL-4 and IL-5 even in response to bacterial antigens, such as PPD or streptokinase, that usually evoke responses with a restricted Th1 profile in nonatopic individuals.[27] Furthermore, allergen-specific TCC derived from polysensitized patients with severe atopy produced very high amounts of IL-4 highly related to the amounts of IL-5, IL-3, and GM–CSF, suggesting that a deregulation of these cytokine gene expressions, clustered on chromosome 5, can be responsible for the atopic phenotype.[28] Indeed a sequence homology has been described between promoter elements of IL-4 and IL-5 genes.[29] Finally, it has recently been shown that cord blood T lymphocytes consistently proliferate in response to Der p I, suggesting the possibility of an *in utero* sensitization to this allergen.[30] Interestingly, CD4 + TCC derived from cord blood showed a different cytokine profile depending on the atopic status of newborns' parents. Der p I-specific TCC derived from cord blood of newborns with nonatopic parents showed a prevalent Th1 profile, whereas when both parents were atopic, newborn CD4 + TCC exhibited a Th0 or Th2 profile.[30]

Taken together, these data suggest that, in addition to the structure of allergens and the type of allergen-presenting cells, the genetic overexpression of some cytokine genes favor the preferential Th2 response in atopic individuals. Further studies are required to clarify whether a deregulation leading to overexpression of IL-4 (and other cytokine) gene is present at levels of intracellular signaling pathways and/or transcription factors and/or promoter elements.

TH2-LIKE CELLS ACCUMULATE IN TARGET ORGANS OF ALLERGIC INFLAMMATION

There is a general consensus that Th2 cells and their cytokines are involved in the pathophysiology of IgE-mediated disorders. Higher proportions of IL-4-producing and lower proportions of IFN-γ-producing TCC were obtained from the PB of patients with severe atopic disease than from nonatopic donors.[8] The majority of TCC derived from the conjunctival infiltrates of patients with vernal conjunctivitis were found to express the Th2 cytokine profile.[31] Using an *in situ* hybridization technique, T cells showing mRNA for Th2-, but not Th1-type, cytokines were found at the site of late-phase reactions in skin biopsies from atopic patients,[3] in mucosal bronchial biopsies or bronchoalveolar lavage from asthmatics,[4,5] and after local allergen challenge in nasal mucosa of allergen-induced rhinitis.[2] Likewise, increased levels of IL-4 and IL-5 were measured in the bronchoalveolar lavage fluid of allergic asthmatics, whereas in nonatopic asthmatics IL-2 and IL-5 were predominant.[5] More recently, in order to assess whether the T-cell response to inhaled allergens induced activation and recruitment of allergen-specific Th2 cells in the airway mucosa of patients with respiratory allergy, biopsy specimens were obtained from the bronchial mucosa of patients with grass-pollen-induced asthma 48 hours after the positive provocation test with the relevant allergen. About one-third of CD4+ clones derived from stimulated mucosae of grass-allergic patients were specific for grass allergens and most of them exhibited a definite Th2 profile; furthermore, they induced IgE production by autologous B cells in the presence of the specific allergen.[2] Taken together, these data suggest that allergen-specific Th2 cells, via their ability to produce IL-4 and IL-5 involved in IgE production and eosinophil response, respectively, may play an important role in the pathophysiology of allergic respiratory disorders. In contrast, the role of CD4+ T cells and T-cell-derived cytokines in the pathogenesis of atopic dermatitis (AD) is still controversial. More than 80 percent of patients with AD have been described as exhibiting elevated levels of serum IgE, with specificity to several allergens. High proportions of Th2-like CD4+ TCC specific for *Dermatophagoides pt.* (Dp) allergen(s) were obtained from the skin lesions of patients with AD, indicating an accumulation or expansion of such T cells in the affected organ.[1] Furthermore, Dp-specific Th2-like clones were also derived from biopsy specimens of intact skin taken after contact challenge with Dp, suggesting that percutaneous sensitization to aeroallergens may play a role in the induction of skin lesions in patients with AD.[32] The majority of TCC derived from the lesional skin of patients with active AD, however, had a Th0-like phenotype and few of them were specific for Dp. Most TCC from lesional skin exhibited also IFN-γ production, and a number of them appeared to be specific for bacterial antigens, suggesting that bacterial infections may complicate the pattern of T-cell responses in affected skin. Finally, the presence of both Dp-specific and Th2-like cells in the skin of AD patients did not always correlate with the presence in the serum of Dp-specific IgE antibodies or elevated serum IgE levels (E. Maggi, unpublished). On the basis of these findings, it is possible to speculate that Th2-like responses against Dp at skin level are involved in the initiation of skin lesions, but the relationship between aeroallergen sensitization and the onset of full-blown lesions remains unclear.

MODULATORY SIGNALS ABLE TO INHIBIT THE Th2 RESPONSE

It has been suggested that, at least in the murine system, Th1 and Th2 cells are repeatedly stimulated memory T cells that have matured into different functional phenotypes from shared pool of precursor cell population. Although in principle Th1 and Th2 cells might arise from distinct precursors, experiments with homogeneous populations of cells from T-cell receptor (TCR) transgenic mice strongly suggest that a single precursor can differentiate into either a Th1 or Th2 phenotype.[33] The recent paper of Reiner *et al.*[34] showing that T cells from mice infected with *Leishmania major* express a restricted TCR repertoire in both progressive infection and protective immunity, regardless of histocompatibility haplotypes, further supports this possibility. According to this model, naive Th precursor (Thp) cells mainly produce IL-2 and progress into early-memory Th0 effector cells following a first activation by the specific antigen.[35] These findings suggest that endogenous IL-12 and IFN-α favor the Th1 development through at least partially different mechanisms.

However, the mechanisms responsible for the differentiation of naive Th cells into the Th1 or Th2 phenotype have not yet been completely clarified. Attention has recently been focused on the possibility that the type of Th response depends upon the nature of antigen-presenting cells (APC) or their products. Although some differences in the response of Th1 and Th2 cells to different APC have been reported,[37] the type of APC *per se* does not critically influence the differentiation of Th precursors into one or another phenotype.[37] Released by APC and/or other cell types during antigen exposure, the role of cytokines appears to be more striking in determining the development of the specific Th1 or Th2 response. With the use of naive, ovalbumin-specific TCR transgenic T cells, it has been shown that heat-killed *Listeria monocytogenes* induced Th1 development *in vitro* through macrophage production of IL-12. The activity of IL-12 is probably related to its ability to promote IFN-γ production by NK cells in a T-cell-independent manner[38] and, in turn, IFN-γ favors the development of Th1 cells. In contrast early IL-4 production at the time of antigen presentation seems to be critical for the maturation of naive Th cells into Th2 cells.[38] Which kind of cells secrete IL-4 for the development of Th2 cells, however, remains unclear at present.

The factors that regulate the development of human Th1 and Th2 clones have been extensively investigated in our laboratory by using peripheral blood lymphocytes cultured with PPD, TES, or allergens in the presence or in the absence of exogenous cytokines or anticytokine antibody. The addition of IL-4 in bulk cultures of PB mononuclear cells stimulated with PPD shifted the differentiation of PPD-specific T cells from a Th1 to a Th0, or even Th2, phenotype.[39] Moreover, IL-4 added in bulk culture before cloning inhibited not only the Th1 differentiation of PPD-specific T cells, but also the development of their cytolytic potential.[39,40] In contrast, early addition of both IFN-γ and anti-IL-4 antibodies induced most of allergen- or TES-specific T cells to differentiate into cytolytic Th0 and Th1, instead of noncytolytic Th2 clones,[40] suggest that the presence of IL-4 or IFN-γ at the time of antigen stimulation of resting T cells have remarkable regulatory effects on their subsequent *in vitro* development into Th1 or Th2 clones. Even though IL-1 does not apparently play any role in the Ag-induced proliferative response of already established human CD4+ T-cell clones, it is required for the *in vitro* development of Th2 clones. Indeed, removal of IL-1 from bulk culture before cloning shifted the differentiation of allergen-specific T cells from the Th2/Th0 to the Th0/Th1 profile (Manetti *et al.*, manuscript in preparation). It is not yet clear whether IL-1 exerts its effect by stimulating early IL-4 production, which in turn induces the Th2 development, or synergizes the effects of IL-4 in regulating the Th cell development.

In contrast we have recently shown that IFN-α and IL-12 have regulatory activity opposite to that of IL-4 on the *in vitro* differentiation of human CD4+ T cells by favoring their development into Th1 clones.[41,42] The inhibitory activity of IL-12 on the development of allergen-specific CD4+ T cells into Th2 cells could be partially prevented by removal from bulk culture before cloning of CD3−CD16+ (NK) cells,[42] whereas the inhibitory activity of IFN-α was not prevented by NK cell removal. Since IFN-α and IL-12 are produced predominantly by macrophages, cells devoted in the processing and presentation of antigen to Th cells, it is reasonable to suggest that, given the capacity of viruses and intracellular bacteria to stimulate macrophage production of IL-12 (that induce IFN-γ secretion by both Th cells and NK cells), Th cells may be simultaneously presented with processed antigen plus cytokines that induce them to differentiate toward a Th1 phenotype.[41] These findings suggest that endogenous IL-12 and IFN-α favor the Th1 development through at least partially different mechanisms.

Even though a highly modulatory effect can be obtained *in vitro* with exogenous cytokines, in human models only secondary responses to common environmental antigens can be assessed. Thus, the question of whether changes induced *in vitro* by cytokines on the profile of antigen-specific human TCC reflect the shifting of a common precursor to one or another phenotype or merely result from selective suppression of clones with already established phenotype remains open. It is of interest, however, that even data obtained in the human models are in favor of a critical regulatory role of cytokines produced by cells of the natural immunity system in determining the nature of the subsequent specific immune response.[41]

How environmental allergens promote the differentiation of Th precursors into Th2 effector cells is less clear. Data obtained so far indicate that the availability of IL-4 and the absence (or low concentrations) of IFN-γ at the time of antigen stimulation are both essential for the development of Th2 responses.[40] A possible explanation would be that allergens and some parasite antigens fail to induce IFN-α and IL-12 production by macrophages and are poor stimulators of NK cells. Under these conditions, a Th1-type response would be hampered and the differentiation of specific Th2 cells would be made possible, provided that some IL-4 is available. Since T cells seem to be unable to differentiate into IL-4-producing cells in the absence of IL-4,[41] IL-4 production by other cell types may be involved. Evidence has been obtained that a small subset of early thymic emigrants in mouse and non-T, non-B cells from both mouse spleen and human bone marrow, probably belonging to the mast cell/basophil lineage, can synthesize IL-4.[43,44] Indeed, IL-4 production by murine non-T, non-B cells is extraordinarily increased during *Nippostrongylus brasiliensis* infection or systemic treatment with anti-IgD antibody,[45] suggesting that these cells may be involved in cytokine production during helminth infections or other situations associated with increased production of IgE antibodies. Although the role of either naive T cells,[43] FcεRI + non-T cells,[44] or mast cells[45] has been suggested, the nature of the cell providing IL-4 that is critical at the time of antigen presentation and recognition in shifting the balance toward the development of Th2 cells, still remains elusive.

The possibility of converting already established TCC to another cytokine profile was also investigated. Whereas IL-4, IL-5, IL-10 do not exert any effect, incubation with IL-12 induced the mRNA expression for, and production of detectable amounts of, IFN-γ in established Th2 clones stimulated with insolubilized anti-CD3 antibody. This change was transient, however, since IFN-γ production declined following removal of IL-12 (Manetti *et al.*, unpublished). A stable change in the cytokine profile of already established TCC can also be obtained upon growth transformation by herpesvirus saimiri (HVS), an oncogenic virus of New World monkeys[46] that is able to transform human T cells and thymocytes to continuous growth. When established human Th1 or Th2 clones were immortalized with HSV, the cytokine activity of Th1 clones was retained and enriched, whereas Th2 clones were switched to a Th0 profile.[47] These data suggest that a given Th phenotype is not absolutely definitive in a given T-cell clone and can be converted into another phenotype. The relevance of these findings in view of possible therapeutic manipulations of Th1- or Th2-mediated disorders is obvious.

CONCLUDING REMARKS

The knowledge of cellular and molecular signals responsible for the regulation of human IgE synthesis has been achieved in the last few years. There is a general consensus that IL-4 and IFN-γ are the main regulatory cytokines of IgE production, with opposite effects; a contact signal, probably due to CD40L–CD40 interaction, however, is needed to induce productive ε-transcripts, leading to IgE synthesis by purified B cells in the presence of IL-4 or IL-13. Convincing evidence is also accumulating to suggest that Th cells producing IL-4 and IL-5, but not, or limited amounts of, IFN-γ that resemble murine Th2 cells accumulate in the blood and/or target organs of patients with helminthic infections or atopic disorders. In addition these cells are easily recruited and expanded by allergen in the airway mucosa and probably play a crucial role in the induction and maintainance of allergic inflammation. In fact these cells can account for both the IgE antibody formation and eosinophilia seen in these patients.

The mechanisms responsible for the preferential expansion of Th2 cells in atopic patients and in patients with helminthic infections are currently under investigation. We have shown that virtually all TCC specific for TES and for purified allergens display the Th2 phenotype of cytokine secretion, whereas the totality of PPD-specific TCC established from the same donors belong to the Th1 cell subset. This finding suggests that different antigens may influence in opposite ways the profile of cytokine secretion of Th cells. It remains to be established whether the preferential ability of helminth component(s) and allergens to expand Th2 cells is related to their molecular structure, to the type of APC involved in their processing, and/or to other microenvironmental influences at the site of immunization.

The reason why environmental allergens induce IgE antibody responses, but only in a minority of individuals (so-called atopics), represents a still more complex question. At least two genetic traits seem to be implied in the control of IgE antibody responses in atopic subjects. First, the responsiveness to individual allergens is controlled by Ir genes linked to the MHC complex. This means that Th cells able to recognize allergen epitopes can be activated only in people possessing appropriate individual sequences in the MHC class II products of APC. This might explain why allergen-specific TCC can be easily derived from allergen-sensitive patients but not from randomly selected nonatopic people. Once recognized, allergens induce the preferential differentiation of Th cells into the Th2 phenotype of cytokine secretion, which may be due to particular features of their structure, to the type of APC involved in their processing, or to other still unknown micro-environmental influences.

The role in the genesis of atopy of additional genes not linked to MHC that control the total serum IgE levels reflecting overall IgE responsiveness has also been suggested; the nature of these genes (probably cytokine genes are involved), as well as the mechanisms by which they exert their activity, are still unknown. Although indirectly, several findings on TCC derived from atopic subjects and from newborns with atopic parents suggest that a deregulation in the production of IL-4 may be responsible for the increase of overall IgE responses in atopic individuals.

Finally, clearcut evidence from studies with both animal and human models suggest that IL-4 can strongly influence activated CD4+ T cells to differentiate into cells that produce the Th2 set of cytokines. In contrast, IFN-α and IL-12 (in part *via* induction of IFN-γ) appear to exert an opposite regulatory effect by favoring the development of Th1-like cells. This suggests that a balance between IL-4 and IFN-α/IFN-γ/IL-12 at the triad (APC/Ag/Th cell) recognition level might play a critical role in determining the cytokine profile of the specific immune response. Better knowledge of the factors modulating the Th2 development provides a means for therapeutical interventions in IgE-mediated disorders, through successful transformation of a Th2-like into a Th1-like response.

REFERENCES

1. VAN DER HEIJDEN, F. L., E. A. WIERENGA, J. D. BOS & M. L. KAPSENBERG. 1991. High frequency of IL-4-producing CD4+ allergen-specific T lymphocytes in atopic dermatitis lesional skin. J. Invest. Dermatol. **97:** 389–394.
2. DEL PRETE, G.-F., M. DE CARLI, P. MAESTRELLI, M. RICCI, L. FABBRI & S. ROMAGNANI. 1993. Allergen exposure induces the activation of allergen-specific Th2 cells in the airway mucosa of patients with allergic respiratory disorders. Eur. J. Immunol. **23:** 1445–1449.
3. KAY, A. B., et al. 1991. Messenger RNA expression of the cytokine gene cluster, interleukin (IL)-3, IL-4, IL-5, and granulocyte/macrophage colony-stimulating factor, in allergen-induced late-phase cutaneous reactions in atopic subjects. J. Exp. Med. **173:** 775–778.
4. HAMID, Q., et al. 1991. Expression of mRNA for interleukin-5 in mucosal bronchial biopsies from asthma. J. Clin. Invest. **87:** 1541–1545.
5. ROBINSON, D. S., et al. 1992. Predominant Th2-like bronchoalveolar T-lymphocyte population in atopic asthma. New Eng. J. Med. **326:** 298–304.
6. DEL PRETE, G.-F., et al. 1988. IL-4 is an essential factor for the IgE synthesis induced in vitro by human T cell clones and their supernatants. J. Immunol. **140:** 4193–4198.
7. GAUCHAT, J.-F., D. LEBMAN, R. L. COFFMAN, H. GASCAN & J. E. DE VRIES 1990. Structure and expression of germline ε transcripts in human B cells induced by interleukin 4 to switch to IgE production. J. Exp. Med. **172:** 463–471.
8. ROMAGNANI, S. 1990. Regulation and deregulation of human IgE synthesis. Immunol. Today **11:** 316–321.
9. PARRONCHI, P., et al. 1990. Non cognate contact-dependent B cell activation can promote IL-4-dependent in vitro human IgE synthesis. J. Immunol. **144:** 2102–2108.
10. JABARA, H. H., S. M. FU, R. S. GEHA & D. VERCELLI. 1990. CD40 and IgE. Synergism between anti-CD40 monoclonal antibody and interleukin 4 in the induction of IgE synthesis by highly purified B cells. J. Exp. Med. **172:** 1861–1866.
11. GAUCHAT, J.-F., et al. 1993. Induction of human IgE synthesis in B cells by mast cells and basophils. Nature **365:** 340–343.
12. MACCHIA, D., F. ALMERIGOGNA, P. PARRONCHI, A. RAVINA, E. MAGGI & S. ROMAGNANI. 1993. Membrane tumor necrosis factor α is involved in the polyclonal B-cell activation induced by HIV-infected human T cells. Nature **363:** 464–466.
13. THYPHRONITIS, G., et al. 1989. IgE secretion by Epstein-Barr virus-infected purified B lymphocytes is stimulated by interleukin 4 and suppressed by interferon γ. Proc. Natl. Acad. Sci. U.S.A. **86:** 5580–5585.
14. WU, C. Y., et al. 1991. Glucocorticoids increase the synthesis of immunoglobulin E by interleukin-4-stimulated human lymphocytes. J. Clin. Invest. **87:** 870–877.
15. MOSMANN, T. R., H. CHERWINSKI, M. W. BOND, M. A. GIEDLIN & R. L. COFFMAN. 1986. Two types of murine helper T-cell clone. I. Definition according to profiles of lymphokine activities and secreted proteins. J. Immunol. **136:** 2348–2357.
16. MOSMANN, T. R. & R. L. COFFMAN. 1989. Heterogeneity of cytokine secretion pattern and functions of helper T cells. Adv. Immunol. **46:** 11–24.
17. SALGAME, P., J. S. ABRAMS, C. CLAYBERGER, H. GOLDSTEIN, J. CONVITT, R. L. MODLIN & B. R. BLOOM. 1991. Differing lymphokine profiles and functional subsets of human CD4 and CD8 T cell clones. Science **254:** 279–281.
18. DEL PRETE, G. F., M. DE CARLI, C. MASTROMAURO, D. MACCHIA, R. BIAGIOTTI, M. RICCI & S. ROMAGNANI. 1991. Purified protein derivative of mycobacterium tuberculosis and excretory-secretory antigen(s) of Toxocara canis expand in vitro human T cells with stable and opposite (type 1 helper or type 2 T helper) profile of cytokine production. J. Clin. Invest. **88:** 346–350.

19. MOSMANN, T. R. & K. W. MOORE. 1991. The role of IL-10 in cross-regulation of TH1 and TH2 responses. Immunoparasitol. Today **12:** 49–53.
20. MAGGI, E., G. F. DEL PRETE, D. MACCHIA, P. PARRONCHI, A. TIRI, I. CHRETIEN, M. RICCI & S. ROMAGNANI. 1988. Profiles of lymphokine activities and helper function for IgE in human T cell clones. Eur. J. Immunol. **18:** 1045–1054.
21. DEL PRETE, G.-F., M. DE CARLI, F. ALMERIGOGNA, M.-G. GIUDIZI, R. BIAGIOTTI & S. ROMAGNANI. 1993. Human IL-10 is produced by both type 1 helper (Th1) and type 2 helper (Th2) T cell clones and inhibits their antigen-specific proliferation and cytokine production. J. Immunol. **150:** 1–8.
22. DEL PRETE, G.-F., M. DE CARLI, M. RICCI & S. ROMAGNANI. 1991. Helper activity for immunoglobulin synthesis of TH1 and TH2 human T cell clones: The help of TH1 clones is limited by their cytolytic capacity. J. Exp. Med. **174:** 809–816.
23. ROMAGNANI, S. 1991. Human TH1 and TH2: Doubt no more. Immunol. Today **12:** 256–257.
24. WIERENGA, E. A., M. SNOEK, C. DE GROOT, I. CHRETIEN, J. D. BOS, H. M. JANSEN & M. KAPSENBERG. 1990. Evidence for compartmentalization of functional subsets of CD4 + T lymphocytes in atopic patients. J. Immunol. **144:** 4651–4656.
25. PARRONCHI, P., *et al.* 1991. Allergen- and bacterial antigen-specific T-cell clones established from atopic donors show a different profile of cytokine production. Proc. Natl. Acad. Sci. U.S.A. **88:** 4538–4542.
26. BAUM, C. G., P. SZABO, G. W. SISKIND, C. G. BECKER, A. FIRPO, C. J. CLARICK & T. FRANCUS. 1990. Cellular control of IgE induction by a polyphenol-rich compound. Preferential activation of Th2 cells. J. Immunol. **145:** 77–83.
28. PARRONCHI, P., *et al.* 1992. Aberrant interleukin (IL)-4 and IL-5 production in vitro by CD4 helper T cells from atopic subjects. Eur. J. Immunol. **22:** 1615–1620.
29. PARRONCHI, P., R. MANETTI, C. SIMONELLI, F. SANTONI RUGIU, M.-P. PICCINNI, E. MAGGI & S. ROMAGNANI. 1991. Cytokine production by allergen (Der pI)-specific CD4 T cell clones derived from a patient with severe atopic disease. Int. J. Clin. Lab. Res. **21:** 186–189.
30. PICCINNI, M.-P., F. MECACCI, S. SAMPOGNARO, R. MANETTI, P. PARRONCHI, E. MAGGI & S. ROMAGNANI. 1993. Aeroallergen sensitization can occur during fetal life. Int. Arch. Allergy Immunol. In press.
31. MAGGI, E., *et al.* 1991. Accumulation of Th2-like helper T cells in the conjunctiva of patients with vernal conjunctivitis. J. Immunol. **146:** 1169–1174.
32. VAN REIJSEN, F. C., C. A. F. M. BRUIJNZEEL-KOOMEN, F. S. KALTHOFF, E. MAGGI, S. ROMAGNANI, J. K. T. WESTLAND & G. C. MUDDE. 1992. Skin-derived aeroallergen specific T cell clones of TH2 phenotype in patients with atopic dermatitis. J. Allergy Clin. Immunol. **2:** 184–189.
33. HSIEH, C. S., A. B. HEIMBERGER, J. S. GOLD, A. O'GARRA & K. H. MURPHY. 1992. Differential regulation of T helper phenotype development by interleukin 4 and 10 in an alpha beta T-cell-receptor transgenic system. Proc. Natl. Acad. Sci. U.S.A. **89:** 6065–6071.
34. REINER, S. L., Z.-E. WANG, F. HATAM, P. SCOTT & R. M. LOCKSLEY. 1993. Th1 and Th2 cell antigen receptors in experimental Leishmaniasis. Science **259:** 1457–1460.
35. SWAIN, S. L. 1991. Regulation of the development of distinct subsets of CD4 + T cells. Immunol. Res. **142:** 14–18.
36. COFFMAN, R. L., R. CHATELAIN, L. M. C. C. LEAL & K. VARKILA. 1991. Leishmania major infection in mice: A model system for the study of CD4 + T-cell subset differentiation. Res. Immunol. **142:** 36–39.
37. CHANG, T.-L., C. M. SHEA, S. URIOSTE, R. C. THOMPSON, W. H. BOOM & A. K. ABBAS. 1990. Heterogeneity of helper/inducer T lymphocytes. III. Responses of IL-2- and IL-4-producing (Th1 and Th2) clones to antigens presented by different accessory cells. J. Immunol. **145:** 2803–2808.
38. SEDER, R. A., W. E. PAUL, M. M. DAVIS & B. F. FAZEKAS DE ST. GROTH. 1992. The presence of interleukin 4 during in vitro priming determines the lymphokine producing potential of CD4 + T cell from T cell receptor transgenic mice. J. Exp. Med. **176:** 1091–1098.

39. MAGGI. E., *et al.* 1992. Reciprocal regulatory role of IFN- and IL-4 on the in vitro development of human TH1 and TH2 clones. J. Immunol. **148:** 2142–2147.
40. PARRONCHI, P., M. DE CARLI, M. P. PICCINNI, D. MACCHIA, E. MAGGI, G.-F. DEL PRETE & S. ROMAGNANI. 1992. IL-4 and IFNs exert opposite regulatory effects on the development of cytolytic potential by TH1 or TH2 human T cell clones. J. Immunol. **149:** 2977–2983.
41. ROMAGNANI, S. 1992. Induction of TH1 and TH2 response: A key role for the "natural" immune response? Immunol. Today **13:** 379–381.
42. MANETTI, R., P. PARRONCHI, M. G. GIUDIZI, M.-P. PICCINNI, E. MAGGI, G. TRIN-CHIERI & S. ROMAGNANI. 1993. Natural killer cell stimulatory factor (NKSF/IL-12) induces TH1-type specific immune responses and inhibits the development of IL-4-producing cells. J. Exp. Med. **177:** 1199–1204.
43. BEN SASSON, S. Z., G. LEGROS, D. H. CONRAD, F. D. FINKELMAN & W. E. PAUL. 1990. Cross-linking Fc receptors stimulate splenic non-B, non-T cells to secrete IL-4 and other lymphokines. Proc. Natl. Acad. Sci. U.S.A. **87:** 1421–1425.
44. PICCINNI, M.-P., *et al.* 1991. Human bone marrow non-B, non-T cells produce interleukin 4 in response to cross-linkage of Fcε and Fcγ receptors. Proc. Natl. Acad. Sci. U.S.A. **88:** 8656–8660.
45. CONRAD, D. H., S. Z. BEN SASSON, G. LEGROS, F. D. FINKELMAN & W. E. PAUL. 1990. Infection with Nippostrongylus brasiliensis or injection of anti-IgD antibodies markedly enhances Fc-ε receptor-mediated interleukin-4 production by non-B, non-T cells. J. Exp. Med. **171:** 1497–1508.
46. BIESINGER, B., I. MULLER-FLECKENSTIN, S. SIMMER, G. LANG, S. WITTMANN, E. PLATZER, R. C. DESROSIERS & B. FLECKENSTEIN. 1992. Stable growth transformation of human T lymphocytes by herpesvirus saimiri. Proc. Natl. Acad. Sci. U.S.A. **89:** 3116–3119.
47. DE CARLI, *et al.* 1993. Immortalization with Herpesvirus Saimiri modulates the cytokine secretion profile of established Th1 and Th2 human T cell clones. J. Immunol. **151:** 5022–5030.

The Role of the Mast Cell in Acute and Chronic Allergic Inflammation

MARTIN K. CHURCH, YOSHIMICHI OKAYAMA, AND
PETER BRADDING

Immunopharmacology Group
Centre Block
Southampton General Hospital
Southampton SO9 4XY
United Kingdom

INTRODUCTION

The mast cell is the primary initiating cell of immediate hypersensitivity reactions. Its ability to bind specific IgE with high affinity and to release its wide array of inflammatory mediators when stimulated immunologically means that it can induce fast and dramatic changes in its local environment. Particular examples of this are the immediate bronchoconstrictor response that follows bronchial allergen challenge, the rhinorrhoea and nasal blockage that follows nasal allergen challenge, and the wheal and flare response that follows injection of allergen into an atopic subject. Thus, to understand the aetiology of allergic disease it is necessary to appreciate some of the biology of the human mast cell.

MAST CELL DEVELOPMENT AND HETEROGENEITY

Mast cells compose a heterogenous population of cells found in high numbers at mucosal surfaces, such as those of the lung, nose, eye, and intestine, and in connective tissues, such as the skin and intestinal submucosa. The predominant mast cell subtypes found at mucosal surfaces and in connective tissue differs from each other in their development, chemical composition, and functionally in their ability to interact with the local environment. Studies with murine mast cells suggest that the presence of IgE complexes, interleukin-3 (IL-3), and colony stimulating factors from fibroblasts and stromal cells, particularly stem cell factor (SCF) stimulate the proliferation of stem cells in the bone marrow. These precursors then migrate, using the blood as a carrier, to their final site of maturation in the tissues. An indication of the functional heterogeneity of mast cells stems from the observations in rodents that parasitic infection stimulates the preferential proliferation of mucosal-type mast cells in the intestinal mucosa.[1] That suppression of T-cell function results in reduction of mucosal mast cell proliferation in parasitic infection[2] strongly suggests that mast cells of this subtype are acting as a part of the immunological defense system. That connective tissue mast cells are neither stimulated to proliferate nor are reduced in number during modulation of T-cell function suggest that their primary role is nonimmunological.

Human mast cells are classified by their neutral protease content, MC_T, containing only tryptase, whereas MC_{TC} contains tryptase, chymase, carboxypeptidase, and cathepsin G.[3–6] While the extrapolation is by no means watertight, many

13

parallels exist between the human MC_T and MC_{TC} mast cell subtypes and rodent mucosal and connective tissue mast cells, respectively. For example, MC_T are preferentially located at mucosal surfaces,[4] increase in numbers in allergic disease,[7-9] and are reduced in number in acquired and chronic immunodeficiency syndromes,[10] suggesting that they depend on immunological factors for their development. In contrast, MC_{TC} are found preferentially at connective tissue sites, are not increased in numbers in areas of heavy T-cell infiltration,[7,9] and are not increased in numbers in immunodeficiency syndromes.[10]

MAST CELLS IN IMMEDIATE ALLERGIC RESPONSES

Immunological stimulation of mast cells at the site of allergic reactions leads to the generation into the local environment of both preformed and newly generated mediators.

Perhaps the most well-known mediator is histamine, a primary amine synthesized from histidine by histidine carboxylase in the Golgi apparatus and transported for storage in specialized secretory granules in combination with the acidic glycosaminoglycans (GAG) of heparin. The histamine content of all tissue associated mast cells is similar, 2–5 pg/cell, while that of the smaller mast cell recovered by bronchoalveolar lavage (BAL) is around 1 pg/cell.[11] Taking into account the mast cell density of the lung, approximately 5×10^3 mast cell/cumin, the enormous histamine storage capacity of this tissue of 10–12 μg/ml is apparent. Following mast cell activation, the granular contents become solubilized and histamine dissociates from the granular matrix by ion exchange with sodium to become free in the extracellular environment. In asthma it induces bronchoconstriction, vasodilation, oedema, mucus secretion, and stimulation of pulmonary reflexes. In rhinitis, histamine plays a major role in rhinorrhoea and a minor one in nasal blockage. In urticaria, histamine induces vasodilation, oedema, and stimulates axon reflexes to induce the characteristic wheal and flare response to allergen challenge.

In addition to preformed mediators, the mast cell may also synthesize newly generated mediators, primarily from arachidonic acid located within the cell membrane. This precursor, liberated by phospholipases, may be acted upon by one of two enzymes, cyclooxygenase and lipoxygenase. In the mast cell, the most abundant, if not the only, prostanoid formed by the cyclooxygenase pathway is PGD_2.[12] Maximal immunological stimulation of isolated human mast cells induces the formation of 100–150 pmol $PGD_2/10^6$ mast cells, some thirty to forty times less than the amount of histamine produced. Once in the extracellular environment, PGD_2 is rapidly metabolized to $9\alpha,11\beta$-PGF_2, a compound with a longer biological half-life but with similar activity to PGD_2.[13,14] In the lung, PGD_2 is a bronchoconstrictor agent with a potency some thirty times greater than histamine,[15] while in the nose and skin it is less effective, contributing to nasal blockage and vasodilation, respectively.[16]

The second arm of the pathway for arachidonate metabolism is the lipoxygenase pathway. In the mast cell, this leads to the production of LTC_4 as the only leukotriene to be synthesized directly by the mast cell.[12] Amounts of leukotriene synthesized by mast cells vary somewhat, skin mast cells generating around 6 pmol/10^6, almost all of which remains as LTC_4, while lung mast cells generate more than 50 pmol/10^6 cells, of which some 80 percent is metabolized extracellularly to LTD_4 and LTE_4. Biologically, the leukotrienes are potent bronchoconstrictor agents and provoke increased permeability of post-capillary venules, which gives them a role also in immediate hypersensitivity reactions in the skin.[17]

A further lipid-derived mediator, platelet activating factor (PAF), also now appears to be generated by the mast cell. This mediator, which is synthesized on demand from alkyl-acyl-glyceryl-phosphoryl-choline, is a weak bronchoconstrictor and vasodilator in the immediate phase of allergic diseases.

MAST CELLS IN CHRONIC ALLERGIC INFLAMMATION

Induction of an allergic response, either naturally or by allergen provocation, is accompanied by an influx of inflammatory cells, of which the eosinophil is characteristically dominant. Furthermore, there is a surge of IgE production from B-lymphocytes following antigen presentation from activated dentritic cells.

Of the mediators discussed thus far, the sulphidopeptide leukotrienes increase the adherence of leukocytes to the vascular endothelium, while PAF is a powerful chemoattractant for both neutrophils and eosinophils. Neither histamine nor eicosanoids, however, can explain the prolonged multiplicity of events that characterize allergic inflammation. The mediators involved in inducing and maintaining such events are the cytokines IL-3, IL-4, and IL-5, which are normally associated with allergic disease.[18] Of these, IL-4 induces the B-cell to switch its production of IgM antibody to IgE and IgG,[19] IL-3 and IL-4 support the differentiation and development of mast cells and basophils,[20] IL-4 increases endothelial cell VACM expression,[21] and IL-5 stimulates the proliferation, migration, and activation of eosinophils.[22] While the TH$_2$-lymphocyte is considered to be a major source of these cytokines, it has recently been discovered that mast cells also could be a source of proinflammatory cytokines.

The first indication that mast cells may be a source of cytokines derived from experiments with Abelson murine leukemia virus-transfected murine cell lines that demonstrated the expression of mRNA and the production of granulocyte-macrophage colony stimulating factor (GM–CSF).[23] Subsequent studies using similar transfected murine mast cell lines suggested that they also had the capacity to produce IL-3 and IL-4, two cytokines associated with IL-5 in the allergic response.[23-25] However, the first cytokine to be unequivocally associated with mast cells was tumor necrosis factor-α (TNF-α), which was identified in IL-3-dependent mast cell lines,[26] rat basophil leukemia cells (RBL),[27] and in rat and mouse peritoneal mast cells.[28,29] Studies in murine mast cells showed that cell activation resulted in stimulation of the production of mRNA for TNF-α[30] and that the cells stored TNF-α within their secretory granules.[28] Extension of these studies into human cells initially used cultured cells to show the presence of mRNA for TNF-α,[31] but then progressed to show generation and release of this cytokine from mature cutaneous mast cells.[32-34]

In situ hybridization studies of biopsies from human asthmatic lung has shown T-lymphocytes, probably of the TH$_2$ subtype, expressing mRNA for IL-4 and IL-5.[18] These cells have negligible capacity to store these cytokines in a preformed form, however, and thus they must be synthesized *de novo* upon cell stimulation. This is a slow process that takes many hours. Thus the possibility that human mast cells may store preformed cytokines ready for rapid release was, indeed, an attractive hypothesis that prompted us to use immunocytochemistry on mucosal biopsies and molecular biological approaches on dispersed cells to examine human mast cell cytokine production in more detail.

In the first of these studies, nasal biopsies from 12 normal and 15 rhinitic subjects were used.[35] Biopsies taken from the inferior or inferomedial edge of the inferior turbinate were fixed immediately in ice-cold acetone containing the protease inhibitors iodacetamide (20 mM) and PMSF (2 mM), stored at $-20°C$ for 24 hours and then processed into glycol methacrylate resin.[36] This resin has the great advantage that it is water soluble, and hence the tissues do not need to be exposed to processing procedures that would destroy sensitive antigenic determinants such as cell surface markers. Furthermore, very thin (2 μm) sections may be cut with excellent morphological preservation, which allows several sections to be cut through a single cell. Hence, adjacent sections may be stained with different antibodies to individual cell markers or constituents and viewed under a camera lucida system to colocalize their expression. The antibodies used for cytokine and cell identification used in this study were 3H4 and 4D9 for IL-4,[36,37] Mab7 and Mab9 for IL-5,[38] 104-B11, 83-E9 and 32112 for IL-6, 4G9/A5/A7 for IL-8, AA1 for mast cells,[39] UCHT1 for pan T-cells, anti-CD$_4$ for the CD$_4^+$ T-cell subset and EG2 for eosinophils.

The results of this study showed cell-associated immunoreactivity with both IL-4 antibodies used. Analysis of sequential sections from five normal subjects stained with 4D9 for IL-4 and AA1 for mast cell tryptase showed that 96–100 percent of IL-4 immunoreactive cells were mast cells, while 40–100 percent of the total number of mast cells contained IL-4. No immunoreactivity for IL-4 was associated with the T-lymphocyte population, again providing evidence of the failure of these cells to store preformed cytokines. Closer analysis of the IL-4 immunoreactivity showed 4D9 to stain only the cytoplasm, while 3H4 gave only a weak cytoplasmic staining and a more dense ring staining around the periphery of the mast cells. That this ring staining was actually inside the cells rather than on the surface of the cells was suggested from fluorescence-activated cell sorting (FACS) analysis of dispersed and purified human skin mast cells, which stained with 3H4 only when permeabilized. In biopsies, only a proportion of the cells stained with both IL-4 antibodies, the majority staining with only one. In normal individuals this cytoplasmic staining with antibody 4D9 was more prevalent with 3H4, giving only occasional positive staining. In rhinitis, however, there was a marked up regulation of 3H4 staining in mast cells, the median number of cells in the submucosa being increased from 14 (range 0–42) to 36 (range 5–73) cells/mm^2 tissue, while the number of cells staining with 4D9 increased to a lesser degree, the normal and rhinitic median values being 22 (range 9–52) and 27 (range 17–59) cells/mm^2 tissue, respectively. Both of these increases are statistically significant at the $P < 0.05$ level. Essentially, similar results were obtained with biopsies from normal and allergic asthmatic subjects.[40]

In vitro studies have also been undertaken to examine the production and release of IL-4 from human mast cells.[41] Using *in situ* hybridization, mRNA for IL-4 has been identified in both human dispersed skin and lung mast cells. Also, using purified mast cell preparations, messenger for IL-4 has been demonstrated by the polymerase chain reaction (PCR) (Okayama and Church, unpublished observations). Immunocytochemistry has shown the presence of IL-4 within both lung and skin mast cells, and with the 4D9 antibody IL-4 immunoreactivity has been localized to the secretory granule of the mast cell (S. Wilson, personal communication). Incubation of mast cells with anti-IgE results in a loss of immunoreactivity in the short term, suggesting the cytokine to be released from the cell. However, attempts to quantitate this by ELISA or by the CT4.Sh cell line bioassay system have proved difficult due to the degradation of IL-4 by the proteolytic enzymes released by the mast cell, as discussed by Tunon de Lara and colleagues elsewhere in this volume.[42]

Using *in situ* hybridization and PCR, we have detected a strong and persistent message for IL-5, which suggests it is a constituent product of mast cells. In nasal biopsies[35] IL-5 immunoreactivity was detected in 9/12 normal individuals and 14/15 rhinitic subjects and was confined to the submucosa. In normal individuals, a median of 50 percent (range 43–50 percent) of IL-5 positive cells were mast cells, while only 19 percent (range 0–38 percent) of mast cells stained positive for IL-5 product. In rhinitis, 75 percent (range 38–87 percent) of IL-5 positive cells were identified as mast cells, with eosinophils also being identified as IL-5-containing cells. The number of mast cells expressing IL-5 also rose to 35 percent (14–60 percent). Interestingly, there was no significant difference between the total number of cells showing IL-5 product between normal and asthmatic subjects.

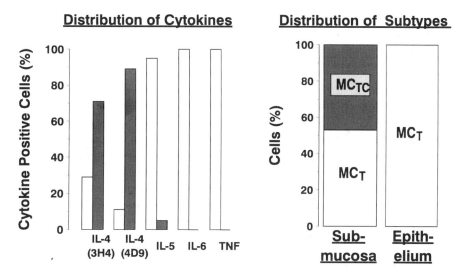

FIGURE 1. The distribution of cytokines in mast cells of nasal biopsies. The **left-hand panel** shows the distribution of cytokines between mast cell subtypes, and the **right-hand panel** the distribution of mast cell subtypes in the submucosa and epithelium. □ indicates MC$_T$ and ■ indicates MC$_{TC}$.

The multifunctional cytokine IL-6 was also observed in mast cells. Like IL-5, a strong persistent message is seen in purified mast cell preparations. In nasal biopsies, almost all the IL-6 immunoreactive cells were shown to be mast cells, the median values for normals and rhinitics being 100 percent (range 77–100 percent) and 95 percent (range 78–100 percent), respectively. In both of these disease groups, about half of the mast cells were shown to contain IL-6 product, the median values for normals and rhinitics being 46 percent (range 0–78 percent) and 58 percent (range 44–71 percent), respectively. There was no apparent up regulation of the number of IL-6 immunoreactive cells in rhinitis when compared to control.

While not examined in the nose, bronchial biopsies have been used to search for and localize TNF-α immunoreactivity.[40] In biopsies from six normal subjects and nine allergic asthmatics, all the TNF-α positive cells were mast cells, with the median number of mast cells showing TNF-α being 13 percent (range 0–27 percent) and 36 percent (range 6–100 percent) in normals and asthmatics, respectively. IL-8 immunoreactivity, although being seen consistently associated with the epithelium, was never seen to be present in mast cells, a finding that contradicts the recent report of IL-8 in the HMC-1 (human mast cell) cell line.[43]

With the knowledge of mast cell heterogeneity, we have recently begun studies to explore whether or not cytokines are preferentially associated with one or other mast cell subtype. In nasal biopsies using specific antibodies to mast cell tryptase and chymase to differentiate the mast cell subtypes, the nasal submucosa was shown to contain 47 percent MC_T and 53 percent MC_{TC} (FIG. 1). By contrast, the epithelium contained only MC_T. Using anticytokine antibodies, an association was made between cytokine content and mast cell subtype in the 269 cells examined in the submucosa. The number of mast cells in the epithelium was too small to obtain reliable results. The results (FIG. 1) showed that IL-4 was expressed in both mast cell subtypes with a degree of selectivity for MC_{TC}. This was a surprising result considering the relationship between IL-4 and the immune system. In contrast, IL-5, IL-6, and TNF-α were almost exclusively localized to the MC_T mast cell subtype.

CONCLUSIONS

While mast cells have been long recognized for their ability to precipitate the early phase of an allergic response, it has only recently been recognized that they may also play a part in the initiation and maintenance of allergic inflammation by the generation of cytokines. Their ability to release preformed cytokines would endow them with the capacity to initiate many immunological events while T-lymphocytes are building up their synthetic capacity following stimulation. Specifically, T-cells, particularly the TH_2 subset of T-cells, requires a pulse of IL-4 to initiate their proliferation and production of IL-4 and IL-5.[44,45] A pulse of IL-5 would help to explain the margination of high numbers of eosinophils that are seen in the blood vessels within minutes of challenge,[46] while the release of the multifunctional cytokines IL-6 and TNF-α would serve to magnify the allergic response.

REFERENCES

1. MILLER, H. R. P., S. J. KING, S. GIBSON, J. F. HUNTLEY, G. F. J. NEWLANDS & R. G. WOODBURY. 1986. Intestinal mucosal mast cells in normal and parasitized rats. In A. D. Befus, J. Bienenstock, and J. A. Denburg, Eds.: Mast Cell Differentiation and Heterogeneity, 239–255. Raven Press. New York.
2. KING, S. J., H. R. MILLER, G. F. NEWLANDS & R. G. WOODBURY. 1986. Depletion of mucosal mast cell protease by glucocorticosteroids: Effect on intestinal anaphylaxis in the rat. Proc. Natl. Acad. Sci. U.S.A. 82: 1214–1218.
3. IRANI, A. A., N. M. SCHECHTER, S. S. CRAIG, G. DEBOIS & L. B. SCHWARTZ. 1986. Two types of human mast cells that have distinct neutral protease compositions. Proc. Natl. Acad. Sci. U.S.A. 83: 4464–4468.
4. IRANI, A. A., T. R. BRADFORD, C. L. KEPLEY, N. M. SCHECHTER & L. B. SCHWARTZ. 1989. Detection of MC_T and MC_{TC} types of human mast cells by immunohistochemistry using new monoclonal anti-tryptase and anti-chymase antibodies. J. Histochem. Cytochem. 37: 1509–1515.

5. IRANI, A. A., S. M. GOLDSTEIN, B. U. WINTROUB, T. BRADFORD & L. B. SCHWARTZ. 1991. Human mast cell carboxypeptidase. Selective localization to MC_{TC} cells. J. Immunol. **147:** 247–253.

6. SCHECHTER, N. M., A. A. IRANI, J. L. SPROWS, J. ABERNETHY, B. U. WINTROUB & L. B. SCHWARTZ. 1990. Identification of a cathepsin G-like proteinase in the MC_{TC} type of human mast cell. J. Immunol. **145:** 2652–2661.

7. IRANI, A. A., S. I. BUTRUS & L. B. SCHWARTZ. 1988. Distribution of T and TC mast cell subsets in vernal conjunctivitis (VC) and giant papillary conjunctivitis (Abstract). NER Allergy Proc. **9:** 451.

8. IRANI, A. A., N. GOLZAR, G. DEBLOIS, B. L. GRUBER & L. B. SCHWARTZ. 1987. Distribution of mast cell subtypes in rheumatoid arthritis and osteoarthritis synovia. Arthritis Rheum. **30:** 66.

9. IRANI, A. A., H. A. SAMPSON & L. B. SCHWARTZ. 1989. Mast cells in atopic dermatitis. Allergy **44**(Suppl. 9): 31–34.

10. IRANI, A. A., S. S. CRAIG, G. DEBLOIS, C. O. ELSON, N. M. SCHECHTER & L. B. SCHWARTZ. 1987. Deficiency of the tryptase-positive, chymase-negative mast cell type in gastrointestinal mucosa of patients with defective T lymphocyte function. J. Immunol. **138:** 4381–4386.

11. FLINT, K. C., K. B. P. LEUNG, F. L. PEARCE, B. N. HUDSPITH, J. BROSTOFF & N. M. I. JOHNSON. 1985. Human mast cells recovered from bronchoalveolar lavage: Their morphology, histamine release and effects of sodium cromoglycate. Clin. Sci. **68:** 427–432.

12. ROBINSON, C., R. C. BENYON, S. T. HOLGATE & M. K. CHURCH. 1989. The IgE- and calcium-dependent release of eicosanoids and histamine from human cutaneous mast cells. J. Invest. Dermatol. **93:** 397–404.

13. HOULT, J. R. S., K. B. BACON, D. J. OSBORNE & C. ROBINSON. 1988. Organ selective conversion of prostaglandin D2 to 9alpha,11beta prostaglandin F2 and its subsequent metabolism in rat, rabbit and guinea pig. Biochem. Pharmacol. **37:** 3591–3599.

14. Beasley, C. R. W., C. Robinson, R. L. Featherstone, J. G. Varley, C. C. Hardy, M. K. Church & S. T. Holgate. 1987. 9-Alpha,11beta-Prostaglandin F2, a novel metabolite of prostaglandin D2, is a potent contractile agonist of human and guinea pig airways. J. Clin. Invest. **79:** 978–983.

15. BEASLEY, C. R. W., J. G. VARLEY, C. ROBINSON & S. T. HOLGATE. 1987. Direct and reflex bronchoconstrictor actions of prostaglandin (PG) D2 and its initial metabolite 9alpha,11beta-PGF2 in asthma. Br. J. Clin. Pharmacol. **23:** 606–607P.

16. NACLERIO, R. M., D. PROUD, S. P. PETERS, G. SILBER, A. KAGEY-KOBOTKA, N. F. ADKINSON & L. M. LICHTENSTEIN. 1986. Inflammatory mediators in nasal secretions during induced rhinitis. Clin. Allergy **16:** 101–110.

17. LEWIS, R. A. & K. F. AUSTEN. 1984. The biologically active leukotrienes. Biosynthesis, metabolism, receptors, functions, and pharmacology. J. Clin. Invest. **73:** 889–897.

18. KAY, A. B. 1991. Lymphocytes-T and their products in atopic allergy and asthma. Int. Arch. Allergy Appl. Immunol. **94:** 189–193.

19. DEL PRETE, G., *et al.* 1988. IL-4 is an essential cofactor for the IgE synthesis induced in vitro by human T-cell clones and their supernatants. J. Immunol. **140:** 4193–4198.

20. TSUJI, K., K. M. ZSEBO & M. OGAWA. 1991. Murine mast cell colony formation supported by IL-3, IL-4, and recombinant rat stem cell factor, ligand for c-kit. J. Cell Physiol. **148:** 362–369.

21. SCHLEIMER, R. P., *et al.* 1992. IL-4 induces adherence of human eosinophils and basophils but not neutrophils to endothelium: Association with expression of VCAM-1. J. Immunol. **148:** 1086–1092.

22. SANDERSON, C. J. 1991. Control of Eosinophilia. Int. Arch. Allergy Appl. Immunol. **94:** 122–126.

23. CHUNG, S. W., P. M. C. WONG, G. SHEN-ONG, S. RUSCETTI, T. ISHIZAKA & C. J. EAVES. 1986. Production of granulocyte-macrophage colony-stimulating factor by Abelson virus-induced tumorigenic mast cell lines. Blood. **68:** 1074–1081.

24. BROWN, M. A., J. H. PIERCE, C. J. WATSON, J. FALCO, J. N. IHLE & W. E. PAUL. 1987. B cell stimulatory factor-1/interleukin-4 mRNA is expressed by normal and transformed mast cells. Cell **50:** 809–818.

25. HUMPHRIES, R. K., S. ABRAHAM, G. KRYSTAL, P. LANSDORP, F. LEMOINE & C. J. EAVES. 1988. Activation of multiple hemopoietic growth factors in Abelson virus transformed myeloid cells. Exp. Hematol. **16:** 774–781.

26. GHIARA, P., D. BORASCHI, L. VILLA, G. SCAPIGLIATI, C. TADDEI & A. TAGLIABUE. 1985. In vitro generated mast cells express natural cytotoxicity against tumor cells. Immunology **55:** 317–324.

27. OKUNO, T., Y. TAKAGAKI, D. H. PLUZNIK & J. Y. DJEU. 1986. Natural cytotoxic (NC) cell activity in basophilic cells: Release of NC-specific cytoxic factor by IgE receptor triggering. J. Immunol. **136:** 4652–4658.

28. Young, J. D. E., C. C. Liu, G. Butler, Z. A. Cohn & S. J. Galli. 1987. Identification, purification and characterization of a mast cell associated cytolytic factor related to tumor necrosis factor. Proc. Natl. Acad. Sci. U.S.A. **84:** 9175–9179.

29. FARRAM, E. & D. S. NELSON. 1980. Mouse mast cells as anti-tumor effector cells. Cell Immunol. **55:** 294–301.

30. GORDON, J. R. & S. J. GALLI. 1990. Mast cells as a source of both preformed and immunologically inducible TNF-alpha/cachetin. Nature **346:** 274–276.

31. STEFFEN, M., M. ABBOUD, G. K. POTTER, Y. P. YUNG & M. A. S. MOORE. 1989. Presence of tumor necrosis factor or a related factor in human basophils/mast cells. Immunology **66:** 445–450.

32. KLEIN, L. M., R. M. LAVKER, W. L. MATIS & G. F. MURPHY. 1989. Degranulation of human mast cells induces an endothelial antigen central to leukocyte adhesion. Proc. Natl. Acad. Sci. U.S.A. **86:** 8972–8976.

33. WALSH, L. J., G. TRINCHIERI, H. A. WALDORF, D. WHITAKER & G. F. MURPHY. 1991. Human dermal mast cells contain and release tumor necrosis factor alpha, which induces endothelial leukocyte adhesion molecule 1. Proc. Natl. Acad. Sci. U.S.A. **88:** 4220–4224.

34. BENYON, R. C., E. Y. BISSONNETTE & A. D. BEFUS. 1991. Tumor necrosis factor-alpha dependent cytotoxicity of human skin mast cells is enhanced by anti-IgE antibodies. J. Immunol. **147:** 2253–2258.

35. BRADDING, P., I. H. FEATHER, S. WILSON, P. G. BARDIN, C. H. HEUSSER, S. T. HOLGATE & P. H. HOWARTH. 1993. Immunolocalization of cytokines in the nasal mucosa of normal and perennial rhinitic subjects: The mast cell as a source of IL-4, IL-5 and IL-6 in human allergic mucosal inflammation. J. Immunol. **151:** 3853–3865.

36. BRITTEN, K. M., P. H. HOWARTH & W. R. ROCHE. 1993. Immunohistochemistry on resin sections: A comparison for resin embedding techniques for small mucosal biopsies. Biotech. Histochem. In press.

37. PASQUALE, C. P., P. M. R. SILVA, M. C. R. LIMA, B. L. DIAZ, J. P. RIHOUX, B. B. VARGAFTIG, R. S. B. CORDEIRO & M. A. MARTINS. 1992. Suppression by cetirizine of pleurisy triggered by antigen in actively sensitized rats. Eur. J. Pharmacol. **223:** 9–14.

38. MCNAMEE, L. A., L. I. FATTAH, T. J. BAKER, T. J. BAINS & P. H. HISSEY. 1991. Production, characterization and use of monoclonal antibodies to human interleukin 5 in an enzyme-linked immunosorbant assay. J. Immunol. Methods. **141:** 81.

39. WALLS, A. F., A. R. BENNETT, H. M. MCBRIDE, M. J. GLENNIE, S. T. HOLGATE & M. K. CHURCH. 1990. Production and characterization of monoclonal antibodies specific for human mast cell tryptase. Clin. Exp. Allergy. **20:** 581–589.

40. BRADDING, P., J. A. ROBERTS, K. M. BRITTEN, S. MONTEFORT, R. DJUKANOVIC, C. H. HEUSSER, P. H. HOWARTH & S. T. HOLGATE. 1993. Interleukins (IL)-4, -5, -6 and TNFα in normal and asthmatic airways: Evidence for the human mast cell as an important source of these cytokines. Submitted for publication.

41. BRADDING, P., et al. 1992. Interleukin 4 is localized to and released by human mast cells. J. Exp. Med. **176:** 1381–1386.

42. TUNON DE LARA, J. M., Y. OKAYAMA, A. R. MCEUEN, C. H. HEUSSER, M. K. CHURCH & A. F. WALLS. 1993. Release and inactivation of interleukin-4 by mast cells. This issue.

43. MÖLLER, A., et al. 1993. Human mast cells produce IL-8. J. Immunol. **151:** 3261–3266.

44. SWAIN, S. L., A. D. WEINBERG, M. ENGLISH & G. HUSTON. 1990. IL-4 directs the development of TH2-like helper effectors. J. Immunol. **145:** 3796–3806.

45. SEDER, R. A., W. E. PAUL, S. Z. BEN SASSON, G. S. LEGROS, A. KAGEY SOBOTKA, F. D. FINKELMAN, J. H. PIERCE & M. PLAUT. 1991. Production of interleukin-4 and other cytokines following stimulation of mast cell lines and in vivo mast cells/basophils. Int. Arch. Allergy Appl. Immunol. **94:** 137–140.

46. DUNN, C. J., G. A. ELLIOT, J. A. OOSTVEEN & I. M. RICHARDS. 1988. Development of a prolonged eosinophil-rich inflammatory leukocyte infiltration in the guinea-pig asthmatic response to ovalbumin inhalation. Am. Rev. Respir. Dis. **137:** 541–547.

Molecular Control of B-Cell Immunopoiesis

J. BANCHEREAU, D. BLANCHARD, F. BRIÈRE,
AND Y. J. LIU

Schering-Plough
Laboratory for Immunological Research
27, chemin des Peupliers
B.P. 11, Dardilly, France

INTRODUCTION

The function of B lymphocytes is to make antibodies in response to all different types of pathogens that invade the organism. B lymphocytes, generated through a process called *lymphopoiesis* in primary lymphoid organs (fetal liver, bone marrow), migrate into peripheral lymphoid organs (lymph nodes, spleen, tonsils) as mature B cells. During antigen-specific immune responses, antigen-specific naive B cells undergo a cascade of events including activation, expansion, mutations, isotype switch, selections, and differentiation into either antibody-secreting plasma cells or memory B cells. These antigen-dependent events occur in different areas of secondary lymphoid organs, as well as other nonlymphoid organs. By opposition to the antigen-independent lymphopoiesis, we propose to call the antigen-dependent events, immunopoiesis. It requires the interaction of B cells with antigens and numerous cell types including T cells, dendritic cells (DC), follicular dendritic cells (FDC), and macrophages. These cells interact with B cells through different cell surface molecules and through the release of polypeptidic mediators called *cytokines*. The present review summarizes the *in vitro* effects of recombinant cytokines on purified human B lymphocytes activated either through their antigen receptors or through their CD40 antigen, an important receptor to a T-cell activation antigen. We then try to integrate these observations into the various *in vivo* sites of B-cell activation.

FUNCTIONAL CONSEQUENCES OF ANTIGEN RECEPTOR ENGAGEMENT

Purified mature B lymphocytes are activated and undergo limited proliferation when triggered through their antigen receptors using immobilized anti-Ig antibodies.[1,2] Particles of *Staphylococcus* aureus strain Cowan (SAC) also appear to act as strong polyclonal activators of B cells, but this may occur through cross-linking of currently unidentified B-cell surface molecules.

IL-2,[3] IL-3,[4] IL-4,[5] IL-10,[6] IL-13,[7] IFNγ[8,9] TNFα and β,[10,11] and High Molecular Weight B-cell growth factor (BCGF) (IL-14?)[12] have been shown to enhance to some extent the proliferation of B cells activated through their antigen receptor (FIG. 1). IL-2 consistently represents one of the most efficient cytokines, particularly after several days of culture, whereas IL-4 inhibits IL-2-dependent B-cell proliferation.[13,14] IL-2 and IL-10 can induce SAC-costimulated or preactivated B

22

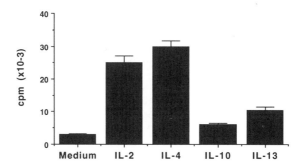

FIGURE 1. Cytokines enhance DNA synthesis of B cells stimulated through their antigen receptor. 5×10^5 purified B cells were cultured in microwells together with 5 μg/ml anti-IgM beads without or with 20 IU/ml IL-2, or 50 ng/ml IL-4, or 100 ng/ml IL-10, or 30 ng/ml IL-13; ^{3}HTdR uptake was measured at day 3.

cells to secrete relatively low levels of IgG, IgA, and IgM, while IL-4 stimulates the production of IgM and IgG by SAC-preactivated B cells.[15]

The limited B-cell growth and differentiation observed following antigen receptor cross-linking led us to hypothesize that the engagement of antigen receptor may essentially represent an activation and/or a selection mechanism for B cells. This implies that other B-cell surface molecules are involved in the massive expansion and differentiation required for the seldom antigen-specific B cells to generate the large amounts of antibodies required to neutralize invading pathogens. In particular, models were established in which activated T cells were shown to induce considerable B-cell proliferation and Ig secretion.[16] This led to the identification of CD40 as a key antigen involved in B-cell growth and differentiation, which is a receptor for CD40-Ligand, an activation antigen of T cells.

FUNCTIONAL CONSEQUENCES OF CD40 ENGAGEMENT

Proliferation of B Lymphocytes

Anti-CD40 antibodies have been isolated for their ability to costimulate with either anti-IgM antibodies or phorbol esters for the proliferation of purified B cells.[17-19] In a soluble form, certain anti-CD40 antibodies can induce some DNA replication in resting B cells.[20,21] B cells cultured with soluble CD40-Ligand (CD40-L) in a monomeric form enter into limited DNA synthesis, but trimeric forms of soluble CD40-L result in quite significant DNA synthesis, particularly in combination with anti-Ig.[22-24] Culture of resting B cells in the CD40 system (anti-CD40 antibody presented by a fibroblastic cell line transfected with FcγRII/CDw32) or on CD40-L transfected cells results in strong and long-lasting B-cell proliferation.[24-30] These culture conditions allow the proliferation of various B-cell subpopulations including naive sIgD$^+$ sIgM$^+$ B cells, germinal center and memory B cells (Arpin and Liu, manuscript in preparation), CD5$^+$, and CD5$^-$ B cells.[31]

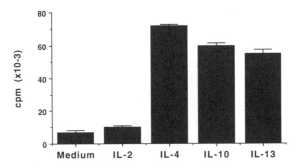

FIGURE 2. Cytokines enhance DNA synthesis of B cells stimulated through their CD40 antigen. 2.5×10^4 purified B cells were cultured on 2.5×10^3 irradiated CDw32 L cells with 0.5 μg mAb 89 with cytokines as in FIGURE 1. ³HTdR uptake was measured at day 6.

Addition of IL-4 to B cells cultured in the CD40 system (FIG. 2), or over CD40-L transfected cells, results in their sustained proliferation,[25,26,30] and this results in the generation of factor-dependent long-term normal B-cell lines. B-cell clones can be generated that contain several hundred cells. IL-13, a cytokine, which shares homology with IL-4,[7,32] can also induce a strong and long-lasting proliferation of B cells stimulated in the CD40 system or with CD40-L transfected cells.[28]

IL-1 and IFNγ enhance the DNA synthesis observed in the CD40 system or with CD40-L transfected cells, with or without IL-4.[30,33] IL-10 appears to be almost as efficient as IL-4 during the first week of culture, but proliferation ceases thereafter. The combination of IL-4 and IL-10 is additive. IL-2 poorly enhances the proliferation of B cells cultured in the CD40 system or with CD40-L transfected cells. Cells cultured in the CD40 system with IL-4 express CD19, CD20, CD40, sIg, high levels of CD23, and HLA class II antigens. Both viral and human IL-10 enhance the proliferation of B cells cultured in the CD40 system or with CD40-L transfected cells.[6,30] B cells cultured in IL-10 differ microscopically from those cultured in IL-4 in that loose aggregates are observed early on, which then yield cultures mostly composed of single large cells. IL-10 upregulates the expression of CD25/Tac on anti-CD40 activated B cells, and accordingly the addition of IL-2 strongly enhances B-cell proliferation.[34]

Differentiation of B Lymphocytes

B cells cultured in the CD40 system or with CD40-L transfected cells, produce marginal amounts of immunoglobulins.[27,30,33,35] However, coculture of human B cells cultured in the CD40 system together with SAC particles produce large amounts of IgM, IgG, and IgA without IgE.[36] Naive sIgD⁺ sIgM⁺ B cells secrete only IgM, whereas sIgD⁻ sIgM⁺ B cells secrete IgG and IgA and lower amounts of IgM. This indicates that the concomitant triggering of sIg and CD40 results in differentiation of human B lymphocytes.

Addition of IL-4 to cells cultured in the CD40 system or on CD40-L transfected cells results in a slight increase in the production of IgM and IgG and in the secretion of IgE following isotype switching[26,27,30,33,35,37–40] (FIG. 3). Addition of IFNγ or IFNα to CD40 activated B cells fails to inhibit IL-4-induced IgE production. Indeed the inhibitory effects of interferons on IL-4-induced IgE production by mononuclear cells[41] may be due to downregulation of CD40-L on IL-4-activated T cells.[29] B cells stimulated through their CD40 antigen secrete IgE and IgG$_4$ in response to IL-13, as a result of isotype switch[28,42] (FIG. 3).

Addition of IL-10 to CD40-activated B lymphocytes results in the production of considerable amounts of IgM, IgG, and IgA without IgE after differentiation into plasma cells (FIG. 3).[6,30] IL-10 induces anti-CD40-activated B cells to secrete IgG$_1$, IgG$_2$, and IgG$_3$. CD40-activated sIgD$^+$ sIgM$^+$ B cells were found to secrete essentially IgM but also IgG$_1$ and IgG$_3$ in response to IL-10, indicating that this cytokine acts as a switch factor for certain IgG subclasses (Brière *et al.*[43] CD40-activated naive sIgD$^+$, sIgM$^+$ B cells cultured with IL-10 also produce low levels of IgA$_1$ and addition of TGFβ induces large amounts of both IgA$_1$ and IgA$_2$, while inhibiting IgM and IgG production[36] (F. Brière, manuscript in preparation). TGFβ is likely to be an IgA-switch factor both in humans and in mice.[44,45] Thus the engagement of CD40 on B cells turns on their isotype switching machinery, the specificity of which is subsequently provided by cytokines (FIG. 4).

Role of CD40 in T-Cell-Dependent B-Cell Activation

It has been shown that activated T cells can induce resting B cells to proliferate and differentiate into Ig-secreting cells (see reference 16, for a review). In particular, the mouse thymoma EL-4 can activate resting human B cells to proliferate,[46] an observation that allowed the cloning of the ligand for CD40.[47] T cells activated with immobilized anti-CD3 antibodies, which mimic T-cell receptor engagement, are able to induce normal B cells to proliferate and secrete Igs.[48,49] Cytokines produced by activated T cells are involved in the growth and differentiation of B cells, but the cell contact cannot be replaced by T-cell supernatants. In contrast, fixed activated T cells or their

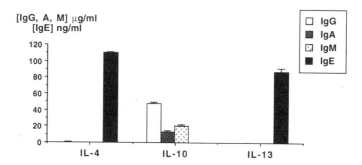

FIGURE 3. Cytokines induce CD40 activated B cells to produce Igs. 2.5×10^4 purified B cells were cultured on 2.5×10^3 irradiated CDw32 L cells with 0.5-μg mAb 89 with cytokines as in FIGURE 1. IgM, IgG, IgA, and IgE were determined by ELISA in day-10 culture supernatants.

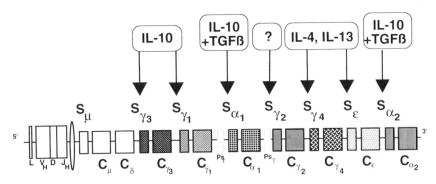

FIGURE 4. Schematic representation of the heavy chain immunoglobulin gene locus in man and cytokines controlling isotype switch. At variance with mice, there is no evidence yet that Interferons can act as IgG switch factors in man. This is consistent with the fact that replication of the common ancestral γ chain into four subclasses occurred independently in mice and man.

membrane-enriched fraction can induce B-cell proliferation, and addition of cytokines can further enhance growth and can induce Ig secretion.[50-53] The CD40-Fc fusion protein inhibits B-cell stimulation induced by activated T cells and their membranes.[27,54] Monoclonal antibodies blocking T-cell-dependent B-cell activation against murine[54] and human[55] activated T cells were in fact specific for CD40-L. In line with these findings, anti-CD40 antibodies strongly block both proliferation and Ig secretion of tonsillar B cells induced by T cells stimulated with immobilized anti-CD3.[56,57] Interestingly, activation of naive sIgD+ sIgM+ B cells is significantly less inhibited by anti-CD40 antibody than that of sIgD- B cells, suggesting that activation of naive B cells may also occur independently of CD40–CD40-L interactions. Anti-CD3 activated T-cell clones isolated from patients suffering from an hyper-IgM syndrome, characterized by mutated nonfunctional CD40-L,[58-62] can induce B cells to proliferate, although the proliferation is more limited than that induced by CD40-L positive T cells. Importantly, naive B cells produce significant amounts of IgM but neither IgG nor IgA even when exogenous IL-10 is further added to cultures. These *in vitro* observations correlate with the hyper-IgM status of patients suffering from mutated-CD40-L and demonstrates the critical role of CD40/CD40-L in isotype switch (Brière and Blanchard, manuscript in preparation). This further indicates that a CD40/CD40-L independent molecular interaction exists between T and B cells. Indeed, this was predicted in other studies indicating that T-cell-dependent B-cell growth and differentiation was essentially dependent on IL-2, whereas B-cell activation induced by CD40 cross-linking resulted in IL-4 and IL-10-dependent B-cell growth and differentiation.[57] This finding is paradoxical in the sense that B cells stimulated through their CD40 antigen virtually do not respond to IL-2 and suggests that another T-cell-dependent signal turns on the B-cell response to IL-2. We are currently searching for B-cell antigens that cross-linking will turn on an IL-2 response.

MOLECULAR CONTROL OF B-CELL IMMUNOPOIESIS: A TENTATIVE SYNTHESIS

Extrafollicular Reaction

It is always difficult and dangerous to try to give *in vivo* biological significance to phenomena that have been observed *in vitro*. This is particularly difficult in the case of human immunology, since studies in man are very quickly limited by ethical considerations. Indeed, it is currently felt that results obtained with human peripheral blood mononuclear cells should be viewed very critically because the quality, proportion, and stage of maturation of immune cells in such suspensions do not reflect those actually involved in immune responses *in vivo*. Nevertheless, we will try to associate the data obtained *in vitro* with purified human B lymphocytes with those obtained by immunohistological analysis of secondary lymphoid organs from human or antigen challenged mice/rats. This synthesis is greatly helped by the finding that mutations in CD40-L gene result in hyper-IgM syndrome. B-cell immunopoiesis can be divided in five different stages that happen in distinct anatomic areas:[63-65] (1) primary and secondary B-cell proliferation and differentiation into plasma blast in extrafollicular areas; (2) blast/centroblast proliferation in the germinal center dark zone; (3) antigen-driven selection in the germinal center basal light zone; (4) proliferation of selected B cells and their differentiation into either memory cells or plasma blasts in the apical light zone; (5) differentiation of plasma blasts into plasma cells in the lymphoid organ medullary cords, bone marrow, or mucosal lamina propria (FIG. 5).

At the site of tissue injury, pathogens/antigens are captured by dendritic cells (DC) (called *Langerhans cells* in the epidermis).[66] The antigen-loaded DCs migrate through lymphatics (they are now called *veiled cells*) into the secondary lymphoid organs (e.g., draining lymph nodes). The arrival of antigen-loaded DC cells (called *interdigitating dendritic cells* at that level) into the paracortical T-cell-rich areas of the lymph nodes results in the shutting of the valvules of the efferent lymphatics. This permits the accumulation of lymphocytes from afferent lymphatics and the selection of antigen-specific T and B cells.[67]

There is no evidence yet that dendritic cells present antigen to B lymphocytes, although it is appealing to speculate that in order to initiate a coordinated T/B cell interaction such DC may present processed antigen to T lymphocytes and unprocessed antigen to B cells. In this case, the antigen could be in the form of immune complexes as shown for follicular dendritic cells (FDC). The interaction between T lymphocytes and dendritic cells results in T-cell activation, characterized by expression of activation antigens such as the CD40-L and secretion of cytokines such as IL-2 and IL-4.[68] The CD40-L readily induced on T cells may directly activate B cells and induce their proliferation and differentiation in an IL-2-dependent fashion.[69] The generated plasma blasts will migrate into the medullary cords following loss of certain adhesion molecules and acquisition of novel ones. Naive B cells expressing sIgM and sIgD will generate plasma cells secreting IgM, characteristic of primary responses. Memory B cells expressing either sIgG or sIgA or sIgE will generate plasma cells producing these isotypes, characteristic of secondary immune responses. At that stage, no somatic mutations have been shown to occur,[70,71] and while isotype switch may occur there in rats/mice, this may be different in man, since the V regions of human IgG and IgA antibodies are in general mutated. This would thus imply that T cells in man do not deliver a CD40-dependent activation to B cells during the extrafollicular reaction nor switch factors such as IL-4, IL-10, or TGFβ. Indeed, CD40/CD40-L interactions

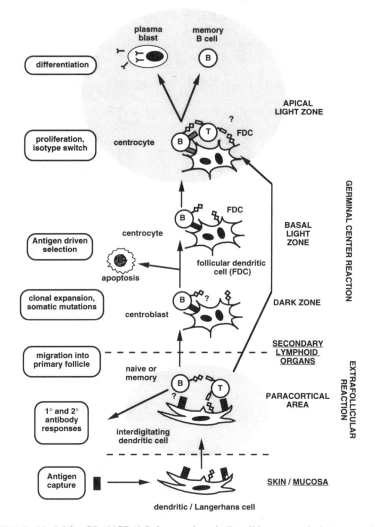

FIGURE 5. Model for CD40/CD40-L interactions in B-cell immunopoiesis (see text). ■ = antigen; ◇◇— = CD40; □ = CD40-L; shaded areas = zones of CD40/CD40-L interactions.

may not be mandatory to initiate the primary B-cell reaction because individuals displaying an altered CD40-L are able to mount an IgM response. This extrafollicular reaction also results in the generation of B-cell blasts and T-cell blasts that will play a key role in the generation of germinal centers.[70] In this respect, CD40-dependent activation of naive B cells is fundamental to launch the germinal center reaction that will lead to the generation of memory B cells. This is demonstrated by the lack of germinal centers in the lymphoid organs of patients with mutated CD40-L.

Proliferation of Blasts and Centroblasts in the Dark Zone

The B-cell blasts generated into the extrafollicular areas migrate, after acquisition of specific adhesion molecules, into primary follicles composed of follicular dendritic cells (FDC) and naive B cells percolating through FDC processes. FDCs most likely represent a stromal element of mesenchymal origin[72] in contrast to dendritic cells, which are of hematopoietic origin.[73] At that level, B-cell blasts undergo extensive proliferation and a few blasts give rise to $\approx 10^4$ cells within 3 days, imposing a cell cycle time of 6–10 hours.[74,75] This constitutes the first stage of germinal center formation, which is thought to end when blasts have filled the FDC network. At that stage, the classical polarization of the germinal center develops, the blasts become centroblasts that constitute the dark zone, and continue to quickly proliferate, but not to increase in numbers. The molecular mechanisms involved in this proliferation remain largely unknown. These mechanisms may involve the production of autocrine high molecular weight BCGF, as deduced from the possible autocrine role of this molecule in lymphoma cell proliferation.[12] Furthermore, FDC processes may provide these B cell blasts or centroblasts with proliferation signals yet to be determined. This stage is characterized by the occurrence of somatic mutations randomly over the whole V region genes following currently undetermined signaling pathways.[76,77] The generated centroblasts further differentiate into nonproliferating centrocytes that form the light zone of the germinal centers. It should be noted that B cells giving rise to memory B cells have been claimed to represent a lineage independent of those giving rise to primary reactions, and that the blasts generating the germinal center reactions would not derive from the extrafollicular foci.[78,79]

Selection and Differentiation of B Lymphocytes in the Light Zone

In the basal light zone centrocytes that reexpress surface Igs are selected by antigen present in the form of immune complexes on FDC processes. Nonselected cells that do not receive signals from their antigen receptor die by apoptosis[80] and are phagocytosed by tingible body macrophages. It is likely that B cells undergoing apoptosis express specific surface antigens that will be recognized by the macrophages and trigger phagocytosis. At that stage, selected B cells may be receptive to the proliferative effect of IL-2 since they have encountered antigen signaling.[81] The selected centrocytes that express Igs of high affinity and high specificity for the eliciting antigen now need to be amplified because they are rare. Furthermore, it is at that stage that isotype switch may occur. Amplification will also lead to the production of either memory cells or plasma cells. These events are thought to occur in the apical light zone and involve T cells that are present at high density at that level. The CD40/CD40-L interaction is most likely to be crucial at that level in turning on the isotype switch machinery, which specificity is given by cytokines such as IL-4/IL-13, IL-10, or TGFβ. In fact, it is economic for the immune system to set up an isotype switch after selection of high affinity mutants rather than at the same time (e.g., in the dark zone) or even earlier (e.g., during the extrafollicular reaction). Indeed, sequencing of a lot of human IgG monoclonal antibodies has shown mutated V genes, whereas IgM antibodies display V genes in a germline configuration. Immunohistology analysis of human tonsils demonstrates the presence of CD40-L positive T cells within the germinal centers.[82] Furthermore, germinal center CD4$^+$ T cells isolated according to CD57 expression display IL-4 and IL-10, which represent switch factors toward IgG_4, IgE, IgG_1,

IgG$_3$, and IgA.[83] CD40 triggering is also likely to be involved in the further differentiation of switched centrocytes. What dictates differentiation of centrocytes into either memory B cells or plasma blasts still remains unclear. Cytokines may be involved in this branching since CD40-activated centrocytes acquire a memory cell phenotype in response to IL-4, as they acquire a plasma blast phenotype in response to IL-10 (Arpin and Liu, manuscript in preparation). Furthermore, circulating antigen itself may skew the differentiation toward plasma blasts that will produce sufficient antibodies to eliminate circulating antigen. Following elimination of free antigen, B cells stop differentiating into plasma blasts and remain in a stand-by situation that is memory. Indeed, the double triggering of CD40 and antigen receptor (with either anti-Ig or SAC particles) has been shown to induce B lymphocytes to differentiate into high rate Ig secreting cells.[36]

Plasma Cell Differentiation

The last important stage to consider in the B-cell natural history is their differentiation into plasma cells. This occurs in three anatomic sites, including the medullary cords of lymph nodes, the mucosal lamina propria, and the bone marrow. It has been estimated that this latter organ produces two-thirds of daily production of IgG and IgA and 20–30 percent of daily IgM secretion. In fact, fairly little is known regarding the molecular control of plasma cell differentiation. It has been claimed that IL-6 plays a crucial role in the development of myelomas and plasmacytomas.[84] Plasma cells of bone marrow can differentiate over bone marrow stroma in an IL-6-dependent fashion and following VLA-4–fibronectin interactions.[85] Recently, plasma blasts generated by anti-CD3-activated T-cell stimulation of B lymphocytes were found to differentiate over bone marrow stroma or synoviocytes and addition of either IL-3 and/or IL-10 has been shown to further enhance Ig secretion (Merville, Dechanet, and Banchereau, manuscript in preparation). Indeed, stimulatory effects of IL-3 on the growth of myeloma progenitors and the growth and differentiation of normal B cells have been reported earlier.[4,86,87]

PERSPECTIVES

The past few years have witnessed immense progress in the understanding of antigen-induced B-cell immunopoiesis, a multistage event occurring in many independent anatomic locations within the organism, involving different cell types and many different molecules. Among the major questions that remain to be addressed are: (1) the nature of CD40–CD40-L independent T/B-cell interactions that permits the differentiation of naive B cells as observed in the hyper-IgM syndrome; (2) the mechanisms controlling the massive proliferation of B-cell blasts and centroblasts in the dark zone; (3) a characterization of the molecular complexes involved in somatic mutations and isotype switch; (4) the mechanisms controlling the migration of the B cells at their various stages of differentiation. This understanding of normal B-cell development should ultimately allow an elucidation of the mechanisms leading to lymphomagenesis/myelomagenesis and autoimmunity, which may then lead to the design of specific therapies.

ACKNOWLEDGMENTS

The authors wish to thank Nicole Courbière for outstanding editorial assistance.

REFERENCES

1. JELINEK, D. & P. E. LIPSKY. 1987. Adv. Immunol. **40:** 1–59.
2. BANCHEREAU, J. & F. ROUSSET. 1992. Adv. Immunol. **52:** 125–251.
3. MINGARI, M. C., F. GEROSA, G. CARRA, R. S. ACCOLLA, A. MORETTA, R. H. ZUBLER, T. A. WALDMANN & L. MORETTA. 1984. Nature **312:** 641–643.
4. XIA, X., L. LI & Y. S. CHOI. 1992. J. Immunol. **148:** 491–497.
5. DEFRANCE, T., *et al.* 1987. J. Immunol. **139:** 1135–1141.
6. ROUSSET, F., *et al.* 1992. Proc. Natl. Acad. Sci. U.S.A. **89:** 1890–1893.
7. MCKENZIE, A. N. J., *et al.* 1993. Proc. Natl. Acad. Sci. U.S.A. **90:** 3735–3739.
8. ROMAGNANI, S., M. G. GIUDIZI, R. BIAGIOTTI, F. ALMERIGOGNA, M. G. MINGARI, E. MAGGI, M. C. LIANG & L. MORETTA. 1986. J. Immunol. **136:** 3513–3516.
9. DEFRANCE, T., J. P. AUBRY, B. VANBERVLIET & J. BANCHEREAU. 1986. J. Immunol. **137:** 3861–3867.
10. KEHRL, J. H., M. ALVAREZ-MON, G. A. DELSING & A. S. FAUCI. 1987. Science **238:** 1144–1146.
11. KEHRL, J. H., A. MILLER & A. S. FAUCI. 1987. J. Exp. Med. **166:** 786–791.
12. AMBRUS, J. L., *et al.* 1993. Proc. Natl. Acad. Sci. U.S.A. **90:** 6330–6334.
13. JELINEK, D. F. & P. E. LIPSKY. 1988. J. Immunol. **141:** 164–173.
14. DEFRANCE, T., B. VANBERVLIET, J. P. AUBRY & J. BANCHEREAU. 1988. J. Exp. Med. **168:** 1321–1337.
15. DEFRANCE, T., B. VANBERVLIET, J. PÈNE & J. BANCHEREAU. 1988. J. Immunol. **141:** 2000–2005.
16. PARKER, D. C. 1993. Annu. Rev. Immunol. **11:** 331–360.
17. VALLÉ, A., C. E. ZUBER, T. DEFRANCE, O. DJOSSOU, M. DERIE & J. BANCHEREAU. 1989. Eur. J. Immunol. **19:** 1463–1467.
18. CLARK, E. A. & J. A. LEDBETTER. 1986. Proc. Natl. Acad. Sci. U.S.A. **83:** 4494–4498.
19. LEDBETTER, J. A., G. SHU, M. GALLAGHER & E. A. CLARK. 1987. J. Immunol. **138:** 788–794.
20. GORDON, J., M. J. MILLSUM, G. R. GUY & J. A. LEDBETTER. 1988. J. Immunol. **140:** 1425–1430.
21. GRUBER, M. F., J. M. BJORNDAHL, S. NAKAMURA & S. M. FU. 1989. J. Immunol. **142:** 4144–4152.
22. ARMITAGE, R. J., T. A. SATO, B. M. MACDUFF, K. N. CLIFFORD, A. R. ALPERT, C. A. SMITH & W. C. FANSLOW. 1992. Eur. J. Immunol. **22:** 2071–2076.
23. LANE, P., T. BROCKER, S. HUBELE, E. PADOVAN, A. LANZAVECCHIA & F. MCCONNELL. 1993. J. Exp. Med. **177:** 1209–1213.
24. HOLLENBAUGH, D., *et al.* 1992. EMBO J. **11:** 4313–4321.
25. BANCHEREAU, J., P. DE PAOLI, A. VALLÉ, E. GARCIA & F. ROUSSET. 1991. Science **251:** 70–72.
26. SPRIGGS, M. K., R. J. ARMITAGE, L. STROCKBINE, K. N. CLIFFORD, B. M. MACDUFF, T. A. SATO, C. R. MALISZEWSKI & W. C. FANSLOW. 1992. J. Exp. Med. **176:** 1543–1550.
27. GRABSTEIN, K. H., C. R. MALISZEWSKI, K. SHANEBECK, T. A. SATO, M. K. SPRIGG, W. C. FANSLOW & R. J. ARMITAGE. 1993. J. Immunol. **150:** 3141–3147.
28. COCKS, B. G., R. DE WAAL-MALEFYT, J.-P. GALIZZI, J. E. DE VRIES & G. AVERSA. 1993. Intern. Immunol. **5:** 657–663.
29. GAUCHAT, J.-F., J.-P. AUBRY, G. MAZZEI, P. LIFE, T. JOMOTTE, G. ELSON & J.-Y. BONNEFOY. 1993. FEBS **3:** 259–266.
30. ARMITAGE, R. J., B. M. MACDUFF, M. K. SPRIGGS & W. C. FANSLOW. 1993. J. Immunol. **150:** 3671–3680.
31. DEFRANCE, T., B. VANBERVLIET, I. DURAND, J. BRIOLAY & J. BANCHEREAU. 1992. Eur. J. Immunol. **22:** 2831–2839.
32. MINTY, A., *et al.* 1993. Nature **362:** 248–250.
33. ROUSSET, F., E. GARCIA & J. BANCHEREAU. 1991. J. Exp. Med. **173:** 705–710.
34. FLUCKIGER, A.-C., P. GARRONE, I. DURAND, J. P. GALIZZI & J. BANCHEREAU. 1993. J. Exp. Med. **178:** 1473–1481.

35. MALISZEWSKI, C. R., K. GRABSTEIN, W. C. FANSLOW, R. ARMITAGE, M. K. SPRIGGS & T. A. SATO. 1993. Eur. J. Immunol. **23:** 1044–1049.
36. DEFRANCE, T., B. VANBERVLIET, F. BRIÈRE, I. DURAND, F. ROUSSET & J. BANCH-EREAU. 1992. J. Exp. Med. **175:** 671–682.
37. JABARA, H. H., S. M. FU, R. S. GEHA & D. VERCELLI. 1990. J. Exp. Med. **172:** 1861–1864.
38. GASCAN, H., J.-F. GAUCHAT, M.-G. RONCAROLO, H. YSSEL, H. SPITS & J. E. DE VRIES. 1991. J. Exp. Med. **173:** 747–750.
39. SHAPIRA, S. K., D. VERCELLI, H. H. JABARA, S. M. FU & R. S. GEHA. 1992. J. Exp. Med. **175:** 289–292.
40. ZHANG, K., E. A. CLARK & A. SAXON. 1991. J. Immunol. **146:** 1836–1842.
41. PÈNE, J., et al. 1988. Proc. Natl. Acad. Sci. U.S.A. **85:** 6880–6884.
42. PUNNONEN, J., G. G. AVERSA, B. G. COCKS, A. N. J. MCKENZIE, S. MENON, G. ZURAWSKI, R. DE WAAL MALEFYT & J. E. DE VRIES. 1993. Proc. Natl. Acad. Sci. U.S.A. **90:** 3730–3734.
43. BRIÈRE, F., C. SERVET-DELPRAT, J. M. BRIDON, J. M. SAINT-REMY & J. BANCHEREAU. 1993. J. Exp. Med. **179:** 757–762.
44. COFFMAN, R. L., D. A. LEBMAN & B. SHRADER. 1989. J. Exp. Med. **170:** 1039–1045.
45. ISLAM, K. B., L. NILSSON, P. SIDERAS, L. HAMMARSTRÖM & C. I. E. SMITH. 1991. Int. Immunol. **3:** 1099–1106.
46. ZUBLER, R. H., C. WERNER-FAVRE, L. WEN, K.-I. SEKITA & C. STRAUB. 1987. Immunol. Rev. **99:** 281–299.
47. ARMITAGE, R. J., et al. 1992. Nature **357:** 80–82.
48. LIPSKY, P. E. 1990. Res. Immunol. **141:** 424–427.
49. NOELLE, R. J. & E. C. SNOW. 1990. Immunol. Today **11:** 361–368.
50. NOELLE, R. J., L. MCCANN, L. MARSHALL & W. C. BARTLETT. 1989. J. Immunol. **143:** 1807.
51. BRIAN, A. A. 1988. Proc. Natl. Acad. Sci. U.S.A. **85:** 564–568.
52. HODGKIN, P. D., L. C. YAMASHITA, R. L. COFFMAN & M. R. KEHRY. 1990. J. Immunol. **145:** 2025–2034.
53. GASCAN, H., et al. 1992. Eur. J. Immunol. **22:** 1133–1141.
54. NOELLE, R. J., M. ROY, D. M. SHEPHERD, I. STAMENKOVIC, J. A. LEDBETTER & A. ARUFFO. 1992. Proc. Natl. Acad. Sci. U.S.A. **89:** 6550–6554.
55. LEDERMAN, S., M. J. YELLIN, A. KRICHEVSKY, J. BELKO, J. J. LEE & L. CHESS. 1992. J. Exp. Med. **175:** 1091–1101.
56. SPLAWSKI, J. B., S.-M. FU & P. E. LIPSKY. 1993. J. Immunol. **150:** 1276–1285.
57. BLANCHARD, D., C. GAILLARD, P. HERMANN, F. FOSSIEZ & J. BANCHEREAU. 1994. Eur. J. Immunol. **24:** 330–335.
58. ALLEN, R. C., et al. 1993. Science **259:** 990.
59. ARUFFO, A., et al. 1993. Cell **72:** 291–300.
60. DISANTO, J. P., J. Y. BONNEFOY, J. F. GAUCHAT, A. FISCHER & G. DE SAINT BASILE. 1993. Nature **361:** 541.
61. KORTHÄUER, U., et al. 1993. Nature **361:** 539–541.
62. FULEIHAN, R., et al. 1993. Proc. Natl. Acad. Sci. U.S.A. **90:** 2170–2173.
63. MACLENNAN, I. C. & D. GRAY. 1986. Immunol. Rev. **91:** 61–85.
64. KROESE, F. G. M., W. TIMENS & P. NIEUWENHUIS. 1990. Reaction patterns of the lymph node. In Current Topics in Pathology, E. Grundman & E. Vollmer, Eds.: 103–148. Springer-Verlag. Berlin.
65. LIU, Y.-J., G. D. JOHNSON, J. GORDON & I. C. M. MACLENNAN. 1992. Immunol. Today **13:** 17–21.
66. STEINMAN, R. M. 1991. Annu. Rev. Immunol. **9:** 271–296.
67. INABA, K., M. D. WITMER & R. M. STEINMAN. 1984. J. Exp. Med. **160:** 858–876.
68. BOGEN, S. A., I. FOGELMAN & A. K. ABBAS. 1993. J. Immunol. **150:** 4197–4205.
69. JACOB, J., R. KASSIR & G. KELSOE. 1991. J. Exp. Med. **173:** 1165–1175.
70. JACOB, J. & G. KELSOE. 1992. J. Exp. Med. **176:** 679–687.
71. MCHEYZER-WILLIAMS, M. G., M. J. MCLEAN, P. A. LALOR & G. J. V. NOSSAL. 1993. J. Exp. Med. **178:** 295–307.
72. SCHRIEVER, F., G. FREEMAN & L. M. NADLER. 1991. Blood **77:** 787–791.

73. Caux, C., C. Dezutter-Dambuyant, D. Schmitt & J. Banchereau. 1992. Nature **360:** 258–261.
74. Liu, Y.-J., D. Y. Mason, G. D. Johnson, S. Abbot, C. D. Gregory, D. L. Hardie, J. Gordon & I. C. M. MacLennan. 1991. Eur. J. Immunol. **21:** 1905–1910.
75. Kroese, F. G. M., A. S. Wubbena, H. G. Seijen & P. Nieuwenhuis. 1987. Eur. J. Immunol. **17:** 1069–1072.
76. Jacob, J., G. Kelsoe, K. Rajewsky & U. Weiss. 1991. Nature **354:** 389–392.
77. Berek, C., A. Berger & M. Apel. 1991. Cell **67:** 1121–1129.
78. Linton, P. J., D. J. Decker & N. R. Klinman. 1989. Cell **59:** 1049–1059.
79. Linton, P. J., D. Lo, L. Lai, G. J. Thorbecke & N. R. Klinman. 1992. Eur. J. Immunol. **22:** 1293–1297.
80. Liu, Y. J., D. E. Joshua, G. T. Williams, C. A. Smith, J. Gordon & I. C. M. MacLennan. 1989. Nature **342:** 929–931.
81. Holder, M. J., Y.-J. Liu, T. Defrance, L. Flores-Romo, T. C. M. MacLennan & J. Gordon. 1991. Int. Immunol. **3:** 1243.
82. Lederman, S., M. J. Yellin, G. Inghirami, J. J. Lee, D. M. Knowles & L. Chess. 1992. J. Immunol. **149:** 3817–3826.
83. Butch, A. W., G.-H. Chung, J. W. Hoffmann & M. H. Nahm. 1993. J. Immunol. **150:** 39–47.
84. Kishimoto, T., S. Akira & T. Taga. 1992. Science **258:** 593–597.
85. Roldan, E., A. Garcia-Pardo & J. A. Brieva. 1992. J. Exp. Med. **175:** 1739–1747.
86. Bergui, L., M. Schena, G. Gaidano, M. Riva & F. Caligaris-Cappio. 1989. J. Exp. Med. **170:** 613–618.
87. Tadmori, W., D. Feingersh, S. C. Clark & Y. S. Choi. 1989. J. Immunol. **142:** 1950–1955.

Modulation by rm Interferon-γ and CD4⁺ T-Lymphocytes of Allergic Eosinophil Accumulation in the Mice Peritoneal Cavity[a]

CLÁUDIA ZUANY-AMORIM,[b] DOMINIQUE LEDUC,[c]
B. BORIS VARGAFTIG,[c] AND MARINA PRETOLANI[c,d]

[b]Fundação Oswaldo Cruz
IOC-Departamento de Fisiologia e Farmacodinâmica
Rio de Janeiro, Brazil

[c]Unité de Pharmacologie Cellulaire
Unité Associée Institut Pasteur
INSERM No. 285
25 Rue du Dr. Roux
75015, Paris, France

INTRODUCTION

Increased evidence suggests that T-lymphocyte activation and eosinophil recruitment are related events in the development of allergic inflammatory reactions. CD4⁺ cells may be divided in two subsets, that is, Th1 and Th2 lymphocytes, according to the pattern of cytokines generated by each cell population. Many of the cytokines released from Th2 CD4⁺ clones, including granulocyte-macrophage colony-stimulating factor (GM-CSF), interleukin (IL)-3, and IL-5, are involved in the eosinophil growth and activation, since they enhance the survival of eosinophils in culture and promote the cytotoxicity and phagocytosis of yeast particles.[1–4] Finally, the role of IL-5 in antigen-induced eosinophil recruitment into the peritoneal cavity[5] or the lung tissue[6] of sensitized mice has been demonstrated.

A reciprocal regulation between Th1 and Th2 clones has been proposed involving the generation of different cytokines from the two T-lymphocyte populations. In particular, interferon-γ (IFN-γ), a cytokine secreted by activated Th1 CD4⁺ cells and natural killer cells, exhibits immunomodulatory effects on various cell types.[7] Accordingly, IFN-γ was shown to inhibit IL-4 generation from Th1 clones and to mediate some effects on B cells, including the switching toward IgE and IgG1 production and the IL-4-induced CD23 expression *in vitro*.[8] Furthermore, the involvement of IFN-γ in the effector T-cell death was reported, suggesting the participation of this cytokine in the mechanisms of self-tolerance.[9] Finally, it was recently reported that IFN-γ suppressed antigen-induced eosinophil recruitment into the mice airways, probably by decreasing the number of CD4⁺ T-lymphocytes.[10]

[a] The work of one of the authors (C.Z.A.) is supported by the Brazilian funding agency CNPq.
[d] To whom correspondence should be addressed.

34

In the present study, we investigated the role of IFN-γ and of CD4$^+$ T lymphocytes in antigen-induced cell accumulation into the peritoneal cavity of sensitized mice. To do so, Balb/c mice sensitized to ovalbumin were treated with IFN-γ or with an anti-IFN-γ antibody, or their CD4$^+$ T lymphocytes were depleted by a specific antibody. Changes in the number of neutrophils and eosinophils in the peritoneal cavity in response to antigen challenge were then evaluated.

MATERIAL AND METHODS

Animals and Sensitization Procedure

Male Balb/c mice aged 8 weeks, weighing approximately 25–30 g raised at the Pasteur Institute (Paris, France) were actively sensitized by a subcutaneous (s.c.) injection of 0.4 ml 0.9% w/v NaCl (saline) containing 100-μg ovalbumin adsorbed in 1.6-mg aluminium hydroxide (16). Seven days later, the animals received the same dose of ovalbumin in the presence of $Al(OH)_3$ and they were used 7 days thereafter.

Antigen-Induced Peritonitis

Peritonitis was induced by the intraperitoneal (i.p.) injection of 0.4 ml of a solution containing either 2.5 or 25-μg ml^{-1} ovalbumin diluted in sterile saline (1 or 10 μg of ovalbumin, as final doses injected per cavity). Control animals received the same volume of sterile saline. At different time intervals after antigen challenge, animals were killed by an overdose of ether and the peritoneal cavity was opened and washed with 3 ml of heparinized saline (10 U ml^{-1}). Around 90 percent of the initial volume was recovered. In rare cases, when hemorrhages were noted in the peritoneal cavity, the animals were discarded.

Leucocyte Analysis

Total leucocytes present in the peritoneal lavages were counted in a Coulter counter ZM (Coultronics, Margency, France) and expressed as numbers of cells ml^{-1}. Differential cell counts were performed after cytocentrifugation (Hettich-Universal) and staining with Diff-Quik stain (Baxter Dade AG, Dudingen). At least 300 cells were counted and results were expressed as number of each cell population ml^{-1}.

In vivo *Treatments*

The dose of 1 μg of ovalbumin and the times of 6 and 24 h after challenge were selected throughout the study. Sensitized mice were treated subcutaneously (s.c.) with rmIFN-γ (5000 U/mouse) or with an anti-IFN-γ antibody (XM G 1.2, 50 μg/mouse) 1 h before and 6 h after the antigen challenge and the animals were killed at 24 h to evaluate the number of infiltrating eosinophils. The immunosuppressive agent FK-506 (2 mg/kg) was administered s.c. 6 h and 5 min before the challenge.

In order to investigate the effect of the different treatments on antigen-induced neutrophil infiltration, sensitized mice were injected s.c. 1 h before and 3 h after ovalbumin administration with 5000 U/mouse rmIFN-γ or with 2 mg/kg FK-506, and they were killed 6 h after the challenge.

rmIFN-γ and the anti-IFN-γ antibody were dissolved in sterile saline containing 0.1 percent human serum albumin (HSA). FK-506 was dissolved in a mixture of ethanol, Tween 80, and saline (1 : 0.2 : 8.8; v/v/v). In control experiments, sensitized mice received s.c. injections of the appropriate vehicles and they were challenged with 1-μg ovalbumin, as previously described.

CD4+ T-Lymphocytes Depletion

In separate experiments, sensitized mice were treated with a specific rat IgG2b antimurine CD4+ T-lymphocyte (GK 1.5; 500 μg/mouse)[11] once a day for two days before and on the day of antigen challenge, and they were killed 6 or 24 h thereafter. GK 1.5 was semipurified from ascitic fluid by 18 percent Na_2SO_4 precipitation followed by gel filtration through a Sepharose 6B column. This fraction had an immunofluorescence titer of 1/350,000, as determined by fluorescence-activated cell sorter (FACS) analysis of thymocyte suspension stained with FITC-labeled GARIg antibody as the second step. The effectiveness of the anti-CD4+ antibody in depleting CD4+ T lymphocytes after a 3-day treatment was determined by FACS analysis. Briefly, spleen cell suspensions were prepared from sensitized mice killed on the day of peritoneal cell washing determination. Ten microliters of 10^8 ml^{-1} splenocytes suspended in minimal essential medium containing 3 percent fetal bovine serum (FBS) and 0.1 percent sodium azide were incubated in 96-well, round-bottomed plates with 50 μl of goat anti-L3T4 (anti-CD4+, YTS 191.1) or anti-Lyt-2 antibody (anti-CD8+, YTS 169.4) conjugated with fluorescein-isothiocyanate (FITC) at optimal dilutions. FACS analysis demonstrated that a 3-day treatment of sensitized mice with GK 1.5 at 500 μg/mouse depleted by 99 percent of the proportion of CD4+ T-cells, without affecting that of CD8+ T-cells.

Materials

Ovalbumin (5× crystallized) was from Immunobiological (Costa Mesa, United States). Heparin was from Choay (Paris, France), and HSA from Bio-Transfusion (Paris, France). Tween-80 was from Fluka Chemika (Buchs, Switzerland). rmIFN-γ and the anti-IFN-γ were from Immugenex (Los Angeles, United States). Goat anti-CD4 (YTS 191.1) and anti-CD8 (YTS 169.4) conjugated with an FITC were purchased from Caltag (San Francisco, United States). FBS and sodium azide were from Mallinckrodt Chemicals (St. Louis, United States). FK-506 was kindly provided by Dr. K. Murato (Fujisawa Pharmaceutical, Osaka, Japan).

Statistical Analysis

Data were analyzed statistically using a microcomputer program and an analysis of variance (ANOVA) followed by Student's t-test for unpaired values. P values of 0.05 or less were considered significant. The results are expressed as means ± SEM of the indicated number of experiments.

RESULTS

Antigen-Induced Cell Accumulation into the Peritoneal Cavity of Sensitized Mice

The i.p. injection of 1 or 10 μg ovalbumin to sensitized Balb/c mice induced a marked and dose-dependent increase in the number of neutrophils, which was detectable 6 h after challenge (FIG. 1a). Ovalbumin administration also induced a dose-dependent eosinophil infiltration, starting at 24 h and reaching a maximum

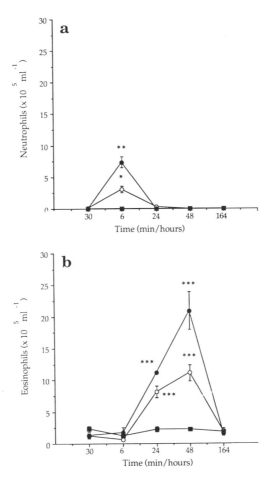

FIGURE 1. Kinetics of antigen-induced neutrophil (**panel a**) and eosinophil (**panel b**) infiltration in the peritoneal cavity of sensitized mice. Cells were enumerated and differentiated at various time intervals (30 min–164 h) after the injection of either saline (■), or 1 (○), or 10-μg (●) ovalbumin. Results are expressed as mean ± SEM (*vertical bars*) of 5–11 experiments. *$P < 0.05$, **$P < 0.01$, and ***$P < 0.001$, as compared to saline-injected animals.

TABLE 1. Effect of the Subcutaneous (s.c.) Administration of 5000 U/Mouse rmIFN-γ on Antigen-Induced Neutrophil and Eosinophil Recruitment into the Peritoneal Cavity of Sensitized Mice

Treatment	Cell Type	
	Neutrophils ($\times$ 10^5/ml)	Eosinophils ($\times$ 10^5/ml)
Saline, s.c.	12.3 $\pm$ 2.5	6.6 $\pm$ 0.7
IFN-γ (5000 U/mouse, s.c.)	9.4 $\pm$ 2.3	2.9 $\pm$ 0.5**

Note. Neutrophil and eosinophil counts in the peritoneal washing were determined 6 h or 24 h after the i.p. administration of 1-μg ovalbumin. Data are expressed as mean $\pm$ SEM of 6–12 experiments.
** $P < 0.01$, as compared to saline-injected mice.

at 48 h. One week later, the eosinophil counts returned to basal levels (FIG. 1b). When nonsensitized mice were challenged i.p. with 10-μg ovalbumin no changes in the number of any cell population was observed (data not shown).

Effect of rmIFN-γ on Antigen-Induced Neutrophil and Eosinophil Recruitment into the Peritoneal Cavity of Sensitized Mice

The s.c. treatment with rmIFN-γ (5000 U/mouse) 1 h before and 6 h after the i.p. injection of 1-μg ovalbumin reduced the eosinophil accumulation into the mice peritoneal cavity by 57 percent ($n = 5$; $P < 0.01$, TABLE 1). In contrast, rmIFN-γ, when administered at the same dose 1 h before and 3 h after the challenge did not modify the neutrophil infiltration into the mice peritoneal cavity (TABLE 1).

Effect of anti-IFN-γ on Antigen-Induced Eosinophil Recruitment into the Peritoneal Cavity of Sensitized Mice

When sensitized mice were pretreated with an anti-IFN-γ antibody, administered s.c. at 50 μg/mouse, 1 h before and 6 h after antigen challenge, a significant increase (54 percent, $n = 12$, $P < 0.05$) in the number of infiltrating eosinophils in response to ovalbumin administration was observed (TABLE 2).

TABLE 2. Effect of the Subcutaneous (s.c.) Administration of 50 μg/Mouse of an Anti-IFN-γ Antibody on Ovalbumin (1-μg)-Induced Eosinophil Recruitment into the Peritoneal Cavity of Sensitized Mice

Treatment	Eosinophils ($\times$ 10^5/ml)
Saline, s.c.	4.8 $\pm$ 0.6
anti-IFN-γ (50 μg/mouse, s.c.)	7.4 $\pm$ 0.9*

Note. Results are expressed as mean $\pm$ SEM of 6–12 experiments.
* $P < 0.05$, as compared to saline-injected mice.

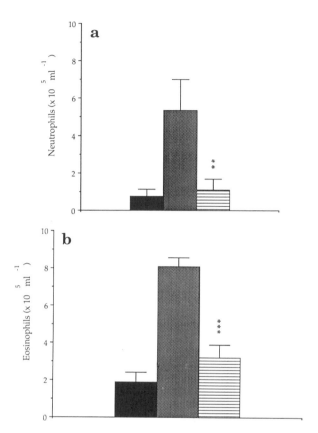

FIGURE 2. Effect of FK-506 on antigen-induced eosinophil accumulation in the peritoneal washing from sensitized mice killed 6 h (**panel a**) or 24 h (**panel b**) after the challenge. Animals were injected i.p. either with saline (■), or with 1-μg ovalbumin (■), and they were treated s.c. with 2 mg kg^{-1} (⊟) FK-506, injected twice, 1 h before and 6 h after antigen challenge, for neutrophil number determination, or 6 h and 5 min before ovalbumin administration, for eosinophil counts. Results are expressed as mean ± SEM (*vertical bars*) of 5–11 experiments. **$P < 0.01$ and ***$P < 0.001$, as compared to antigen-challenged untreated mice.

Effect of FK-506 on Antigen-Induced Eosinophilia into the Peritoneal Cavity of Sensitized Mice

Eosinophilia induced by the i.p. injection of 1-μg ovalbumin was significantly inhibited by the treatment of sensitized mice with 2 mg kg^{-1} FK-506, administered s.c. 6 h and 5 min before the challenge (FIG. 2b). Indeed, a 60 percent reduction in the number of eosinophils was observed ($n = 11$, $P < 0.001$). Contrary to what we have observed with IFN-γ, the treatment with 2 mg/kg FK-506 was also very effective in decreasing neutrophil accumulation induced by antigen challenge (FIG. 2a).

Effect of the in vivo *Depletion of CD4⁺ T Cells on Antigen-Induced Eosinophilia into the Peritoneal Cavity of Sensitized Mice*

The *in vivo* depletion of CD4$^+$ T lymphocytes following the i.v. treatment with 500 μg/mouse/per day for 3 days of GK 1.5 suppressed antigen-induced eosinophil and neutrophil infiltration in the peritoneal cavity of sensitized mice ($n = 6$; $P < 0.001$, for both groups, TABLE 3). Under these conditions, treatment of sensitized mice with a rat IgG2b isotype did not modify the increased numbers of the different cell populations induced by antigen challenge (data not shown).

TABLE 3. Effect of the Intravenous (i.v.) Administrations of an Anti-CD4$^+$ Antibody (GK 1.5, 500 μg/Mouse/Day for 3 Days) on Antigen-Induced Neutrophil and Eosinophil Accumulation into the Peritoneal Cavity of Sensitized Mice

	Cell Type	
Treatment	Neutrophils ($\times$ 10^5/ml)	Eosinophils ($\times$ 10^5/ml)
Saline, i.v.	7.5 ± 1.5	11.8 ± 1.9
GK 1.5 3 × 500 μg/mouse, i.v.	2.5 ± 1.1***	3.1 ± 0.5***

Note. Neutrophil and eosinophil counts in the peritoneal washing were determined 6 or 24 h after the i.p. administration of 1-μg ovalbumin. Results are expressed as mean ± SEM of 6 experiments.
*** $P < 0.001$, as compared to saline-treated mice.

DISCUSSION

In the present study, the role of IFN-γ and of CD4$^+$ T lymphocytes in the antigen-induced cell accumulation in the peritoneal cavity of sensitized Balb/c mice was investigated. The administration of rmIFN-γ markedly reduced eosinophil, but not neutrophil infiltration, suggesting that this cytokine may play a role in the regulation of allergic eosinophilia. Furthermore, pretreatment with an anti-IFN-γ antibody enhanced significantly antigen-induced eosinophil infiltration into the peritoneal cavity, further supporting the concept that inhibition of the endogenous production of Th1-derived cytokines, such as IFN-γ, may result in an enhanced Th2 response.

The inhibition of allergic eosinophilia by IFN-γ seems paradoxical because of the well-documented ability by this cytokine to display proinflammatory activities, such as the increase of monocyte-macrophage functions and vascular permeability.[12] However, a number of experimenters report evidence of an inhibitory effect of IFN-γ in various models of allergic and nonallergic inflammation. Thus, Wahl et al.[13] showed that IFN-γ markedly reduced mononuclear cell recruitment accompanying bacterial cell wall-induced arthritis in mice. Interestingly enough, Iwamoto *et al.*[10] recently showed that the administration of IFN-γ to sensitized mice suppressed antigen-induced eosinophil recruitment into the airways. This phenomenon was accompanied by a decrease in the number of CD4+ T lymphocytes, one of the major source of eosinophilotactic cytokines in the airways. Among CD4+ T lymphocytes, Th1 and Th2 subsets are distinguished on the basis of the cytokines they secrete *in vitro*. Thus, Th1 clones mainly produce IFN-γ, TNF-β, and IL-2, whereas Th2 clones generate IL-4 and IL-5. Both cell types, however, are able to secrete IL-3 and GM-CSF,[14,15] which are involved in monocyte-macrophage and eosinophil proliferation and chemotaxis[2,4,16] in various species, including mice. Since IL-5 is unique in selectively promoting the proliferation and differentiation of the eosinophil lineage and in increasing their survival,[17] an effect of IFN-γ on the generation of IL-5 from activated Th2 T lymphocytes may be proposed as one of the mechanisms involved in the inhibition of allergic eosinophilia in mice. Accordingly, it was recently demonstrated that the incubation with IFN-γ suppressed the proliferation of Th2 clones.[18] Furthermore, Schandené *et al.*[19] reported that IFN-γ inhibited the *in vivo* generation of IL-5 accompanying the Omenn's syndrome.

In the present study we demonstrated that the effect of IFN-γ was selectively directed against eosinophils, since the neutrophil infiltration observed 6 h after ovalbumin administration was unaffected by IFN-γ. Since the depletion of the animals in CD4+ T lymphocytes was equally effective in inhibiting antigen-induced neutrophil and eosinophil recruitment in the peritoneal cavity of sensitized mice, it is likely that the reduction in the number of CD4+ T lymphocytes as the mechanism of action of IFN-γ[10] does not account alone for the lack of effect on neutrophil recruitment we have observed. Indeed, the incubation of monocytes and neutrophils with IFN-γ decreases the *in vitro* monocyte, but not neutrophil migration,[20] suggesting that inhibition by IFN-γ of antigen-induced eosinophil, but not neutrophil recruitment, might be the consequence of a direct effect on eosinophil chemotaxis and/or on the expression of adhesion proteins selectively involved in the eosinophil transmigration through the endothelial cell wall. For example, the $\alpha_4\beta_1$ integrin VLA-4 is expressed on eosinophils and other leucocytes, but not on neutrophil surface.[21] Accordingly, it has been recently demonstrated that the local or systemic pretreatment of guinea pigs with an anti-VLA-4 antibody inhibited allergic and nonallergic eosinophil accumulation in the skin.[22] The ability of IFN-γ to interfere with the expression of VLA-4 adhesion molecule, however, requires further investigation.

In the present study we also demonstrate that pretreatment of sensitized mice with the immunosuppressive agent FK-506 or with the specific antibody directed against CD4+ T-lymphocytes suppressed both neutrophil and eosinophil infiltration into the mice peritoneal cavity induced by antigen challenge. The mechanism of the inhibition of cell recruitment observed with FK-506 was not elucidated yet. However, FK-506 was shown to decrease *in vitro* T-cell and mast cell cytokine production,[23–35] suggesting that it may prevent the *in vivo* generation of those cytokines responsible for both eosinophil and neutrophil infiltration following antigen challenge.

In conclusion, our results demonstrate that allergic eosinophilia in mice can be modulated by IFN-γ, a Th1-derived cytokine, and by suppressing CD4+ lymphocytes either with a specific antibody or with an immunosuppressive drug, such as FK-506. Since antigen stimulation leads to the generation of a large variety of cyokines, their determination in biological fluids and tissues and the correlation between their presence and the different cell types involved will be an important step for further understanding the mechanisms of allergic inflammation.

ACKNOWLEDGMENTS

The authors wish to thank Dr. G. Bordenave and Miss C. Denoyelle (Department of Immunology, Institut Pasteur, Paris, France) for help in the fluorescent analysis of lymphocytes and CD4$^+$ cells exhaustion.

REFERENCES

1. ROTHENBERG, M. E., W. F. OWEN, D. S. SILBERSTEIN, J. WOODS, R. J. SOBERMAN, K. F. AUSTEN & R. L. STEVENS. 1988. Human eosinophils have prolonged survival, enhanced functional properties, and become hypodense when exposed to human interleukin 3. J. Clin. Invest. **81:** 1986–1992.
2. ROTHENBERGH, M. E., J. PETERSEN, R. L. STEVENS, D. S. SILBERSTEIN, D. T. MAC-KENZIE, K. F. AUSTEN & W. F. OWEN. 1989. IL-5-dependent conversion of normo-dense human eosinophils to the hypodense phenotype uses 3T3 fibroblasts for enhanced viability accelerated hypodensity, and sustained antibody-dependent cytotoxicity. J. Immunol. **143:** 2311–2316.
3. LOPEZ, A. F., C. J. SANDERSON, J. R. GAMBLE, H. D. CAMPBELL, I. YOUNG & M. A. VADAS. 1988. Recombinant human interleukin-5 is a selective activator of human eosinophil function. J. Exp. Med. **167:** 219–224.
4. SILBERSTEIN, D. S., W. F. OWEN, J. C. GASSON, J. F. DIPERSIO, D. W. GOLDE, J. C. BINA, R. SOBERMAN & K. F. AUSTEN. 1989. Enhancement of human eosinophil cytotoxicity and leukotriene synthesis by biosynthetic (recombinant) granulocyte-macrophage colony-stimulating factor. J. Immunol. **137:** 3290–3294.
5. KANETO, M., Y. HITOSHI, K. TAKATSU & S. MATSUMOTO. 1991. Role of interleukin-5 in local accumulation of eosinophils in mouse allergic peritonitis. Int. Arch. Allergy Appl. Immunol. **96:** 41–45.
6. OKUDAIRA, H., M. NOGAMI, D. MATSUZUKI, M. SUKO, S. KASUYA & K. TAKATSU. 1991. T-cell-dependent accumulation of eosinophils in the lung and its inhibition by monoclonal anti-interleukin-5. Int. Arch. Allergy Appl. Immunol. **94:** 171–173.
7. TRINCHIERI, G. & B. PERUSSIA. 1985. Immune interferon: A pleiotropic lymphokine with multiple effects. Immunol. Today **6:** 131–135.
8. TAN, H., L. K. LEBECK & S. L. NEHLSEN-CANNARELLA. 1992. Regulatory role of cytokines in Ig-E mediated allergy. J. Leukoc. Biol. **52:** 115–118.
9. LIU, Y. & C. A. JANEWAY, JR. 1990. Interferon γ plays a critical role in induced cell death of effector T cell: A possible third mechanism of self-tolerance. J. Exp. Med. **172:** 1735–1739.
10. IWAMOTO, I., H. NAKAJIMA, H. ENDO & S. YOSHIDA. 1993. Interferon γ regulates antigen-induced eosinophil recruitment into the mouse airways by inhibiting the infiltration of CD4$^+$ T cells. J. Exp. Med. **177:** 573–576.
11. DIALYNAS, D. P., Z. S. QUAN & K. A. WALL. 1983. Characterization of the murine T cell surface molecule, designated L3T4, identified by monoclonal antibody GK 1.5: Similarity of L3T4 to the human Leu3/T4 molecule. J. Immunol. **131:** 2445–2451.
12. ABE, Y., S. SEKIYA, T. YAMASITA & F. SENDO. 1990. Vascular hyperpermeability induced by tumor necrosis factor and its augmentation by IL-1 and IFN-γ is inhibited by selective depletion with a monoclonal antibody. J. Immunol. **145:** 2902–2907.
13. WAHL, S. M., J. B. ALLEN, B. OHURA, D. E. CHENOWET & R. HAND. 1991. IFN-γ inhibits inflammatory cell recruitment and the evolution of bacterial cell wall-induced arthritis. J. Immunol. **146:** 95–100.
14. MOSMANN, T. R., H. CHERWINSKI, M. W. BOND, M. A. GIEDLIN & R. A. COFFMAN. 1986. Two types of murine helper T-cell clone. I. Definition accordingly to profiles of lymphokines activities and secreted proteins. J. Immunol. **136:** 2348–2354.
15. CHERWINSKI, H., J. SCHUMACHER, K. BROWN & T. MOSMANN. 1987. Two types of mouse helper T cell clone. III. Further differences in lymphokines synthesis between

Th1 and Th2 clones revealed by RNA hybridization, functionally monospecific bio-assays, and monoclonal antibodies. J. Exp. Med. **166:** 1229–1232.

16. LOPEZ, A. F., *et al.* 1987. Stimulation of proliferation, differentiation and function of human cells by primate interleukin 3. Proc. Natl. Acad. Sci. U.S.A. **84:** 2761–2765.

17. SANDERSON, C. J. 1992. Interleukin-5, eosinophils, and disease. Blood **79:** 3101–3109.

18. GAJEWSKI, T. F. & F. W. FITCH. 1988. Anti-proliferative effect of IFN-γ in immune regulation, I. IFN-γ inhibits the proliferation of Th2 but not Th1 murine helper T lymphocyte clones. J. Immunol. **140:** 4245–4252.

19. SCHANDENÉ, L., *et al.* 1993. T helper type 2-lyke cells and therapeutic effects of interferon-γ in combined immunodeficiency with hypereosinophilia (Omenn's syndrome). Eur. J. Immunol. **23:** 56–60.

20. GRANSTEIN, R. D., M. R. DEAK, S. L. JACQUES, T. J. MARGOLIS, D. BLOTTE, WHITAKER, F. H. LONG & E. P. AMENTO. 1989. The systemic administration of gamma interferon inhibits collagen synthesis and acute inflammation in a murine skin wounding model. J. Invest. Dermatol. **93:** 18–24.

21. WALSH, G. M., J. J. MERMOD, A. HARTNELL, A. B. KAY & A. J. WARDLAW. 1991. Human eosinophil, but not neutrophil, adherence to IL-1-stimulated human umbilical vascular endothelial cells is $\alpha_4\beta_1$ (very late antigen-4) dependent. J. Immunol. **146:** 3419–3425.

22. WEG, V. B., T. J. WILLIAMS, R. R. LOBB & NOURSHARGH. 1993. A monoclonal antibody recognizing very late activation antigen-4 inhibits eosinophil accumulation *in vivo.* J. Exp. Med. **177:** 561–566.

23. SAWADA, S., G. SUZUKI, Y. KAWASE & F. TAKAKU. 1987. Novel immunosuppressive agent, FK-506. In vitro effects on the cloned T cell activation. J. Immunol. **139:** 1797–1803.

24. SIERKIERKA, J. J., S. H. Y. HUNG, M. POE, C. S. LIN & N. H. SIGAL. 1989. A cytosolic binding protein for the immunosuppressant FK-506 had peptidylpropyl isomerase activity but is distinct from cyclophilin. Nature **3:** 755–757.

25. HATFIELD, S. M. & N. W. ROEHM. 1992. Cyclosporine and FK-506 inhibition of murine mast cell cytokine production. J. Pharmacol. Exp. Ther. **260:** 680–688.

Regulation of IgE Production by β_2-Adrenoceptor Agonists

O. COQUERET, V. LAGENTE,[a] C. PETIT FRÈRE,
P. BRAQUET, AND J.-M. MENCIA-HUERTA[b]

Institut Henri Beaufour
91952 Les Ulis
France

INTRODUCTION

B lymphocytes represent the effector cell of the humoral limb of the immunity because they produce antibodies directed against various antigens. Immature B cells differentiate in antibody-secreting cells in two steps. The first step is independent of the presence of the antigen and occurs primarily in the bone marrow where immunoglobulin gene rearrangement occurs. The second step is antigen-dependent and leads to the differentiation of mature B lymphocytes into memory B cells. This second process happens mostly in secondary lymphoid organs, such as lymph nodes, tonsils, spleen, Peyer's patches, and is characterized by cell proliferation and affinity maturation through somatic hypermutation.

It is now well established that T lymphocytes and T-cell-derived soluble factors play an important role in B-lymphocyte differentiation. Indeed, cellular interactions are an important feature of B-cell differentiation since T and B cells must physically interact to initiate this process.[1] These interactions between T and B lymphocytes are mediated by cell-surface molecules such as major histocompatibility complex (MHC) class II antigens or LFA-1 (lymphocyte-function-associated antigen) molecules, as well as by soluble factors such as cytokines.[1-3] However, the mechanisms that regulate the extent of the interaction between B and T cells remain uncertain. One possible nonlymphoid mechanism implicated in the regulation of immunoglobulin production involves the autonomic nervous system. Indeed, primary and secondary lymphoid organs are innervated by norepinephrine-containing nerve fibers that enter the vasculature and distribute to the parenchyma.[4] It has also been shown that lymphocytes express β_2 adrenoceptors.[5-7] These findings suggest that β_2-adrenoceptor agonist may play a role in the regulation of B-cell function.

The effects of adrenergic and noradrenergic components on T and B lymphocytes have already been investigated. Stimulation of β_2 adrenoceptors induced an increase of intracellular cyclic adenosine monophosphate (cAMP) levels, an effect associated with a decrease of the proliferation of human T cells in response to mitogenic stimuli.[8] Particularly, isoproterenol has been shown to inhibit the production of IL-2 and to block the expression of its receptor on activated T cells, suggesting a cAMP-induced inhibition of lymphokine production.[8] In the mouse, β_2-adrenoceptor agonists have been shown to enhance the proliferation and differentiation of LPS-stimulated B lymphocytes[9] and to enhance the number of cells secreting antibodies directed against the T-dependent antigen, TNP-KLH.[10] In

[a] Current address: Faculté de Pharmacie, 35000 Rennes, France.
[b] To whom correspondence should be addressed.

this latter case, β_2-adrenoceptor stimulation results in an increase of both the amount of specific IgM and the number of B lymphocytes secreting anti-TNP IgM. No effect of β_2-adrenoceptor agonists on MHC class II expression was noticed, suggesting that these phenomena are unrelated to an increase of the number of T/B cell interactions.[10] This effect was rather related to an increase of the number of B-lymphocyte precursors and not to the proliferation of a given population of B cells already activated to differentiate into immunoglobulin-secreting cells.

Due to their relaxing effect on bronchial smooth muscle cells, inhaled β_2-adrenoceptor agonists are the main bronchodilator drugs used in the symptomatic treatment of asthma. They are usually safe and well tolerated, but increasing evidence indicates that their repeated administration produces various side effects.[11,12] Given the effect of these drugs on murine B-lymphocyte differentiation, it was of interest to investigate the action of these compounds on Ig production in humans. Indeed, part of the reported deleterious effect of β_2-adrenoceptor agonists in asthma might be explained by an increase of IgE-dependent processes.

EFFECTS OF β_2-ADRENOCEPTOR AGONISTS ON IgE PRODUCTION IN HUMAN *IN VITRO*

Addition of salbutamol or fenoterol to human peripheral blood mononuclear cells (PBMC) induced a dose-dependent increase in IgE production, such an effect

TABLE 1. Effect of Salbutamol in the Presence or in the Absence of D,L-Propranolol and Butoxamine on IgE Production and on the Number of IgE-Secreting Cells

Agonist	IgE (pg/ml)	IgE-Secreting Cells (Number/1×10^5 Cells)
None	150	17
IL-4 (30 U/ml)	650	19
IL-4 + salbutamol (10 nM)	1075	38
IL-4 + salbutamol + propranolol	325	25
IL-4 + salbutamol + butoxamine	250	21

being observed only when IgE production was initiated by IL-4 (TABLE 1). No effect of these drugs on IgG, IgM, or IgA production was observed. This effect appears to be mediated via β_2 receptors, since the addition of propranolol or butoxamine into the incubation medium blocked the potentiating effect of these compounds on the IL-4-driven IgE production (TABLE 1).

Elisaspot experiments demonstrated that in the presence of IL-4, salbutamol induced an increase of the number of IgE-secreting cells and that this effect was mediated via β_2-adrenoceptors (TABLE 1). No effect of salbutamol on cell proliferation or viability was noticed. Thus, the effect of salbutamol on IgE production might not be explained by the proliferation of a subpopulation of B cells already committed into IgE-secreting cells.

Surface antigens of cells, such as CD21, CD23, LFA-1, ICAM-1, have been shown to play a role in the interactions between B and T cells. The effect of salbutamol might be explained by an increase in the expression of cell-surface antigens involved in the interaction between B and T cells. As assessed by flow cytometry, however, no effect of salbutamol on CD21, CD23, LFA-1, ICAM-1, and MHC class II expression, in the presence or in the absence of IL-4, was observed. This suggests that the effect of salbutamol could not be merely attributed to an increase of the number of T/B cell interactions.

T-cell-derived soluble factors, such as IL-4, IL-6, and IFN-γ, have been shown to be implicated in the regulation of IgE production in humans.[2,3] It has been shown that IL-4 induces IgE secretion from human PBMC, whereas such production is inhibited by IFN-γ.[2] Results also suggested that IL-6 might potentiate the effect of IL-4.[3] When PBMC were added with phytohemagglutinin-A (PHA) in the presence of salbutamol, a slight and nonsignificant increase in IL-4 production was noticed and no effect on IL-6 production was observed. By contrast, a significant decrease of IFN-γ production was observed, both in the presence or in the absence of PHA. Moreover, when added in the presence of IL-4, salbutamol potentiated the inhibitory effect of IL-4 on IFN-γ release. Therefore, the enhanced IgE synthesis could be explained by an inhibition of the production of IFN-γ.

It has been hypothesized that the soluble form of the low-affinity receptor for IgE (CD23) plays a role in the regulation of IgE synthesis in humans.[13] In the presence of IL-4, salbutamol induced an increase of the release of this soluble fragment, and this effect was maximal after 11 days in culture. Since no effect of salbutamol on the cell-surface expression of CD23 was noticed, the drug may accelerate the processing of the molecule. Given the fact that the influence of this fragment on IgE production is controversial, however, this may not be the only explanation for the observed enhancing effect of salbutamol.

EFFECTS OF β_2-ADRENOCEPTOR AGONISTS ON IgE PRODUCTION IN THE MOUSE

A similar effect of salbutamol was also observed *in vitro* in the mouse. Indeed, when LPS-preactivated B lymphocytes were added with salbutamol and IL-4, an increase of IgE production was noticed as compared to the effect of IL-4 alone. No effect was observed when the drug was added alone to the culture, and a similar effect was observed in the presence or in the absence of macrophages. These results suggested a direct effect of β_2-adrenoceptor agonists on B lymphocytes. No effect of this drug on IgG$_1$ production and on the expression of CD23 on B lymphocytes was noted.

In order to evaluate the *in vivo* effect of salbutamol on IgE production, Balb/c mice were sensitized with ovalbumine (OA) and treated with a daily injection of salbutamol (1 mg/kg). This treatment induced an increase in the production of both total and specific IgE. No effect of this drug on the basal level of IgE in nonsensitized animals was observed. As assessed by flow cytometry, salbutamol did not increase the *in vivo* expression of lymphocyte surface-associated molecules, such as Thy-1, CD8, CD4, B220, and LECAM. A slight decrease of the percentage of CD23$^+$ splenocytes was observed. Thus, the induction of these molecules is unlikely to be the mechanism by which salbutamol induces an enhanced IgE production.

In the mouse, two types of murine T helper cells have been described, based on the pattern of cytokine production.[14] Th1 cells secrete IL-2 and IFN-γ, whereas Th2 cells secrete IL-4, IL-5, and IL-10. IL-4 and IFN-γ have been shown to regulate IgE production both *in vitro* and *in vivo,* whereas IL-10 inhibits Th1 functions and IFN-γ production.[15,16] Salbutamol induced an increase of the *ex vivo* release of IL-4, IL-5, IL-6, and IL-10 from concanavalin-A activated splenocytes (TABLE 2). This effect of salbutamol was observed both in sensitized and nonsensitized mice. By contrast, no effect of β_2-adrenoceptor agonists treatment on IL-2

TABLE 2. Effect of Salbutamol on the Cytokine Release from Con-A-Activated Murine Splenocytes

Treatment	Cytokines Release					
	IL-2 (ng/ml)	IFN-γ (U/ml)	IL-4 (pg/ml)	IL-5 (pg/ml)	IL-6 (U/ml)	IL-10 (U/ml)
Medium	11.9 ± 1	35 ± 4	287 ± 49	29 ± 11	97 ± 37	9 ± 1
Salbutamol (1 mg/kg)	11.3 ± 1	99 ± 10	459 ± 69	114 ± 12	380 ± 95	32 ± 2
OA (10 μg)	13.3 ± 1	63 ± 8	333 ± 66	168 ± 15	166 ± 37	22 ± 2
OA + Salbutamol	13.1 ± 1	63 ± 8	521 ± 120	324 ± 69	343 ± 83	31 ± 4

and IFN-γ release was noted. Thus, the effect of salbutamol could be explained at least by an increase of the release of cytokines from Th2-type lymphocytes.

POSSIBLE MECHANISMS OF ACTION OF SALBUTAMOL ON IgE PRODUCTION

It remains to be determined which cell type among lymphocytes and macrophages is the target of β-adrenoceptor agonists. The results obtained *in vitro* in the mouse indicated that salbutamol may exert a direct effect on B lymphocytes. Since the levels of expression of CD23 and IgG_1 secretion in the mouse are not modified *in vitro* by salbutamol, it is unlikely that this drug exerts its effect via an increase of the release of IL-4 from B lymphocytes. In addition, the fact that *in vitro* cultures are performed in the presence of IL-4 does not allow an accurate investigation of the role of this cytokine. In humans, B and T lymphocytes express β_2 adrenoceptor, leaving open the possibility that salbutamol exerts its effects through both cell types. Thus, experiments in humans should be performed using purified B lymphocytes in the presence of anti-CD40 antibodies[17] and IL-4 to determine whether these drugs act directly on these cells. It is more likely that the present results suggest that β_2-adrenoceptor agonists exert their effect through the modulation of cytokine production from T cells. *In vivo* in the mouse, the effect of salbutamol could be explained by an increase in the levels of IL-4, IL-5, and IL-10. Particularly, in the light of recent works, the effect of salbutamol on IL-10 production indicate that this drug may inhibit Th1 functions. In humans, the effects of β_2-adrenoceptor agonists on IFN-γ synthesis may indicate that salbutamol mediates its *in vitro* effects through T lymphocytes. This is in keeping with previous studies that have reported a direct effect of salbutamol on human T-cell clones.[7] Experiments are currently conducted in the laboratory to investigate the effects of this drug on IL-10 production. Because the existence of Th2-type lymphocytes in human is still controversial, it might be of interest to determine whether T cells that express β_2-adrenoceptors produce the same pattern of cytokine as compared to the ones that do not.

CONCLUSION

The concentrations of β_2-adrenoceptor agonists used in this study are within the range of concentrations to which lymphocytes may be exposed *in vivo*. Locally, norepinephrine-containing nerves have been shown to release high levels of norepinephrine,[18] and administered β_2-adrenoceptor agonists used in the treatment of asthma yield plasma concentrations ranging from 1×10^{-5} M to 1×10^{-6} M. Since the concentrations used in these studies are physiologically relevant, the present results suggest that the local release of norepinephrine, or the exposure to therapeutic agents may profoundly influence antibody production. Thus, salbutamol can function as an immunomodulator through its capacity to enhance IgE production and to increase or repress the production of selected cytokines. Given the clinical importance of β_2-adrenoceptor agonists in the symptomatic treatment of asthma, further studies are now required to determine whether these drugs exhibit the same effects in humans, particularly in asthmatic patients.

REFERENCES

1. VERCELLI, D., H. H. JABARA, K. ARAI & R. S. GEHA. 1989. Induction of human IgE synthesis requires interleukin-4 and T/B cells interactions involving the T cell receptor/CD3 complex and MHC class II antigens. J. Exp. Med. **169:** 1295–1307.
2. PÈNE, J., *et al.* 1988. IgE production by normal human lymphocytes is induced by interleukin 4 and suppressed by interferons gamma and alpha and prostaglandin E2. Proc. Natl. Acad. Sci. U.S.A. **85:** 6880–6884.
3. VERCELLI, D., H. H. JABARA, K. ARAI, T. YOKOTA & R. S. GEHA. 1989. Endogenous interleukin 6 plays an obligatory role in interleukin 4-dependent human IgE synthesis. Eur. J. Immunol. **19:** 1419–1424.
4. FELTEN, D. L., S. Y. FELTEN, S. L. CARLSON, J. A. OLSCHOWKA & S. LIVNAT. 1985. Noradrenergic and peptidergic innervation of lymphoid tissue. J. Immunol. **135:** 755s.
5. LANDMANN, R. M. A., E. BURGISSER, M. WESP & F. R. BÜHLER. 1984. Beta-adrenergic receptors are different in subpopulations of human circulating lymphocytes. J. Recept. Res. **4:** 37–50.
6. POCHET, R., G. DELESPESSE, P. W. GAUSSET & H. COLLET. 1979. Distribution of beta-adrenergic receptors on human lymphocyte subpopulations. Clin. Exp. Immunol. **38:** 578–584.
7. DAILEY, M. O., J. SCHREURS & H. SHULMAN. 1988. Hormone receptors on cloned T lymphocytes. J. Immunol. **140:** 2931–2936.
8. R. D. FELDMAN, G. W. HUNNINGHAKE & W. L. MCARDLE. 1987. β_2-adrenergic receptor-mediated suppression of interleukin 2 receptors in human lymphocytes. J. Immunol. **139:** 3355–3359.
9. KOUASSY, E., Y. S. LI, W. BOUKHRIS, I. MILLET & J. P. REVILLARD. 1988. Opposite effects of the catecholamines dopamine and norepinephrine on murine polyclonal B-cell activation. Immunopharmacology **16:** 125–137.
10. SANDERS, V. M. & F. E. POWELL-OLIVER. 1992. β_2-adrenoceptor stimulation increases the number of antigen-specific precursor B lymphocytes that differentiate into IgM-secreting cells without affecting burst size. J. Immunol. **148:** 1822–1828.
11. WOOLCOCK, A. J. 1990. β-agonists and asthma mortality. Drugs **40**(5): 653–656.
12. SPITZER, W. O., *et al.* 1992. The use of β-agonists and the risk of death and near death from asthma. New Eng. J. Med. **326:** 501–506.
13. SARFATI, M. & G. DELESPESSE. 1988. Possible role of human lymphocyte receptor for

IgE (CD23) or its soluble fragments in the *in vitro* synthesis of human IgE. J. Immunol. **141:** 2195–2199.

14. MOSMANN, T. R., H. CHERWINSKY, M. W. BOND, M. A. GIEDLIN & R. L. COFFMAN. 1986. Two types of murine helper T cells clones. I. Definition according to profile of lymphokines activities and secreted proteins. J. Immunol. **136:** 2348.

15. FINKELMANN, F. D., I. M. KATONA, J. F. URBAN, C. M. SNAPPER, J. OHARA & W. E. PAUL. 1986. Suppression of *in vivo* polyclonal IgE responses to the lymphokine B cell stimulatory factor-1. 1986. Proc. Natl. Acad. Sci. U.S.A. **83:** 9675–9678.

16. FIORENTINO, D. F., A. ZLOTNIK, P. VIEIRA, T. R. MOSMANN, M. HOWARD, K. W. MOORE & A. O'GARRA. 1991. IL-10 acts on the antigen-presenting cell to inhibit cytokine production by Th1 cells. J. Immunol. **146:** 3444–3451.

17. HAIFA, H., F. SHU MAN, G. RAIF & D. VERCELLI. 1991. CD40 and IgE: Synergism between anti-CD40 monoclonal antibody and Interleukin 4 in the induction of IgE synthesis by highly purified human B cells. J. Exp. Med. **172:** 1861–1864.

18. FELTEN, D. L., K. D. ACKERMAN, S. J. WIEGAND & S. Y. FELTEN. 1987. Noradrenergic sympathetic innervation of the spleen. J. Neurosci. Res. **18:** 28.

Release and Inactivation of Interleukin-4 by Mast Cells[a]

J. M. TUNON de LARA,[b,c,e] Y. OKAYAMA,[c]
A. R. McEUEN,[c] C. H. HEUSSER,[d] M. K. CHURCH,[c]
AND A. F. WALLS[c]

[b]Service des Maladies Respiratoires
CHU de Bordeaux
Hôpital du Haut Lévêque
33604 Pessac, France

[c]Immunopharmacology Group
Southampton General Hospital
Tremona Road
Southampton SO9 4XY, England

[d]Ciba-Geigy
CH-4002 Basel
Switzerland

INTRODUCTION

Mast cells have long been recognized as critical effectors of IgE-dependent immediate hypersensitivity reactions.[1] More recently, mast cells have been shown to be involved in a wide variety of immunological responses, including the production and the release of multifunctional cytokines.[2] *In vitro* stimulation of mouse mast cells induces the expression of messenger RNA (mRNA) for, and the secretion of interleukin-1 (IL-1), -3, -4, -5, -6, granulocyte-macrophage colony stimulating factor (GM-CSF), interferon-γ (IFN-γ), and tumor necrosis factor-α (TNF-α).[3-5] In humans, mast cells isolated from skin have also been demonstrated to contain TNF-α.[6] Moreover, there is a growing body of evidence suggesting that they can be a source of different cytokines including GM-CSF, IL-3, IL-4, and IL-5.[7]

This latter group of cytokines is also generated by Th2-lymphocytes (along with IL-6 and IL-10), and could be particularly important in the control of the allergic response.[8] GM-CSF and IL-3 are factors involved in the growth and differentiation of basophils and eosinophils. IL-5 stimulates both the differentiation and the activation of eosinophils. IL-4 is responsible, among other actions, for the isotype switching of B cells to IgE synthesis. These cytokine-mediated effects, which promote an immediate hypersensitivity response, can be opposed to those of the cytokines generated by Th1-lymphocytes (i.e., IL-2, TNF-β, INF-γ) that are involved in delayed-type hypersensitivity. T cells of Th2 phenotype could

[a] One of the authors (J.M.T.L.) received a scholarship Lavoisier from the Ministère des Affaires Etrangères, Paris, France, and was supported by a grant from the Institut Pneumologique d'Aquitaine. Financial support from the National Asthma Campaign and the Medical Research Council, United Kingdom, is gratefully acknowledged.

[e] To whom correspondence should be addressed.

thus play a major role in the allergic response to an antigen, although the mechanism determining the selection of the Th2 subset remains unclear. Nevertheless, it has been demonstrated both *in vivo* and *in vitro* that IL-4 is required for lymphocytes to secrete Th2 cytokine profile, including IL-4 itself.[9,10] By their capacity to generate cytokines, mast cells could provide T lymphocytes with a local pulse of IL-4 that might initiate the development of the Th2 phenotype.

PRODUCTION OF IL-4 BY MAST CELLS

The first evidence for IL-4 production by mast cells was provided by experiments performed in mast cell lines. Some unstimulated IL-3-dependent mast cell lines are known to transcribe low levels of mRNA for IL-4, although they do not secrete detectable amounts of this cytokine.[11] The activation of nontransformed murine mast cell lines by cross-linking FcεRI or using a calcium ionophore can significantly increase the expression of mRNA for IL-4 along with that for IL-3, IL-5, IL-6, and GM-CSF.[3] Moreover, both of these types of activation can induce a delayed release of IL-4, commencing after 1 h and maximum at 4–6 h following the stimulation. Non-B non-T cells with mast cell/basophil characteristics isolated from mouse spleen can also generate IL-4 upon IgE-dependent activation.[12] These results have been confirmed with human non-B non-T cells derived from bone marrow and stimulated through their Fcε or Fcγ receptors.[13]

In contrast, little is known about cytokine generation in human mature basophils or mast cells. Nevertheless, immunocytochemical methods have revealed the presence of IL-4 in human mast cells purified from both skin and lung tissues.[14] Furthermore, IL-4 has been localized to mast cells in the respiratory tract of rhinitic and asthmatic patients. In a preliminary study, the challenge of purified lung mast cells was found to provoke the release of IL-4 along with histamine. Subsequently, we have been able to apply *in situ* hybridization and polymerase chain reaction (PCR) technology to demonstrate increased expression of IL-4 mRNA in human skin mast cells following activation by anti-IgE in the presence of stem cell factor.[15] Recently, it has been demonstrated that human peripheral blood basophils can produce IL-4 upon an IgE-dependent activation.[16] This IL-4 generation is observed when basophils, like some murine mast cell lines, are primed by IL-3, a cytokine also reported to potentiate the release of leukotriene C4 by basophils. The time course of IL-4 production by basophils is different from that of degranulation, indicating that IL-4 is not released as a preformed mediator but is newly synthesized in the presence of IL-3.

Taken together, these observations provide strong evidence that human mast cells are capable of transcribing mRNA for IL-4 and may secrete this cytokine under conditions that remain to be clearly defined. Nevertheless, the results of studies with rodent mast cells, spleen or bone marrow non-B non-T cells, human mature mast cells, or basophils, all suggest that the main trigger for IL-4 production is the activation of the IgE receptor that is expressed on these different cell types.

RELEASE OF IL-4 BY HUMAN MAST CELLS

Although the high-affinity receptor for IgE is expressed by all human mast cells, different subsets have been distinguished by their composition of proteases and tissue distribution.[17] For example, a differential distribution of tryptase and chymase has been used to classify mast cells on an immunocytochemical basis, with those containing both tryptase and chymase being termed MC_{TC}, while those containing tryptase alone are termed MC_T. This division bears some relationship with the mucosal and connective tissue distribution of mast cells: in the bronchial mucosa, the majority are of the MC_T type while the majority of those of the skin are of the MC_{TC} subset. In addition, a functional heterogeneity has been found when comparing the reponses of these different subsets to IgE or nonimmunological stimuli.[18]

It is thus important to analyze the cytokine production by the different subpopulations of human mast cells. For this purpose, we investigated the capacity of human skin and lung mast cells to release IL-4 following either IgE receptor stimulation or direct activation using a calcium ionophore.

Mast cells were dispersed from foreskin or lung tissue following surgery, using collagenase and hyaluronidase. Skin mast cells were purified using a discontinuous Percoll gradient (mast cell purity >85 percent) and lung mast cells using an immunomagnetic procedure with anti-c-kit monoclonal antibody YB5B8 (a gift from L. Ashman, Melbourne, Australia) coupled to Dynabeads (mast cell purity >75 percent). Purified mast cells were challenged with anti-IgE and IL-4 was measured in the supernatants by a specific ELISA within the first hour and at 2, 4, and 6 hours. As a control of mast cell activation, histamine release was measured in the supernatants using a spectrofluorometric procedure.

Following anti-IgE activation of purified lung mast cells, IL-4 release was detectable in 6 out of 10 experiments (FIG. 1). This generation of IL-4 occurred after 2 h of incubation in four cases and during the first 30 min in the two other cases. The mean quantity of IL-4 released was 6.4 ± 3.6 ng/10^6 lung mast cells, and there was a corresponding histamine release of 17 ± 6 percent of the total cellular histamine. The calcium ionophore ionomycin (3 μM) did not, however, induce any significant release of IL-4 (0.45 ± 0.2 ng/10^6 lung mast cells), although it provoked a substantial release of histamine (57 ± 24 percent). These results confirm that lung mast cells can release IL-4 following IgE-mediated activation, although this property appears to be restricted to a subgroup of subjects. The kinetics of IL-4 release and the lack of any response to calcium ionophore do not, however, support the hypothesis that IL-4 is stored within the mast cell granules.

In contrast to lung mast cells, purified skin mast cells did not release detectable amounts of immunoreactive IL-4 after activation with either anti-IgE or the calcium ionophore. Even with a sensitive bioassay with an IL-4 sensitive cell line termed CTh4S,[19] no IL-4 was detected. This apparent discrepancy between immunocytochemical studies and the experiments in which mast cells were challenged *in vitro* could be related to either a lack of response to IgE-mediated activation, or the degradation of IL-4 by proteases released along with the cytokine.

We have found that the IL-4 sensitive cell line CTh4S might be cocultured with human skin mast cells in the presence of low concentrations of stem cell factor. Preliminary results demonstrate that the proliferation of the CTh4S cells is enhanced following activation with anti-IgE (Okayama, unpublished data). This proliferation was inhibited by 8F12, an anti-IL-4 monoclonal antibody[16] known to affect the functional properties of this cytokine (unpublished results). This observation suggests that IL-4 may be inactivated by skin-mast-cell-derived proteases liberated following an IgE-mediated stimulation.

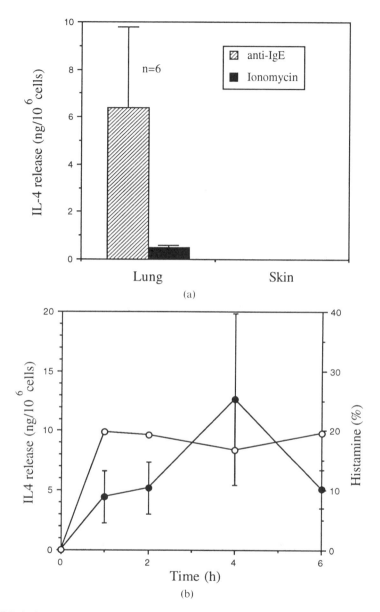

FIGURE 1. IL-4 release by human mast cells. (**a**) Mean concentrations of IL-4 released following activation of lung and skin mast cells with either anti-IgE or ionomycin (3 μM). (**b**) The time course of both IL-4 (*closed symbols*) and histamine (*open symbols*) release by purified lung mast cells.

REGULATION OF IL-4 ACTIVITY BY MAST CELL PROTEASES

A characteristic feature of mast cells are the electron-dense granules in which are packaged the preformed mediators that are released into the external microenvironment following cell activation. Of these, the most abundant constituents are the neutral proteases that coexist with heparin proteoglycan, forming a crystalline complex. The major proteases that have been purified from human mast cells are tryptase, chymase, and carboxypeptidase. Tryptase is present in all mast cells at all anatomical sites investigated,[20,21] whereas chymase[17] and carboxypeptidase[22] are restricted to the MC_{TC} subpopulation. Mast cells of this subpopulation might also contain a protease with antigenic and enzymological similarities to neutrophil cathepsin-G,[23] but this enzyme has yet to be isolated from human mast cells. Although the precise role of these proteases in allergic disease remains to be elucidated, their proteolytic properties could confer on mast cells a role in controlling the bioavailability of cytokines. It has recently been shown that human mast cell chymase can convert inactive IL-1β to an active IL-1,[24] and cathepsin-G derived from neutrophils has been found to inactivate TNF.[25] We have investigated the ability of human mast cell proteases to degrade IL-4.

Mast cells were purified as previously described and lysed by two freeze–thaw cycles. Lysates were then incubated with human recombinant IL-4 (a gift from Ciba-Geigy, Basel, Switzerland) at 37°C and the IL-4 concentrations were measured by ELISA or by bioassay with the CTh4S cell line.

Following incubation of IL-4 with lysates of purified mast cell, we observed a concentration-dependent decrease in immunoreactive IL-4 by ELISA (FIG. 2(a)). This effect, however, was strongly dependent on cell type since skin mast cell lysates could degrade 20 pg of IL-4/min/10^4 cells, while the catalysis rate obtained with lung mast cell lysate was less than 5 pg/min/10^4 cells (FIG. 2(b)). The decrease in IL-4 concentration was accompanied by a loss of functional activity as measured by the CTh4S line. The effect of time and the concentration of skin mast cell lysates were similar with both assays. To identify the mast cell proteases responsible for the IL-4 catalysis, we next determined the inhibitor profile of the reaction. FIGURE 3 indicates that inhibitors of chymotryptic activity (e.g., SBTI, aprotinin, chymostatin) could prevent the degradation of IL-4, while tryptase inhibitors (e.g., TPCK, TLCK) failed to diminish the reaction.

These preliminary results suggest that IL-4 can be degraded by the chymotryptic proteases contained within skin mast cells and can explain the difficulties we have experienced in measuring IL-4 in supernatants from activated skin mast cells. The much less efficient degradation of IL-4 by lung mast cell lysates, on the other hand, accords with the lower proportion of mast cells of phenotype MC_{TC} in this tissue, and may be related to the relative persistence of IL-4 in supernatants of challenged lung mast cells. It should be kept in mind, however, that IL-4 release by lung mast cells was restricted to a number of subjects whose characterization remains to be established. For example, the allergic status of the donors of mast cells could not be determined in the experiments involving IL-4 release or degradation. We can speculate that this factor is of importance regarding the generation of IL-4 and its bioavailability. It will be important to identify and characterize further the chymotryptic proteases responsible for the catalysis of IL-4.

CONCLUSION

There is compelling evidence that human mast cells can produce IL-4, a cytokine that is required for lymphocytes to secrete cytokines of the Th2 profile,

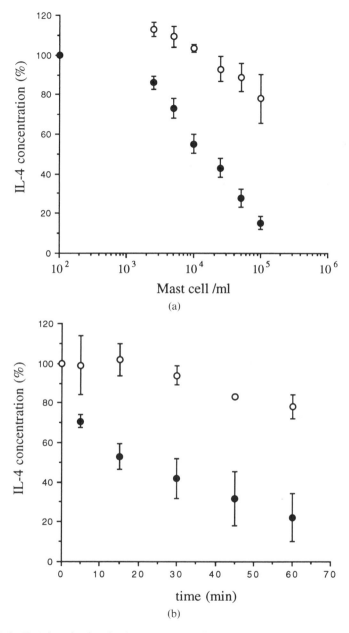

FIGURE 2. IL-4 inactivation by human mast cell lysates. (**a**) The effect of increasing concentrations of skin or lung mast cell lysates on IL-4 detection by ELISA. (**b**) Time-course of IL-4 inactivation by skin or lung mast cell lysates. (*Key: Closed symbols* represent skin mast cells; *open symbols* represent lung mast cells.)

including IL-3, GM-CSF, IL-5, IL-6, IL-10, and IL-4 itself. By initiating this response, mast cells could make an important contribution in the development of allergic diseases, which is additional to their well-established role as effectors of IgE-dependent immediate hypersensitivity. Apparent differences between lung and skin mast cells in their ability to release IL-4 *in vitro* appear to be related to IL-4 degradation by chymotryptic proteases that are coreleased by skin mast cells. As major sources of extracellular proteases, mast cells could also have important roles in controlling the bioavailability of IL-4 and other cytokines at sites of inflammation. The IgE response to an antigen is under the control of IL-4, and it is tempting to speculate that the differences in proteases content between lung and skin mast cells could reflect differences between routes of sensitization. Inhaled antigens may thus induce an IgE-mediated response, while contact antigens in

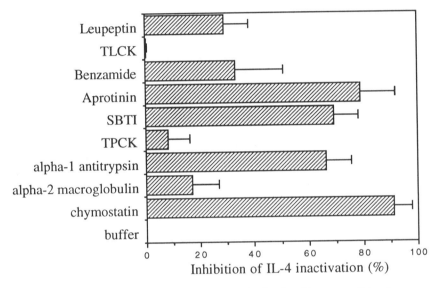

FIGURE 3. Inhibitor profile for IL-4 inactivation by skin mast cell lysates.

skin could initiate delayed hypersensitivity responses. Further studies are required to investigate this possible association.

REFERENCES

1. SCHWARTZ, L. B. & K. F. AUSTEN. 1984. Structure and function of the chemical mediators of mast cells. Prog. Allergy **34:** 271–321.
2. GORDON, J. R., P. R. BURD & S. J. GALLI. 1990. Mast cells as a source of multifunctional cytokines. Immunol. Today **11:** 458–464.
3. PLAUT, M., J. H. PIERCE, C. J. WATSON, J. HANLEY-HYDE, R. P. NORDAN & W. E. PAUL. 1989. Mast cell lines produce lymphokines in response to cross linkage of FcεRI or to calcium ionophores. Nature **339:** 64–67.

4. BURD, P. R., *et al.* 1989. Interleukin 3-dependent and -independent mast cells stimulated with IgE and antigen express multiple cytokines. J. Exp. Med. **170:** 245–257.
5. GORDON, J. R. & S. J. GALLI. 1990. Mast cells as a source of both preformed and immunologically inductible TNF-α/cachectin. Nature **346:** 274–276.
6. WALSH, L. J., G. TRINCHIERI, H. A. WALDORF, D. WHITAKER & G. F. MURPHY. 1991. Human dermal mast cells contain and release tumor necrosis factor α which induces endothelial leukocyte adhesion molecule. 1. Proc. Natl. Acad. Sci. U.S.A. **88:** 4220–4224.
7. HOLGATE, S. T. & M. K. CHURCH. 1992. The mast cell. Br. Med. Bull. **48:** 40–50.
8. ROMAGNANI, S. 1991. Human Th1 and Th2 subsets: Doubt no more. Immunol. Today **12:** 256–257.
9. LE GROS, G., S. Z. BEN-SASSON, R. SEDER, F. D. FINKELMAN & W. E. PAUL. 1990. Generation of interleukin 4 (IL-4)-producing cells in vivo and in vitro: IL-2 and IL-4 are required for in vitro generation of IL-4-producing cells. J. Exp. Med. **172:** 921–929.
10. KOPF, M., G. LE GROS, M. BACHMANN, M. C. LAMERS, H. BLUETHMANN & G. KOHLER. 1993. Disruption of the murine IL-4 gene blocks Th2 cytokine responses. Nature **362:** 245–248.
11. BROWN, M. A., J. H. PIERCE, C. J. WATSON, J. FALCO, J. N. IHLE & W. E. PAUL. 1987. B cell stimulatory factor-1/interleukin-4 mRNA is expressed by normal and transformed mast cells. Cell **50:** 809–818.
12. BEN-SASSON, S. Z., G. LE GROS, D. H. CONRAD, F. D. FINKELMAN & W. E. PAUL. 1990. Cross-linking Fc receptors stimulates splenic non B, non T-cells to secrete interleukin 4 and other lymphokines. Proc. Natl. Acad. Sci. U.S.A. **87:** 1421–1425.
13. PICCINNI, M. P., *et al.* 1991. Human bone marrow non B, non T-cells produce interleukin 4 in response to cross-linkage of Fcε and Fcγ receptors. Proc. Natl. Acad. Sci. U.S.A. **88:** 8656–8660
14. BRADDING, P., *et al.* 1992. Interleukin 4 is localized to and released by human mast cells. J. Exp. Med. **176:** 1381–1386.
15. OKAYAMA, Y., *et al.* 1993. Expression of IL-4 mRNA in human dermal mast cells in response to Fc receptor cross linkage in the presence of SCF. J. Allergy Clin. Immunol. **91:** 256.
16. BRUNNER, T., C. H. HEUSSER & C. A. DAHINDEN. 1993. Human peripheral blood basophils primed by interleukin 3 (IL-3) produce IL-4 in response to immunoglobulin E receptor stimulation. J. Exp. Med. **177:** 605–611.
17. IRANI, A. A., N. M. SCHECHTER, S. CRAIG, G. DEBLOIS & L. B. SCHWARTZ. 1986. Two types of human mast cells that have distinct neutral protease compositions. Proc. Natl. Acad. Sci. U.S.A. **83:** 4464–4468.
18. LOWMAN, M. A., P. H. REES, R. C. BENYON, M. K. CHURCH & S. T. HOLGATE. 1988. Human mast cell heterogeneity: Histamine release from mast cells dispersed from skin, lung, adenoids, tonsils and intestinal mucosa in response to IgE-dependent and non immunological stimuli. J. Allergy Clin. Immunol. **81:** 590–597.
19. HU-LI, J., J. OHARA, C. WATSON, W. TSANG & W. E. PAUL. 1989. Derivation of a T cell line that is highly responsive to IL-4 and IL-2 (CT.4R) and of an IL-2 hyporesponsive mutant of that line (CT.4S). J. Immunol. **142:** 800–807.
20. CRAIG, S. S., G. DEBLOIS & L. B. SCHWARTZ. 1986. Mast cells in human keloid, small intestine and lung by an immunoperoxydase technique using a murine monoclonal antibody against tryptase. Am. J. Pathol. **124:** 427–435.
21. WALLS, A. F., D. B. JONES, J. H. WILLIAMS & M. K. CHURCH. 1990. Immunohistochemical identification of mast cells in formaldehyde-fixed tissue using monoclonal antibodies specific for tryptase. J. Pathol. **162:** 119–126.
22. IRANI, A. A., S. M. GOLDSTEIN, B. U. WINTROUB, T. BRADFORD & L. B. SCHWARTZ. 1991. Human mast cell carboxypeptidase selective localisation to MC$_{TC}$ cells. J. Immunol. **147:** 247–253.
23. SCHECHTER, N. M., A. M. A. IRANI, J. L. SPROWS, J. ABERNETHY, B. WINTROUB & L. B. SCHWARTZ. 1990. Identification of a cathepsin G-like proteinase in the MC$_{TC}$ type of human mast cell. J. Immunol. **145:** 2652–2661.

24. MIZUTANI, H., N. SCHECHTER, G. LAZARUS, R. A. BLACK & T. S. KUPPER. 1991.
      Rapid and specific conversion of precursor interleukin 1β (IL-1β) to an active IL-1
      species by human mast cell chymase. J. Exp. Med. **174:** 821–825.
25. SCUDERI, P., P. A. NEZ, M. L. DUERR, B. J. WONG & C. M. VALDEZ. 1991. Cathepsin
      G and leucocyte elastase inactivate human tumor necrosis factor and lymphotoxin.
      Cell. Immunol. **135:** 299–313.

Differentiation of Human Mast Cells from Bone-Marrow and Cord-Blood Progenitor Cells by Factors Produced by a Mouse Stromal Cell Line

MICHEL AROCK,[a,e] FLORENCE HERVATIN,[b]
JEAN-JACQUES GUILLOSSON,[a]
JEAN-MICHEL MENCIA-HUERTA,[c]
AND DOMINIQUE THIERRY[d]

[a]Faculté de Pharmacie
Laboratoire d'Hématologie
4 Avenue de l'Observatoire
75006 Paris, France

[b]Commissariat à l'Energie Atomique
DSU
DPTE
91191 Saclay, France

[c]Institut H. Baufour
1 Avenue des Tropiques
91952 Les Ulis Cedex, France

[d]Section autonome de Radiobiologie appliquée à la médecine
Institut de Protection et de Sureté Nucléaire
Fontenay-aux-roses
92260 BP 06, France

INTRODUCTION

Growth and differentiation of hematopoietic (progenitor) cells is regulated by a complex network of cytokines and a variety of microenvironmental factors.[1-3] In contrast to the murine system, the human progenitors can only be maintained for a limited period of time when cultured on a layer of normal human marrow stromal cells (i.e., in the Dexter system). Under these conditions, the number of surviving progenitors declines in a few weeks and these cells disappear completely in less than 8 weeks.[4] Normal bone-marrow-derived stroma can be replaced by different mouse stromal cell lines that support self-renewal of murine hematopoietic progenitors.[5-9] The mechanism by which these cells support the growth of progenitors is undetermined since they synthesize various cytokines, such as interleukin-1 (IL-1), granulocyte-macrophage colony stimulating factor (GM–CSF), and IL-6, known to act on progenitor cells' survival and differentiation.[10-12] On the other hand, direct contact between these stromal cells and hematopoietic progenitors appears important for the self-renewal of the latter cells. Among

[e] To whom correspondence should be addressed.

these stromal cell lines, MS-5 (a lipoblast line) is one of the most efficient in supporting human hematopoiesis *in vitro*.[13,14]

During the last decades, great efforts have been made to identify the factors controlling growth and differentiation of human mast cells. In contrast to the situation in the murine system,[15,16] IL-3 is not sufficient to grow or differentiate normal human mast cells from bone-marrow cultures.[17] More recently, the growth of human mast cells was induced in long-term cord-blood-cell cultures by the use of a fibroblast cell line (3T3) layer[18,19] or in long-term bone-marrow cultures in the presence of recombinant human stem cell factor (SCF).[20] In these different systems, the development of mast cells is accompanied by a rapid loss of the self-renewal capacity of the hematopoietic stem cells. The present study was designed to evaluate whether the culture of human-bone-marrow- or cord-blood-derived progenitors in the presence of MS-5 would induce continuous differentiation of human mast cells in long-term cultures, as well as survival of undifferentiated progenitors.

MATERIALS AND METHODS

MS-5 Cell Line

The mouse stromal cell line MS-5 was kindly provided by Dr. K. J. Mori (Department of Biology, Niigata University, Niigata, Japan) and was cultured in complete Iscove modified Dulbecco's medium (IMDM) containing 1 percent L-glutamine, 0.5 percent vitamins, 1 percent essential and nonessential aminoacids, 1 percent penicillin/streptomycin solution (all from Gibco, Paisley, UK), and 20 percent pretested horse serum (HS) (Biological Industries, Illkirch, France). Every 3 to 4 days, the cells were treated with trypsin and diluted one-third to one-quarter in new flasks in fresh medium. For the preparation of conditioned medium (CM), confluent layers of MS-5 cells were incubated for 7 days and the culture medium was harvested and centrifuged. Cell-free supernatants were then passed through a 0.45-μm filter and stored at $-20°$ until use.

Positive Selection of Bone-Marrow and Cord-Blood CD34+ Progenitor Cells

Bone-marrow (BM) or cord-blood (CB) mononuclear cells (MNC) were obtained by centrifugation on Ficoll gradients (density: 1077 g/ml, Sigma, St. Louis, Missouri) of BM or CB samples obtained from normal donors after their informed consent. Cells expressing the CD34 surface antigen were selectively removed from MNC by rosetting with CD34 monoclonal antibodies-bearing magnetic beads (Dynabeads CD34, Dynal, Biosys SA, Compiègne, France) and separated by attraction to a rare-earth magnet. After selection, the beads were detached from the CD34+ cells by the means of Detachabead (Dynal) and removed magnetically. In some experiments, the purity of the enriched cell population was assessed upon staining with My10 antibody (HPCA-1) and isotype-specific secondary antibody, followed by fluorescence-activated cell sorter (FACS) analysis. In these experiments, cells were consistently >85 percent CD34+.

Normal Human Bone-Marrow-Derived Stromal Monolayers

Normal bone-marrow mononuclear cells (2.10^6/ml) were seeded in complete IMDM containing 10 percent pretested fetal calf serum (FCS, Biological Industries,

Illkirch, France), 10 percent HS, and 1.10^{-6} M hydrocortisone (Sigma, St. Louis, Missouri). Cells were incubated at 37°C (5 percent CO_2 in air) for one week. The nonadherent elements were then harvested and stromal layers were fed with fresh medium and cultured for another week. After this 2-week incubation period, the stromal cell layers obtained were used as normal bone-marrow-derived microenvironment.

Culture of BM- or CB-Derived CD34+ Cells in the Presence of Stromal Cells or CM

BM- or CB-derived CD34+ cells were seeded at 5.10^4/ml on confluent monolayers of MS-5 cells or normal human-bone-marrow-derived stromal cells in complete IMDM supplemented with 10 percent FCS and 10 percent HS (5 percent CO_2 in air). After gentle agitation, half of the supernatant was replaced each week by fresh medium and nonadherent cells were removed, counted, and aliquots were used for subsequent cytological and mediator analysis as well as for clonogenic assays. In some experiments, BM- or CB-derived CD34+ cells were seeded at 5.10^4/ml in complete IMDM supplemented with 50 percent MS-5 CM and fed with fresh medium every week. In both experiments, cultures were driven for up to 12 weeks.

Assay for Clonogenic Cells

Nonadherent BM-derived cocultured cells were assayed for their clonogenic capability using a classical semisolid culture method. Briefly, 5.10^3 cells were seeded in 35-mm Petri dishes in 1-ml complete IMDM containing 0.9 percent methylcellulose (Methocel MC, Fluka Chemie AG, Buchs, Switzerland), 20 percent FCS, 1 percent deionized BSA, and 200 U/ml recombinant human GM–CSF (a gift from Sandoz Biotechnology, Basel, Switzerland; specific activity 5.10^6 U/mg). The cultures were then incubated at 37°C (5 percent CO_2 in air) for 10 to 12 days. At the end of the incubation period, colonies were scored under an inverted microscope.

Cytological and Immunocytochemical Staining

Each week, nonadherent cells were collected and used to perform cytocentrifuge preparations that were stained with May Grumwald-Giemsa or with 0.5 percent toluidine blue solution (0.5 N HCl; 2 hours at room temperature). Alternatively, cytocentrifuge preparations were subjected to immunohistochemical labeling using murine monoclonal antitryptase antibody conjugated to alkaline phosphatase (G3-AP, 6 μg/ml). With this technique, tryptase-containing granules are stained in blue.[21]

The percent of metachromatic or tryptase + cells was evaluted by differential counts on 300 cells under a light microscope.

Measurement of Histamine

Histamine in cell lysates and in cell-free supernatants was measured by a specific radioimmunoassay (RIA; Immunotech, Marseille, France).

RESULTS

Enhanced Survival of Clonogenic Cells by Coculture with MS-5 Monolayers

Normal human purified CD34+ cells were cocultured under the same experimental conditions either on confluent monolayers of MS-5 cells or in the presence of normal human BM-derived stromal cells. The number of nonadherent cells and of clonogenic elements was evaluated at weekly intervals. The results of these evaluations are shown in FIGURE 1 for cellularity and FIGURE 2 for clonogenicity. Data demonstrated no significant differences between MS-5 monolayers and BM-derived stroma concerning the number of viable nonadherent cells remaining in culture. An initial conservation of the number of viable cells was observed between day 0 and day 28 in both culture conditions, followed by a slow decrease leading to the disappearance of nonadherent cells between week 10 and week 12. Concerning the number of clonogenic cells evaluated in a CFU–GM assay, the data demonstrated a significant difference between BM-derived CD34+ cells cultured on MS-5 monolayers and the same elements cultured on BM-derived stroma. Indeed, the number of CFU–GM obtained between week 1 and week 6 was at least tenfold higher in the MS-5 coculture as compared to cultures on BM-derived stroma (BM-ds). At week 6, nearly all the CFU–GM had disappeared on BM-ds, whereas the number of CFU–GM obtained on MS-5 monolayers represented at least 1 percent of the nonadherent cells and remained stable until week 12. Similar results were observed with CB-derived CD34+ cells.

Development of Human Mast Cells from CD34+ Cells

BM- or CB-derived CD34+ cells were cultured for up to 12 weeks on MS-5 monolayers or on human BM-derived stroma. When cultured on BM-derived

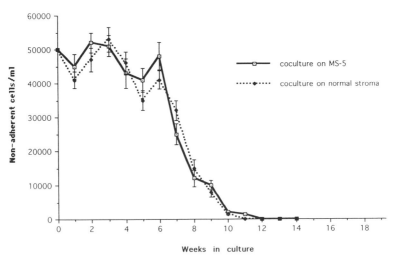

FIGURE 1. Effect of the nature of stromal cell layers on the development of nonadherent cells from bone-marrow-derived CD34+ cells. CD34+ cells were seeded at 5.10^4/ml on confluent monolayers of stromal cells ($n = 4$ in each condition).

stroma cells, the CD34+ cells gave rise, after a 6 week culture period, to terminally differentiated myeloid elements (primarily neutrophils and macrophages) with less than 2 percent mast cells (MCs). On the contrary, when CD34+ cells were cultured on MS-5 monolayers, MCs in low numbers (less than 5 percent of total cells) appeared at week 2 and represented, at week 8, as much as 70 percent of total cells when derived from BM precursors or 30 percent of total cell counts when initiated from CB progenitors (FIG. 3). At this stage, the other elements present in the cultures were essentially immature granulocytes (myeloblasts and promyelocytes). Cultured MCs typically appeared as large mononuclear cells with small, densely packed purple granules. To confirm the nature of these granulated cells, metachromatic staining as well as immunological revelation of tryptase + cells was performed. The proportion of metachromatically stained elements and of tryptase + cells in the cultures was in agreement with the proportion of mast cells identified by May Grünwald-Giemsa staining. The evolution of the percent tryptase positive cells from BM- or CB-derived CD34+ cells is shown in FIGURE 4.

Effect of MS-5 Conditioned Medium on the Growth of MCs

Development of mast cells from BM- or CB-derived CD34+ cells cultured on MS-5 monolayers suggested the possibility that mast cell growth factor(s) (MCGFs) might be synthesized and released by this stromal cell line. To assess this possibility, BM-derived CD34+ cells were cultured in the presence of 50 percent MS-5 CM for up to 8 weeks. Under this experimental condition, the development of MCs was similar to the growth of these cells when cultured on MS-5 monolayers.

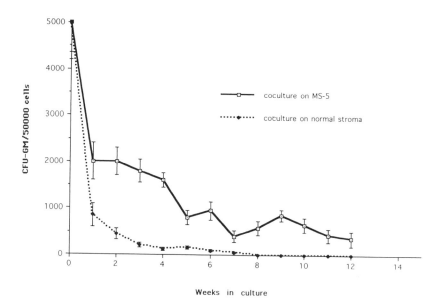

FIGURE 2. Effect of the nature of stromal cell layers on the time course of clonogenic cells from bone-marrow-derived CD34+ cells. CD34+ cells were seeded at 5.10^4/ml on confluent monolayers of stromal cells ($n = 4$ in each condition).

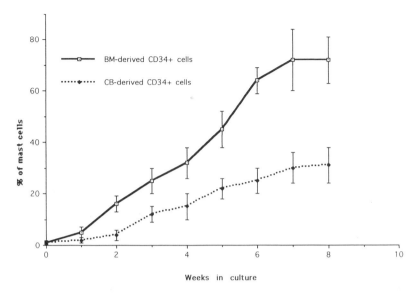

FIGURE 3. Development of mast cells from BM- or CB-derived CD34+ cells cocultured on confluent MS-5 layers for up to 8 weeks ($n = 4$ in each condition). Results are expressed as the mean ± sd of the percent of mast cells morphologically identifiable by M.G.G. staining.

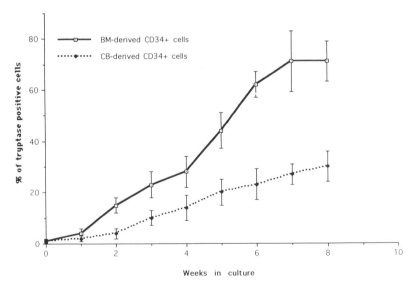

FIGURE 4. Time course of tryptase positive cell development from BM- or CB-derived CD34+ cells cocultured on confluent MS-5 monolayers for up to 8 weeks. Each data point represents the mean ± sd ($n = 4$ in each condition).

Particularly, the time course of the appearance of MCs was identical as was the maximal percentage of these cells. These results confirmed that intimate contact between CD34+ cells and MS-5 monolayer was not mandatory to the growth and differentiation of MCs and that MCGF(s) is (are) present in MS-5 conditioned medium at significant levels.

Effect of MS-5 CM on Formation of Histamine in Long-Term Culture

To quantify the time-course appearance of histamine in CD34+ cells cultured in the presence of MS-5 CM, this mediator was measured at weekly intervals in whole cell suspensions for up to 8 weeks. The data presented in FIGURE 5

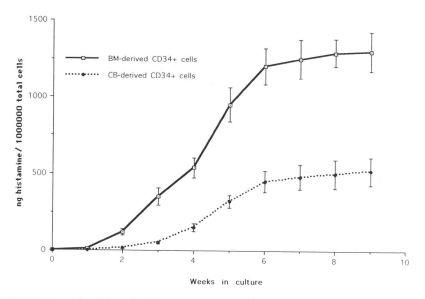

FIGURE 5. Levels of histamine in cell extracts (ng/10⁶ cells) obtained by long-term culture of BM- or CB-derived CD34+ cells in the presence of 50 percent MS-5 CM. Each data point represents the mean ± sd ($n = 4$ in each condition).

demonstrated a time-dependent increase of cellular histamine levels, corresponding to the regular increase of the percent of identifiable mast cells in such cultures.

DISCUSSION

The growth and differentiation of hematopoietic cells is controlled by various cytokines. In the murine system, stromal cells are capable of sustaining long-term hematopoiesis *in vitro,* as well as continuous differentiation of committed progenitors. On the other hand, in the rodent system, a number of cytokines (IL-3, IL-4, IL-9, IL-10, and stem cell factor (SCF)) induces or promotes the growth of MCs.[22,23] In humans, MC growth is not induced from bone-marrow progenitors by these cytokines, except for SCF. Induction of differentiation of human mast cells may be obtained under long-term culture conditions, particularly by the use of stromal cells. Stromal cells are known to produce cytokines such as SCF, and it has been recently demonstrated that this cytokine induces differentiation of human MCs in long-term cultures.[20] However, whether SCF is indeed the only critical factor for stromal-cell-dependent MC differentiation remains unknown. Alternatively, additional (stromal-cell-derived) MC growth factors (such as NGF in the murine system) can be produced,[24] and the stromal cell line, MS-5, is known to produce soluble factors capable of stimulating murine as well as human granulocyte colony formation from bone-marrow cells in a semisolid culture and to sustain murine as well as human hematopoiesis in long-term cultures.[13,14] In contrast, SCF does not exhibit such an activity on bone-marrow cells, and is unable to sustain long-term hematopoiesis in liquid cultures.[25] Under our culture conditions, MS-5 cells were able to sustain long-term hematopoiesis from human CB- or BM-derived CD34+ cells, as well as the terminal differentiation of these purified progenitors into mast cells. The latter result indicates that these cells derive directly from multipotential precursors, a fact that is poorly documented in the human system.

Because direct contact between CD34+ cells and the MS-5 cell layer is not mandatory for mast cell growth in our culture system, this activity is certainly due to a soluble factor(s) that remains to be characterized. The human mast cell differentiation assay presented here might represent a useful tool for studying the maturation pathway, as well as the reactivity (in terms of cytokine production) of these cells.

SUMMARY

Human bone-marrow or cord-blood progenitors (i.e., CD34+ cells) are easily purified by immunological methods and can be cultured on normal human-bone-marrow stromal cells for limited periods of time. Under these culture conditions, the number of progenitors declines in a few weeks and these cells disappear completely in less than 8 weeks. This fact suggests that this culture system is deprived of growth factor(s) able to support the self-renewal of stem cells. We have developed the culture of immunomagnetically purified human-bone-marrow- or cord-blood-derived CD34+ cells on a supportive mouse lipoblastic stromal cell line, MS-5. The long-term survival of clonogenic cells was analyzed in these cultures and compared with the results obtained by culture on human-bone-marrow stromal cells. The results demonstrated that only coculture of CD34+ cells on MS-5 layers allows the survival of clonogenic progenitors for at least 12 weeks. Cytospin smears were regularly performed and cell morphology was examined after classical staining methods (i.e., M.G.G. and toluidine blue staining). Histologic analysis demonstrated the growth of mast-cell-like metachromatic cells after the second week of incubation on MS-5 layer. The highest percentage of these cells was observed after 8 weeks, and averaged about 30 percent for cord-blood cells and 70 percent for bone-marrow cells. To further confirm the nature of the metachromatic cells obtained under this culture condition, immunohistochemical staining of tryptase was performed on the same samples. The results demonstrated similar percentages of tryptase+ cells and of metachromatic elements. Measurement of cellular histamine demonstrated that culture of CD34+ cells on MS-5 monolayers induced the formation and increase of this mediator. To determine whether the contact between MS-5 layers and CD34+ cells was an absolute requirement for the development of mast cells, CD34+ cells were cultured in the presence of MS-5 conditioned medium. This condition allowed the development of similar percentage of mast cells when compared with the coculture experiments, indicating that a soluble factor was involved in mast cell differentiation. Whatever the soluble factor(s) responsible for this mast cell growth activity, our culture system allows us to obtain significant amounts of highly enriched normal human mast cell populations useful for further studies on the reactivity of this cell subset.

REFERENCES

1. CLARK, S. C. & R. KAMEN. 1987. The human hematopoietic colony stimulating factors. Science **236:** 1228–1237.
2. SIEFF, C. A. 1987. Hematopoietic growth factors. J. Clin. Invest. **79:** 1549–1558.
3. METCALF, D. 1989. The molecular control of cell division, differentiation, commitment and maturation in hemopoietic cells. Nature **339:** 27–31.
4. DEXTER, T. M., T. D. ALLEN & L. G. LAJTHA. 1977. Conditions controlling the proliferation of haematopoietic stem cells in vitro. J. Cell Physiol. **91:** 335–344.
5. KODAMA, H., Y. AMAGAI, H. KOYAMA & S. SAKAI. 1982. A new preadipose cell line derived from newborn mouse calvaria can promote the differentiation of pluripotent hemopoietic stem cells in vitro. J. Cell Physiol. **112:** 89–95.
6. KODAMA, H., H. SUDO, H. KOYAMA, S. KASAI & S. YAMAMOTO. 1984. In vitro hemopoiesis within a microenvironment created by MC3T3-G2/PA6 preadipocytes. J. Cell Physiol. **118:** 233–241.
7. JOHNSON, A. & K. DORSHKIND. 1986. Stromal cells in myeloid and lymphoid long-term bone marrow cultures can support multiple hemopoietic lineages and modulate their production of hemopoietic growth factors. Blood **68:** 1348–1354.
8. COLLINS, L. S. & K. DORSHKIND. 1987. A stromal cell line from myeloid long-term bone marrow cultures can support myelopoiesis and B lymphopoiesis. J. Immunol. **138:** 1082–1088.
9. HUNT, P., D. ROBERTSON, D. WEISS, D. RENNICK, F. LEE & O. N. WITTE. 1987. A single bone marrow-derived stromal cell type supports the in vitro growth of early lymphoid and myeloid cells. Cell **48:** 997–1007.
10. MIYANOMAE, T., H. TSURUSAWA, J. FUJITA & K. J. MORI. 1982. Role of the stromal cells in the regulation of granulopoiesis in long-term bone marrow culture: Effect of conditioned medium on granulopoiesis in vitro. Biomedicine **36:** 14–18.
11. GODARD, C. M., Y. L. AUGERY, M. GINSBOURG & C. JASMIN. 1983. Established cell lines of mouse marrow adherent cells producing differentiation factor(s) for the granulocyte-macrophage lineage. In Vitro **19:** 897–903.
12. SONG, Z. X., R. K. SHADDUCK, D. J. INNES, A. WAHEED & P. J. QUESENBERRY. 1985. Hemopoietic factor production by a cell line (TC-1) derived from adherent murine marrow cells. Blood **66:** 273–282.
13. ITOH, K., H. TEZUKA, H. SAODA, M. KONNO, K. NAGATA, T. UCHIYAMA, H. UCHINO & K. J. MORI. 1989. Reproducible establishment of hemopoietic supportive stromal cell lines from murine bone marrow. Exp. Hematol. **17:** 145–153.
14. MIYASHITA, M., K. SUGIMOTO, J. SUZUKI, S. TANIGUCHI, K. ARAMAKI & K. J. MORI. 1991. Hierarchical regulation of interleukin production: Induction of interleukin 6 (IL-6) production from bone marrow cells and stromal cells by interleukin 3 (IL-3). Leukemia Res. **15:** 1125–1131.
15. RAZIN, E., C. CORDON-CARDO & R. A. GOOD. 1981. Growth of a pure population of mouse mast cells in vitro with conditioned medium derived from concanavalin A-stimulated splenocytes. Proc. Natl. Acad. Sci. U.S.A. **78:** 2559–2563.
16. IHLE, J. N., *et al.* 1983. Biologic properties of homogenous interleukin 3. J. Immunol. **131:** 282–287.
17. VALENT, P., J. BESEMER, C. SILLABER, D. MAURER, J. H. BUTTERFIELD, K. KISHI,

K. Lechner & P. Bettelheim. 1990. Failure to detect interleukin-3 binding sites on human mast cells. J. Immunol. **145:** 3432–3438.

18. Furitsu, T., H. Saito, A. Dvorak, L. B. Schwartz, A. A. Irani, J. F. Burdick, K. Ishizaka & T. Ishizaka. 1989. Development of human mast cells in vitro. Proc. Natl. Acad. Sci. U.S.A. **86:** 10039–10043.

19. Irani, A. A., S. S. Craig, G. Nilsson, T. Ishizaka & L. B. Schwartz. 1992. Characterization of human mast cells developed in vitro from fetal liver cells cocultured with murine 3T3 fibroblasts. Immunology **77:** 136–144.

20. Valent, P., et al. 1992. Induction of differentiation of human mast cells from bone marrow and peripheral blood mononuclear cells by recombinant human stem cell factor/Kit-ligand in long-term culture. Blood **80:** 2237–2245.

21. Irani, A. A., N. M. Schechter, S. S. Craig, G. Deblois & L. B. Schwartz. 1986. Detection of MCT and MCTC type human mast cells by immunohistochemistry using new monoclonals anti-trypase and anti-chymase antibodies. J. Histochem. Cytochem. **37:** 1509–1515.

22. Galli, S. J. 1993. New concepts about the mast cell. New Eng. J. Med. **328:** 257–265.

23. Thompson-Snipes, L., V. Dhar, M. W. Bond, T. R. Mosmann, K. W. Moore & D. M. Rennick. 1991. Interleukin 10: A novel stimulatory factor for mast cells and their progenitors. J. Exp. Med. **173:** 507–510.

24. Matsuda, H., Y. Kannan, H. Ushio, Y. Kiso, T. Kanemoto, H. Suzuki & Y. Kitamura. Nerve growth factor induces development of connective tissue-type mast cells in vitro from murine bone marrow cells. J. Exp. Med. **174:** 7–14.

25. Wineman, J. P., S. I. Nishikawa & C. E. Müller-Sieburg. 1993. Maintenance of high levels of pluripotent hematopoietic stem cells in vitro: Effect of stromal cells and c-Kit. Blood **81:** 365–372.

Cytokines and Airway Inflammation

P. H. HOWARTH,[a] P. BRADDING, D. QUINT,
A. E. REDINGTON, AND S. T. HOLGATE

University Medicine
Level D, Centre Block
Southampton General Hospital
Tremona Road
Southampton SO9 4XY
United Kingdom

INTRODUCTION

Cytokines are low-molecular-weight glycoproteins released by one cell and active either on themselves (autocrine) or on another cell population (paracrine) to modify cell function. They thus mediate communication both between cells of the immune system and between these cells and noninflammatory structural cells. Cytokines were originally described on the basis of their functional activity, but are now classified into a variety of families, the numerical positioning in the families reflecting their order of discovery. The increasing identification of cytokine genes and gene clusters along with the realization that cytokines often have multiple biological actions has, however, questioned the rationale of these present classifications. The interleukins are numbered 1 to 13, with the recently identified interleukin-13 (IL-13)[1] genetically encoded for chromosome 5q clustered with the genes for IL-3, IL-4, IL-5, and granulocyte-macrophage colony stimulating factor,[2] all cytokines relevant to allergic airways inflammation. The interferons (IFNs) and tumor necrosis factors (TNFs) are similar to the interleukins but are classified separately, as are the chemokines, an expanding family of recently discovered small molecular-weight cytokines, such as regulated and normal T-lymphocytes expressed and secreted (RANTES), which share many properties. Colony stimulating factors act on immature haemopoietic cells to enhance growth while also exerting proliferative actions on mature cell populations and possessing interleukinlike activity.

While the discovery of cytokines that regulate cell function relevant to airway inflammation, and thus clinical disease expression, generated the hope that modification of a single cytokine might provide global control of the disease process, it is now appreciated that cytokines exhibit both pleotropy and multiplicity of actions and that differing cytokines interact both synergistically and antagonistically. There is thus redundancy in the system and the net effect at any one time will depend upon the local balance of cytokine expression. This is evident with the regulation of IgE production by B-cells. Although the initiation of B-cell IgE synthesis is dependent upon IL-4, it is also enhanced by IL-5, IL-6, and IL-13, whereas the actions of these cytokines are opposed by interferon (IFN)γ, IL-8, and IL-12.[1,3–7] The relative regulation of B-cells by these cytokines at any one time determines the net balance between activation or repression of gene expression for IgE mRNA.

---

[a] To whom correspondence should be addressed.

Thus to understand the relevance of cytokines to the mucosal inflammation that characterizes both asthma and rhinitis, changes in the nonstructural cell populations are described and the potential role of cytokines to these changes detailed. The current *in vivo* evidence for cytokine synthesis, storage, and release within the airways is then discussed along with the available information concerning cytokine cell provenances.

MUCOSAL INFLAMMATION AND AIRWAYS DISEASE

Both asthma and rhinitis are now appreciated to be airway disorders associated with mucosal inflammation. In the upper airways this is predominantly seen in allergic rhinitis, but is evident within the lower airways in both allergic and non-allergic forms. Abnormalities of cell accumulation and cell activation have been described for a number of nonstructural cell types, including mast cells, eosinophils, T-lymphocytes, and macrophages.

Although not a reported finding in all studies there is a consensus for an increase in mast cells within the epithelium in both the upper and lower airways in rhinitis and asthma.[8-11] This is paralleled within the lower airways by increased recovery of mast cells from the airway lumen by bronchoalveolar lavage (BAL).[12] These recovered mast cells are in a heightened state of activation, having both an increased spontaneous and stimulated release of histamine.[13,14] Consistent with this, elevated levels of mast cell mediators are identified in BAL fluid recovered from asthmatic airways.[15-17] There is also evidence of eosinophil airway accumulation and activation in both asthma and rhinitis.[18,19] Nasal biopsies taken out of season and in season in patients with seasonal allergic rhinitis identify an accumulation of eosinophils in both the epithelium and lamina propria.[20,21] These cells are in an activated state, as identified by transmission electronmicroscopic evidence of ultrastructural granular changes. This is supported by an increased recovery of the eosinophil activation product, eosinophil cationic protein (ECP), in nasal lavage during symptom expression.[22] Similarly the eosinophils recruited into the airways in asthma are in an activated state and stain positively with the monoclonal antibody EG2, which is considered to recognize the activated form of ECP within the cells.[18]

These changes in mast cells and eosinophils represent the primary numerical cellular changes within the airways in asthma and rhinitis. Acute changes in neutrophils are described following allergen exposure in the lower airways,[23] and we have recently identified similar findings within the upper airways. A neutrophil accumulation is not, however, a feature of chronic airway inflammation in asthma,[24] and is only encountered in chronic rhinitis when aetiologies additional to allergens are relevant. Within the lavage the alveolar macrophage is the major cell population, accounting for 80–90 percent of the total cell population. This does not vary between asthmatics and nonasthmatics except when the percentage decreases due to a marked increase in eosinophils. Similarly, while T-lymphocytes represent the commonest nonconstituatory cell population within the airway epithelium, detailed immunohistochemical studies of CD3, CD4, and CD8 cell populations in biopsies[24] and flow cytometric analysis of the same subpopulations in BAL[25] have not identified any consistent increase in either the total cell population or an alteration in the subset balance. The T-lymphocytes in asthma are, however, in an activated state with enhanced expression of the cell surface markers IL-2 (CD25), HLA-DR, and VLA-1 on BAL T-lymphocytes,[25,26] and an increase in CD25$^+$ cells has been reported in mucosal biopsies from asthmatic subjects.[27]

CYTOKINES AND MAST CELL PROLIFERATION,
DIFFERENTIATION, AND ACTIVATION

Mast cells are derived from $CD34^+$ pluripotential progenitor cells within the bone marrow.[28] Although not identifiable in the peripheral blood on morphological grounds, these progenitor cells are considered to migrate to tissues where they undergo a process of maturation and differentiation. The mast cells within the respiratory tract can be characterized on the basis of their neutral protease content. The MC_T phenotype, which contains tryptase as the only neutral protease, is prominent at mucosal surfaces, while the MC_{TC} phenotype, which contains tryptase, chymase, and carboxy-peptidase as its neutral proteases, is prevalent at connective tissue sites. It is uncertain whether these differences reflect the existence of distinct subsets, derived from committed phenotypes or whether they reflect mast cells at either differing stages of maturation or of functional activation, in response to local cytokine stimulation. The latter is more probable, especially as a degranulation gradient has been described within the airway wall.[29]

The processes of mast cell proliferation within the bone marrow and maturation/differentiation at tissue sites are regulated by cytokines. This has best been defined with murine mast cells. Culture of murine bone marrow for several weeks with IL-3 results in a population of immature mast cells that resemble the human equivalent of the MC_T mast cell. These cells are designated bone-marrow-derived cultured mast cells (BMCMC). Consistent with this, IL-3 administration *in vivo* to mice results in a proliferation of immature mast cells.[30] This effect of IL-3 does, however, appear species specific, as culture of human bone marrow with IL-3 does not result in the generation of immature mast cell colonies. This may be explained by the fact that human mast cells do not possess IL-3 receptors.[31] It is now also apparent that the microenvironment is critical to mast cell development, as coculture of immature murine mast cells with murine 3T3 fibroblasts allows the mast cells to mature and adopt a MC_{TC}-like phenotype. Furthermore, coculture with 3T3 fibroblasts maintains the viability of mature mast cells.[33] Similarly coculture of murine 3T3 fibroblasts with human cord blood mononuclear cells results in the development of mast cells with the characteristics of MC_{TC} cells.[34] Two factors that may be derived from fibroblasts contribute to this development, stem cell factor (SCF) and nerve growth factor (NGF). The recent cloning of SCF has enabled the demonstration of the relevance of this cytokine. Injection of recombinant rat (rr) SCF^{164} (equivalent to the soluble form of SCF) into S1/S1^d mice, which lack mast cells due to a SCF gene mutation, corrects the deficiency. Systemic administration of SCF to rats results in a proliferation of both mucosal and connective tissue mast cell populations.[35] Similarly *in vitro* administration of rr SCF^{164} to an IL-3-dependent BMCMC line generates mature connective-tissue-like mast cells.[36] Human SCF has also been cloned and stimulates mast cell development from human cord blood mononuclear cells. These mast cells possess an immature phenotype, indicating that factors additional to SCF are required for their full development. One fibroblast factor that contributes to this with murine cells is NGF. With human cells, however, this cytokine favors the generation of basophils, which are derived from a distinctly different lineage, rather than mast cells. It may be that cell–cell contact with fibroblasts is an important aspect of cell development/maturation and that sole exposure to soluble cytokine rather than a transmembrane bound form is insufficient.

Other cytokines that have been considered of potential relevance to mast cell growth are IL-4, IL-9, IL-10, transforming growth factor β, and the interferons. Although IL-4 promotes the development of IL-3-dependent BMCMC and synergizes with IL-3 in inducing the proliferation of mature murine peritoneal mast cells,[37] it confoundingly appears to exert an inhibitory effect on human mast cells differentiation.[38] No published information is available on the effects of either IL-9 or IL-10 on human mast cells, although these cytokines are both growth factors for murine cells.[39,40] Similarly there have been no studies on human mast cells of the effects of TGFβ and the interferons, both factors which in murine cell lines inhibit the proliferation of IL-3 dependent BMCMC.[41]

In addition to these actions on mast cell maturation and differentiation, there is also evidence that cytokines may either induce mast cell degranulation *per se* or prime mast cells to enhance their release to immunological stimuli. Both IL-1 and SCF have been shown to prime human lung mast cells for increased mediator release in response to IgE-dependent activation,[42,43] while IL-1 and TNFα have been shown to directly induce histamine release from adenoidal and dermal mast cells, respectively.[44,45] The difficulty in studying these effects, however, is illustrated by the report that while SCF has no direct effect on mediator release from BMCMC *in vitro*, the *in vivo* administration of this cytokine induces activation of dermal mast cells.[46]

It is thus apparent that much remains to be established concerning the role of cytokines on human mast cell proliferation and activation. It is, however, also apparent that the balance of growth promoting and growth inhibiting cytokines at differing levels within the airways could influence the expansion of the mast cell population at one site, for example, epithelium, while cell numbers within an alternative site within the mucosa, for example, lamina propria, were unaltered. Furthermore, the demonstration that sequential and competitive interactions between differing cytokines determine the neutral proteases phenotype of BMCMC[47] allows a mechanism for the selective promotion of MC_T or MC_{TC} subtypes, while a local cytokine gradient within the airways could also contribute to the described degranulation gradient for mast cells.

CYTOKINES AND EOSINOPHIL MATURATION, ACTIVATION, AND TISSUE ACCUMULATION

Three cytokines of the IL-4 family, IL-3, IL-5, and granulocyte-macrophage colony stimulating factor (GM–CSF), have recurring relevance to tissue eosinophilia in airway inflammation.

Studies on human bone marrow *in vitro* establish that IL-3, IL-5, and GM–CSF are all capable of stimulating eosinophil production.[48,49] Of these cytokines, only IL-5 is selective for eosinophil progenitors, as IL-3 and GM–CSF also promote neutrophil and macrophage development. These three cytokines, however, interact with respect to eosinophils, as IL-3 and GM–CSF both increase the number of IL-5-responsive eosinophil colony-forming cells, while IL-5 promotes the generation of mature eosinophils from these precursors. Interleukins 3 and 5, along with GM–CSF, also influence eosinophils to adopt a hypodense phenotype *in vitro*.[50,51] Circulating hypodense eosinophils are a feature of asthma and are associated with a heightened state of eosinophil activation, demonstrating enhanced LTC_4 production, superoxide generation, and Ig-dependent cytotoxicity.[52–54]

For tissue recruitment eosinophils have to be immobilized on the vascular endothelium at the site of allergic inflammation, to permit transendothelial migration. This process involves the interaction between specific adhesion molecules

TABLE 1. Cytokine Regulation and Ligand Association for Leucocyte Endothelial Adhesion Molecules

LECAM	Cytokine Regulators					Ligand/Epitope
	IL-1	IFN-γ	TNFα	IL-4	IL-4 + TNFα	
P-selectin	+	?	+	?	?	Sialyl-Lewis^x
E-selectin	+	–	+	–	–	Sialyl-Lewis^x
ICAM-1	+	+	+	–	+	LFA-1, Mac-1
VCAM-1	+	–	+	+	+ +	VLA-4

Key: + = enhanced expression; – = no influence.

expressed on the vascular endothelium and their complementary ligands on the eosinophil cell surface. Four pairs of leucocyte endothelial adhesion molecules (LECAMs) are considered relevant to allergic inflammation, two selectins, *P*-selectin and *E*-selectin, and two members of the immunoglobulin supergene family, intercellular adhesion molecule-1 (ICAM-1) and vascular cell adhesion molecule-1 (VCAM-1). Of these, *P*-selectin (CD62) is stored preformed in Weibel-Palladie bodies in vascular endothelial cells and mobilized to the cell surface by exposure to histamine, PAF, and leukotriene C_4. This response is rapid, while enhanced production of *P*-selectin and the generation of the other LECAMs is under cytokine regulation and require *de novo* protein synthesis.[55] Four cytokines are of particular reference, IL-1, IL-4, TNFα, and IFN-γ, and the net effect on LECAM expression will depend upon relative balance of stimulation (TABLE 1). In this respect the effect of IL-4 is interactive with that of TNFα, as their effects are additive on VCAM-1 expression, while IL-4 downregulates the influence of TNFα on *E*-selectin expression.[56] Cytokines might also regulate eosinophil-endothelial adhesion by modulating the expression of the cell surface ligands. Interleukins-3 and -5, GM–CSF, and TNFα have all been shown to increase Mac-1 (CD11b/CD18) expression on eosinophils through regulation of the CD11b α chain.[57] It is now appreciated, however, that change in the cell surface expression of these ligands is not the only regulatory event, as β_2-integrins, such as LFA-1 and Mac-1, can be expressed on the cell surface in either active or inactive forms.[58] The change from inactive to active occurs through a structural conformational change. The local factors that regulate this change have been imprecisely defined, but it appears that *E*-selectin itself[59] and the chemokines IL-8 and macrophage inflammatory protein (MIP)-1β are all capable of triggering this process.[60] These chemokines can be presented to the eosinophil not as soluble forms but bound to proteoglycans, such as CD44, on the luminal surface of the vascular endothelium. By this means the eosinophil–endothelial adherence is enhanced in a specific rather than random manner, and is not at the vagaries of factors that influence blood flow and hence the local concentration of soluble cytokine.

Once firm endothelial adherence has occurred and transendothelial migration achieved through a CD18-dependent process, the directed movement of eosinophils toward the airway lumen will depend upon a chemotactic gradient. Although the cytokines IL-3, IL-5, and GM–CSF are only weakly chemotactic themselves,[61,62] they have the ability, at low concentrations, to prime eosinophils such that this cell has an increased chemotactic response to platelet activating factor (PAF) and leukotriene (LT)B_4 and responds chemotactically to IL-8.[62,63] Other chemokines, such as RANTES, and novel chemotactic factors, such as lymphocyte chemotactic factor (LCF), are now also known to be eosinophil chemoattractants, as is IL-2.[64-66] The presence of eosinophils within the tissue will depend not only upon their recruitment but also on their tissue survival. Eosinophils undergo a process of controlled cell death (apoptosis), in which there is degradation of DNA by endogenous nucleases, and subsequent removal by macrophages. The survival of eosinophils is increased *in vitro* by IL-3, IL-5, and GM–CSF,[67-70] and for IL-5 this has been demonstrated to be due to inhibition of apoptosis.[71]

It is thus apparent that cytokines have the potential to regulate the airway accumulation of eosinophils through the stimulation of their progenitors, by inducing their endothelial adherence, promoting chemotaxis, priming the cell for activation, and also by prolonging tissue survival.

EVIDENCE FOR CYTOKINE GENERATION/STORAGE/RELEASE *IN VIVO* IN ASTHMA AND RHINITIS

Sampling of the airways by lavage and biopsy has allowed direct investigation of cytokine expression in relationship to disease activity in asthma and rhinitis. Such studies have addressed either the presence of mRNA for cytokines, indicative of the potential for their generation, or the presence of generated cytokine as either stored product within cells or as the released form in biological fluid.

Two approaches have been applied to the investigation of cytokine mRNA expression within the airways. The first is to take whole biopsy samples, extracting the mRNA, generating cDNA with reverse transcriptase, amplifying the cDNA message by the polymerase chain reaction in the presence of oligonucleotide primers, and detecting the reaction product on an agarose gel, containing ethidium bromide, under UV transillumination. This technique is a very sensitive method for detecting gene expression, but does not identify the cell provenance. The second technique is that of *in situ* hybridization. By this method, mRNA expression is investigated using antisense- (complementary to mRNA) and sense- (having identical sequence to mRNA) labeled oligonucleotide probes or riboprobes, with the presence of positive antisense binding being detected by the method of labeling. This method is less sensitive than the PCR techniques, but has the potential advantage of enabling the cell provenance for a positive signal to be identified, provided that an additional method for cell identification or cell purification can be incorporated. Using the PCR technique on biopsies from the upper and lower airways from patients with allergic rhinitis ($n = 11$) and asthma ($n = 10$), and from nonatopic control subjects ($n = 12$), we have demonstrated that IL-4 and IL-5 are preferentially expressed in both asthma and rhinitis, that IFN-γ is present in both disease and nondisease status, that GM–CSF has increased expression in asthma but not rhinitis, and that no signal is apparent for either IL-2 or IL-3 in any of the samples investigated with the probes employed (TABLE 2). Studies using *in situ* hybridization have confirmed the IL-5 message within bronchial biopsies from asthmatics[72] and have demonstrated, following acute allergen challenge in the upper airways, an increase in mRNA expression for IL-4, IL-5, GM–CSF, and in this instance, also IL-3.[73] A close correlation was found 24 hours following challenge between IL-5 mRNA expression and the presence of eosinophils. It is not possible, however, from these *in situ* studies in biopsies to assess the cell source for these cytokines, but the increased expression of IL-3, IL-4, IL-5, and GM–CSF following the challenge is consistent with activation of

TABLE 2. Cytokine Gene Expression in Mucosal Biopsies Assessed by PCR Technique

	Percentage of Biopsies Positive					
	IL-2	IL-3	IL-4	IL-5	GM–CSF	IFN-γ
Nasal Biopsies						
Nonrhinitic	0	0	0	0	0	100
($n = 7$)						
Rhinitic	0	0	82	73	0	82
($n = 11$)						
Bronchial Biopsies						
Nonasthmatic	0	0	40	0	20	100
($n = 5$)						
Asthmatic	0	10	90	60	50	90
($n = 10$)						

the TH$_2$-lymphocytes subpopulation. Supportive of this has been the findings from the same researchers that in atopic asthma there is an increase in the proportion of cells recovered by bronchoalveolar lavage with positive *in situ* hybridization signals for IL-2, IL-3, IL-4, IL-5, and GM–CSF in comparison with nonsmoking, nonatopic control subjects, but no difference in the IFN-γ mRNA message.[74] Cell separation identified that the IL-4 and IL-5 mRNA in lavage could be colocalized to CD$_2$+ T-lymphocytes. An increase in cells recovered with mRNA signals for IL-4, IL-5, and GM–CSF, but not IL-2, IL-3, or IFN-γ, has also been repeated 24 hours following allergen challenge within the lower airways, which supports the concept of allergen-induced activation of TH$_2$-like cells.[75] In this instance, however, no cell separation was undertaken to identify the cell provenance for the gene expression. It is thus apparent that gene expression for IL-4, IL-5, and GM–CSF is selectively upregulated in both tissue and lavage cells in atopic asthma and that there is also evidence of a potential enhancement of IL-2 and IL-3 generation by lavage cells. This potential has to be interpreted in association with the findings from studies investigating the presence of cytokine product, as gene activation does not invariably lead to the transcription of protein.

Immunohistochemical techniques have been used to investigate the presence and localization of cytokines within biopsy samples and immunoenzymatic and bioassay techniques employed to measure free cytokine levels in lavage fluid. Positive immunohistochemical staining for IL-4, IL-5, IL-6, and TNFα has been reported in biopsies from both the upper and lower airways.[76,77] Irrespective of disease status, with an increase in IL-4 and TNFα immunoreactive cells in asthma, and IL-4 positive cells in rhinitis. In addition there is increased GM–CSF and IL-8 immunoreactivity within the airway epithelium in asthma.[78,79] Dual immuno-histochemical staining and immunostaining of adjacent 2-μm tissue sections with cell colocalization by the camera-lucida system has identified that tissue mast cells are the major cell type containing preformed IL-4, IL-5, IL-6, and TNFα, with eosinophils also demonstrating positive immunostaining for IL-5 and to a lesser extent IL-4.[76,77,80] No cytokine product has been identified in tissue T-lymphocytes.

We have observed distinct patterns of immunostaining with two separate mono-clonal antibodies (MoAb's) directed against IL-4. One MoAb, 4D9, demonstrates intracellular mast cell staining, while the other MoAb, 3H4, gives a peripheral

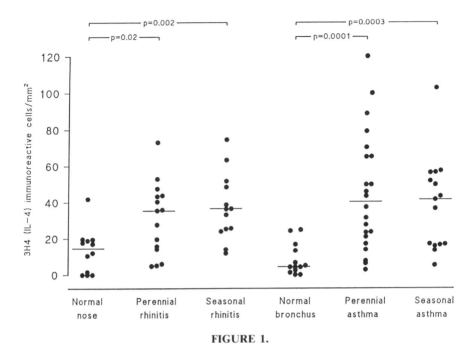

FIGURE 1.

ring pattern of immunostaining. This characteristic pattern of immunoreactivity with MoAb 3H4 is enhanced in both allergic asthma and rhinitis (FIG. 1). In comparison with normal controls there is an increase in tissue mast cell immunoreactivity to MoAb 3H4 in perennial and seasonal rhinitis and perennial and seasonal asthma. The findings in seasonal rhinitics outside the pollen season are intermediate between normal controls and those findings in active rhinitis. We have found that therapy with the inhaled topical corticosteroid, fluticasone propionate, used prophylactically, prevents the seasonal increase in 3H4 immunoreactivity in association with a reduction in eosinophil accumulation. The interpretation of this pattern of IL-4 immunoreactivity is at present undetermined. The peripheral cellular immunoreactivity cannot be attributed to cell surface binding of IL-4 to IL-4 receptors, as these would be evident also on other cell types as well as in normal airways, but could be accounted for by active IL-4 secretion, with the secreted form of IL-4 undergoing a structural conformational change, such that an epitope not exposed in the tertiary structure of the stored form is available in the secreted form for recognition by MoAb 3H4. In support of this interpretation, a similar distinct pattern of immunoreactivity has been described with two antibodies against transforming growth factor (TGF)β_1 with macrophages.[81] One MoAb stains the stored form and the other stains the secreted extracellular form. It is possible that the secreted form of IL-4, while not bound to IL-4 receptors, is in fact presented in association with the plasma membrane and involved in cell–cell contact interactions rather than released free into the surrounding extracellular fluid. Again there would be a precedent for this, with monocyte–macrophage cell surface presentation of IL-1α and TNFα.

Consistent with the concept of active IL-4 secretion in asthma and rhinitis one study has reported elevated levels of immunoreactive IL-4 in bronchoalveolar lavage fluid from atopic asthmatics in association with increased levels of IL-5.[82] This pattern differed from those findings in nonatopic asthma, in which elevated levels of IL-5 and IL-2 but not IL-4 were reported. One further study in patients with atopic asthma failed to identify elevated levels of IL-4, but the levels reported were all below the sensitivity of the assay used and thus difficult to interpret.[83] This study did, however, identify elevated levels of IL-6, GM–CSF, and TNFα in asthma in relationship to disease expression but not IL-1α, IL-1β, or IL-2. The IL-6 and GM–CSF immunoreactivity in this instance may be derived from epithelial cells, as GM–CSF immunoreactivity has been demonstrated in bronchial biopsies from asthmatics[78] and asthmatic epithelial cells in culture have been shown to generate IL-1, IL-6, GM–CSF, and IL-8.[84,85] Alternative sources for the GM–CSF could either be alveolar macrophages, since macrophages from asthmatics spontaneously generate GM–CSF *in vitro*,[86] or eosinophils, since this cell population has now been identified as capable of generating IL-1, IL-3, IL-5, IL-6, IL-8, GM–CSF, TNFα, and MIP-1α.[87–93]

CYTOKINE MODEL OF AIRWAY INFLAMMATION

The presence of stored cytokine product in mast cells suggests that in the acute allergic reaction the initial cytokine response within the airways will be mast cell derived. The release of IL-4 and TNFα will initiate leucocyte recruitment through upregulation of leucocyte endothelial cell adhesion molecules. This recruitment will be enhanced by the corelease of IL-1 from airway macrophages. Macrophages from asthmatics have been reported to exhibit an increased spontaneous release of IL-1 *in vitro*,[94] and there is evidence of macrophage activation during the immediate airway response to allergen.[73] Interleukin-4 may favor the subsequent involvement of TH$_2$-like lymphocytes, since IL-4 promotes the development of TH$_2$ lymphocytes and is required for their initial activation burst.[95,96] Activated T-lymphocytes will generate IL-3, IL-4, IL-5, and GM–CSF, all cytokines relevant to allergic inflammation. The temporal occurrence of TH$_2$ activation following airway challenge in the nose and lower airways suggests that cytokine release from this cell population leads to the perpetuation of the airway inflammatory response. Interleukins 3 and 5 and GM–CSF produced by this cell population along with IL-4, would all contribute to continuing eosinophil recruitment, priming, and activation. Granulocyte-macrophage colony stimulating factor generation from both epithelial and fibroblast sources will also contribute to the maintenance of the tissue eosinophilia through prolongation of their tissue survival. Cytokines might also serve a moderating function, to limit the consequences of the airway inflammation, as TNFα has been demonstrated to upregulate the epithelial generation of inducible nitric oxide synthase, the enzyme responsible for the synthesis of the bronchodilator nitric oxide.

In chronic allergic airways inflammation there is evidence of ongoing tissue mast cell cytokine secretion of IL-4, increased IL-4, and IL-5 mRNA expression in lavage T-lymphocytes, and evidence of epithelial generation of GM–CSF. It is thus probable that all three of these cell types—mast cells, T-lymphocytes, and epithelial cells—will contribute to the cytokine regulation of chronic airways disease. Interleukin-4, in addition to its effects on IgE synthesis, will upregulate low-affinity IgE receptor expression on nonmetachromatic cells, such as macrophages and eosinophils, expanding the range of cells directly capable of interacting with allergen. Activation of these and other cell types generating the cytokine pool within the airways contribute to the structural changes of myofibroblast proliferation, collagen deposition, and smooth-muscle hyperplasia and smooth-muscle hypertrophy, which are features of chronic asthma.

REFERENCES

1. PUNNONEN, J., et al. 1993. Interleukin 13 induces interleukin-1 independent IgG4 and IgE synthesis and CD23 expression by human B cells. Proc. Natl. Acad. Sci. U.S.A. **90:** 3730–3734.

2. BOULAY, J. L. & W. E. PAUL. 1993. The putative lymphokine P600 is a member of the IL-4 family. J. Immunol. **150:** 11A.

3. DEL PRETE, G., et al. 1988. IL-4 is an essential factor for the IgE synthesis induced in vitro by human T cell clones and their supernatants. J. Immunol. **140:** 4193–4198.

4. PENE, J., et al. 1988. Interleukin 5 enhances interleukin 4-induced IgE production by normal human B cells. The role of soluble CD23 antigen. Eur. J. Immunol. **18:** 929–935.

5. VERCELLI, D., H. H. JABARA, K. ARAI, T. YOKOTA & R. S. GEHA. 1989. Endogenous IL-6 plays an obligatory role in IL-4-induced human IgE synthesis. Eur. J. Immunol. **19:** 1419–1424.

6. KIMATA, H., A. YOSHIDA, C. ISHIOKA, I. LINDLEY & H. MIKAWA. Interleukin 8 (IL-8) selectively inhibits immunoglobulin E production induced by IL-4 in human B cells. J. Exp. Med. **176:** 1227–1231.

7. KINIWA, M., M. GATELEY, R. CHIZZONITE, C. FARGEAS & G. DELEPESSE. 1992. Recombinant interleukin-12 suppresses the synthesis of immunoglobulin E by interleukin-4 stimulated human lymphocytes. J. Clin. Invest. **90:** 262–266.

8. LAITINEN, L. A., A. LAITINEN & T. HAAHTELA. 1993. Airway mucosal inflammation even in patients with newly diagnosed asthma. Am. Rev. Respir. Dis. **147:** 697–704.

9. PESCI, A., et al. 1993. Histochemical characteristics and degranulation of mast cells in epithelium and lamina propria of bronchial biopsies from asthmatic and normal subjects. Am. Rev. Respir. Dis. **147:** 684–689.

10. ENERBACK, L., U. PIPKORN & G. GRANERUS. 1986. Intraepithelial migration of nasal mucosal mast cells in hay fever. Int. Arch. Allergy Appl. Immunol. **80:** 44–51.

11. VIEGAS, M., E. GOMEZ, J. BROOKS & R. J. DAVIES. 1987. The effect of the pollen season on nasal mast cell numbers. Br. Med. J. **294:** 414.

12. TOMIOKA, M., et al. 1984. Mast cells in bronchoalveolar lumen of patients with bronchial asthma. Am. Rev. Respir. Dis. **129:** 1000–1005.

13. FLINT, K. C., et al. 1985. Bronchoalveolar mast cells in extrinsic asthma: A mechanism for the initiation of antigen specific bronchoconstriction. Br. Med. J. **291:** 923–926.

14. WARDLAW, A. J., et al. 1988. Eosinophils and mast cells in bronchoalveolar lavage in subjects with mild asthma. Relationship to bronchial reactivity. Am. Rev. Respir. Dis. **137:** 62–69.

15. LIU, M. C., et al. 1990. Evidence for elevated levels of histamine, prostaglandin D_2 and other bronchoconstricting prostaglandins in the airways of subjects with mild asthma. Am. Rev. Respir. Dis. **142:** 126–132.

16. WENZEL, S. C., A. A. FOWLER & L. B. SCHWARTZ. 1988. Activation of pulmonary mast cells by bronchoalveolar allergen challenge: In vivo release of histamine and tryptase in atopic subjects with and without asthma. Am. Rev. Respir. Dis. **137:** 1002–1008.

17. CASALE, T. B., et al. 1987. Elevated bronchoalveolar lavage fluid histamine levels in allergic asthmatics are associated with methacholine bronchial hyperresponsiveness. J. Clin. Invest. **79:** 1197–1203.

18. DJUKANOVIC, R., *et al.* 1990. Quantification of mast cells and eosinophils in the bronchial mucosa of symptomatic atopic asthmatics and healthy control subjects using immunohistochemistry. Am. Rev. Respir. Dis. **142:** 863–871.
19. PIPKORN, U., G. KARLSSON & L. ENERBACK. 1988. The cellular response of the human allergic mucosa to natural allergen exposure. J. Allergy Clin. Immunol. **83:** 1046–1054.
[References 20, 21, 22 not provided by the author.]
23. METZGER, W. J., H. B. RICHERSON, K. WORDEN, M. MONICK & G. W. HUNNINGHAKE. 1986. Bronchoalveolar lavage of allergic asthmatic patients following allergen provocation. Chest **89:** 477–483.
24. BRADLEY, B. L., *et al.* 1991. Eosinophils, T-lymphocytes, mast cells, neutrophils, and macrophages in bronchial biopsy specimens from atopic subjects without asthma and normal control subjects and relation to bronchial hyperresponsiveness. JACI **88:** 661–674.
25. HOWARTH, P. H., *et al.* 1991. Airway inflammation and atopic asthma: A comparative bronchoscopic investigation. Int. Arch. Allergy Appl. Immunol. **94:** 266–269.
26. WALKER, C., *et al.* 1992. Allergic and non-allergic asthmatics have distinct patterns of T-cell activation and cytokine production in peripheral blood and bronchoalveolar lavage. Am. Rev. Respir. Dis. **146:** 109–115.
27. AZZAWI, M., *et al.* 1990. Identification of activated T-lymphocytes and eosinophils in bronchial biopsies in stable atopic asthma. Am. Rev. Respir. Dis. **142:** 1402–1413.
28. KIRSCHENBAUM, A. S., S. W. KESSLER, J. P. GODD & D. D. METCALF. 1991. Demonstration of the origin of human mast cells from CC34+ bone marrow progenitor cells. J. Immunol. **146:** 1410–1414.
29. BRADDING, P. Interleukins (IL)-4, -5, -6 and TNFα in normal and asthmatic airways: Evidence for the human mast cell as an important source of these cytokines. Am. J. Respir. Cell Mol. Biol. In press.
30. METCALF, D., *et al.* 1986. Effects of purified bacterially synthesised murine mutli-CSF (IL-3 on haematopoiesis in normal adult mice). Blood **68:** 46–57.
31. VALENT, P., *et al.* 1990. Failure to detect IL-3-binding sites on human mast cells. J. Immunol. **145:** 3432–3437.
32. LEVI-SCHAFFER, E., K. F. AUSTEN, P. M. GRAVELLESE & R. L. STEVENS. 1986. Coculture of interleukin 3-dependent mouse mast cells with fibroblasts results in a phenotypic change of the mast cells. Proc. Natl. Acad. Sci. U.S.A. **83:** 6485–6488.
33. LEVI-SCHAFFER, F., *et al.* 1985. Fibroblasts maintain the phenotype and viability of the rat heparin-containing mast cell *in vitro*. J. Immunol. **135:** 3454–34??.
34. FURITSU, T., *et al.* 1989. Development of human mast cells *in vitro*. Proc. Natl. Acad. Sci. U.S.A. **86:** 10039–10043.
35. TSAI, M., *et al.* 1991. The rat *c-kit* ligand, stem cell factor induces the development of connective tissue-type and mucosal mast cells *in vivo*. Analysis by anatomical distribution, histochemistry, and protease phenotype. J. Exp. Med. **174:** 125–131.
36. TAKAGI, M., *et al.* 1992. Stimulation of mouse connective tissue-type mast cells by haematopoietic stem cell factor, a ligand for the *c-kit* receptor. J. Immunol. **148:** 3446–3453.
37. HAMAGUCHI, Y., *et al.* 1987. Interleukin-4 as an essential factor for *in vitro* clonal growth of murine connective tissue-type mast cells. J. Exp. Med. **165:** 268–273.
38. NILSSON, G., A.-M. IRANI & L. B. SCHWARTZ. 1993. Regulation of growth and differentiation of human mast cells *in vitro*. Allergy **16:** 109.
39. HUTMER, L., *et al.* 1990. Mast cell growth enhancing activity (MEA) is structurally related and functionally identical to the novel mouse T cell growth factor P40/TCGFIII (Interleukin-9). Eur. J. Immunol. **20:** 1413–1416.
40. THOMPSON-SNIPES, L., *et al.* 1991. Interleukin 10: A novel stimulatory factory for mast cells and their progenitors. J. Exp. Med. **73:** 507–510.
41. BROIDE, D. H., S. I. WASSERMAN, J. ALVARO-GRACIA, N. J. ZVAIFLER & G. S. FIRESTEIN. 1989. Transforming growth factor-β1 selectivity inhibits IL-3-dependent mast cell proliferation without affecting mast cell function or differentiation. J. Immunol. **143:** 1591–1597.
42. SALARI, H. & M. CHAN-YEUNG. 1989. Interleukin-1 potentiates antigen-mediated arachidonic acid metabolite formation in mast cells. Clin. Exp. Allergy **19:** 637–641.

43. BISCHOFF, S. C. & C. A. DAHINDEN. 1992. *C-kit* ligand: A unique potentiator of mediator release by human lung mast cells. J. Exp. Med. **173:** 237–244.

44. SUBRAMANIAN, N. & M. A. BRAY. 1987. Interleukin-1 releases histamine from human basophils and mast cells *in vitro*. J. Immunol. **138:** 271–275.

45. VAN OVERVELD, F. J., PH. G. JORENS, M. RAMPART, W. DE BACKER & P. A. VERMEIRE. 1991. Tumour necrosis factor stimulates human skin mast cells to release histamine and tryptase. Clin. Exp. Allergy **21:** 711–714.

46. WERSHIL, B. K., M. TSAI, E. N. GEISSLER, K. M. ZSEBO & S. J. GALLI. 1992. The rat *c-kit* ligand, stem cell factor, induces *c-kit* receptor-dependent mouse mast cell activation *in vivo*. Evidence that signalling through the *c-kit* receptor can induce expression of cellular function. J. Exp. Med. **175:** 245–255.

47. GURISH, M. E., *et al.* 1992. Differential expression of secretory granule proteases in mouse mast cells exposed to interleukin 3 and *c-kit* ligand. J. Exp. Med. **175:** 1003–1012.

48. CLUTTERBUCK, E. J., E. M. A. HIRST & C. J. SANDERSON. 1989. Human interleukin-5 (IL-5) regulates the production of eosinophils in human bone marrow cultures: Comparison and interaction with IL-1, IL-3, IL-6 and GM-CSF. Blood **73:** 1504–1506.

49. CLUTTERBUCK, E. J. & E. J. SANDERSON. 1990. Regulation of human eosinophil precursor production by cytokines: A comparison of recombinant human interleukin-1 (rhIL-1), rhIL-3, rhIL-5, rhIL-6 and granulocyte-macrophage colony-stimulating factor. Blood **75:** 1774–1779.

50. OWER, W. F., JR., *et al.* 1987. Regulation of human eosinophil viability, density and function by granulocyte/macrophage colony-stimulating factor in the presence of 3T3 fibroblasts. J. Exp. Med. **166:** 129–141.

51. ROTHENBERG, M. E., *et al.* 1988. Human eosinophils have prolonged survival, enhanced functional properties, and becomes hypodense when exposed to human interleukin 3. J. Clin. Invest. **81:** 1886–1922.

52. KAJITA, T., Y. YUI & H. MITA. 1985. Release of leukotriene C4 and its relation to the cell density. Int. Arch. Allergy Appl. Immunol. **78:** 406–410.

53. PINCUS, S. H., W. R. SCHOOLEY, A. M. DINAPOLI & S. BRODER. 1981. Metabolic heterogeneity of eosinophils from normal and hypereosinophilic patients. Blood **58:** 1175–1180.

54. OWEN, W. F., *et al.* 1989. Interleukin 5 and phenotypically altered eosinophils in the blood of patients with the idiopathic hypereosinophilic syndrome. J. Exp. Med. **170:** 343–348.

55. MONTEFORT, S., S. T. HOLGATE & P. H. HOWARTH. 1993. Leucocyte-endothelial adhesion molecules and their role in bronchial asthma and allergic rhinitis. Eur. Respir. J. **6:** 1044–1054.

56. THORNHILL, M. H., *et al.* 1991. Tumour necrosis factor combines with IL-4 or IFN-γ to selectively enhance endothelial adhesiveness for T-cells. J. Immunol. **146:** 592–598.

57. THORNE, K. J. I., B. A. RICHARDSON, G. MAZZA & A. E. BUTTERWORTH. 1990. A new method for measuring eosinophil activating factors, based on the increased expression of CR3 α chain (CD11b) on the surface of activated eosinophils. J. Immunol. Methods **133:** 47–54.

58. SMYTH, S. S., C. C. JONECKIS & L. V. PARISE. 1993. Regulation of vascular integrins. Blood **81:** 2827–2843.

59. LO, S. K., *et al.* 1991. Endothelial-leucocyte adhesion molecule-1 stimulates the activity of leucocyte integrins CR3 (CD11b/CD18, Mac-1, $\alpha m \beta 2$) on human neutrophils. J. Exp. Med. **173:** 1493–1500.

60. TANAKA, Y., D. H. ADAMS & S. SHAW. 1993. Proteoglycans on endothelial cells present adhesion-inducing cytokines to leucocytes. Immunol. Today **14:** 111–115.

61. WANG, J. M., *et al.* 1989. Recombinant human interleukin-5 is a selective eosinophil chemoattractant. Eur. J. Immunol. **19:** 701–705.

62. WARRINGA, R. A. J., *et al.* 1991. Modulation and induction of eosinophil chemotaxis by granulocyte-macrophage colony-stimulating factor and interleukin-3. Blood **77:** 2694–2700.

63. WARRINGA, R. A. J., *et al.* 1992. Modulation of eosinophil chemotaxis by interleukin-5. Am. J. Respir. Cell Mol. Biol. **7:** 631–636.

64. KAMEYOSHI, Y., *et al.* 1992. Cytokines RANTES released by thrombin-stimulated platelets is potent attractant for human eosinophils. J. Exp. Med. **176:** 587–592.

65. RAND, T. H., W. W. CRUIKSHANK, D. M. CENTER & P. F. WELLER. 1991. Lymphocyte chemotactic factor and other CD4-binding ligands elicit eosinophil migration. J. Exp. Med. **173:** 1521–1528.

66. RAND, T. H., D. S. SILBERSTEIN, H. KORNFELD & P. F. WELLER. 1991. Human eosinophil express functional interleukin 2 receptors. J. Clin. Invest. **88:** 825–832.

67. OWEN, W. F., JR., *et al.* 1987. Regulation of human eosinophil visibility, density and function by granulocyte/macrophage colony-stimulating factor in the presence of 3T3 fibroblasts. J. Exp. Med. **166:** 129–141.

68. ROTHENBERG, M. E., *et al.* 1988. Human eosinophils have prolonged survival, enhanced functional properties, and become hypodense when exposed to human interleukin 3. J. Clin. Invest. **81:** 1886–1922.

69. LOPEZ, A. F., *et al.* 1986. Recombinant human granulocyte-macrophage colony-stimulating factor stimulates *in vitro* mature human neutrophil and eosinophil function, surface receptor expression and survival. J. Clin. Invest. **78:** 1220–1228.

70. TAI, P.-C., L. SUN & C. J. F. SPRY. 1991. Effects of IL-5, granulocyte/macrophage colony-stimulating factor (GM-CSF) on the survival of human blood eosinophils *in vitro*. Clin. Exp. Immunol. **85:** 312–316.

71. STERN, M., L. MEAGHER, J. SAVILL & C. HASLETT. 1992. Apoptosis in human eosinophils. Programmed cell death in the eosinophil leads to phagocytes by macrophages and is modulated by IL-5. J. Immunol. **148:** 3543–3549.

72. HAMID, Q., *et al.* 1991. Expression of mRNA for interleukin-5 in mucosal bronchial biopsies from asthma. J. Clin. Invest. **87:** 1541–1546.

73. DURHAM, S. R., *et al.* 1992. Cytokine messenger RNA expression for IL-3, IL-4, IL-5 and granulocyte/macrophage colony-stimulating factor in the nasal mucosa after local allergen provocation: Relationship to tissue eosinophils. J. Immunol. **148:** 2390–2394.

74. ROBINSON, D. S., *et al.* 1992. Predominant Th2 like bronchoalveolar T-lymphocyte population in atopic asthma. New Eng. J. Med. **326:** 298–304.

75. ROBINSON, D. S. Activation of CD4+ T cells and increased IL-4, IL-5 and GM-CSF mRNA positive cells in bronchoalveolar lavage fluid (BAL) 24 hours after allergen inhalation challenge of atopic asthmatic patients. J. Allergy Clin. Immunol. In press.

76. BRADDING, P., *et al.* Immunolocalisation of cytokines in the nasal mucosa of normal and perennial rhinitic subjects: The mast cell as a source of IL-4, IL-5 and IL-6 in human allergic mucosal inflammation. J. Immunol. In press.

77. BRADDING, P., *et al.* Interleukins (IL-)-4, -5, -6 and TNFα in normal and asthmatic airways: Evidence for the human mast cell as an important source of these cytokines. Am. J. Cell Respir. Cell Mol. Biol. In press.

78. SOUSA, A. R., *et al.* 1993. Detection of GM-CSF in asthmatic bronchial epithelium and decrease by inhaled corticosteroids. Am. Rev. Respir. Dis. **147:** 1557–1561.

79. REDINGTON, A. E., *et al.* 1993. Bronchial epithelial cytokine production in asthmatics and non-asthmatics. Thorax. In press.

80. BRADDING, P., *et al.* 1992. Interleukin 4 immunoreactivity is localised to and released by human mast cells. J. Exp. Med. **176:** 1381–1386.

81. FLANDERS, K. C., *et al.* 1989. Transforming growth factor β_1: Histochemical localisation with antibodies to different epitopes. J. Cell Biol. **108:** 653–660.

82. WALKER, C., *et al.* 1992. Allergic and non-allergic asthmatics have distinct patterns of T-cell activation and cytokine production in peripheral blood and bronchoalveolar lavage. Am. Rev. Respir. Dis. **146:** 109–115.

83. BROMIDE, D. H., *et al.* 1992. Cytokines in symptomatic asthma airways. J. Allergy Clin. Immunol. **89:** 958–967.

84. MATTOLI, S., *et al.* 1990. Bronchial epithelial cells exposed to isocyanates potentiate activation and proliferation of T-cells. Am. J. Physiol. **259:** L320–L327.

85. CROMWELL, O., *et al.* 1992. Expression and generation of interleukin-8, IL-6 and granulocyte-macrophage colony-stimulating factor by bronchial epithelial cells and enhancement by IL-1β and tumour necrosis factor-α. Immunol. **77:** 330–337.

86. HOWELL, C. J., *et al.* 1989. Identification of an alveolar macrophage-derived activity in bronchial asthma that enhances leukotriene C4 generation by human eosinophils stimulated by ionophore A23187 as a granulocyte-macrophage colony-stimulating factor. Am. Rev. Respir. Dis. **140:** 1340–1347.

87. WELLER, P. F., *et al.* 1993. Accessory cell function of human eosinophils HLA-DR dependent, MHC-restricted antigen-presentation and IL-1α expression. J. Immunol. **150:** 2554–2562.

88. KITA, H., *et al.* 1991. GM-CSF and interleukin 3 release from human peripheral blood eosinophils and neutrophils. J. Exp. Med. **174:** 745–748.

89. DESREUMAUX, P., *et al.* 1992. Interleukin-5 messenger RNA expression by eosinophils in the intestinal mucosa of patients with coeliac disease. J. Exp. Med. **175:** 293–296.

90. HAMID, Q., *et al.* 1992. Human eosinophils synthesise and secrete interleukin-6 *in vitro.* Blood **80:** 1496–1501.

91. BRAUN, R. K., *et al.* 1992. Human peripheral blood eosinophils have the capacity to produce IL-8 (Abstr.). FASEB J. **6:** 3912.

92. MOQBEL, R., *et al.* 1991. Expression of mRNA for the granulocyte/macrophage colony-stimulating factor (GM-CSF) in activated human eosinophils. J. Exp. Med. **174:** 749–52.

93. COSTA, J. J., *et al.* 1993. Human eosinophils can express the cytokines tumour necros factor α and macrophage inflammatory protein-1α. J. Clin. Invest. **91:** 2673–2684.

94. PUJOL, J.-L., B. COSSO, J. CLOT, F.-B. MICHEL & P. GODARD. 1990. Interleukin-1 release by alveolar macrophages in asthmatic patients and healthy subjects. Int. Arch. Allergy Appl. Immunol. **91:** 207–210.

95. SWAIN, S. L., A. D. WEINBERG, M. ENGLISH & G. HUSTON. 1990. IL-4 directs the development of TH₂-like helper effectors. J. Immunol. **145:** 3796–3806.

96. LE GROS, G., S. Z. BEN-SASSON, R. SEDER, F. D. FINKELMAN & W. E. PAUL. 1990. Generation of interleukin-4 (IL-4) producing cells *in vivo* and *in vitro:* IL-2 and IL-4 are required for *in vitro* generation of IL-4 producing cells. J. Exp. Med. **172:** 921–929.

Growth and Colony-Stimulating Factors Mediate Eosinophil Fibroblast Interactions in Chronic Airway Inflammation[a]

J. GAULDIE, G. COX, M. JORDANA, I. OHNO,
AND H. KIRPALANI

Departments of Pathology, Medicine, and Pediatrics
McMaster University
Hamilton, Ontario, Canada L8N 3Z5

INTRODUCTION

In many states of chronic tissue inflammation in the airways, such as seen in asthma, chronic rhinitis, nasal polyposis, and to some extent pulmonary fibrosis, there is a notable accumulation of eosinophilic granulocytes that have been implicated in the reactivity of the tissue and that likely contribute to tissue destruction and remodeling. Nasal polyps are grapelike structures of unknown etiology that arise from the posterior and sphenoid sinus mucosae and cause nasal obstruction.[1-3] Nasal polyposis occurs equally in normal individuals and in patients with atopic reactivity. This disorder shares a number of tissue features similar to those described for asthma, including the prevalence of eosinophils, varying degrees of basement membrane thickening, and fibrosis in the stroma.[2-5] The ease of access to tissue makes the nasal polyp an interesting and highly rewarding paradigm for the examination of eosinophil accumulation and the determination of mechanisms whereby these cells are maintained in an activated state within the tissue. We and others have recently reported that human airways tissue structural cells (TSC), specifically fibroblasts and epithelial cells, influence the biology of myeloid cells through the release of various cytokines.[6] Proliferation of stem cells and differentiation along the granulocyte pathway appear to be controlled by a series of growth factors that, by the nature of the assays used to describe them, are termed colony-stimulating factors (CSF).[7-9] The CSFs are further defined by the types of granulocyte colonies they induce in culture, and include macrophage CSF (M–CSF, also termed CSF-1), neutrophil granulocyte CSF (G–CSF), and granulocyte-macrophage CSF (GM–CSF).[10-12] These colony-stimulating factors are now known to be released from stromal cells within the tissue,[13-16] particularly after stimulation of these cells by inflammatory cytokines such as interleukin-1 (IL-1) and tumor necrosis factor (TNF),[17-23] products of activated monocytes, in a network of cells and cytokines.[24] GM–CSF in particular can modulate the behavior of eosinophils *in vitro* and can play a profound role in regulating the tissue presence of these cells.[25-29] In turn, eosinophils in the tissue can be shown to release a series of

[a] This work was supported by MRC Canada, the Ontario Thoracic Society, and Astra Draco Sweden. One of the authors (G.C.) is a Parker B. Francis Fellow in Pulmonary Research.

growth factors, including transforming growth factor-β (TGF-β),[30,31] and platelet-derived growth factor (PDGF), which have a profound impact on the behavior and differentiation of tissue cells.[32-36] We have used the nasal polyp to determine the presence of many of these important cytokines and the cellular source within the polyp, and have now documented a number of important autocrine and paracrine interactions resulting in the presence of activated myeloid cells as well as altered phenotypes of tissue structural cells.

MATERIAL AND METHODS

Tissues

Nasal polyp tissues were obtained from patients undergoing polypectomies for nasal obstruction. Control normal tissue was obtained from the inferior turbinate of patients at the time of surgery for submucosal resection. Tissue was immediately rinsed with Ham's F12 medium and sections removed and frozen in liquid nitrogen for subsequent extraction of mRNA in 4 M guanadinium isothiocyanate (ISCN). For *in situ* hybridization and immunohistochemistry, a small (20–30 mg) piece of tissue was fixed for 24 hours in 4 percent paraformaldehyde in 0.01 M phosphate-buffered saline (PBS), 4°C and then stored in 70 percent ethanol prior to embedding in paraffin.[37]

Colony-Stimulating Factor Production by Tissue Fibroblasts

Epithelial cells and fibroblast lines that were established by outgrowth from nasal tissues as previously described were cultured in the presence or absence of 10 ng/ml of recombinant human IL-1β.[16,38] Supernatants were harvested, filtered, and assayed for CSF activity by bioassay and immunoassay (Quantikine RMD, Minneapolis).

RNA Analysis

Cells were suspended in 4 M guanidinium ISCN prior to extraction by phenol chloroform, and in some instances poly A$^+$ RNA was prepared prior to Northern gel analysis. For GM–CSF determination, a 600-bp fragment of human GM–CSF cDNA (GI Institute) and for TGF-β examination, a 640-bp fragment of porcine TGF-β1 cDNA (K. Flanders, NIH, Bethesda) was labeled by random priming with ^{32}P dCTP for use in Northern gel analysis and with ^{35}S dCTP for *in situ* hybridization.

In situ *Hybridization*

In situ hybridization was performed as previously described.[37] In short, sections of nasal polyps were dewaxed and pretreated with carbol Chromotrope (1.25 percent Chromotrope 2R) to block nonspecific reactions with eosinophils prior to hybridization overnight with the appropriate probes and then again immersed in carbol Chromotrope to stain eosinophils prior to autoradiography and counterstaining with hematoxylin-eosin.

Immunohistochemistry

Sections were examined for the presence of cytokines using specific antibodies for GM–CSF, TGF-β1, and PDGF. In brief, after blocking of endogenous peroxidase, dewaxed sections were stained with primary antibody and then Avidin peroxidase complexes with visualization with diaminobenzidine and hydrogen peroxide.

RESULTS AND DISCUSSION

Colony-Stimulating Factor Produced by Polyp Structural Cells

We established a series of primary fibroblast lines and primary epithelial cell cultures from nasal polyps as well as from control tissue of the inferior turbinate of the nares. Supernatants of these cell lines cultured with or without the addition of IL-1 showed the presence of significant levels of all three CSFs (TABLE 1).

TABLE 1. Content of Colony-Stimulating Factors GM–CSF, G–CSF, and M–CSF in Conditioned Medium

Cell Source	GM–CSF (pg/ml)	G–CSF (ng/ml)	M–CSF (ng/ml)
Nasal polyp epithelial cell	$489 \pm 118 \; n = 10$	$1.63 \pm 0.26 \; n = 6$	$<0.8 \; n = 3$
Nasal polyp fibroblast	$663 \pm 258 \; n = 12$	$0.6 \pm 0.3 \; n = 5$	$5.0 \pm 0.0 \; n = 2$
Normal nasal epithelial cell	$126 \pm 35 \; n = 3$	$1.08 \pm 0.24 \; n = 5$	$1.0 \pm 0.1 \; n = 2$
Normal nasal fibroblast	$194 \pm 69 \; n = 5$	$1.3 \pm 0.9 \; n = 5$	$4.8 \pm 0.8 \; n = 2$

Fibroblast lines established from nasal polyp releases significantly more CSF under control or stimulated conditions than lines established from the inferior turbinate and this was also the case for epithelial cell cultures. When freshly isolated peripheral blood eosinophils were placed in culture in the presence of these structural cell supernatants, there was a striking maintenance of cell survival and viability. Normally eosinophils will die in culture over a period of 2 or 3 days. Fibroblast supernatant and epithelial cell supernatant maintained eosinophil viability up to 7 days. This maintenance of viability was abrogated only when we added a neutralizing antibody to GM–CSF. Thus, structural cells in the nasal polyp, including the fibroblast and epithelial cell, release GM–CSF both spontaneously and upon stimulation by inflammatory cytokines such as IL-1, and this GM–CSF can act upon eosinophils to maintain viability and induce a state of activation. This activation (but not degranulation) can be detected in the nasal polyp by staining with an immunohistochemical reagent for EG2, a granule-associated marker for an activated eosinophil.

When we stained nasal polyp sections with antibody to GM–CSF, a large number of cells were seen to be positive, including epithelial cells and interstitial fibroblasts. Thus, within the tissue, the structural cells appear intrinsically activated to release colony-stimulating factors that can directly impact on the accumulation and activation of eosinophils in tissue.

Growth Factors Produced by Eosinophils in Nasal Polyps

There are several cytokines that have a profound impact on the behavior of structural cells such as fibroblasts. These include a series of growth factors such as transforming growth factor-β and platelet-derived growth factor. PDGF induces a major proliferative response in the fibroblast,[39] while TGF-β modulates collagen gene expression in these same cells.[40] When we probed the nasal polyp tissue by in situ hybridization techniques for cells actively producing RNA for TGF-β and PDGF, the eosinophil was shown as one of the major cellular sources for active expression of mRNA for these growth factors (FIG. 1). Previous studies have demonstrated that eosinophils are capable of releasing a factor that mediates fibroblast proliferation.[41] It is likely that this factor is PDGF, and our demonstration of eosinophils being positive for PDGF mRNA in the nasal polyp is further evidence that the eosinophil in the tissue can release cytokines that modulate fibroblast behavior. TGF-β has been shown to be present in a number of tissues exhibiting fibrosis. Immunohistochemical staining of the polyp showed a broad distribution of TGF-β associated with the matrix throughout the tissue. Whether the eosinophil is the major source of this TGF-β is unclear since this cytokine can also induce TGF-β expression of autocrine production by fibroblasts. Given that the in situ analysis demonstrates the eosinophil as being one of the major sources of TGF-β mRNA, however, this is further evidence that the eosinophil produces factors that profoundly affect the behavior of the fibroblast.

One further surprising finding occurred when we examined the nasal polyp tissue by in situ hybridization for cells actively producing GM–CSF mRNA. Once again, we found that the eosinophil was one of the major sources for the production of this particular cytokine. Thus, while many of the structural cells produced GM–CSF, the eosinophil that had entered the tissue and was now under the influence of this CSF was also a producer of the same factor in an autocrine fashion. Further evidence that these nasal polyp eosinophils were actively producing GM–CSF came when we isolated these cells from the nasal polyp and placed them in culture. Instead of dying as would be the case for peripheral blood eosinophils, the nasal polyp eosinophils remained viable in culture and again this viability was abrogated only when we added a neutralizing antibody to GM–CSF.

The fact that eosinophils in the tissue are actively producing GM–CSF could have a further feedback effect on the structural cells. Previous studies from Gabbiani's group have demonstrated that in vivo, GM–CSF was able to induce a myelofibroblastlike phenotype in fibroblasts and they were able to show the presence of fibroblast staining for smooth-muscle-specific actin by immunohistochemistry.[42] When we examined the nasal polyp with antibody to smooth-muscle actin, the majority of the fibroblasts throughout the polyp as well as the smooth-muscle cells of the vessels were highly positive for smooth-muscle actin. Thus, the GM–CSF produced by the eosinophil may have induced the smooth-muscle actin-positive phenotype in the fibroblast in the polyp.

Steroid Modulation of Cell/Cytokine Interaction

One of the most powerful inhibitors of cytokine production by inflammatory cells and structural cells is the use of corticosteroid. Monocytes and fibroblasts treated with dexamethasone are no longer stimulated by either LPS or IL-1 to produce cytokines such as GM–CSF. Moreover, we have shown that eosinophils treated with corticosteroids are no longer responsive to the viability enhancing activity of GM–CSF.[43] Thus, one would expect that treatment of nasal polyps

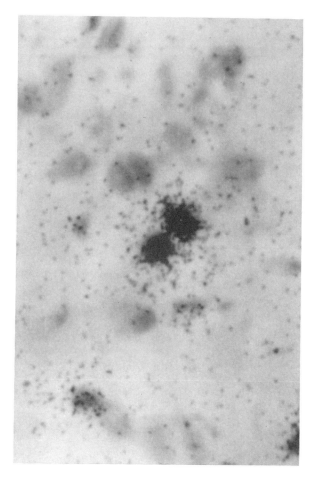

FIGURE 1. Autoradiogram of a section from a nasal polyp tissue. Example of sections that were pretreated with chromotrope 2R, hybridized with the TGF-β1 cDNA probe, and counterstained with chromotrope 2R. Note a positive hybridization signal only on positively counterstained cells (eosinophils). (Magnification: 1000×.)

with topical steroid would reduce the presence of cells actively making various cytokines and modulate the structure or content of the nasal polyp. Jerry Dolovich and Manel Jordana in some preliminary studies have treated nasal polyps with topical budesonide, a powerful corticosteroid, and have been able to show a dramatic reduction in the presence of GM–CSF by immunohistochemistry. Moreover, in nasal polyps that have been subjected to extended topical steroid treatment with budesonide, fibroblasts no longer stain positive for smooth-muscle actin, implying that the myelofibroblast phenotype has reverted to a normal fibroblast. Whether the steroid interferes with the ability of the fibroblast to respond to GM–CSF in a manner similar to that of the eosinophil is unknown. Apparent use of steroid decreases inflammatory cytokine production and presence, however, and results in the modulation of the fibroblast phenotype and decreases the presence of activated eosinophils in the nasal polyp.

CONCLUSIONS

If we examine the nasal polyp as a paradigm of chronically inflammed tissue involving eosinophil infiltration and fibroblast proliferation, we can demonstrate that the fibroblast produces cytokines that have a profound impact on the accumulation and activation of the eosinophil. In turn, as the eosinophil enters the tissue, it becomes an equivalent effector cell and releases its own cytokines, which in turn can affect the behavior of the fibroblast. Induction of new phenotype behavior can be the result of a network of autocrine and paracrine systems in which the fibroblast and eosinophil contribute to the chronic activation of the tissue. Interruption of this chronic activation by drugs such as steroids can result in the downregulation of the cytokine networks, and if they are used over a prolonged period of time, may introduce a measure of normal cell function into these chronically inflamed tissues. The network of eosinophil and fibroblast is but one example of similar networks that occur in a variety of other tissues. It is clear, however, when one considers allergic diseases, such as asthma, that involve tissue eosinophils, many of these same mechanisms that we have documented in the nasal polyp might play a role in the induction of hyperreactivity and contribute directly to the chronic nature of inflammatory diseases in the airways.

REFERENCES

1. CONNELL, J. T. 1979. Nasal hypersensitivity. *In* Comprehensive Immunology, Vol. 6, S. Gupta and R. A. Good, Eds.: 397–426. Plenum. New York.
2. CAUNA, N., K. H. HINDERER, G. W. MANZETTI & E. W. SWANSON. 1972. Fine structure of nasal polyps. Ann. Otol. **81:** 41–58.
3. KAKOI, H. & F. HIRAIDE. 1987. A histological study of formation and growth of nasal polyps. Acta Otolaryngol. **103:** 137–144.
4. ROCHE, W. R., J. H. WILLIAMS, R. BEASLEY & S. T. HOLGATE. 1989. Subepithelial fibrosis in the bronchi of asthmatics. Lancet **i:** 520–524.
5. DJUKANOVIC, R., J. WILSON, K. M. BRITTEN, S. J. WILSON, A. F. WALLS, W. R. ROCHE, P. H. HOWARTH & S. T. HOLGATE. 1990. Quantitation of mast cells and eosinophils in the bronchial mucosa of symptomatic atopic asthmatics and healthy control subjects using immunohistochemistry. Am. Rev. Respir. Dis. **142:** 863–871.
6. GAULDIE, J., M. JORDANA, G. COX, T. OHTOSHI, J. DOLOVICH & J. DENBURG. 1991. Fibroblasts and other structural cells in airways inflammation. Am. Rev. Respir. Dis. **145:** 514–517.
7. METCALF, D. & N. A. NICOLA. 1983. Proliferative effects of purified granulocyte colony-stimulating factor (G-CSF) on normal mouse hemopoietic cells. J. Cell. Physiol. **228:** 810–815.

8. METCALF, D. 1985. The granulocyte-macrophage colony-stimulating factors. Science **229:** 16–22.
9. CLARK, S. C. & R. KAMEN. 1987. The human hematopoietic colony-stimulating factors. Science **236:** 1229–1237.
10. METCALF, D. 1986. The molecular biology and functions of the granulocyte-macrophage colony-stimulating factors. Blood **67:** 257–267.
11. SONODA, Y., Y.-C. YANG, G. G. WONG, S. C. CLARK & M. OGAWA. 1988. Analysis in serum-free culture of the targets of recombinant human hemopoietic growth factors: Interleukin 3 and granulocyte/macrophage-colony-stimulating factor are specific for early developmental stages. Proc. Natl. Acad. Sci. U.S.A. **85:** 4360–4364.
12. WONG, G. G., *et al.* 1987. Human CSF-1: Molecular cloning and expression of a 4 kb cDNA encoding the hematopoietin and determination of the complete amino acid sequence of the human urinary protein. Science **235:** 1504–1508.
13. VANCHERI, C., *et al.* 1991. Neutrophilic differentiation induced by human upper airway fibroblast-derived granulocyte/macrophage colony-stimulating factor (GM-CSF). Am. J. Respir. Cell Mol. Biol. **4:** 11–17.
14. SMITH, S. M., D. K. P. LEE, J. LACY & D. L. COLEMAN. 1990. Rat tracheal epithelial cells produce granulocyte/macrophage colony-stimulating factor. Am. J. Respir. Cell Mol. Biol. **2:** 59–68.
15. OHTOSHI, T., C. VANCHERI, G. COX, J. GAULDIE, J. DOLOVICH, J. A. DENBURG & M. JORDANA. 1991. Monocyte-macrophage differentiation induced by human upper airway epithelial cells. Am. J. Respir. Mol. Biol. **4:** 255–263.
16. COX, G., J. GAULDIE & M. JORDANA. 1992. Bronchial epithelial cell-derived cytokines (G-CSF and GM-CSF) promote the survival of peripheral blood neutrophils *in vitro.* Am. J. Respir. Cell Mol. Biol. **7:** 507–513.
17. BAGBY, G. C., C. A. DINARELLO, P. WALLACE, C. WAGNER, S. HEFENEIDER & E. MCCALL. 1986. Interleukin 1 stimulates granulocyte macrophage colony-stimulating activity release by vascular endothelial cells. J. Clin. Invest. **78:** 1316–1321.
18. BROUDY, V. C., K. KAUSHANSKY, J. M. HARLAN & J. W. ADAMSON. 1987. Interleukin-1 stimulates human endothelial cells to produce granulocyte-macrophage colony-stimulating factor and granulocyte colony-stimulating factor. J. Immunol. **139:** 464–468.
19. BROUDY, V. C., K. KAUSHANSKY, G. M. SEGAL, J. M. HARLAN & J. W. ADAMSON. 1987. Tumor necrosis factor type stimulates human endothelial cells to produce granulocyte/macrophage colony-stimulating factor. Proc. Natl. Acad. Sci. U.S.A. **83:** 7467–7471.
20. SEELENTAG, W. K., J. J. MERMOD, R. MONTESANO & P. VASSALLI. 1987. Additive effects of interleukin 1 and tumour necrosis factor-alpha on the accumulation of the three granulocyte and macrophage colony-stimulating factor mRNAs in human endothelial cells. EMBO J. **6:** 2261–2265.
21. SEELENTAG, W. K., J. MERMOT & P. VASSALLI. 1989. Interleukin 1 and tumor necrosis factor-α additively increase the levels of granulocyte-macrophage and granulocyte colony-stimulating factor (CSF) mRNA in human fibroblasts. Eur. J. Immunol. **19:** 209–212.
22. MUNKER, R., J. GASSON, M. OGAWA & H. P. KOEFFLER. 1986. Recombinant human tumor necrosis factor induces production of granulocyte-monocyte colony stimulating factor mRNA and protein from lung fibroblasts and vascular endothelial cells in vitro. Nature **323:** 79–82.
23. MARINI, M., M. SOLOPERTO, M. MEZZETTI, A. FASOLI & S. MATTOLI. 1991. Interleukin-1 binds to specific receptors on human bronchial epithelial cells and upregulates granulocyte/macrophage colony-stimulating factor synthesis and release. Am. J. Respir. Cell Mol. Biol. **4:** 519–524.
24. ARAI, K.-I., F. LEE, A. MIYAJIMA, S. MIYATAKE, N. ARAI & T. YOKOTA. 1990. Cytokines: Coordinators of immune and inflammatory responses. Annu. Rev. Biochem. **59:** 783–836.
25. OWEN, W. F., JR., M. F. ROTHENBERG, D. S. SILBERSTEIN, J. C. GASSON, R. L. STEVENS, K. F. AUSTEN & R. J. SOBERMAN. 1987. Regulation of human eosinophil

viability, density, and function by granulocyte-macrophage colony-stimulating factor in the presence of 3T3 fibroblasts. J. Exp. Med. **166:** 129–141.

26. LOPEZ, A. F., *et al.* 1986. Recombinant human granulocyte-macrophage colony-stimulating factor stimulates *in vitro* mature human neutrophil and eosinophil function, surface receptor expression and survival. J. Clin. Invest. **78:** 1220–1228.

27. ROSE, R. M., *et al.* 1992. The effect of aerosolized recombinant human granulocyte macrophage colony-stimulating factor on lung leukocytes in nonhuman primates. Am. Rev. Respir. Dis. **146:** 1279–1286.

28. SILBERSTEIN, D. S., *et al.* 1986. Regulation of human eosinophil function by granulocyte-macrophage colony-stimulating factor. J. Immunol. **137:** 3290–3294.

29. VANCHERI, C., J. GAULDIE, J. BIENENSTOCK, G. COX, R. SCICCHITANO, A. STANISZ & M. JORDANA. 1989. Human lung fibroblast-derived granulocyte-macrophage colony stimulating factor (GM-CSF) mediates eosinophil survival *in vitro*. Am. J. Respir. Cell Mol. Biol. **1:** 289–295.

30. WONG, D. T., *et al.* 1990. Human eosinophils express transforming growth factor α. J. Exp. Med. **172:** 673–681.

31. OHNO, I., *et al.* 1992. Eosinophils in chronically inflamed human upper airway tissues express transforming growth factor β1 gene (TFGβ1). J. Clin. Invest. **89:** 1662–1668.

32. KHALIL, N., O. BEREZNAY, M. SPORN & A. H. GREENBERG. 1989. Macrophage production of transforming growth factor β and fibroblast collagen synthesis in chronic pulmonary fibrosis. J. Exp. Med. **170:** 727–737.

33. MARTINET, Y., W. N. ROM, G. R. GROTENDORST, G. R. MARTIN & R. G. CRYSTAL. 1987. Exaggerated spontaneous release of platelet-derived growth factor by alveolar macrophages from patients with idiopathic pulmonary fibrosis. New Eng. J. Med. **317:** 202–209.

34. HOYT, D. G. & J. S. LAZO. 1988. Alterations in pulmonary mRNA encoding procollagens, fibronectin and transforming growth factor precede bleomycin-induced pulmonary fibrosis in mice. J. Pharmacol. Exp. Ther. **246:** 765–771.

35. FABISIAK, J. P. & J. KELLEY. 1992. Platelet-derived growth factor. *In* Cytokines of the Lung, J. Kelley, Ed.: 3–40. Dekker. New York.

36. KELLEY, J. 1992. Transforming growth factor-β. *In* Cytokines in the Lung, J. Kelley, Ed.: 101–138. Dekker. New York.

37. OHNO, I., R. LEA, S. FINOTTO, J. MARSHALL, J. DENBURG, J. DOLOVICH, J. GAULDIE & M. JORDANA. 1991. Granulocyte/macrophage colony-stimulating factor (GM-CSF) gene expression by eosinophils in nasal polyposis. Am. J. Respir. Cell Mol. Biol. **5:** 505–510.

38. JORDANA, M., J. SCHULMAN, C. MCSHARRY, L. B. IRVING, M. T. NEWHOUSE, G. JORDANA & J. GAULDIE. 1988. Heterogeneous proliferative characteristics of human adult lung fibroblast lines and clonally derived fibroblasts from control and fibrotic tissue. Am. Rev. Respir. Dis. **137:** 579–584.

39. RAINES, E. W., D. F. BOWEN-POPE & R. ROSS. 1990. Platelet-derived growth factor. *In* Handbook of Experimental Pharmacology, Vol. 95, Peptide Growth Factors and Their Receptors, M. B. Sporn and A. B. Roberts, Eds.: 173–262. Springer-Verlag. Heidelberg.

40. RAGHU, G., S. MASTA, D. MEYERS & A. S. NARAYANAN. 1989. Collagen synthesis by normal and fibrotic human lung fibroblasts and the effect of transforming growth factor-β. Am. Rev. Respir. Dis. **140:** 95–100.

41. PINCUS, S. A., S. H. RAMESH & D. J. WYLER. 1987. Eosinophils stimulate fibroblast DNA synthesis. Blood **70:** 572–574.

42. RUBBIA-BRANDT, L., A. SAPPINO & G. GABBIANI. 1991. Locally applied GM-CSF induces the accumulation of smooth muscle actin containing fibroblasts. Virchows Arch. (B) **60:** 73–82.

43. COX, G., T. OHTOSHI, C. VANCHERI, J. A. DENBURG, J. DOLOVICH, J. GAULDIE & M. JORDANA. 1991. Promotion of eosinophil survival by human bronchial epithelial cells and its modulation by steroids. Am. J. Respir. Cell Mol. Biol. **4:** 525–531.

RANTES, A Novel Eosinophil–Chemotactic Cytokine

JENS-MICHAEL SCHRÖDER, YOSHIKAZU KAMEYOSHI,
AND ENNO CHRISTOPHERS

Department of Dermatology
University of Kiel
24105 Kiel, Germany

INTRODUCTION

The development of inflammation in common is known to involve a series of cellular events controlled by a variety of mediators. Leukocytes, once activated in the circulation, adhere to the inner wall of mainly capillary vessels, and then migrate to the inflammatory focus. Signal substances for leukocytes to migrate to an inflammatory focus usually are chemotactic factors. Recruitment of leukocytes from the vascular lumen into the inflamed tissue is one example of an inflammatory event that is mediated via a cascade of specifically induced signals.

Initiation of this process can be caused by local decrease of blood flow and leukocytosis in regional vessels. Thereafter inflammatory cells and the endothelium of the vessel interact in a reversible manner through the expression of adherence proteins. Adherence proteins are expressed in both endothelium and leukocytes. This initial interaction between inflammatory cells and the endothelium is truly important; however, it only represents one of many proximal events in the inflammatory cascade.

Although the mechanisms of adherence of inflammatory cells to the endothelium is becoming increasing clear, the remaining events necessary to move leukocytes from a local vessel into an area of inflammation still remain an enigma.

This enigma includes the movement of leukocytes between endothelial cells and the ability of these cells to recognize gradients of chemotactic factors either in the fluid phase (chemotaxis) or on surfaces (haptotaxis).

CHEMOTACTIC FACTORS

A number of chemotactic agents have been identified in the past that possess potent activity to recruit leukocytes. The majority of these factors are relatively short acting and include leukotriene B_4 (LTB_4), platelet activating factor (PAF), complement fragment C5a, and bacteria-derived formylated methionylpeptides.

In a number of inflammatory diseases, including so-called neutrophilic dermatoses (such as psoriasis), as well as some lung diseases, including also lung giant cell carcinoma, predominantly neutrophilic granulocytes are found in the affected tissues. In a number of inflammatory diseases other leukocyte forms and subtypes, depending upon the disease and its stage, are representative. The pattern of leukocyte infiltration into affected tissues appears to be determined by the local liberation of leukotactic mediators.

All chemotaxins just mentioned are chemotactic for different leukocyte types

91

and subsets, and represent pan-leukotactic rather than leukocyte-selective factors. It appears to be difficult to explain the selective appearance of different leukocyte forms in affected tissues of different inflammatory diseases. Therefore it has been suggested that apart from pan-leukocyte chemotactic factors mediators that have leukocyte-selective chemotactic properties also exist.

CHEMOKINES: A NOVEL FAMILY OF LEUKOCYTE-SELECTIVE ATTRACTANTS

This working hypothesis was originally confirmed with the characterization of a novel neutrophil-chemotactic cytokine,[1-4] later termed Interleukin-8 (IL-8),[5] which in contrast to known leukocyte attractants, does not show significant chemotactic activity for monocytes[1,2] or eosinophils[1] *in vitro*. IL-8 represents a member of a superfamily of low molecular-weight chemotactic cytokines (now termed *chemokine family*[6]) that is structurally characterized by the presence of four cysteines in the same relative position (FIG. 1). Another member is referred to as *monocyte chemotactic protein-1* (MCP-1), which is a selective attractant for monocytes without any chemotactic properties for neutrophils, eosinophils, or lymphocytes.[7]

Apart from these two chemotactic cytokines others were reported to be preferential or selective chemotaxins for neutrophils (besides IL-8, there are also NAP-2,

```
              1      10       20        30        40        50        60        70        80
NAP-2             ...AELRCMCIKTTSG-IHP-KNIQSLEVIGK-GTHCNQV-EVIATL-KDGRKICLDPDAPRIKK-IVQKKLAGDESAD
hNAP-1/IL-8    AVLPRSAKELRCQCIKTYSKPFHP-KFIKELRVIES-GPHCANT-EIIVKL-SDGRELCLDPKENWVQR-VVEKFLKRAENS
hMGSA/GROα     ASVATELRCQCLQTLQG-IHP-KNIQSVMVKSP-GPHCAQT-EVIATL-KNGRKACLNPASPIVKK-IIEKMLNSDKSN
hGROβ          ASPL-----------------L--------K-------------------KNGQ--------M----------KNG---
hGROγ          ASVA-----------------L--------R-------------------K--------MVQ------ILNKGSTN
hENA-78        AGPAAAVLRELRCVCLQTTQG-VHP-KMISNLQVFAI-GPQCSKV-EVVASL-KNGKEICLDPEAPFLKK-VIQKILDGGNKEN
hGCP-2         GPVSAVLTELRCTCLRVTLR...

              1      10       20        30        40        50        60        70        80
hMIP-1α/LD-78     ADTPTAC-CFSYTSRQI-PQNFIAD-Y-FETSSQ-CSKP-GVIF-LTKRSRQVCADPSEEWVQKYV--SDLELSA
hI309          VDSKSMQVPFSRC-CFSFAEQEI-PLRAILC-Y-RNTSSI-CSNE-GLIF-KLKRGKEACALDTVGWVQRHR--KMLRHCPSKRK
hMIP-1β/ACT-2  ...APMGSDPPTSC-CFSYTARKL-PRNFVVD-Y-YETSSL-CSQP-AVVF-QTKRSKQVCADPSESWVQEYV--YDLELN
hRANTES/       SPYSSDTTPC-CFAYIARPL-PRAHIKE-Y-FYTSGK-CSNP-AVVF-VTRKNRQVCANPEKKWVREYI--NSLEMS
hMCP-1/MCAF    QPDAINAPVTC-CYNFTNRKI-SVQRLAS-YRRITSSK-CPKE-AVIF-KTIVAKEICADPKQKWVQDSM--DHLDKQTQTPKT
hMCP-2         DSVSIPITC-CFNVINRKI-PIQRLES-YTRITNIQ-CPKE-AVIF-KT--GKEVCADPKERWVRDSMKHLDQIFQNLKP
hMCP-3         KSTTC-CYRFINKKI-PKQRLES-YRRTTSSH-CPRE-AVIF-K----DKEICADPTQKWVQDFMKHLDKKTQTPKL
```

FIGURE 1. Chemotactic cytokines (Chemokines). Amino acid sequence alignment of different members of the IL-8 supergene family. The single letter code for amino acids is used; hNAP-2 = human neutrophil activating protein 2;[42] hIL-8 = human interleukin 8;[35-37] hMGSA/groAlpha = human melanoma growth stimulatory activity/groAlpha;[44,45] hgroBeta = human groBeta; hgroGamma = human groGamma;[46] hENA-78 = human epithelial cell derived neutrophil activating protein 78;[46] hGCP-2 = human granulocyte chemotactic protein 2;[59] hMIP-1Alpha = human macrophage inflammatory protein 1Alpha;[47] hI-309 = human I-309;[48] hMIP-1Beta = human macrophage inflammatory protein 1Beta;[47] h RANTES = human cytokine "Regulated and normal T-lymphocyte expressed and secreted";[24] hMCP-1/MCAF = human monocyte chemotactic protein 1/monocyte chemotactic and activation factor;[7] MCP-2 and MCP-3 = monocyte chemotactic proteins 2 and 3.[49] Note the same relative position of four cysteines (*shaded area*).

TABLE 1. Leukotactic Properties of Chemokines

Chemokine	Chemotactic[a] for	Not Chemotactic[a] for	Reference
IL-8	Neu, Lym, Bas	Eos, Mono	35–37
NAP-2	Neu	Eos, Mono	43
GroAlpha	Neu	Eos, Mono	44, 45
GroBeta	Neu	?	46
GroGamma	Neu	?	46
ENA-78	Neu	Eos, Mono	46
GCP-2	Neu	Mono	50
MCP-1	Mono	Neu, Eo, Ly	7, 36
MCP-2	Mono	Neu	49
MCP-3	Mono	Neu	49
MIP-1Alpha	Ly, Eo	Neu	26, 47
MIP-1Beta	Ly	Neu, Eo	26, 47
RANTES	Ly, Mo, Eo	Neu	22, 26, 27, 32
I-309	Mo	Neu	48

[a] Neu = neutrophils; Lym = lymphocytes; Bas = basophils; Eos = eosinophils; Mono = monocyte.

gro-Alpha, Beta, Gamma, ENA-78, GCP-2), monocytes (besides MCP-1, there are also I-309, MCP-2, MCP-3, RANTES), memory T-lymphocytes (RANTES), other T-lymphocyte-subsets (IL-8, MIP-1 Alpha, MIP-1 Beta), and basophils (IL-8) (TABLE 1). Eosinophils (Eos) were not originally reported to be attracted by chemokines, making it attractive to hypothesize whether a member of the chemokine family could be a preferential or selective Eo-chemotaxin.

EOSINOPHIL-CHEMOTACTIC FACTORS

In the past a number of Eo-attractants have been identified. The complement fragment C5a (fifth component of complement) represents a potent, and *in vitro,* very efficient (percentage of input migrating cells in the cell migration assay system) chemotaxin for human eosinophils.[8] As mentioned earlier, it is also a powerful chemotaxin for neutrophils, monocytes, and lymphocytes.

It has long been suggested that leukotriene B_4 (LTB_4) is an important chemotactic factor for eosinophils. In guinea pigs it indeed elicits high chemotactic responses.[9] Human eosinophils, however, respond poorly to LTB_4.[10] Later the platelet activating factor (PAF) was identified as the most efficient chemotactic factor for human eosinophils, albeit attracting neutrophils as well.[11]

In recent studies we observed that eosinophils are capable of producing their own chemotaxin when incubated with exogenous arachidonic acid.[12] This lipidlike chemotaxin, which was originally called "*eosinophil chemotactic lipid* (ECL),[12] we recently have structurally characterized as identical with the eicosanoid 5-oxo-15-hydroxy-eicosatetraenoic acid (5-oxo-15-HETE).[13] 5-oxo-15-HETE represents a novel Eo-chemotaxin, which seems to be more potent and of similar efficacy as found for PAF.[11] In addition it appears to bind to a different, so far unknown type of chemotaxin-receptor.[12]

Apart from lipidlike Eo-attractants and C5a, other proteinaceous Eo-chemotaxins have also been detected: interleukin 5 (IL-5), which originally was described as T-cell-replacing factor and is known to stimulate bone-marrow precursor cells to differentiate into mature eosinophils, shows selective chemoattractant properties for human eosinophils.[14] In a similar manner, granulocyte-macrophage colony-stimulating factor (GM–CSF) and interleukin 3 (IL-3) also represent selective eosinophil attractants;[15,16] however, in our hands these attractants are less efficient (percentage input migrated cells) than the other chemotaxins. Another protein-aceous Eo-attractant, called lymphocyte-derived chemotactic factor (LCF), originally detected as lymphocyte and monocyte chemotaxin, which binds to CD4, has been reported to represent a powerful and selective Eo-attractant, which does

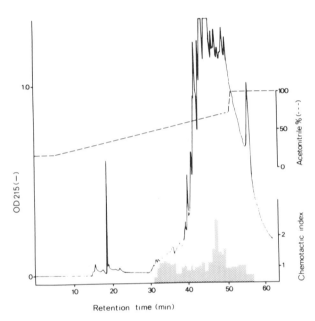

FIGURE 2. Preparative reversed phase (RP-8) HPLC of a supernatant of lymphocyte prepa-rations. Peripheral blood mononuclear cell preparations obtained after Ficoll centrifugation of human blood were separated and the lymphocyte preparations were stimulated with Concanavalin A (10 μg/ml) for 48 h and supernatants were separated by preparative RP-8 HPLC. Human eosinophil chemotactic activity (shaded area) was tested in aliquots of each fraction using the indirect cell-counting method recently described.[1]

not attract neutrophils.[17] Its molecular structure, however, as yet has not been reported. All these chemotactic cytokines have relative molecular masses > 15 kD.

As reported earlier members of the family of chemokines show molecular masses between 6 and 10 kD. The findings that members of the C–X–C-chemokine family represent neutrophil-selective attractants and members of the C–C-chemo-kine family are selective attractants for monocytes and/or lymphocyte subsets, but not for neutrophils, raised the question whether this supergene family also contains chemotactic cytokines for eosinophils, thus completing the spectrum of leukocyte-selective attractants.

SUPERNATANTS OF LYMPHOCYTE-CELL PREPARATIONS CONTAIN EO-CHEMOTACTIC PROTEINS

In order to test the working hypothesis that, besides IL-8[1] or MCP-1,[18] peripheral blood mononuclear cell (PBMC) preparations also secrete Eo-chemotactic cytokines, PBMC-preparations were stimulated for 48 h with bacterial lipopolysaccharide (1 μg/ml) together with concanavalin A (10 μg/ml).

Supernatants of PBMC-preparations were separated by preparative reversed-phase HPLC and analyzed for Eo-chemotactic activity using purified human Eo-preparations.

Fractions eluting at 60 percent acetonitrile showed a single peak of Eo-chemotatic activity. When analyzed for its M_r by the use of size exclusion-HPLC, biological activity came from the column in fractions corresponding to an M_r near 8 kD, exactly in the same fractions where IL-8 elutes. In order to evaluate the cellular origin of the 8-kD eosinophil chemotactic protein, supernatants of purified, LPS-stimulated monocytes were analyzed. Under conditions known to elicit maximum release of neutrophil-chemotactic IL-8, no eosinophil chemotactic activity could be detected. Indeed preparations of lymphocytes obtained after elutriation of mononuclear cells released Eo-chemotactic proteins when incubated for 2 days in the presence of Con A, as shown by preparative RP-HPLC analyses (FIG. 2). These preparations usually contained variable numbers of platelets.

EO-CHEMOTACTIC PROTEINS RELEASED FROM PLATELETS

Since platelets are known to be a rich source of some members of the IL-8 family—such as platelet factor 4,[19] a structurally related attractant we termed NAP-4[20] and platelet basic protein or its truncation products, connective tissue activating peptide (CTAP) III and β-thromboglobulin,[21] we investigated whether platelets contain Eo-chemotactic proteins. When lysates of platelets were analyzed for Eo-chemotaxins, strong Eo-chemotactic activity could be detected. To evaluate whether Eo-chemotactic activity is also released from platelets upon physiologic stimulation, platelets were stimulated with thrombin. Consequently, the majority of Eo-chemotactic activity was detected in supernatants after incubation with 1 U/ml thrombin for 15 min.[22]

When these supernatants were separated by TSK-2000-size exclusion HPLC, a major peak of Eo-chemotactic activity appeared in fractions corresponding to an M_r near 8 kD. Furthermore the elution behavior of this activity indicated that it does not come from the highly efficient Eo-chemotaxin PAF,[11] which is known to be produced by platelets[23] and which elutes from the TSK-2000 HPLC column at a different time. Furthermore, PAF can be easily diafiltered through a YM-5 Amicon membrane, which is used for concentrating supernatants of thrombin-stimulated platelets.

For purification of Eo-chemotactic proteins, supernatants were applied to a preparative RP-8 reversed-phase HPLC column after acidification with trifluoroacetic acid (TFA), and proteins were eluted with an increasing gradient of acetonitrile containing 0.1 percent TFA.

Fractions were tested for Eo-chemotaxis using the indirect cell counting Boyden chamber technique with purified human Eos as described.[12] A single peak of biological activity was obtained, which usually coeluted with a small peak absorbing at 215 nm appearing between the two major peaks of connective tissue activat-

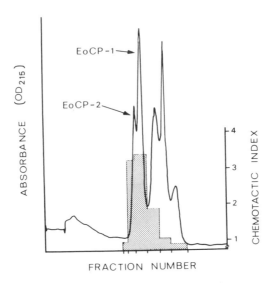

FIGURE 3. Cyanopropyl-RP-HPLC of partially purified platelet-derived Eo-chemotaxins. Purified platelets were stimulated for 30 min with thrombin (1 U/ml), and supernatants were separated by preparative RP-8 HPLC followed by CN–HPLC. Proteins were eluted with a gradient of *n*-propanol containing 0.1 percent TFA. Eosinophil-chemotactic activity in the fractions is presented by the shaded area. Note the presence of a broad peak of Eo-chemotactic activity.

ing peptide III (CTAP III) and platelet factor 4 (PF4) (data not shown). Fractions eluting from RP-8-HPLC were further purified by the use of cyanopropyl (CN) reversed-phase HPLC with *n*-propanol as eluent. Eo-chemotactic activity was present in two early eluting peaks absorbing at 215 nm (FIG. 3). When necessary these fractions were collected and contaminating high molecular mass proteins were separated by TSK-2000-size exclusion HPLC.

Final purification was achieved by the use of narrow-pore RP-18-HPLC. Eo-chemotactic activity eluted in two peaks absorbing at 215 nm tentatively termed Eo-chemotactic protein 1 (EoCP-1), the earlier eluting compound representing a broadened peak, and EoCP-2, the later eluting compound, representing a sharp peak.[22] Upon SDS-PAGE analysis the mobility of EoCP-2 is identical with that seen for Ser-IL-8_{72},[22] whereas EoCP-1, the quantitatively predominant Eo-chemotaxin in platelet supernatants, shows a higher mobility with a calculated M_r of 7 kD,[22] when the Tricine method without urea was used.

The molecular weight of both EoCP-1 and EoCP-2 was determined by electrospray mass spectrometry (ESP-MS). Whereas EoCP-1 revealed a calculated molecular mass of $8,355 \pm 10$, for EoCP-2 the molecular mass was determined to be $7,862.8 \pm 1.1$.[22]

CYTOKINE RANTES IS AN EO-ATTRACTANT

When both EoCP-1 and EoCP-2 were analyzed by gas-phase amino-acid sequencing in both preparations, a single sequence was obtained. As shown in

FIGURE 4, this sequence is identical for both preparations. However, in the EoCP-1-preparation residue numbers 4 and 5 could not be determined, whereas in EoCP-2 at the same position, two serine residues were detected.

Both amino-acid sequences are identical to that deduced from a cytokine cDNA termed RANTES[24] (*r*egulated *a*nd *n*ormal *T*-cell *e*xpressed and *s*ecreted). The calculated molecular weight of RANTES is 7,847.03, which differs from EoCP-1 by 508 mass units and from EoCP-2 by 15.8 mass units. Since *N*-glycosylation sites are absent from RANTES, most likely serine residues in EoCP-1 are *O*-glycolysated, which leads to broadening of the RP–HPLC peak. In EoCP-2 the difference of 15.8 mass units can be accounted for by the assumption of oxidation having taken place. Since the mass difference corresponds to that of a single oxygen, oxidation on the single methionine residue number 67 most likely could have taken place. Oxidation of methione is very common, especially in the case of samples that have been exposed to the atmosphere before analyses. Both forms of natural RANTES cytokine forms were analyzed for Eo-chemotactic properties and showed similar potency in eliciting Eo-chemotaxis when the Boyden chamber method was used (FIG. 5). It is interesting to note that chemotactic efficacy, the number of Eos having migrated through the chemotaxis filter per time unit, varied depending upon the donor for both forms of RANTES, which could come from nonresponding cells recently detected upon ultrastructural analyses of RANTES-stimulated Eos.[25]

Since half-maximal chemotactic stimulation is identical for both natural forms of RANTES, derivatization at serine residue numbers 4 and 5 appears not to affect potency and efficacy of Eo-chemotactic stimulation. Since recombinant RANTES is now commercially available, this preparation was also tested for eosinophil chemotactic properties.

Similarly, rRANTES induces chemotactic responses in human eosinophils with similar ED_{50} and efficacy as seen for natural forms.[22,26] When both natural RANTES forms were tested for neutrophil chemotaxis, neither the RANTES preparations nor rRANTES showed any significant neutrophil chemotactic activity (data not shown), in accordance with previous findings with rRANTES.[27] In support of the observation that rRANTES also attracts human monocytes, both natural RANTES forms were found to be chemotactic for monocytes (our unpublished results).

When rRANTES was tested for Eo-chemokinetic activity using a checkerboard analysis in a Boyden chamber migration assay system, significant chemokinetic

```
HuMIP-1α    ADTPTAC-CFSYTSRQI-PQNFIAD-Y-FETSSQ-CSKPGVIF-LTKRSRQVCADPSEEWVQKYV--SDLELSA

HuMIP-1β    APMGSDPPTSC-CFSYTARKL-PHNFVVD-Y-YETSSL-CSQPAVVF-QTKRGKQVCADPSESWVQEYV--YDLELN

MCP-1/MCAF  QPDAINAPVTC-CYNFTNRKI-SVQRLAS-YRRITSSK-CPKEAVIF-KTIVAKEICADPKQKWVQDSM--DHLDKQTQTPKT

I-309       VDSKSMQVPFSRC-CFSFAEQEI-PLRAILC-Y-RNTSSI-CSNEGLIF-KLKRGKEACALDTVGWVQRHR--KMLRHCPSKRK

RANTES      SPYSSDTTPC-CFAYIARPL-PRAHIKE-Y-FYTSGK-CSNPAVVF-VTRKNRQVCANPEKKWVREYI--NSLEMS

EoCP-1      SPYXXDTTPX-XFAYIA

EoCP-2      SPYSSDTTPX-XFAYIARPL-PRAXXXE-Y-FYXXG
```

FIGURE 4. Amino acid sequence alignments of Eo-chemotactic proteins (EoCPs). EoCP sequences were experimentally determined; the other sequences are cDNA derived. The single-letter code for amino acids is used. X stands for amino acids that could not be determined. Note the identity of both EoCP sequences with that of cytokine RANTES.

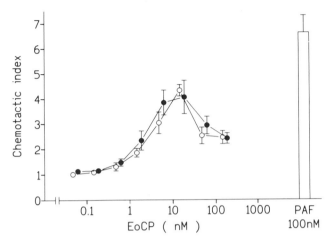

FIGURE 5. Eo-chemotactic activity of both natural forms of RANTES. Platelet-derived RANTES, EoCP-1 (–●–), and EoCP-2 (–○–), were investigated for Eo-chemotactic activity. Chemotactic index represents the quotient of Eos migrating under stimulatory conditions and random migration. One-hundred nanomolar concentration of PAF were used as positive control.

activity was detected at concentrations higher than 50 ng/ml, which is similar to the concentration eliciting significant Eo-chemotaxis (TABLE 2).

The migratory response, however, at chemokinetic stimulation is lower than that seen at chemotactic stimulation. Therefore RANTES is a chemotactic rather than chemokinetic cytokine, which is supported by recent investigations.[26]

Cross-desensitization studies of Eo-chemotaxis revealed that pretreatment of human eosinophils with RANTES reduces chemotactic responses only to RANTES, not, however, to other chemotaxins such as C5a or PAF (TABLE 3), which is consistent with the hypothesis that RANTES binds to a separate receptor on human eosinophils. A C–C chemokine receptor was recently cloned that binds human RANTES as well as other chemokines, such as human macrophage inflammatory protein-1 Alpha (MIP-1 Alpha), human macrophage inflammatory protein-1 Beta (MIP-1 Beta), and human monocyte chemotactic protein-1 (MCP-1).[28,29] Similar or possibly identical receptors were identified on human

TABLE 2. Checkerboard Analysis of Eo-Chemotactic Activity of rRANTES

rRANTES in Lower Chamber (ng/ml)	rRANTES in Upper Chamber (ng/ml)				
	0	10	25	50	100
0	1.0	0.9	0.9	0.9	1.2
10	0.8	1.0	1.0	1.0	1.1
25	1.1	1.0	1.1	1.3	1.4
50	2.0	1.6	1.6	1.8	1.4
100	2.5	2.6	2.6	2.6	1.6

Note: Results are expressed as migration index of an experiment performed in duplicate. A representative out of three experiments is shown.

TABLE 3. Cross-Desensitization of Eo-Chemotactic Responses toward RANTES and Other Chemotaxins

Preincubation with	Stimulation with		
	rRANTES [1 μg/ml]	C5a [1 ng/ml]	PAF [50 ng/ml]
rRANTES [2 μg/ml]	**9**	202	144
rC5a [2 ng/ml]	92	**22**	95
PAF [100 ng/ml]	69	123	**16**

Note: Data represent percentage of net Eo-chemotaxis of buffer pretreated cells. Note the presence of strong desensitization only with homolog chemotaxins (data shown in boldface).

monocytes[30] and monocytic cells.[31] The gene for this receptor was mapped to human chromosome 3p21. The receptor is a member of the G-protein-coupled receptor superfamily. It has 33 percent amino-acid identity with receptors for IL-8 and may be a human homologue to a product of US 28, an open reading frame of human cytomegalovirus suggesting a role of these chemokines in viral immunity.[28,29]

POSSIBLE ROLE OF RANTES IN EOSINOPHILIC INFLAMMATION

RANTES was originally identified as an apparently T-lymphocyte-specific inducible gene, which was found to be expressed by cultured T-cell lines that were antigen-specific and growth factor dependent.[24] RANTES mRNA expression has been found to be inducible in peripheral blood leukocyte preparations. It is therefore likely, but yet not proved, that supernatants of stimulated lymphocytes contain Eo-chemotactic RANTES. The absence of 8-kD Eo-chemotactic proteins in supernatants of stimulated human monocytes points toward a lack of RANTES mRNA expression in monocytes, which is supported by polymerase chain reaction (PCR) investigations using RANTES-specific primers.[32]

Eosinophils or products of Eos are found in a variety of inflammatory conditions including late phase reactions, allergic diseases, and asthma [for review see reference 33]. Release of toxic substances such as cationic Eo granule proteins, which are released in low amounts by cytochalasin-B-treated eosinophils *in vitro*,[26] and peptidoleukotrienes are believed to be important in Eo-derived inflammatory reactions. The finding of predominantly Eos, and only to a lesser extent neutrophils in such inflammatory diseases led to the hypothesis of a local production of Eo-selective or preferential (relative to neutrophils) attractants in the tissues. Eo-chemotactic cytokines such as GM–CSF, IL-5, IL-3, and LDCF have been suggested to be important for tissue infiltration by Eos.

The cytokine RANTES has now been detected as a potent and selective Eo-chemotaxin[22,26,34] and has already been described as a memory T-lymphocyte-selective (CD45 RO +) chemotactic factor.[27] Therefore this cytokine could be of particular importance in inflammatory processes in which both memory

T-lymphocytes and eosinophils are present in affected tissues, such as asthma, atopic dermatitis, and allergic late phase reactions.

The finding that human platelets represent a source of preformed RANTES is unexpected and fits well with previous observations that other members of the chemotactic cytokine family, such as platelet factor 4 and connective-tissue-activating peptide III, are stored in the α-granules of platelets. These cytokines, however, belong to the C–X–C branch of the family.[35-37] Therefore cytokine RANTES represents the first example of a C–C branch member, which is also stored in platelets.

The biological significance of Eo-chemotactic RANTES in platelets is as yet speculative. Nevertheless, the release of RANTES upon physiological stimulation with thrombin serves as additional evidence for a contribution of platelets to inflammatory reactions.[38]

It was suggested by guinea pig models that platelets are a prerequisite component in allergic asthma, since platelet depletion reduces eosinophil infiltration into the lung following PAF—or allergen—exposure to sensitized animals.[39] Similarly, PAF antagonists or PGI_2 pretreatment produced similar inhibitory activities.

Moreover bronchial eosinophil accumulation was reduced without a significant change in neutrophil infiltration after antigen challenge in thrombocytopenic allergic rabbits compared to control animals.[40] Clinical observations, such as elevation of plasma platelet factor 4[41] or β-thromboglobulin[41] also suggest platelet activation associated with allergen exposure in allergic asthmatics.[41,42]

It is therefore tempting to speculate that after antigen challenge in the lung, RANTES produced and released by infiltrated T-lymphocytes and/or platelets and possibly also by other cells might play a role for selective eosinophil infiltration being released directly or indirectly possibly via PAF- or antigen-stimulation *in vivo*.

REFERENCES

1. SCHRÖDER, J.-M., U. MROWIETZ, E. MORITA & E. CHRISTOPHERS. 1987. Purification and partial biochemical characterization of a human monocyte-derived neutrophil-activating peptide that lacks Interleukin 1 activity. J. Immunol. **139:** 3474–3483.
2. YOSHIMURA, T., K. MATSUSHIMA, S. TANAKA, E. A. ROBINSON, E. APPELLA, J. J. OPPENHEIM & E. J. LEONARD. 1987. Purification of a human monocyte-derived neutrophil chemotactic factor that shares sequence homology with other host defense cytokines. Proc. Natl. Acad. Sci. U.S.A. **84:** 9233–9237.
3. WALZ, A., P. PEVERI, H. ASCHAUER & M. BAGGIOLINI. 1987. Purification and amino acid sequencing of NAF, a novel neutrophil-activating factor produced by monocytes. Biochem. Biophys. Res. Commun. **149:** 755–761.
4. VAN DAMME, J., J. VANN BEEUMEN, G. OPDENAKKER & A. BILLIAU. 1988. A novel, NH_2-terminal sequence-characterized human monokine possessing neutrophil chemotactic, skin reactive and granulocytosis-promoting activity. J. Exp. Med. **167:** 1364–1376.
5. WESTWICK, J., S. W. LI & R. D. CAMP. 1989. Novel neutrophil stimulating peptides. Immunol. Today **10:** 146–147.
6. LINDLEY, I. J. D., J. WESTWICK & S. L. KUNKEL. 1993. Nomenclature announcement—the chemokines. Immunol. Today **14:** 24.
7. LEONARD, E. J. & T. YOSHIMURA. 1990. Human monocyte chemoattractant protein-1 (MCP-1). Immunol. Today **11:** 97–101.
8. KAY, A. B., H. S. SHIN & K. F. AUSTEN. 1973. Selective attraction of eosinophils and synergism between eosinophil chemotactic factor of anaphylaxis (ECF-A) and a fragment cleaved from the fifth component of complement (C5a). Immunology **24:** 969–976.

9. CZARNETZKI, B. M., W. KÖNIG & L. M. LICHTENSTEIN. 1976. Eosinophil chemotactic factor (ECF). I. Release from polymorphonuclear leukocytes by the calcium ionophore A 23187. J. Immunol. **117:** 229–234.

10. MORITA, E., J.-M. SCHRÖDER & E. CHRISTOPHERS. 1989. Differential sensitivities of purified human eosinophils and neutrophils to defined chemotaxins. Scand. J. Immunol. **29:** 709–716.

11. WARDLAW, A. J., R. MOQBEL, O. CROMWELL & A. B. KAY. 1986. Platelet-activating factor. A potent chemotactic and chemokinetic factor for human eosinophils. J. Clin. Invest. **78:** 1701–1712.

12. MORITA, E., J.-M. SCHRÖDER & E. CHRISTOPHERS. 1990. Identification of a novel and highly potent eosinophil chemotactic lipid in human eosinophils treated with arachidonic acid. J. Immunol. **144:** 1893–1900.

13. SCHWENK, U., E. MORITA, R. ENGEL & J.-M. SCHRÖDER. 1992. Identification of 5-Oxo-15-hydroxy-6,8,11,13-eicosatetraenoic acid as a novel and potent human eosinophil chemotactic eicosanoid. J. Biol. Chem. **267:** 12482–12488.

14. WANG, J. M., A. RAMBALDI, A. BIONDI, Z. G. CHEN, C. J. SANDERSON & A. MANTOVANI. 1989. Recombinant human interleukin 5 is a selective eosinophil chemoattractant. Eur. J. Immunol. **19:** 701–705.

15. WARRINGA, R. A. J., L. KOENDERMAN, P. T. M. KOK, J. KREUKMIET & P. L. B. BRUIJNZEEL. 1991. Modulation and induction of eosinophil chemotaxis by granulocyte-macrophage colony stimulating factor and interleukin-3. Blood **77:** 2694–2700.

16. KAMEYOSHI, Y., E. MORITA, J.-M. SCHRÖDER & E. CHRISTOPHERS. 1992. Recombinant human interleukin-3 is a chemoattractant for human eosinophils, but not for neutrophils. Submitted for publication.

17. RAND, T. H., W. W. CRUIKSHANK, D. M. CENTER & P. F. WELLER. 1991. CD4-mediated stimulation of human eosinophils: Lymphocyte chemoattractant factor and other CD4-binding ligands elicit eosinophil migration. J. Exp. Med. **173:** 1521–1528.

18. YOSHIMURA, T., N. YUHKI, S. K. MOORE, E. APPELLA, M. I. LERMAN & E. J. LEONARD. 1989. Human monocyte chemoattractant protein-1 (MCP-1): Full-length cDNA cloning, expression in mitogen-stimulated blood mononuclear leukocytes, and sequence similarity to mouse competence gene JE. FEBS Lett. **244:** 487–493.

19. DEUEL, T. F., R. M. SENIOR, D. CHANG, D. L. GRIFFIN, R. L. HEINRIKSON & E. T. KAISER. 1981. Platelet factor 4 is chemotactic for neutrophils and monocytes. Proc. Natl. Acad. Sci. U.S.A. **78:** 4584–4587.

20. SCHRÖDER, J.-M., M. STICHERLING, N.-L. M. PERSSOON & E. CHRISTOPHERS. 1990. Identification of a novel platelet-derived neutrophil-chemotactic polypeptide with structural homology to platelet factor 4. Biochem. Biophys. Res. Commun. **172:** 898–904.

21. CASTOR, C. W., J. W. MILLER & D. A. WALZ. 1983. Structural and biological characteristics of connective tissue activating peptide (CTAP-III), a major human platelet-derived growth factor. Proc. Natl. Acad. Sci. U.S.A. **80:** 765–769.

22. KAMEYOSHI, Y., A. DÖRSCHNER, A. I. MALLET, E. CHRISTOPHERS & J.-M. SCHRÖDER. 1992. Cytokine RANTES released by thrombin-stimulated platelets is a potent attractant for human eosinophils. J. Exp. Med. **176:** 587–592.

23. CHIGNARD, M., J. P. LE CONEDIC, B. B. VARGAFTIG & J. BENVENISTE. 1980. Platelet-activating factor (PAF-acether) secretion from platelets: Effect of aggregating agents. Br. J. Haematol. **46:** 455–464.

24. SCHALL, T. J., J. JONGSTRA, B. J. DYER, J. JORGENSEN, C. CLAYLBERGER, M. M. DAVIS & A. M. KRENSKY. 1988. A human T cell-specific molecule is a member of a new gene family. J. Immunol. **141:** 1018–1025.

25. KAPP, A., W. CZECH, J. KRUTMANN & G. ZECK-KAPP. 1993. Differential regulation of eosinophil activation by cytokines—The role of GM-CSF, IL-5 and RANTES (Abstract). Arch. Derm. Res. **285:** 97.

26. ROT, A., M. KRIEGER, T. BRUNNER, S. C. BISCHOFF, T. J. SCHALL & C. A. DAHINDEN. 1992. RANTES and macrophage inflammatory protein 1 alpha induce the migration and activation of normal human eosinophil granulocytes. J. Exp. Med. **176:** 1489–1495.

27. SCHALL, T. J., K. BACON, K. J. TOY & D. V. GOEDDAL. 1990. Selective attraction of monocytes and T lymphocytes of the memory phenotype by cytokine RANTES. Nature (London) **347:** 669–671.

28. NEOTE, K., D. DiGREGORIO, J. Y. MAK, R. HORUK & T. J. SCHALL. 1993. Molecular cloning, functional expression, and signaling characteristics of a C-C chemokine receptor. Cell **72:** 415–425.

29. GAO, J. L., D. B. KUHNS, L. TIFFANY, D. MCDERMOTT, X. LI, U. FRANCKE & P. M. MURPHY. 1993. Structure and functional expression of the human macrophage inflammatory protein 1alpha/RANTES receptor. J. Exp. Med. **177:** 1421–1427.

30. WANG, J. M., B. SHERRY, M. J. FIVASH, D. J. KELVIN & J. J. OPPENHEIM. 1993. Human recombinant macrophage inflammatory protein-1 alpha and -beta and monocyte chemotactic and activating factor utilize common and unique receptors on human monocytes. J. Immunol. **150:** 3022–3029.

31. WANG, J. M., D. W. MCVICAR, J. J. OPPENHEIM & D. J. KELVIN. 1993. Identification of RANTES receptors on human monocyte cells: Competition for binding and desensitization by homologous chemotactic cytokines. J. Exp. Med. **177:** 699–705.

32. KIENE, P., M. MENKE, E. CHRISTOPHERS & J.-M. SCHRÖDER. 1993. Detection of RANTES mRNA by the polymerase chain reaction (Abstract). Arch. Derm. Res. **285:** 96.

33. LEIFERMAN, K. M. 1991. A current perspective on the role of eosinophils in dermatologic diseases. J. Am. Acad. Dermatol. **24:** 1101–1112.

34. ALAM, R., S. STAFFORD, P. FORSYTHE, R. HARRISON, D. FAUBION, M. A. LETTBROWN & J. A. GRANT. 1993. RANTES I a chemotactic and activating factor for human eosinophils. J. Immunol. **150:** 3442–3448.

35. BAGGIOLINI, M., A. WALZ & S. L. KUNKEL. 1989. Neutrophil-activating peptide-1/interleukin 8, a novel cytokine that activates neutrophils. J. Clin. Invest. **84:** 1045–1049.

36. SCHALL, T. J. 1991. Biology of the RANTES/SIS cytokine family. Cytokine **3:** 165–183.

37. SCHRÖDER, J.-M. 1992. Chemotactic cytokines in the epidermis. Exp. Dermatol. **1:** 12–19.

38. PAGE, C. P. 1989. Platelets as inflammatory cells. Immunopharmacology **17:** 51–59.

39. LELLOUCH-TUBIANA, A., J. LEFORT, M.-T. SIMON, A. PFISTER & B. B. VARGAFTIG. 1988. Eosinophil recruitment into guinea pig lungs after PAF-acether and allergen administration. Modulation by prostacyclin, platelet depletion, and selective antagonists. Am. Rev. Respir. Dis. **137:** 948–954.

40. COYLE, A. J., C. P. PAGE, L. ATKINSON, R. FLANAGAN & W. J. METZGER. 1990. The requirement for platelets in allergen-induced late asthmatic airway obstruction. Eosinophil infiltration and heightened airway responsiveness in allergic rabbits. Am. Rev. Respir. Dis. **142:** 587–593.

41. KNAUER, K. A., L. M. LICHTENSTEIN, N. F. ADKINSON, JR. & I. F. FISH. 1981. Platelet activation during antigen-induced airway reactions in asthmatic subjects. New Eng. J. Med. **304:** 1404–1407.

42. GRESELE, P., S. GRASSELLI, T. TODISCO & G. G. NENCI. 1985. Platelets and asthma. Lancet, **ii:** 347.

43. WALZ, A., B. DEWALD, V. VON TSCHARNER & M. BAGGIOLINI. 1989. Effects of the neutrophil-activating peptide NAP-2, platelet basic protein, connective tissue-activating peptide III, and platelet factor 4 on human neutrophils. J. Exp. Med. **170:** 1745–1750.

44. SCHRÖDER, J.-M., N. PERSSOON & E. CHRISTOPHERS. 1990. Lipopolysaccharide-stimulated human monocytes secrete apart from NAP-1/IL-8 a second neutrophil-activating protein: NH$_2$-terminal aminoacid sequence-identity with melanoma growth stimulatory activity (MGSA/gro). J. Exp. Med. **171:** 1091–1100.

45. MOSER, B., I. CLARK-LEWIS, R. ZWAHLEN & M. BAGGIOLINI. 1990. Neutrophil-activating properties of the melanoma growth-stimulatory activity. J. Exp. Med. **171:** 1797–1802.

46. WALZ, A., R. BURGENER, B. CAR, M. BAGGIOLINI, S. L. KUNKEL & R. M. STRIETER. 1991. Structure and neutrophil-activating properties of a novel inflammatory peptide (ENA-78) with homology to IL-8. J. Exp. Med. **174:** 1355–1363.

47. TAUB, D., K. CONLON, A. R. LLOYD, J. J. OPPENHEIM & D. J. KELVIN. 1993. Preferential migration of activated CD4$^+$ and CD8$^+$ T-cells in response to MIP-1alpha and MIP-1beta. Science **260:** 355–358.
48. MILLER, M. D. & M. S. KRANGEL. 1992. The human cytokine I-309 is a monocyte chemoattractant. Proc. Natl. Acad. Sci. U.S.A. **89:** 2950–2954.
49. VAN DAMME, J., P. PROOST, J.-P. LENAERTS & G. OPDENAKKER. 1992. Structural and functional identification of two human tumor-derived monocyte chemotactic proteins (MCP-2 and MCP-3) belonging to the chemokine family. J. Exp. Med. **176:** 59–65.
50. PROOST, P., C. D. WOLF-PEETERS, R. CONINGS, G. OPDENAKKER, A. BILLIAU & J. VAN DAMME. 1993. Identification of a novel granulocyte chemotactic protein (GCP-2) from human tumor cells. J. Immunol. **150:** 1000–1010.

Interleukin-1 Receptor Antagonist Inhibits Pulmonary Hypertension Induced by Inflammation[a]

NORBERT F. VOELKEL[b] AND RUBIN TUDER[c]

[b]Division of Pulmonary and Critical Care Medicine
University of Colorado Health Sciences Center
Denver, Colorado 80202

[c]Department of Pathology
University of Colorado Health Sciences Center
Denver, Colorado 80202

INTRODUCTION

Structural alterations of the lung vessels can occur in each part of the vascular tree including the lung capillaries. In addition to the well-established forms of angitis, there is increasing evidence that inflammatory mechanisms defined by cell–cell interactions and mediator release are part of chronic pulmonary vascular disorders associated with the development of pulmonary hypertension.[1-3] Patients with chronic obstructive pulmonary diseases and patients with a smoking history demonstrate muscularization of their pulmonary small arteries[4] and intravascular cell aggregates consisting of neutrophils, monocytes, and platelets—aided perhaps by alveolar macrophages—these cells could provide the cytokines and growth factors involved in the structural alterations characteristic for chronic pulmonary hypertensive states.[5]

In this study we examine the hypothesis that interleukin-1 (IL-1) plays an important part in the development of chronic pulmonary hypertension and in the vascular remodeling process that accounts for the structural alterations of hypertensive lung vessels. We take the view that the 17,000 Dalton polypeptide, which is synthesized in two major species, IL-α and IL-β acts on the lung vessels either directly or in combination with lipid mediators. Our approach is to examine in two accepted experimental models of chronic pulmonary hypertension[2,3] whether treatment with the interleukin-1 receptor antagonist (IL-1ra)[6,7] prevents development of pulmonary hypertension. The monocrotaline (MCT) rat model[8] represents the paradigm of inflammatory pulmonary hypertension, whereas the model of chronic hypoxia exposure represents a *per se* noninflammatory model of hypertension.[9]

Our rationale for such a pharmacological approach stems from the combination of several pertinent facts regarding the action of interleukin-1. This cytokine acts as a procoagulant, stimulates the production of collagen in fibroblasts,[10] it is produced by endothelial cells *in vitro*,[11] and it is mitogenic for fibroblasts and vascular smooth-muscle cells.[12-14] Moreover, the actions of IL-1 and of platelet activating factor (PAF) and of eicosanoids are apparently intertwined such that the inhibition of the action of PAF or of eicosanoid synthesis may result in the inhibition of synthesis of action of IL-1.[15,16] Finally, it has been shown that mono-

[a] This work has been supported by a grant from the American Heart Association.

cyte and endothelial cell IL-1 production can be stimulated oxygen dependently, during hypoxia and reoxygenation;[17,18] therefore, IL-1 could play a role in the vascular remodeling that occurs in the lungs during chronic hypoxia.

METHODS

We used male Sprague-Dawley rats weighing 250–280 g for the monocrotaline studies. Rats received one single subcutaneous injection (60 mg/kg) of the alkaloid monocrotaline.[2] One group of rats received injections of twice-daily IL-1ra (Synergen, Boulder, Colorado) in a dose of 2-mg/kg i.p. Since antibodies can develop in animals after prolonged administration of this human IL-1ra, the treatment period did not exceed 2 weeks. Rats were exposed to a simulated altitude of 16,000 feet in a hypobaric chamber for 3 weeks to induce chronic pulmonary hypertension. Control animals for both study designs received twice-daily injections of IL-1ra (2 mg/kg).

Measurement of Pulmonary Artery Pressure

At the end of a 3-week period the rats were weighed and anesthetized and a catheter was advanced into the main pulmonary artery through the jugular vein. The catheter was connected to a pressure transducer, and mean pulmonary artery pressure was measured and recorded. Following the recording of the pulmonary artery pressure, a blood sample was withdrawn through the catheter for measurement of the hematocrit. Thereafter the animal was killed, the heart and lungs were excised and weighed. The free wall of the right heart ventricle was dissected and the weight ratio of right ventricle over left ventricle plus septum RV/(LV + S) was calculated.[2,3]

IL-1 Radio Immunoassay

The rat lungs were dissected free of large conducting airways and rapidly frozen in liquid nitrogen for the measurement of IL-1α. Lung homogenate was centrifuged and the precipitate was used for measurement of IL-1α. A commercially obtainable RIA kit containing a rat-specific IL-1α antibody was used for these measurements.

Lung Histology and Immunohistology

Lung tissue sections were either prepared for routine histology or frozen sections of agarose-inflated lungs were used for immune histology. A polyclonal rabbit anti-rat IL-1α antibody was used for immune localization of IL-1α in lung tissues. IL-1 generated by incubating rat spleen with endotoxin was used as a blocking antigen to assure the specificity of the immune localization.

Northern Blot Procedures for IL-1 and IL-1ra

Total RNA was isolated from rat lung tissues, fractionated by formaldehyde gel electrophoresis, and transferred onto Nytran membranes. Human cDNA probes for IL-1α and IL-1ra were used, and a mouse cDNA probe for β-actin. The hybridizations with IL-1ra or IL-1 cDNAs were performed under low-stringency conditions.

RESULTS

Both the subcutaneous injection of monocrotaline and the 3-week hypoxia exposure generated pulmonary hypertension (the mean PAP ranged from 31 to 44 mm/Hg in the monocrotaline group and from 21 to 32 mm/Hg in the chronic hypoxic exposure group). Thus the monocrotaline-induced pulmonary hypertension in this particular comparative study was more severe than that produced by chronic hypoxia. Control animals treated for 2 weeks with s.c. injections of IL-1ra had a mean PAP range from 18 to 21 mm/Hg. Two weeks of treatment with IL-1ra reduced the PAP pressure in the MCT-treated animals (PAP pressure range 22–30 mm/Hg), but had no effect on the hypoxia-induced pulmonary hypertension (PAP pressure range 25–42 mm/Hg). In fact, there was a trend for the IL-1ra treatment to augment the hypoxia-induced pulmonary hypertension.

TABLE 1.

	n	RV/(LV + S)	Lung Wet Weight (g)
MCT	6	0.335 ± 0.027	2.73 ± 0.30
MCT + IL-ra	6	0.240 ± 0.022^a	2.35 ± 0.18
IL-ra	6	0.221 ± 0.009^a	1.70 ± 0.15^a

^{a} $p < 0.05$ different from MCT.

TABLE 1 shows the effect of IL-1ra treatment on the right heart hypertrophy. IL-1ra treatment reduced the right heart hypertrophy in the monocrotaline, but not in the hypoxia-challenged rats. The effect of IL-1ra treatment on rat lung weight in the MCT group was not statistically significant.

Since IL-1α mRNA was increased only during the first 3 days of chronic hypobaric hypoxia exposure (FIG. 1), and since treatment with IL-1ra had no effect on the hypoxia-induced pulmonary hypertension, tissue measurements for IL-1α were only performed with the lungs from the MCT-treated animals. MCT treatment generated measurable levels of IL-1α throughout the 3-week observation period, whereas IL-1α levels were below the assay detection limit in all control rat lungs and in most of the lungs obtained from IL-1ra-treated MCT rats. Although MCT caused IL-1α synthesis in rat lungs, the levels were small in comparison to the levels measured 2 hours after *in vivo* endotoxin (*S. enteritidis*) challenge.

IL-1α staining of smooth muscle cells was observed in lungs from control and MCT (day 3 after MCT) rats. Ubiquitous staining of alveolar septum cells and enhanced staining of bronchial smooth-muscle cells were found in lungs from endotoxin-treated rats.

Low-level expression of IL-1α and IL-1ra was present in lungs from control rats. MCT treatment caused a 40 percent increase in IL-1α mRNA and a 110 percent increase in IL-1ra mRNA.

Rat Lung IL-1α mRNA
During Chronic Hypoxia

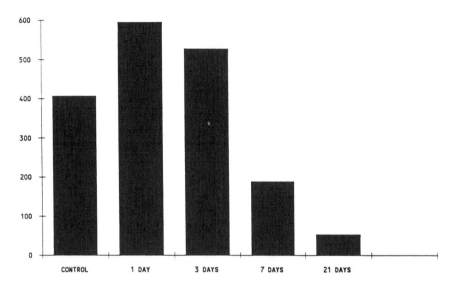

FIGURE 1. Rat lung tissue was homogenized and the RNA was extracted. A human cDNA probe was used for Northern hybridization under low stringency conditions. The figure shows the change in lung tissue IL-1α mRNA from rats exposed to 16,000 feet in a hypobaric pressure chamber for 3 weeks. The density of the IL-1α hybridization signal was measured using a densitometer and corrected for the density obtained for the GAPDH ("housekeeping gene") signal.

DISCUSSION

The main results of this study are that a 2-week treatment with IL-1ra inhibits the development of pulmonary hypertension and right heart hypertrophy in the monocrotaline—but not in the hypoxia model—IL-1α increases in lung tissue following MCT treatment of rats. This increase in IL-1α is inhibited by IL-1ra treatment. Immune staining of control, monocrotaline- and endotoxin-treated rat lungs show low-level expression of IL-1α in alveolar septum cells and in smooth-muscle cells.[19] The lack of effect of IL-1ra treatment in the chronic hypoxia pulmonary hypertension model can perhaps be explained by a nonsustained expression of the IL-1α gene in lung tissue through the course of the hypoxic exposure.

Pulmonary vascular remodeling is a complex process involving several cell types and a multitude of growth-promoting signals. We have previously shown that chronic treatment with PAF antagonists caused a drastic reduction of the lung vasculature in these two rat models of chronic pulmonary hypertension. Because of the interaction between PAF, lipoxygenase-derived metabolites, and prostaglandins, we wished to probe both of these models for a potential role of IL-1. Although twice-daily i.p. injections of IL-1ra had a clear effect on the development of pulmonary hypertension in the MCT model, there was no reduction in pulmonary hypertension—in fact, a distinct trend toward higher pulmonary arterial pressures—in the chronically hypoxic rats. Although hypoxia and reoxygenation have been shown to mediate induction of IL-1α in endothelial cells in culture and likewise in human monocytes,[17,18] our data indicate that—at least on the lung tissue level—IL-1α message is only initially expressed and then suppressed during the chronic phase of hypoxic exposure (from day 7 to day 21 of high-altitude exposure). The reasons for such an adaptive process of IL-1α gene expression in the lung are not clear. It is, however, of interest that IL-1α can induce formation of nitric oxide,[20,21] an important modulator of pulmonary vascular tone and perhaps vascular remodeling. We find it tempting to speculate that IL-1ra treatment of the chronically hypoxic rats may have inhibited nitric oxide formation in the lungs, and perhaps caused the trend toward higher pulmonary arterial pressure values in the IL-1ra-treated animals.

In the aggregate our studies show that IL-1 may be an important factor in the network of inflammatory activities regulating the adaptive processes of the lung circulation. IL-1α is widely distributed among the lung cells. Our data with endotoxin-challenged rats indicate that IL-1α can be rapidly expressed in alveolar cells and muscle cells of veins and bronchi. *In situ* hybridization studies using a human IL-1α cDNA probe show a surprising absence of signal in large-vessel endothelium. It is likely therefore that IL-1 participates in indirect ways in the pulmonary vascular remodeling.[19]

ACKNOWLEDGMENT

The authors wish to thank Dr. William Arend for his helpful suggestions for providing the cDNA probes and Dr. J. Vanice, Synergen, Boulder, Colorado, for generously providing the IL-1ra.

REFERENCES

1. SELBY, C., E. DROST, S. LANNAN, P. K. WRAITH & W. MACNEE. 1991. Neutrophil retention in the lungs of patients with chronic pulmonary disease. Am. Rev. Respir. Dis. **143:** 1359–1364.
2. ONO, S., J. Y. WESTCOTT & N. F. VOELKEL. 1992. PAF antagonists inhibit pulmonary vascular remodeling induced by hypobaric hypoxia in rats. J. Appl. Physiol. **73**(3): 1084–1092.
3. ONO, S. & N. F. VOELKEL. 1991. PAF antagonists inhibit monocrotaline-induced lung injury and pulmonary hypertension. J. Appl. Physiol. **71**(6): 2483–2492.
4. HALE, K. A., S. L. WING, B. A. GOSNELL & D. E. NIEWOEHNER. 1984. Lung disease in long-term cigarette smokers with and without chronic air-flow obstruction. Am. Rev. Respir. Dis. **130:** 716–721.
5. VOELKEL, N. F., J. CZARTOLOMNA, J. SIMPSON & R. C. MURPHY. 1992. FMLP causes

eicosanoid-dependent vasoconstriction and edema in lungs from endotoxin-primed rats. Am. Rev. Respir. Dis. **145:** 701–711.

6. AREND, W. P., H. G. WELGUS, R. C. THOMPSON & S. P. EISENBERG. 1990. Biological properties of recombinant human monocyte-derived interleukin 1 receptor antagonist. J. Clin. Invest. **85:** 1694–1697.
7. AREND, W. P. 1991. Interleukin 1 receptor antagonist. J. Clin. Invest. **88:** 1445–1451.
8. KAY, J. M. & D. HEATH. 1969. Crotalaria Spectabilis, The Pulmonary Hypertension Plant. Springfield, Ill. Thomas.
9. RABINOVITCH, M., W. GAMBLE, A. S. NADAS, O. S. MIETTINEN & L. REID. 1979. Rat pulmonary circulation after chronic hypoxia: Hemodynamic and structural features. Am. J. Physiol. **236:** H818–H826.
10. SAMPSON, P. M., C. L. ROCHESTER, B. FREUNCHLLICH & J. A. ELIAS. 1992. Cytokine regulation of human lung fibroblast hyaluran (hyaluronic acid) production. J. Clin. Invest. **90:** 1492–1503.
11. WARNER, S. J. C., K. R. AUGER & P. LIBBY. 1987. Recombinant human interleukin 1 induces interleukin 1 production by adult human vascular endothelial cells. J. Immunol. **139:** 1911–1917.
12. RAINES, E. W., S. K. DOWER & R. ROSS. 1989. Interleukin-1 mitogenic activity for fibroblasts and smooth muscle cells is due to PDGF-AA. Science **243:** 393–396.
13. LIBBY, P., S. J. C. WARNER & G. B. FRIEDMAN. 1988. Interleukin 1: A mitogen for human vascular smooth muscle cells that induces the release of growth-inhibitory prostanoids. J. Clin. Invest. **81:** 487–498.
14. LIBBY, P., J. M. ORDOVAS, L. K. BIRINYI, K. R. AUGER & C. A. DINARELLO. 1986. Inducible interleukin-1 gene expression in human vascular smooth muscle cells. J. Clin. Invest. **78:** 1432–1438.
15. VALONE, F. H. & L. B. EPSTEIN. 1988. Biphasic platelet-activating factor synthesis by human monocytes stimulated with IL-1-β tumor necrosis factor, or IFN-γ[1]. J. Immunol. **141**(11): 3945–3950.
16. DINARELLO, C. A., I. BISHAI, L. J. ROSENWASSER & F. COCEANI. 1984. The influence of lipoxygenase inhibitors on the in vitro production of human leukocytic pyrogen and lymphocyte activating factor (interleukin-1). J. Immunopharm. **6**(1): 43–50.
17. KOGA, S., et al. 1992. Synthesis and release of interleukin 1 by reoxygenated human mononuclear phagocytes. J. Clin. Invest. **90:** 1007–1015.
18. SHREENIWAS, R., et al. 1992. Hypoxia-mediated induction of endothelial cell interleukin-1α. J. Clin. Invest. **90:** 2333–2339.
19. VOELKEL, N. F., R. TUDER, J. BRIDGES & W. P. AREND. Interleukin-1 receptor antagonist treatment reduces pulmonary hypertension generated in rats by monocrotaline. Submitted for publication in Am. J. Respir. Cell Mol. Biol.
20. BEASLEY, D., J. H. SCHWARTZ & B. M. BRENNER. 1991. Interleukin 1 induces prolonged L-arginine-dependent cyclic guanosine monophosphate and nitrite production in rat vascular smooth muscle cells. J. Clin. Invest. **87:** 602–608.
21. CORBETT, J. A., M. A. SEETLAND, J. R. LANCASTER, JR. & M. L. McDaniel. 1993. A 1-hour pulse with IL-1β induces formation of nitric oxide and inhibits insulin secretion by rat islets of Langerhans: Evidence for a tyrosine kinase signaling mechanism. FASEB J. **7:** 369–374.

Qualitative and Quantitative Analysis of Cytokine Transcripts in the Bronchoalveolar Lavage Cells of Patients with Asthma[a]

SHAU-KU HUANG,[b,e] GUHA KRISHNASWAMY,[c]
SONG-NAN SU,[d] HUI-QING XIAO,[b] AND MARK C. LIU[b]

[b]The Johns Hopkins Asthma and Allergy Center
5501 Hopkins Bayview Circle
Baltimore, Maryland 21224-6801

[c]Division of Allergy and Clinical Immunology
East Tennessee State University
Johnson City, Tennessee 37601

[d]Department of Medical Research
Taipei Veterans General Hospital
Taipei, Taiwan

INTRODUCTION

Bronchial asthma is typically associated with bronchial hyperreactivity to a variety of stimuli, such as inhaled allergens.[1] Studies of the inflamed asthmatic airways have demonstrated the presence of eosinophils and activated T-lymphocytes infiltrating the bronchial mucosa.[1,2] It has been suggested that this inflammatory state is a consequence of the elaboration of various proinflammatory cytokines and mediators in the asthmatic airways.[1-3] It has also become evident that a network of cytokines control the chronic inflammatory state.[3] Further understanding of the molecular pathogenesis of asthma is thus intimately linked to identifying the types and sources of these cytokines coupled with functional studies of their respective roles in inducing asthma.

Using the technique of in situ hybridization, mRNAs for granulocyte-macrophage colony stimulating factor (GM–CSF), interleukin-2 (IL-2), IL-3, IL-4, and IL-5 have been found in the infiltrating cells of asthmatic airways.[4] The expression of IL-3, 4, and 5 mRNAs suggested that Th2 cells were involved, a phenomenon also observed in studies of the cutaneous and nasal late phase responses.[5,6] Although informative, these studies using the techniques of in situ hybridization as well as ELISA/bioassay for the various cytokines can be extremely laborious, time-consuming, and an accurate quantitation of cytokine mRNAs is not possible, particularly for the purpose of monitoring the efficacy of therapeutic intervention.

Since its introduction, the polymerase chain reaction (PCR) has been used

[a] This work was supported by a Postdoctoral Fellowship from the Irvington Institute for Medical Research and by a Scholar in Allergy Award from Merrell Dow-AAAI (both to S.-K.H.).

[e] To whom correspondence should be addressed.

extensively to analyze gene expression. Recently, it has also been used to analyze expression of cytokine genes in cells and tissues.[7–11] Quantitative PCR analyses have also been used successfully in several studies of the steady-state mRNA level.[12–15] We have used RT–PCR to analyze the expression of a panel of cytokine genes in mild allergic asthmatics, as well as to quantitate the amount of IL-5 mRNA in the bronchoalveolar lavage (BAL) cells of allergic asthmatics following challenge with a relevant allergen.[16]

MATERIALS AND METHODS

Patients, Bronchoalveolar Lavage, and Segmental Allergen Challenge

The presence and severity of asthma was determined by clinical history, pulmonary function testing, and bronchial provocation with methacholine, using previously established techniques.[17] The presence or absence of atopy was defined by skin testing to a panel of common aeroallergens. The asthmatic patients were all atopic, as determined by positive skin testing and history. Their asthma was mild. None of the patients had asthma symptoms at the time of BAL or segmental allergen challenge. The control individuals had no history of asthma, normal FEV_1 values, and negative bronchoprovocation testing; they were also skin-test negative. All asthmatic and normal subjects were nonsmokers.

BAL was performed in accordance with the guidelines recommended by an NIH workshop for use in individuals with asthma. After medical evaluation, lavage was performed only on subjects with FEV_1 greater than 60 percent of predicted values. BAL was performed in each lung segment as described.[16] In provocation studies, four asthmatic subjects underwent segmental challenge with short ragweed antigen as described.[16] BALs from these patients were performed 18 to 24 h after allergen challenge.

RNA Extraction, Reverse Transcription, and PCR Amplification

BAL cells obtained from lung lavages were washed in ice-cold phosphate-buffered saline (PBS) and total cellular RNA was extracted by the RNAzol[B] technique.[18] The resulting RNA was quantitated using spectrophotometry. The integrity of the RNA was assessed by electrophoresis of the RNA samples in a 2 percent ethidium bromide-stained agarose gel, and observing the intact 28S and 18S ribosomal RNA bands. An aliquot of total cellular RNA (1 μg or otherwise indicated) was then reverse-transcribed to cDNA, and PCR was performed in the presence of specific primers for the various cytokines as described.[16,19] The specificity of amplification was checked by assessing whether a fragment of the expected size had been obtained. Equal amounts of the PCR-amplified products (10 μl) were run on a 3 percent (2-g Nusieve GTG and 1-g Sigma agarose) ethidium bromide-stained gel. The identity of each fragment was confirmed by Southern blotting or restriction enzyme digestion of the fragments.

Competitive RT–PCR for Quantitation of IL-5 mRNA

To quantitate the level of steady-state IL-5 transcripts, a competitive PCR assay[16] was performed using a modified IL-5 cRNA as an internal standard (IS).

The standard was comprised of a plasmid construct (pSP64) containing IL-5 Bam HI-cDNA fragment inserted with a 93-bp Sty I-SV40 DNA fragment. RT–PCR of the IS results in a fragment of 387 bp, while test RNA amplification results in a fragment of 294 bp, allowing the two products to be separated by agarose gel electrophoresis. By mixing the cRNA standard with test RNA followed by reverse transcription and amplification of both templates in the same tube, all variables related to the integrity of RNA, conditions of reverse transcription, and PCR amplification are internally controlled and equally affect both RNA samples. The same approach was used for competitive PCR analysis of IL-5 transcripts in the asthmatic BALs.

The competitive PCR assay was performed as follows: an aliquot of the test RNA (100–200 ng) from either normal saline- or ragweed-challenged site, and varying concentrations of the IS cRNA (0.001–1.0 pg) were reverse-transcribed to cDNA in the same tube. The conditions for reverse transcription (carried out in the Cetus thermocycler) were the same as described earlier.

RESULTS

1. *Qualitative PCR analysis of cytokine transcripts from BAL cells of asthmatic and nonasthmatic individuals.* Using the RT–PCR technique, we analyzed the profiles of cytokine-gene and IL-2R gene expression in BAL cells from five normal subjects and six patients with mild asthma, and examined whether qualitative differences between asthmatic and nonasthmatic control BALs could be seen. We found that the distribution of the various cell types in the BAL cells of asthmatic and control individuals was similar, except for a slight preponderance of eosinophils and epithelial cells in the asthmatic BALs (data not shown). The marginal elevation of these cell types is probably a reflection of the mild nature of the disease, as judged by the pulmonary function tests and bronchoprovocation data.

The purified RNA from the BAL samples was reverse-transcribed and the resulting cDNA was amplified (under the same conditions for both control and asthmatic samples) using specific primers. Results[16] showed that asthmatics expressed a variety of transcripts for IL-1β (6 out of 6; 6/6), IL-2 (1/6), GM–CSF (5/6), IFN-γ (4/6), TNF-α (3/6), IL-5 (5/6), IL-6 (5/6), IL-8 (6/6), and IL-2R (6/6). Surprisingly, nonasthmatics also expressed similar overall profiles, including IL-1β (5/5), IL-2 (1/5), GM–CSF (4/5), IFN-γ (4/5), TNF-α (0/5), IL-5 (4/5), IL-6 (4/5), IL-8 (5/5), and IL-2R (4/5). Overall, no qualitative differences could be seen between controls and asthmatic BALs, except, perhaps, in the transcripts for TNF-α. This may reflect the mild nature of asthma in the patient population studied, or there may be a quantitative difference, but the qualitative PCR analysis failed to detect it. To investigate the latter possibility, we compared the relative amount of cytokine transcripts after varying the cycle numbers in the PCR. The results, however, showed no differences in the relative intensities of the amplified cytokine fragments in the asthmatic and nonasthmatic groups. This prompted us to employ a *quantitative* PCR technique to analyze the steady-state IL-5 transcripts in the allergen-challenged BALs from four additional asthmatic patients, and to identify the cellular source of IL-5 transcripts (see below).

2. *Enhanced expression of IL-5 mRNA in challenged asthmatic lungs: Analysis by quantitative PCR.* Since quantitative differences in mRNA expression of the various cytokines could exist, in the absence of demonstrable differences on phenotyping by a qualitative PCR technique. we have developed a quantitative

PCR technique for measurement of minute (pg) amounts of IL-5 mRNA based on competition of the test RNA with a known quantity of an internal cRNA standard. We chose IL-5 because of its role in the regulation of eosinophil activation and in the pathogenesis of allergic inflammation.[20-22]

We applied this quantitative technique to analyze the level of IL-5 mRNA, before and after allergen challenge, in the total RNAs obtained from the BAL cells of four asthmatic individuals.[16] One hundred to 200 ng of each RNA sample was mixed with varying amounts of internal standard cRNAs and subjected to reverse transcription. PCR was carried out in the presence of a trace amount of ^{32}P-dCTP- and IL-5-specific primers. First, analysis of the cellular compositions in BALs showed that there were large increases in the percentage of eosinophils following allergen challenge, with inconsistent changes in the neutrophil population and slight decreases in lymphocyte percentage (TABLE 1). Using a PCR approach, we found that while the prechallenge (control) BAL cells expressed no detectable IL-5 transcripts, there were IL-5 mRNAs in the cells from allergen-challenged

TABLE 1. The Percentage of Lymphocytes, Neutrophils, and Eosinophils in the Pre- and Post-Ag-Challenged BALs

Subjects		% of Cell Population			Total Number of Cells
		Lymphocyte	Neutrophil	Eosinophil	
550	Saline	13.0	7.2	1.2	16×10^6
	Antigen	7.4	10.8	49.8	73×10^6
568	Saline	11.2	14.4	1.4	18×10^6
	Antigen	9.0	5.4	78.2	224×10^6
573	Saline	11.6	20.0	0.4	17×10^6
	Antigen	10.4	16.6	27.2	36×10^6
617	Saline	13.8	4.2	1.0	7×10^6
	Antigen	11.5	8.1	72.2	78×10^6

Note: Four asthmatic subjects (patients 550, 568, 573, and 617) underwent segmental challenge with short ragweed antigen by instilling a total dose of 100 protein nitrogen units (PNU) in 5-ml normal saline into one airway segment. Sham challenge was performed with 5-ml normal saline in another airway segment. BALs from these patients were performed 18 to 24 h after allergen challenge. The BAL fluids were centrifuged (600 ×g for 15 minutes at 20°C). The differential cell counts were performed on cytospin preparations of BAL cells stained with Diff-Quik (Harleco). Five-hundred cells were enumerated.

sites for all patients studied (data not shown; see reference 16). To determine quantitatively the level of transcripts, the competitive PCR assays were performed. Representative results are shown in FIGURE 1, while the control sample of patient 568 expressed no detectable IL-5 mRNA in 1 μg of total RNA (FIG. 1A); following allergen challenge, BAL cells expressed 0.8 pg per 1 μg of total BAL RNAs. The input of RNA was equal in all circumstances, and at the exponential phase of amplification, the intensity of β-actin PCR product was similar between challenged and unchallenged samples.[16]

In order to determine the cellular source of the IL-5 transcripts in the ragweed-challenged BALs, the BAL cells collected from the Ag-challenged sites of three patients were separated into two fractions, eosinophils (>76 percent pure in all three samples) and mononuclear cells. Total cellular RNAs were extracted using RNAzol. A competitive PCR analysis of IL-5 transcripts was performed (described earlier) to determine quantitative difference. FIGURE 1B shows representative results. While the eosinophil fraction of patient 550 expressed less than 0.15 pg of IL-5 transcripts/1-μg total eosinophil RNA, the monoclear cell fraction expressed 4 pg of IL-5 mRNA/1 μg of total mononuclear-cell RNA. Equal amplification of β-actin from both eosinophil and mononuclear fractions was observed. A similar pattern was observed for other patients studied.[16] These experiments suggest that the predominant source of IL-5 mRNA in the BAL cells of asthmatics is the mononuclear cells (presumably the T cells).

DISCUSSION

By combining both qualitative and quantitative assays using the RT–PCR, we have analyzed a panel of steady-state mRNAs for various cytokines and the IL-

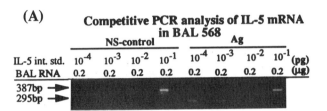

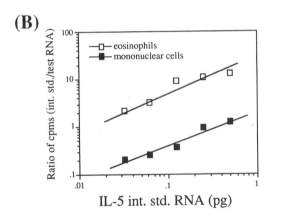

FIGURE 1. (A) Competitive PCR analysis of IL-5 transcripts in saline and allergen-challenged BAL samples of patient 568. RNA was extracted from the cells, using RNAzol containing guanidine isothiocyanate. For competitive PCR analysis, 200 ng of RNAs was mixed with varying amounts of IL-5 internal standard cRNA as indicated. The mixed RNA was reverse-transcribed into cDNA in the presence of oligo-d(T) as a primer, reverse transcriptase (2.5 U/μl), RNasin (1 U/μl), dNTPs (1 mM each), and MgCl$_2$ (5 mM). The resulting cDNA was then amplified using IL-5-specific primers. PCR-amplified products were analyzed in a 3% agarose gel stained with ethidium bromide. (B) Quantitative PCR analysis of IL-5 transcripts in eosinophils and mononuclear cells of allergen-challenged BAL samples of patient 550. For competitive PCR analysis, 100 ng of RNAs was mixed with varying amounts of IL-5 internal standard cRNA as indicated. PCR was carried out in the presence of trace amount of ^{32}P-dCTP and IL-5 primers. The ratio of radioactivity (cpm), corrected for the difference in the molecular weight between wild type and modified IL-5 amplified fragment, was plotted against varying amounts of input internal standard cRNAs as indicated.

2R in the BAL cells from asthmatic subjects or patients challenged with ragweed allergen. In our study population, no qualitative difference could be seen in the cytokine profile of BAL cells in allergic asthmatic and normal subjects. The expression of both Th1 and Th2 cytokine mRNAs in BAL cells in individuals we studied suggests that these cytokines are involved in the normal maintenance of lung homeostasis, and that the failure to detect differences using PCR may be due to the mild nature of the disease in the asthmatic subjects examined. This is supported by the low eosinophil counts in the study subjects that is consistent with mild asthma.[23]

Since we used unfractionated BAL cells for the qualitative PCR study, the cell sources for these cytokine transcripts, even in normal BALs, are multiple. Thus these cytokine transcripts could represent activation of T cells, mast cells, alveolar macrophages, eosinophils, or even bronchial epithelial cells. Using similar PCR-based techniques, we have found expression of transcripts for IL-1β, IL-2R, GM–CSF, IL-5, and even IL-8 from highly purified and activated eosinophils (unpublished data). Similarly, we have found that human respiratory epithelium constitutively expresses transcripts for IL-1β, IL-6, IL-8, and GM–CSF (Krishnaswamy *et al.,* manuscript in preparation). Thus, the cellular localization of this cytokine profile would be important, since the selective recruitment of activated T cells and eosinophils along with the epithelial damage seen in asthma could contribute to quantitatively larger amounts of proinflammatory cytokines in the asthmatic airways. The constitutive expression of cytokine mRNAs by epithelial cells could also explain the prominent expression of multiple cytokine mRNAs in the BAL cells of the control subjects.

Our results vary from those of Robinson *et al.,* who found a predominant expression of Th2 associated cytokines in atopic asthma, using the technique of *in situ* hybridization.[4] These investigators also found expression of various cytokine mRNAs in nonasthmatics, but significantly higher numbers of BAL cells expressed the cytokine mRNAs for IL-2, IL-3, IL-4, IL-5, and GM–CSF in asthmatic individuals. The most likely reason for our not finding a difference in the pattern of cytokine mRNAs between asthmatic and normal individuals is that the disease was mild or quiescent in our patient population. Thus, qualitatively, the expression of cytokine mRNAs by the asthmatics may have been no different from the controls. Using a population with more severe asthma may provide better discrimination. This is also supported by the fact that allergen challenge, which induces acute symptomatology and an active inflammatory response in the challenged lungs, resulted in an upregulation of IL-5 mRNAs. These results suggest that the severity or extent of inflammation associated with disease may be an important variable in determining the expression of cytokine genes.

We have demonstrated the use of an internal standard to accurately quantitate IL-5 mRNA levels in the BAL cells of asthmatic individuals. Using this technique, we have shown that the predominant cell source for IL-5 mRNA in the BAL cells of asthmatics is the mononuclear rather than in the eosinophil fraction. These data are consistent with mononuclear cells playing an important role in the pathogenesis of the inflammatory response in atopic asthma. Further time-course studies are needed to confirm our findings. Our study also demonstrates that the technique of quantitative PCR, using a competitive template as an internal standard, can provide an efficient, rapid, and economical way to measure cytokine-gene expression in inflammatory airway diseases. Quantitative PCR amplification of cytokine mRNAs in BAL cells, in combination with immunohistochemistry or ELISA for the cell-associated or secreted proteins, could provide powerful insights into the molecular pathogenesis of allergic inflammatory and other lung diseases, and will assist in the molecular classification of these diseases.

ACKNOWLEDGMENTS

We thank Dr. Thorunn Rafnar for advice during this study.

REFERENCES

1. METZGER, W. J., G. W. HUNNINGHAKE & H. B. RICHERSON. 1985. Late asthmatic responses: Inquiry into mechanisms and significance. Clin. Rev. Allergy **3:** 145–165.
2. BRADLEY, B. L., *et al.* 1991. Eosinophils, T-lymphocytes, mast cells, neutrophils and macrophages in bronchial biopsy specimens from atopic subjects with asthma: Comparison with atopic subjects without asthma and normal control subjects and relationship to bronchial hyperresponsiveness. J. Allergy Clin. Immunol. **88:** 661–674.
3. JOHNSTON, S. L. & S. T. HOLGATE. 1990. Cellular and chemical mediators—Their roles in allergic diseases. Curr. Opin. Immunol. **2:** 513–524.
4. ROBINSON, D. S., *et al.* 1992. Predominant T_{H2}-like bronchoalveolar T-lymphocyte population in atopic asthma. New Eng. J. Med. **326:** 298–304.
5. KAY, A. B., *et al.* 1991. Messenger RNA expression of the cytokine gene cluster, interleukin 3 (IL-3), IL-4, IL-5 and granulocyte-macrophage colony stimulating factor in allergen-induced late-phase cutaneous reactions in atopic subjects. J. Exp. Med. **173:** 775–778.
6. DURHAM, S. R., *et al.* 1992. Cytokine mRNA expression for IL-3, IL-4, IL-5 and granulocyte-macrophage colony stimulating factor in the nasal mucosa after local allergen provocation: Relationship to tissue eosinophilia. J. Immunol. **148:** 2390–2394.
7. DESREUMAUX, P., *et al.* 1992. Interleukin 5 messenger RNA expression in the intestinal mucosa of patients with Coeliac disease. J. Exp. Med. **175:** 293–296.
8. PETER, J. B. 1991. The polymerase chain reaction: Amplifying our options. Rev. Infect. Dis. **13:** 166–171.
9. EHRLICH, H. A., D. GELFAND & J. J. SNINSKY. 1991. Recent advances in the polymerase chain reaction. Science **252:** 1643–1650.
10. BRENNER, C. A., A. W. TAM, P. A. NELSON, E. G. ENGLEMAN, N. SUZUKI, K. E. FRY & J. W. LARRICK. 1989. Message amplification phenotyping (MAPPing): A technique to simultaneously measure multiple mRNA's from small numbers of cells. Biotechniques **7:** 1096.
11. EHLERS, S. & K. A. SMITH. 1991. Differentiation of T cell lymphokine gene expression: The in vitro acquisition of T cell memory. J. Exp. Med. **173:** 25–36.
12. WANG, A. M., M. V. DOYLE & D. F. MARK. 1989. Quantitation of mRNA by the polymerase chain reaction. Proc. Natl. Acad. Sci. U.S.A. **86:** 9717–9721.
13. LI, B., P. K. SEHAJPAL, A. KHANNA, H. VLASSARA, A. CERAMI, K. H. STENZEL & M. SUTHANTHIRAN. 1991. Differential regulation of transforming growth Factor β and Interleukin 2 in human T cells: Determination by usage of novel competitor DNA constructs in the quantitative polymerase chain reaction. J. Exp. Med. **174:** 1259–1262.
14. FELDMAN, A. M., P. E. RAY, M. S. COLLEEN, J. A. MERCER, W. MINOBE & M. R. BRISTOW. 1991. Selective gene expression in failing human heart: Quantification of steady-state levels of messenger RNA in endomyocardial biopsies using the polymerase chain reaction. Circulation **83:** 1866–1872.
15. GILLILAND, G., S. PERRIN, K. BLANCHARD & F. BUNN. 1990. Analysis of cytokine mRNA and DNA: Detection and quantitation by competitive polymerase chain reaction. Proc. Natl. Acad. Sci. U.S.A. **87:** 2725–2729.

16. KRISHNASWAMY, G., M. KUMAI, M. LIU, S.-N. SU, B. STEALEY, D. G. MARSH & S. K. HUANG. 1993. Expression of multiple cytokine mRNAs in the bronchoalveolar lavage cells of asthmatics and non-asthmatics: Analysis by the polymerase chain reaction. Am. J. Respir. Cell Mol. Biol. **9:** 279.
17. LIU, M. C., *et al.* 1991. Immediate and late inflammatory responses to ragweed antigen challenge of the peripheral airways in allergic asthmatics. Am. Rev. Respir. Dis. **144:** 51–58.
18. CHOMCZYNKI, P. & N. SACCI. 1987. Single-step method of RNA isolation by acid guanidinium thiocyanate-phenol-chloroform extraction. Anal. Biochem. **162:** 156–160.
19. KUMAI, M., G. KRISH, D. G. MARSH & S. K. HUANG. 1993. Modulating effect of human monocyte Fc receptor on allergen-induced T-cell responses. Immunology **79:** 174–177.
20. LOPEZ, A. F., *et al.* 1988. Recombinant human IL-5 is a selective activator of human eosinophils. J. Exp. Med. **167:** 219.
21. ROTHENBERG, M., J. PETERSON, R. L. STEVENS, D. S. SILBERSTEIN, D. T. MCKENZIE, K. F. AUSTEN & W. F. OWEN. 1989. IL-5-dependent conversion of normodense eosinophils to the hypodense phenotype uses 3T3 fibroblasts for enhanced viability, accelerated hypodensity and sustained antibody-dependent cytotoxicity. J. Immunol. **143:** 2311–2316.
22. WANG, J. M., A. RAMBALDI, A. BIONDI, Z. G. CHEN, C. J. SANDERSON & A. MONTOVANI. 1989. Recombinant human IL-5 is a selective eosinophil chemoattractant. Eur. J. Immunol. **19:** 701–705.
23. BOUSQUET, J., *et al.* 1990. Eosinophilic inflammation in asthma. New Eng. J. Med. **323:** 1033–1038.

The Three-Dimensional Structure of Human Interleukin-5 at 2.4-Angstroms Resolution: Implication for the Structures of Other Cytokines

T. N. C. WELLS,[a] P. GRABER,[a] A. E. I. PROUDFOOT,[a]
C. Y. AROD,[a] S. R. JORDAN,[b] M. H. LAMBERT,[b]
A. M. HASSEL,[b] AND M. V. MILBURN[b]

[a]Glaxo Institute for Molecular Biology
14 Chemin des Aulx
1228 Plan-les-Ouates
Geneva, Switzerland

[b]Glaxo Research Institute
Department of Structural and Biophysical Chemistry
5 Moore Drive
Research Triangle Park, North Carolina 27709

THE THREE-DIMENSIONAL STRUCTURE OF HUMAN INTERLEUKIN-5

Interleukin 5 (IL-5) is a specific cytokine involved in the development and differentiation of eosinophils. It plays an important role in diseases associated with increased levels of eosinophils, such as asthma and atopic dermatitis.[1,2] We have solved the three-dimensional structure of human IL-5 to a resolution of 2.4 Å using X-ray crystallographic techniques. The molecule is a dimer of identical subunits that are joined together by disulphide bridges. The crystal structure reveals a novel two-domain structure where each domain of the protein is a 4-helical bundle containing two short stretches of beta sheet. These domain structures show a high degree of similarity to the cytokine fold, which has already been described in Interleukin-2 and -4, granulocyte, and granulocyte-macrophage colony stimulating factors, and porcine and human growth hormones. This high degree of similarity within known cytokine structures has led us to make predictions of the structures of cytokines for which no three-dimensional information is available. Furthermore, it provides the molecular basis for the design of agonists and antagonists of IL-5, which will be important in the therapy of eosinophil mediated diseases.

IL-5 is a T-cell-derived cytokine that causes eosinophilpoesis and activation of eosinophils. In order to investigate its biology and its role in models of asthmatic inflammation, we have produced the protein in large quantities. A synthetic gene for human IL-5 was overexpressed in *E. coli*, where the protein forms inclusion bodies. This protein can then be subsequently renatured under carefully controlled conditions of protein concentration and buffer redox potential to give large quantities of active protein.[3] Unlike the natural human IL-5, the *E. coli* derived material is not glycosylated. It is of equal potency, however, showing that glycosylation is not required for biological activity. We mapped the positions of the disulphide

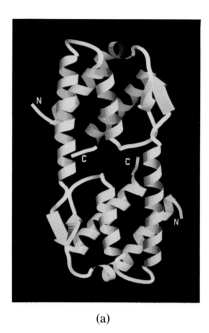

(a)

FIGURE 1. (a) Ribbon tracing of IL-5 that shows the novel dimer configuration. One chain is shown in *green* and the other in *purple,* and the four α-helices and two β-strands are clearly visible in each domain. The structure contains two domains related to each other by a twofold axis of symmetry, and the viewing direction is along this twofold axis. **(b)** A chain tracing of the backbone α-carbon residues for one of the IL-5 monomers shown in *red* with every tenth residue labeled in *green.*

bonds[4] and found that the molecule adopts an antiparallel disulphide linked topology. This means that the cysteine-44 of one subunit bonds to cysteine-86 on the other subunit, giving two disulphide bonds per dimer. The protein was cystallized[5] by the hanging drop vapor diffusion method. The crystallization conditions were 100 mM tris-HCl, pH 8.5, 200–250-mM sodium acetate, and 26–30 percent PEG 4000, with incubation at 22°C. Parallelepiped crystals grew to dimensions of 0.6 × 0.4 − 1.0 mm in about 4 weeks. Protein from the crystals was analyzed by N-terminal sequencing and mass spectrometry, confirming the presence of the N-terminal methionine, and that some oxidation and formylation of the protein had occurred.[6]

The protein structure was solved using multiple isomorphous replacement data collected using five heavy atom derivatives. Three of these used conventional heavy atom soaks (K_2PtCl_6, $NaAuCl_4$, and K_3IrCl_6). For the last two, however, we used protein expressed in a methionine auxotroph of *E. coli,* grown on a medium enriched with seleno-L-methionine.[7] This protein had selenomethionine incorporated into the two methionine residues in the IL-5 sequence; Met-1 and Met-107 at an efficiency of over 90 percent. This selenomethionine protein is fully

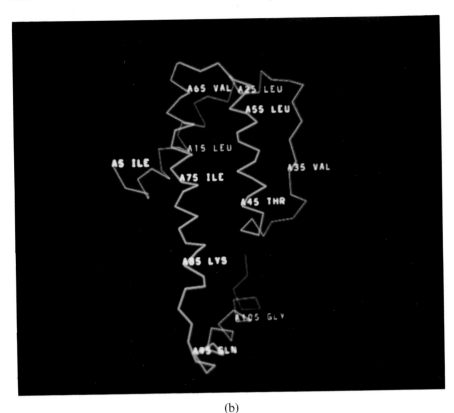

(b)

FIGURE 1. *Continued.*

active in a cell-differentiation assay, in fact showing slightly more activity than its sulphur-containing counterpart. The change of sulphur for the heavier atom selenium provided a derivative protein that gave useful phasing information. In addition, the clear selenium peaks in the difference Patterson allowed immediate identification of the position of Met-107 and thus the C-terminal helices.

The crystal structure of IL-5[8] shows an intimated dimer configuration in which each domain contains secondary structural elements from both chains (FIG. 1). The core of IL-5 is two left-handed bundles of four α-helices laid end to end, with two short antiparallel β-strands packed on opposite sides of the dimer. Starting with the amino terminus, one polypeptide chain of IL-5 forms three α-helices (A, B, and C) and one β-strand ($\beta1$), all tightly packed together. From this point (Cys-86) the backbone crosses into the other half of the dimer to form a second β-strand ($\beta2'$) and a fourth helix (helix D'). These two pieces of secondary structure pack against the other monomer chain to complete a bundle of four helices and a two-strand antiparallel β-sheet. From this structure it can be seen why the IL-5 molecule is unstable as a monomer, since many hydrophobic residues that are normally present in the core of the dimer would be exposed to solvent (FIG. 2).

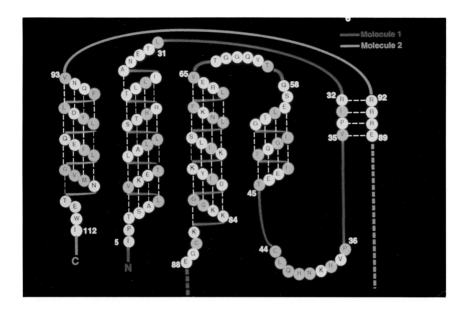

FIGURE 2. Schematic representation of the secondary structure of IL-5 shown for one of the IL-5 domains. An IL-5 domain is made up from part of one monomer chain shown in *red* and the other monomer chain shown in *green*. The amino acids are color coded in terms of the side chain solvent accessible surface, with buried residues in *orange,* intermediately exposed residues in *yellow,* and solvent exposed residues in *blue*. The *thin dashed lines* show the hydrogen bonds that contribute to the overall secondary structure.[8]

The IL-5 monomer and dimer have solvent accessible surface areas of 9300 A^2 and 11,500 A^2, respectively. This implies that an extremely large proportion of the monomer surface area (about 7000 A^2) is at the interface between the two monomer chains.

Even more surprisingly the two domains of the IL-5 dimer are homologous to the known X-ray crystallographic and NMR structures of granulocyte-macrophage[9] and macrophage[10] colony stimulating factors (GM–CSF and M–CSF), IL-2, and IL-4,[11,12] and is similar to the human and porcine growth hormones,[13,14] even though these proteins do not share any significant sequence similarity (FIG. 3). The structure for the IL-5 domain shows two different key differences from the other four α-helical bundle proteins. First, the two pairs of helices (A, D' and B, C) are at an angle of approximately 40°C to each other, which is atypical for these protein bundles. Second, the connectivity of the four helices in IL-5 is up-up-down-down. More frequently, in other noncytokine folds that contain four α-helical bundles, the joining sections between the helices are shorter and lead to an up-down-up-down arrangement of the helices. The connectivity seen in IL-5 is the most common connectivity seen in cytokines, however, and therefore is presumably important in receptor binding.

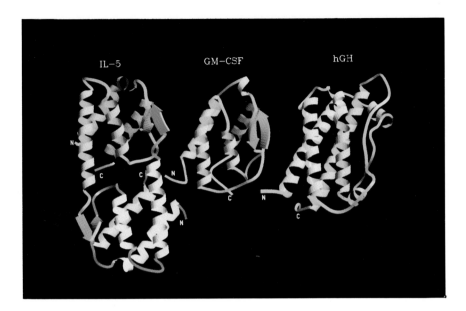

FIGURE 3. Comparison of the three-dimensional structures of IL-5, GM–CSF, and hGH. All three molecules are shown with the helical bundles in approximately the same orientation.

To date very few experiments have been carried out relating the sequence of IL-5 to its function, and therefore the receptor binding site is not well characterized. The human and murine sequences show 70 percent similarity, but display some species-specific activity.[15] Experiments with chaemeric proteins formed from the human and mouse genes for IL-5 have implied that the C-terminal 36 amino acids are crucial for the activity of the protein. In this region there are only eight residues that differ between the two species, of which only three changes are nonconservative amino acid substitutions—at positions 81, 84, and 94.[8] In the human IL-5, glycine-81 and lysine-84 are part of the C-terminal of the third helix, and changes here would probably produce little structural perturbation. Conversely, Asn-94 lies at the N-terminal end of the final helix and substitution here could lengthen the β-sheet containing the loop connecting the third and fourth helices. The role of the C-terminus in the biological activity of IL-5 is also implied from experiments involving the CNBr digestion of the protein.[16] This leaves a molecule that lacks the last eight amino acids from the C-terminal (after Met-107). From the crystal structure we can see that the two C-terminal helices, implicated in receptor binding, are close to one another in space. This means that there are two almost identical helix surfaces on the same side of the dimer molecule. The residues that are exposed are Asp-98, Gln-101, Glu-102, Gly-105, and Asn-108, all of which are prime candidates for being in the receptor binding site. The importance of these residues is currently being tested by site-directed mutagenesis.

PREDICTIONS FOR THE STRUCTURES OF OTHER CYTOKINES

As has already been discussed, the four α-helical bundles with up-up-down-down connectivity is a common topology for many cytokines. In fact, the novel dimeric structure of IL-5 is a dramatic example of the way that proteins can evolve toward the same fold from a completely different starting point. To date six structures of cytokines are known that have this fold—IL-2, IL-4, M–CSF, GM–CSF, growth hormone, and IL-5. There are, however, many cytokines for which the three-dimensional structure is not known. We therefore attempted to address the question: Is it likely that any of the cytokines for which a three-dimensional structure is not available will look like any of the cytokines for which structures have already been solved? We aligned several of the sequences of cytokines whose tertiary structure is not known with the sequences of the known cytokine 4-helical bundle structures. Since there is little primary sequence homology between the cytokines, we calculated an alignment based on two factors. First, the primary sequence alignment was calculated using a Neddleman–Wunsch algorithm. Second, the secondary structures were predicted for the cytokines and were represented in terms of α-helices, β-sheets, and coil secondary structures.[17] The alignments were then carried out to optimize a composite score made up of the primary and secondary structural similarities. The score for these alignments were then normalized by carrying out 141 further alignments with sequences of equal length randomly selected from the Brookhaven protein data bank, and were then expressed as a normalized Z-score. This score shows how much better the fit is compared to the randomly selected sequences, and is expressed in numbers of standard deviations above the mean.[8] These scores therefore give evidence for similar tertiary structures when the Z-value is greater than 3.5.[8]

These results can be seen in TABLE 1, where for each sequence used, the cytokine fold that has the highest similarity is shown along with its Z-score. The amino acid sequences and predicted secondary structures of IL-6, IL-7, IL-10, IL-11, stem cell factor (SCF), and erythropoietin (EPO) align particularly well with one or more of the known cytokine structures, suggesting that these cytokines adopt the four α-helical bundle topology. IL-3 and LIF give much lower scores, and so no prediction can be made. As a control, IL-1β and IL-8 show very low scores; this is consistent with their known three-dimensional structures that are not α-helical bundles. This commonality among the tertiary structures of so many cytokines has important implications for molecular recognition, and the design of antagonists. The calculations show that IL-5 is most highly homologous with IL-4, for which antagonists have already been made.[18] It will be interesting to see if similar mutants made in IL-5 will also have antagonistic properties.

FUTURE POSSIBILITIES

One of the key reasons to study IL-5 is to identify ways of inhibiting its action *in vivo*. Therapeutically, it would be hoped that an IL-5 receptor antagonist would prevent eosinophilic influx into the inflamed tissues, and that this would prevent the normal onset of inflammation. To date, four possible approaches to block the receptor–ligand interaction have been considered.

(i) Using monoclonal antibodies directed against IL-5 to lower the amount of free IL-5 present in the inflamed tissue.[19]

TABLE 1. Predictions of Three-Dimensional Structures of Cytokines

Query Sequence	Tertiary Structure	Number of Residues Used in Alignment	Z-Scores					
			IL-2	IL-4	IL-5	GM-CSF	M-CSF	GH
IL-1β	β-barrel	153	-0.55	-0.83	-0.67	-0.80	0.04	-0.29
IL-2	4α-2β	133	—	3.25	0.65	1.49	1.56	1.74
IL-3	Unknown	133	1.86	0.49	0.89	1.61	2.43	2.66
IL-4	4α-2β	129	**4.37**	—	**4.95**	2.33	2.69	2.38
IL-5	4α-2β	115	1.27	**4.38**	—	0.32	2.58	0.35
IL-6	Unknown	183	2.04	1.50	1.71	0.95	**3.58**	2.15
IL-7	Unknown	129	**4.72**	2.69	1.46	0.92	2.33	2.86
IL-8	1α-4β	72	1.18	1.33	-0.12	-0.19	0.95	0.50
IL-10	Unknown	161	**3.71**	2.86	0.97	2.87	0.82	1.75
IL-11	Unknown	182	1.88	1.02	**4.34**	**3.97**	1.08	2.77
GM-CSF	4α-2β	127	2.46	0.99	2.51	—	3.27	1.01
G-CSF	Unknown	174	1.14	0.26	0.32	2.29	0.26	2.30
M-CSF	4α-2β	150	2.19	1.90	2.86	3.18	—	1.84
GH	4α	191	1.79	1.26	0.52	0.70	1.37	—
LIF	Unknown	179	0.82	-0.02	0.82	1.92	0.78	2.32
SCF	Unknown	164	1.67	2.38	1.02	0.20	**6.35**	0.57
EPO	Unknown	166	0.55	2.89	0.55	**3.55**	0.55	1.36

(ii) A soluble portion of the alpha chain of the IL-5 receptor can be produced recombinantly, containing the extracellular domain of the protein. This protein may be produced *in vivo* by alternative splicing[20] and has a high affinity for IL-5. The role of this protein *in vivo* may be to act as a control mechanism on the amount of IL-5 present at the site of inflammation, and so addition of a soluble IL-5-receptor alpha subunit may act as an alternative to antibody therapy.[21]

(iii) Site-directed mutagenesis could be used to produce a protein with IL-5 antagonist properties. This approach requires the production of a protein that can still bind to the IL-5 receptor but is unable to induce signaling. It is unlikely, however, that a single-point mutation will destroy all of the agonist properties of a protein ligand. In the case of IL-4, a residue at the end of the C-terminal helix, tyrosine 124, is critically important for the activity of that protein. Mutation of this residue to an aspartic acid[22] produced a highly potent (subnanomolar) inhibitor, which shows only very weak agonist (<0.5 percent maximal response). A similar aromatic amino acid, tryptophan 110 occurs in the C-terminal region of IL-5.

The key question here is how to identify which part of the proteins is important in the binding of the receptor. There are two principal routes to finding this out, both of which are synergistic. First, if the structure of the receptor ligand complex were known, then sterically blocking the effector binding site could result in an antagonist, as has been shown for human growth hormone.[23] Since the subunit of the IL-5 receptor binds IL-5 with a nanomolar dissociation constant, it should be possible to produce crystals of IL-5 complexed with a soluble IL-5R-alpha chain. Currently, the limitation here is the supply of the soluble receptor. Although the receptor can be expressed in *E. coli,* we have experienced great difficulties in obtaining active refolded material (unpublished data). An alternative approach has been to produce the protein as a secreted product in bacculovirus infected insect cells.[24]

Second, in the absence of a receptor ligand complex structure, the amino acids that contribute to surface charge could be systematically removed and replaced with noncharged amino acids using site-directed mutagenesis.[25,26] This will tell us whether the region responsible for pharmacological activity was localized, as in the case of fibrinogen[27] and IL-8,[28] or whether it was distributed over a large area of the protein surafce, as has been shown for IL-1.[29]

In inflammatory diseases such as asthma, the use of a whole protein as a therapeutic agent is especially attractive. There exists the possibility of nebulizing such a protein directly onto the surface of the lung—and this bypasses many of the normal bioavailability problems associated with using proteins as therapeutic agents.

(iv) If the pharmacophore is localized, such that only a limited amount of the protein surface is absolutely required for the interaction, the possibility exists that peptides can be made that mimic the three-dimensional conformation of the active region. This has already been achieved for the fibrinogen pharmacophore (arginine–glycine–aspartate) where cyclic peptides have been made that inhibit platelet aggregation with high potency. If the pharmacophore is found to be similarly localized in IL-5, then once the relative locations of the important groups in the pharmacophore are known, it should be possible to design nonpeptide mimetics with IL-5 antagonist properties. Such an approach might eventually lead to an orally active molecule.

These types of experiments will help us not only to understand the interaction of IL-5 with its receptor, but will eventually help to delineate the important signaling pathways in inflammatory cell types such as eosinophils. This in turn will be important for the development of new therapeutic agents in diseases such as asthma that involve this important protein.

ACKNOWLEDGMENT

We would like to thank Nadine Huber for help in preparing this manuscript.

REFERENCES

1. SANDERSON, C. J. 1990. *In* Advances in Pharmacology, Vol. 23: 163–177. Academic Press. New York.
2. TAKATSU, K. 1992. Curr. Opin. Immunol. **4:** 200–206.
3. PROUDFOOT, A. E. I., D. FATTAH, E. H. KAWASHIMA, A. BERNARD & P. T. WINGFIELD. 1990. Biochem. J. **270:** 356–361.
4. PROUDFOOT, A. E. I., G. J. DAVIES, G. TURCATTI & P. T. WINGFIELD. 1991. FEBS Lett. **283:** 61–64.
5. HASSEL, A. M., T. N. C. WELLS, P. GRABER, A. E. I. PROUDFOOT, R. J. ANDEREGG, W. BURKHART, M. V. MILBURN & S. R. JORDAN. 1993. J. Mol. Biol. **229:** 1150–1152.
6. ROSE, K., P.-O. REGAMEY, R. ANDEREGG, T. N. C. WELLS & A. E. I. PROUDFOOT. 1992. Biochem. J. **286:** 825–828.
7. GRABER, P., A. R. BERNARD, A. M. HASSELL, M. V. MILBURN, S. R. JORDAN, A. E. I. PROUDFOOT, D. FATTAH & T. N. C. WELLS. 1993. Eur. J. Biochem. **212:** 751–755.
8. MILBURN, M. V., A. M. HASSELL, M. H. LAMBERT, S. R. JORDAN, A. E. I. PROUDFOOT, P. GRABER & T. N. C. WELLS. 1993. Nature **363:** 172–176.
9. DIEDERICHS, J., T. BOONE & P. A. KARPLUS. 1991. Science **254:** 1779–1782.
10. PANDIT, J., A. BOHM, J. JANCARIK, R. HALENBECK, K. KOTHS & S.-H. KIM. 1992. Science **258:** 1358–1362.
11. BAZAN, J. F. & D. B. MCKAY. 1992. Science **257:** 410–413.
12. SMITH, L. J., C. REDEFIELD, J. BOYD, G. M. P. LAWRENCE, R. G. EDWARDS, R. A. G. SMITH & C. M. DOBSON. 1992. J. Mol. Biol. **224:** 899–904.
13. DE VOS, A. M., M. ULTSCH & A. A. KOSSIAKOFF. 1992. Science **255:** 306–312.
14. ABDEL-MEGUID, S. S., H.-S. SHEIEH, W. W. SMITH, H. E. DAYRINGER, B. N. VIOLAND & L. A. BENTLE. 1987. Proc. Natl. Acad. Sci. U.S.A. **84:** 6434–6439.
15. MCKENZIE, A. N. J., S. C. BARRY, M. STRATH & C. J. SANDERSON. 1991. EMBO J. **10:** 1193–1199.
16. KODDAMA, S., N. TSURUOKA & M. TSUJIMOTO. 1991. Biochem. Biophys. Res. Commun. **178:** 514–518.
17. LAMBERT, M. H. & H. A. SCHERAGA. 1989. J. Comp. Chem. **10:** 770–797.
18. KRUSE, N., T. LEHRNBECHER & W. SEBALD. 1991. FEBS Lett. **286:** 58–60.
19. DEVOS, R., W. FIERS & J. TAVERNIER. 1993. European Patent Application 0-533-006-A1.
20. TAVERNIER, J., T. TUYPENS, G. PLAETINCK, A. VERHEE, W. FIERS & R. DEVOS. 1992. Proc. Natl. Acad. Sci. U.S.A. **89:** 7041–7045.
21. DEVOS, R., W. FIERS, G. PLAETINCK, J. TAVERNIER & J. VAN DER HEYDEN. 1992. European Patent Application 0-492-214-A2.
22. KRUSE, N., H.-P. TONY & W. SEBALD. 1992. EMBO J. **11:** 3237–3244.
23. FUH, G., B. C. CUNNINGHAM, R. FUKUNGA, S. NAGATA, D. GOEDDEL & J. A. WELLS. 1992. Science **256:** 1677–1680.
24. DEVOS, R., *et al.* 1993. J. Biol. Chem. **268:** 6581–6587.
25. BEDOUELLE, H. & G. WINTER. 1986. Nature **320:** 371–374.
26. CUNNINGHAM, B. C., P. JHURANI, P. NG & J. A. WELLS. 1989. Science **243:** 1330–1336.

27. D'souza, E. E., M. H. Ginsberg & E. F. Plow. 1991. Trends Biochem. Sci. **16:** 246–250.
28. Hebert, C. A., R. V. Vitangcol & J. B. Baker. 1991. J. Biol. Chem. **268:** 18989–18994.
29. Labriola-Tomkins, E., *et al.* 1991. Proc. Natl. Acad. Sci. U.S.A. **88:** 11182–11186.

Interactions between Respiratory Epithelial Cells and Cytokines: Relationships to Lung Inflammation[a]

KENNETH B. ADLER,[b] BERNARD M. FISCHER,[b]
DAVID T. WRIGHT,[b] LEAH A. COHN,[b]
AND SUSANNE BECKER[c]

[b]Department of Anatomy, Physiological Sciences, and
Radiology
College of Veterinary Medicine
North Carolina State University
Raleigh, North Carolina 27606

[c]TRC Environmental Corporation
6320 Quadrangle Drive
Chapel Hill, North Carolina 27514

INTRODUCTION

Respiratory airways, both extrapulmonary (trachea and bronchi) and intrapulmonary, are lined by epithelium. Thus, epithelial cells become the first points of contact for a variety of inhaled antigens, particulates, or other noxious or potentially toxic or hazardous agents, many of which can alter the natural and finely tuned milieu present in the airways. In terms of inflammatory reactions, epithelial cells lining the respiratory airways can be considered to function in two major capacities as both "target" cells and "effector" cells. As target cells, epithelia can respond to a number of different exogenous, as well as endogenously produced, agents or mediators by alterations in their defense function: secretion of mucus, efficiency of ciliary beating (and thus mucociliary clearance), and ion transport related to fluid absorption/secretion. As effector-type cells, epithelia can respond to these endogenous or exogenous stimuli by synthesizing and/or releasing a number of secondary mediators of inflammation [e.g., eicosanoids, oxygen free radicals, platelet-activating factor (PAF), cytokines] that can contribute to local inflammatory responses, as well as diffuse away and influence structure and function of neighboring cells and tissues. Complex interrelationships have developed related to the ability of epithelial cells to respond to inflammatory stimuli and communicate with each other and other cell types throughout the respiratory system in an autocrine-, paracrine-, endocrine-, and/or exocrine-type capacity.

Over the last 5–10 years a novel group of inflammatory mediators, collectively labeled "cytokines" have been described. These are pluripotent agents produced

[a] This work was supported in part by Grant HL 36982 from the National Institutes of Health, a grant from the state of North Carolina, and grants from Hoffmann La Roche, Inc., Nutley, N.J., and Glaxo, Inc., RTP, North Carolina. Although the research in this article has been supported in part by the Health Effects Laboratory, U.S. Environmental Protection Agency, through Contract 68-DO-0110 to TCR Environmental Corporation, it has not been subjected to agency review and therefore does not necessarily reflect the views of the agency and no official endorsement should be inferred. Mention of trade names or commercial products does not constitute endorsement or recommendation for use.

and secreted by a wide variety of cell types, including endothelial and epithelial cells, macrophages, and monocytes.[1-4] They include the interleukins, interferons, tumor necrosis factor, transforming growth factors, and others. In the lung and respiratory tract, cytokines are involved in the pathogenesis of a number of lesions associated with initiation and propagation of inflammatory reactions and ultimately with the development of disease. In this report, complex interactions that may occur between cytokines and epithelial cells of the respiratory airways are described.

AIRWAY EPITHELIA AS "TARGET" CELLS

Mucociliary Escalator/Apparatus

The nasal, tracheal, and bronchial airways are lined by a well-differentiated pseudostratified ciliated columnar epithelium. It consists mainly of ciliated, goblet (mucus producing), and basal cells. Ciliated and goblet cells form the mucociliary apparatus that serves as one of the primary defenses of the respiratory tree and lung against inhaled microbes, particulates, and other foreign substances. Beating of the cilia in a coordinated manner moves such foreign substances caught in the mucous layer up and out of the airways. In certain diseases, such as asthma and cystic fibrosis, aberrations in this apparatus may be involved in the pathogenesis. During airway inflammation, cytokines often are present at inflammatory sites, and can be key components in perturbation of the epithelium and persistence of inflammatory reactions. In this situation, cytokines can directly or indirectly alter the mucociliary apparatus by affecting ciliary beating or mucus secretion.

PAF is a potent inflammatory mediator produced by a wide variety of cells, including macrophages, neutrophils, endothelium, and epithelium.[5-8] Work from this laboratory and others have demonstrated that PAF stimulates release of mucinlike glycoproteins.[9-11] In rodent tracheal explants 10^{-4} M PAF induced significant increases in mucin production and corresponding increases in sulfopeptidyl leukotrienes (C_4, D_4, and E_4). Both the PAF receptor antagonist, Ro 19-3704, and the mixed cyclo- and lipoxygenase inhibitor nordihydroguiaretic acid (NDGA) blocked the PAF-induced increase in mucin secretion.[9] In addition, studies with guinea pig tracheal epithelial cells in organotypic culture demonstrated a similar reaction to PAF, with an increase in production in 15-, 12-, and 5-hydroxy eicosatetraenoic acids (HETEs). This PAF-induced mucin hypersecretion was inhibitable by the same PAF receptor antagonists.[10] Exogenously administered HETEs can induce mucin hypersecretion.[10,12]

PAF and 15-HETE each may act by activating phospholipase C. Both cause increased production of inositol polyphosphates in airway epithelium,[12,13] and down-regulation of protein kinase C (PKC) abolishes 15-HETE-induced mucous secretory activity.[12] Larivee *et al.*[11] recently demonstrated that the PKC-zeta isozyme appears to be a key factor in PAF-induced mucin secretion in feline tracheal epithelial cell cultures, with PAF inducing translocation of this isozyme from the cytosolic to the membrane fraction. Phorbol ester [phorbol myristate acetate (PMA)] alone was insufficient to increase mucin release, even though it induced translocation of PKC activity to the membrane fraction.[11] Interestingly enough, PKC-zeta is a calcium and diacylglycerol independent isozyme.[14-17] Thus, PAF stimulation of mucin secretion by airway epithelial cells appears to be a lipoxygenase-dependent process linked to activation of phospholipase C, with resultant hydrolysis of membrane phosphoinositides to inositol polyphosphates and activation of PKC.

Other cytokines have been shown to induce mucus glycoprotein (MGP) secretion by airway epithelial cells, such as tumor necrosis factor-alpha (TNF) and interleukin-1β (IL-1β). TNF (20 ng/ml) stimulates MGP secretion within one hour of exposure, peaking at 8 hours.[18] A similar concentration of IL-1β induced significant increases in MGP secretion at 8 hours only.[19]

TNF and IL-1β also can affect ciliary beat frequency in an indirect manner. In the unstimulated epithelium, TNF had no effect on bioelectrical properties of tracheal epithelial cells, but after isoproterenol-induced β-adrenergic receptor stimulation of the epithelium, TNF attenuated epithelial bioelectric properties.[20] The synthesis of endothelin, a potent vasoconstrictor and bronchoconstrictor, in tracheal epithelial cells can be regulated by inflammatory cytokines such as TNF and IL-1β. Both agents stimulated increased synthesis of endothelin, with IL-1β effects being more persistent than those of TNF.[21] Endothelin, in turn, increased ciliary beat frequency in these cells. These endothelin-induced effects can be attenuated by indomethacin, calcium deficiency, and inhibition of chloride ion transport.[22] Endothelin also has been shown to increase hydrolysis of PIP_2 to inositol polyphosphates, but does not appear to activate PKC.[23,24]

Thus, function and control of the epithelial mucociliary apparatus may be altered by cytokines produced as a result of airway inflammation. (See TABLE 1 for summary.)

Surfactant

Surfactant is produced by epithelial cells deeper in the airways and in the alveoli. Surfactant, composed of proteins and phospholipids, is important for the maintenance of normal alveolar function and gas exchange. In very premature infants inadequate amounts of surfactant is often a major problem affecting normal respiration. Ballard et al.[26] examined the effects of interferon-gamma (IFN-γ) on alveolar cells from fetal lungs. IFN-γ, dexamethasone, and the combination of the two all increased the content of surfactant protein A (SP-A). IFN-γ plus dexamethasone appeared to act synergistically to produce about a 10-fold increase in SP-A content. IFN-γ also stimulated SP-A mRNA, but had no effect on other surfactant proteins.[26]

Unlike its stimulatory effect on mucin production, TNF decreased mRNA levels and expression of both SP-A and SP-B in human pulmonary adenocarcinoma cell lines. Twenty-five ng/ml (500 U/ml) of TNF was enough to cause almost complete inhibition of SP-A mRNA.[27] In an alveolar epithelial cell line, IFN-γ increased SP-A content, similar to that described for fetal tissue. TNF did not affect cell growth or viability.[27]

During airway inflammation, the epithelial cells can come into contact with infiltrating leukocytes, and can respond in a variety of ways. There are several ways in which epithelial cells may potentiate or exacerbate the inflammatory reaction, such as increased expression of adhesion molecules and release of reactive oxygen species. These cells have other protective mechanisms that can be upregulated during an inflammatory response, such as antioxidant enzyme systems (see TABLES 2–5).

TABLE 1. Cytokine Effects on the Mucociliary Apparatus and Surfactant Proteins

Effect on	Cytokines Involved	Mechanism or Inhibitors	References
Mucin/mucus glycoprotein secretion	PAF (+) TNF-α (+) IL-1β (+) C3a (+)	PAF: 1. PKC-zeta 2. Lipoxygenase-dependent, 15-HETE	Larivée, 1993 (PAF, PKC; FTEC)[11] Adler, 1992 (PAF, lipoxygenase; GPTE)[9] Levine, 1993 (TNF-α; human bronchi)[18] Levine, 1993 (IL-1β, human bronchi)[19]
Ciliary beat frequency; short circuit current; and potential difference	Endothelin (+)	ET-1: Increases IP$_3$ Endothelin: Inhibited by indomethacin, Ca^{++} deficient media and Cl$^-$ ion transport inhibitors	Marom, 1985 (C3a; human airway)[25] Nally, 1992 and 1993 (ET-1; bovine and human bronchi)[23,24] Tamaoki, 1991 (ET; CTE)[22]
Endothelin-1 and precursor synthesis	TNF-α (NC or −) TNF-α (+) TGFβ (+) IL-1 (+) IL-8 (+) IL-6 (+)		Sato, 1989 (TNF-α, CTE)[20] Endo, 1992 (GPTE)[21]
Surfactant proteins	GM-CSF (+) Proteins: IFN-γ (+) TNF-α (−)		Ballard, 1990 (IFN-γ; human fetal alv. epithel. cells)[26] Wispé, 1990 (TNF-α, H441-4 cells)[27]
mRNA	mRNA: IFN-γ (+) TNF-α (−)		

Abbreviations: PAF = platelet activating factor; (+) = increase; (−) = decrease; (nc) = no change or no effect; TNF-α = tumor necrosis factor-alpha; IL-1β = Interleukin-1beta; ET or ET-1 = endothelin or endothelin-1; CTE = canine tracheal epithelium; IFN-γ = interferon-gamma; H441-4 = human pulmonary adenocarcinoma cell line with morphologic features of epithelial cells; FTEC = feline tracheal epithelial cells; GPTE = guinea pig tracheal epithelial cells; human fetal alv. epithel. cells = human fetal alveolar epithelial cells; PKC = protein kinase C; 15-HETE = 15-hydroxy eicosatetraenoic acid; TGFβ = transforming growth factor beta.

TABLE 2. Cytokine Effects on Adhesion Molecules, Integrins, Extracellular Matrix Components, and Leukocyte Chemotaxis to the Airway Epithelium

Effect on	Cytokines Involved	Mechanism or Inhibitors	References
ICAM expression	ICAM: IL-1β (+) TNF-α (+) IFN-γ (+)		ICAM: Wegner, 1990 (IL-1β, TNF-α, IFN-γ; MBEC)[28] Tosi, 1992 (IL-1β, TNF-α; HTEC, 9HTEo$^-$)[29]
PMN adherence	PMN: IL-1β (+ or −) TNF-α (+ or −)	In primary canine tracheal epithelium these cytokines cause decreased PMN adherence; however, promoted PMN adherence to human cells	Subauste, 1993 (IFN-γ, TNF-α; BEAS-2B)[31] Look, 1992 (IFN-γ, HTEC, BEAS-2B)[30] PMN: Tosi, 1992 (IL-1β, TNF-α; HTEC, 9HTEo$^-$)[29] Schroth, 1992 (IL-1β, TNF-α; CTEC)[32]
Leukocyte chemotaxis	LPS (+, PMNs) TNF-α (+, MCP-1) IL-1β (+, MCP-1) (Tachykinins − +, PMNs) PAF (+, EOS)	LPS and PMNs: DBcAMP, PGE$_2$, and antioxidants (DMSO) attenuated LPS-induced PMN chemotaxis PAF and EOS: PKC activation (by PMA) is necessary for a significant response	Koyama, 1991 (LPS, PMNs; BBEC)[33] Standiford, 1991 (IL-1β, TNF-α, MCP-1; A549 cells)[34] Von Essen, 1992 (tachykinins, PMNs, BBEC)[35] Masuda, 1993 (PAF, EOS; HTEC)[36]
Integrin expression	TGFβ1 (+)		Sheppard, 1992 (GPTE)[37]
Laminin expression and mRNA	IFN-α and γ (+)		Maheshwari, 1991 (IFN-α and γ, laminin; A549 cells)[38]
Fibronectin mRNA	IFN-γ (+)		Maheshwari, 1990 (IFN-γ, fibronectin; A549 cells)[39]
Migration to fibronectin and defect repair	TNF-α (+, migration) TNF-α (−, proliferation, defect repair)		Ito, 1993 (TNF-α; BBEC)[40]

Abbreviations: LPS = lipopolysaccharide; MCP-1 = monocyte chemoattractant protein-1; PMNs = neutrophils; EOS = eosinophils; ICAM = intercellular adhesion molecule; BBEC = bovine bronchial epithelial cells; MBEC = monkey bronchial epithelial cells; HTEC = human tracheal epithelial cells; 9HTEo$^-$ = human tracheal epithelial cell line; BEAS-2B = human bronchial epithelial cell line; A549 = Type II epithelial cell line; CTEC = canine tracheal epithelial cells; PMA = phorbol myristate acetate, a phorbol ester; TGFβ1 = transforming growth factor beta one; IFN-α = interferon-alpha. For other abbreviations, please see those listed with TABLE 1.

TABLE 3. Cytokine Effects on Antioxidant Enzymes, Eicosanoids, and Smooth-Muscle Contraction

Effect on	Cytokines Involved	Mechanism or Inhibitors	References
Antioxidant enzyme gene expression/mRNA	Mn-SOD: LPS (+), TNF-α (+), IL-1 (+); Cu/Zn-SOD: These cytokines have no effect	LPS affects are inhibitable by actinomycin	Wispé, 1990 (TNF-α, Mn-SOD; H441-4 cells)[27]; Visner, 1990 (LPS, TNF-α, IL-1, Mn-SOD, Cu/Zn-SOD; L2 cells)[48]
PLA$_2$ gene expression and activity	cPLA$_2$: IFN-γ (+), TNF-α (NC), IL-6 (NC), IL-1 (NC)	cPLA$_2$: IFN-γ stimulated cPLA$_2$ gene expression blocked by PKC and Ca^{++}/calmodulin-dependent PK inhibitors, but not by cyclo-heximide (Wu, 1993)	cPLA$_2$: Miyashita, 1993 (TNF-α, IL-6, IL-1, BET-1A)[49]; Wu, 1993 (IFN-γ; BEAS-2B)[50]
Arachidonic acid release	[^{3}H]-AA release: IL-5 (+), IFN-γ (+)	[^{3}H]-AA: IL-5 effects blocked by EGTA and PLA$_2$ inhibitors	[^{3}H]-AA and 15-HETE: Wu, 1993 (IFN-γ; BEAS-2B)[51]
Eicosanoid production	15-HETE: IFN-γ (+), IL-5 (+)	15-HETE: IFN-γ had no effect on 15-LO activity; IL-5 + Ca^{++} ionophore enhance 15-HETE release	Wu, 1993 (IL-5, BEAS-2B)[52]
Epithelium-dependent smooth muscle contraction	IL-1β (−, ACh-dependent contraction); IL-2 (+, airway spasms); IFN-γ (−, airway spasms)	IL-1β induces release of EpDRF (Tamaoki, 1993); PGE$_2$ and PGI$_2$ are major components of EpDRF (Prie, 1990)	Tamaoki, 1993 (IL-1β; canine bronchial segments)[53]; Prie, 1990 (PGE$_2$ and I$_2$; guinea pig tracheas and bronchi)[54]; Munakata, 1993 (IL-2, IFN-γ; guinea pig airway strips)[55]

Abbreviations: Mn-SOD = manganese super oxide dismutase; Cu/Zn-SOD = copper/zinc super oxide dismutase; L2 = rat pulmonary epithelial-like cell line; BET-1A = human airway (bronchial) epithelial cell line; cPLA$_2$ = cytosolic phospholipase A2; IL-5, -6, -1, -2 = interleukin-5, -6, -1, -2; ^{3}H-AA = tritiated arachidonic acid; PK = protein kinase; 15-LO = 15-lipoxygenase; EGTA = ethylene glycol-bis(β-aminoethyl ether) N,N,N',N'-tetraacetic acid; ACh = acetyl choline; GM–CSF = granulocyte/macrophage colony stimulating factor; EpDRF = epithelium-derived relaxing factor; PGE$_2$, I$_2$ = prostaglandin E2, I2. For other abbreviations see those listed for TABLES 1 and 2.

TABLE 4. Cytokine Effects on Airway Epithelial Class I and II Antigen Expression, Complement Components, and Coagulation System

Effect on	Cytokines Involved	Mechanism or Inhibitors	References
Complement Components	C3: IL-4 (+) IL-1α (+) IFN-γ (+ or NC) IL-1β (+) IL-2 (+) IFN-α (−) C5: IL-4 (−) IL-1α (−) IFN-α (−) IL-1β (−) IFN-γ (−) IL-2 (−)		Rothman, 1990 (IFN-α and γ, IL-1α and β, IL-2, C3 and C5; A549 cells)[56] Khirwadkar, 1993 (IL-4, IFN-γ, C3 and C5; A549 cells)[57]
Class I and II antigen expression	IFN-γ (+) (Also enables treated cells to present antigen to autologous T cells, but at a lower efficiency than monocytes) TNF-α (NC)		IFN-γ: Harbeck, 1988 (class II; rat Type II cells)[58] Rossi, 1990 (class II, human ciliated bronchial epithelial cells)[59] Momburg, 1986 (class I; mouse BEC)[60] Mezzetti, 1991 (antigen presentation; HBEC)[61] Spurzem, 1992 (TNF-α, class II; BBEC)[62]

Coagulation system	TF Procoagulant Activity: TGFβ (+)		TF: Johnson, 1993 (TNF-α, TGFβ; HPEC)[63]
	TNF-α (+)		PA: Johnson, 1993 (TNF-α, TGFβ, t-PA: HPEC)[63]
	Plasminogen activator activity (fibrinolytic activity):		Marshall, 1992 (IL-1β, TNFα, u-PA; A549)[64,65]
	IL-1β (+, u-PA)		Gross, 1990 (LPS, TNFα, u-PA; rat Type II cells)[66]
	TNF-α (+, u-PA and t-PA)	PA expression: Inhibitable by glucocorticoids; not linked to PKC or cAMP (Marshall, 1992)	PA mRNA: Marshall, 1992[64,65]
	LPS (+, u-PA)		Gross, 1990[66]
	TGFβ (−)		PAI: Marshall, 1992 (IL-1β, TNF-α, NC; TGFβ, +)[64,65]
	PA mRNA: IL-1β (+, u-PA)		Johnson, 1993 (TNF-α, TGFβ, +)[66]
	TNF-α (+, u-PA)		
	PA inhibitor activity, mRNA, and protein:		
	IL-1β (NC)		
	TNF-α (NC or sl. +)		
	TGFβ (+, PAI-1)		

Abbreviations: IL-4, -1α = interleukin-4, -1alpha; HBEC = human bronchial epithelial cells; mouse BEC = mouse bronchial epithelial cells; TF procoagulant activity = tissue factor procoagulant activity; u-PA = urokinase-type plasminogen activator; t-PA = tissue plasminogen activator; PA = plasminogen activator; PAI = plasminogen activator inhibitor; cAMP = cyclic adenosine 3′,5′-monophosphate; HPEC = human tracheal epithelial cell line. Please see other tables for other abbreviations not listed here.

TABLE 5. Other Cytokine Effects on Airway Epithelium

Effect on	Cytokines Involved	Mechanism of Inhibitors	References
Mink lung epithelial cell lines proliferation	TGFβ1 (−) TNF-α (−)	TGFβ1 inhibition negated by pertussis-toxin-sensitive G protein (Howe, 1990)	Howe, 1990 (TGFβ1; CCL64 cell line)[67] Kelley, 1992 (TGFβ, TNF-α; Mv1Lu cell line)[68]
Human small cell bronchial carcinoma	IFN-β and IFN-γ treatment provides a slight increase in response rate when used with other chemotherapy agents (adriamycin + cyclophosphamide + vincristine)		Zabel, 1990 (human)[69]

Note: Please see other tables for abbreviations.

Adhesion Molecule Expression and Leukocyte Interactions

Recently, intercellular adhesion molecule-1 (ICAM-1) has been reported to be of potential importance in the pathogenesis of asthma.[28] In a primate model of asthma, IL-1β, TNF, and IFN-γ all increased ICAM-1 surface expression in a primate bronchial epithelial cell line and whole primate trachea sections. ICAM-1 expression was most intense at the basolateral aspect of the epithelium, enabling infiltrating leukocytes to adhere to the epithelium.[28] Similar work has been done with human tissues and cell lines. Both TNF and IL-1β increased surface ICAM-1 expression in primary human tracheal epithelial cells, and this in turn supported adherence of neutrophils.[29] In the transformed human bronchial epithelial cell line BEAS-2B, however, only IFN-γ increased ICAM-1 expression.[30,31] Subauste *et al.*[31] did note that there was some increased expression of ICAM-1 in response to TNF, but the response reached its peak early in the time course of exposure (4 hours). However, the combination of TNF and IFN-γ appeared to have an additive effect.[31] In contrast, TNF and IL-1β decreased neutrophil adherence to canine tracheal epithelium.[32] Other effects of these proinflammatory cytokines have been described in relation to their effects on leukocyte chemotaxis toward the airway epithelium (see TABLE 2).

Reactive Oxygen Species and Cellular Protective Mechanisms

Reactive oxygen species include such agents as hydrogen peroxide, superoxide anion, hydroxyl radical, ozone, and nitrogen dioxide. Work from this laboratory and others has shown that proinflammatory agents like PAF and PKC activators (PMA) can stimulate the production of hydrogen peroxide by tracheal and bronchial epithelial cells.[41-43] Inactivation of PKC inhibited both PAF- and PMA-induced hydrogen peroxide release by guinea pig tracheal epithelial cells.[41,42] (It is important to note that hydrogen peroxide can be converted to the very reactive hydroxyl radical that can cause further aberrations in epithelial homeostasis.) Previous work from this laboratory has shown that reactive oxygen species stimulate secretion of mucus glycoproteins by explant and cell cultures of rodent trachea.[44,45] The superoxide generating system of purine + xanthine oxidase can activate phospholipase C in guinea pig tracheal epithelial cells *in vitro,* resulting in production of inositol polyphosphate and PKC activation and translocation.[46] Ozone, an oxidant pollutant, also has profound effects on airway epithelium. Ozone-exposed nasal epithelium demonstrates a dramatic increase in DNA synthesis, as compared to air-exposed cells; TNF, IL-1β, and lipopolysaccharide (LPS) each were able to attenuate the ozone-induced increase in DNA synthesis.[47] It appears in this case that these cytokines might be serving a protective function, although the exact mechanism of protection is not known. Relatedly, many of these proinflammatory cytokines may have beneficial effects in the airways. A human pulmonary adenocarcinoma cell line incubated with TNF demonstrates increased levels of manganese superoxide dismutase (Mn–SOD) mRNA.[27] A similar phenomenon has been demonstrated in a rat pulmonary epithelial cell line: LPS, IL-1, and TNF induced increases in Mn–SOD mRNA but had no effect on Cu/Zn–SOD mRNA. The LPS-induced increase was inhibitable by actinomycin, a protein synthesis inhibitor[48] (see TABLE 3).

Cytokines and Eicosanoids

As mentioned earlier, PAF-induced mucin secretion appears to be partially dependent on lipoxygenase metabolism of arachidonic acid. Other investigators have shown that cytokines are able to control eicosanoid synthesis at the level of phospholipase A_2 (PLA_2), an enzyme that catalyzes the release of arachidonic acid from membrane lipids and thus serves as the rate-limiting enzyme in oxidation reactions of arachidonic acid. PLA_2 has two forms: cytosolid ($cPLA_2$) and secretory ($sPLA_2$). TNF, IL-1, and IL-6 all had no effect on $cPLA_2$ gene expression in BET-1A cells.[49] However, IFN-γ induced $cPLA_2$ gene expression and caused an increase in cellular PLA_2 protein levels and enzyme activity in human tracheal epithelial cells *in vitro*. The IFN-γ-induced gene expression was blocked by a variety of PKC inhibitors and one calcium/calmodulin-dependent protein kinase inhibitor, but not by the protein synthesis inhibitor, cycloheximide.[50] In another report, IFN-γ was shown to increase 15-HETE levels, with no effect on 15-lipooxygenase activity. However, there was a corresponding increase in arachidonic acid release in response to IFN-γ stimulation indicating a $cPLA_2$ dependent mechanism.[51] 15-HETE is important in PAF-mediated mucin secretion, which was further linked to PKC.[10,12] In addition, IL-5 exposure of human tracheal epithelium induces increased arachidonic acid release, and, in combination with calcium ionophore, enhanced 15-HETE release[52] (see TABLE 3). Thus, the interplay between cytokines and arachidonate metabolites appears to involve a finely tuned system where cytokines stimulate arachidonic acid release through upregulation of $cPLA_2$ synthesis and enzymatic activity. This in turn leads to increased production of stimulatory eicosanoids (e.g., 15-HETE) that may be further regulated by PKC, to lead ultimately to increased secretion of mucus.

AIRWAY EPITHELIA AS "EFFECTOR" CELLS

Production of Cytokines

The production of cytokines in injured or diseased airways has classically been considered a function of stimulated macrophages.[70] Recently, however, it has become apparent that stromal cells and respiratory epithelial cells have the ability to synthesize and release inflammatory cytokines, such as IL-1, IL-6, IL-8, and growth factors that modulate differentiation of inflammatory cells, such as GM–CSF, G–CSF, and M–CSF. In human bronchial cell lines, Mattoli et al.[71] first described the production of IL-1α, IL-1β, and IL-6 following exposure to toluidine isothiocyanate. Both IL-1 and IL-6 were secreted between 48 hours and 6 days of culture.[72] In a study by Takizawa et al.[73] IL-6 was found to be produced in both primary bronchial epithelial cell cultures and in the BEAS-2B cell line in the absence of specific stimulation. Henke et al.[74] compared production of IL-1β, IL-6, and IL-8 in supernatants of primary cultures of nasal epithelium obtained from normals and individuals with the disease, cystic fibrosis (CF). IL-1 was not detected in the culture supernatants, while IL-6 and IL-8 were produced spontaneously by both normal and CF epithelium. CF epithelial cells produced 4 to 5 times the amount of IL-6 as normal epithelial cells, however, although approximately the same levels of IL-8. Nakamura et al.[75] reported that epithelial lining fluid from CF individuals induced IL-8 gene expression in the BET-1A human bronchial epithelial cell line, and suggested that neutrophil elastase in the fluid was the predominant inducer of IL-8 in CF. GM–CSF has been found to be produced spontaneously by airway epithelial cells *in vitro*.[76] Studies from our laboratory have demonstrated IL-8, but not IL-6, gene expression in isolated human nasal epithelial cells.[77] When placed into culture, both nasal and bronchial epithelial cells demonstrated expression of genes for IL-1, IL-6, and GM–CSF, with release of immunoreactive IL-6 and GM–CSF, but not IL-1β, into the medium. Relatedly, it has been suggested that IL-6 is an autocrine regulator of epithelial cell growth.[73]

Regulation of Airway Epithelial Cell Cytokines Production by Cytokines

Production of cytokines by airway epithelial cells, like many other cell types, appears susceptible to regulation by IL-1 and TNF. The A549 type II cell-like tumor line responded to both IL-1 and TNF, but not to endotoxin (LPS), by increasing IL-8 mRNA and protein levels.[78] In a study by Nakamura *et al.*,[79] utilizing the BET-1A and HS-24 bronchial epithelial cell lines, the IL-8 response to TNF was shown to be controlled in the 5' flanking region by a response element located between base pairs -130 to -112 relative to the transcription start site. In freshly isolated nasal epithelial cells, TNF and IL-1 stimulation resulted in increased IL-8 mRNA and protein, but IL-1 or IL-6 protein was not secreted within 24 hours after stimulation. *In situ* hybridization studies demonstrated expression of IL-6 and IL-8 mRNAs in primary airway epithelial cell cultures, with TNF and IL-1 inducing increased expression of these genes in a concentration-dependent manner.[80] Airway epithelial cells do not produce IL-6, IL-8, or GM–CSF in response to IL-6, although the cells do express receptors for IL-6.[81]

In a recent study conducted on individuals exposed to LPS-contaminated grain dust, we compared levels of IL-1, IL-6, and IL-8 mRNA in tracheal epithelial biopsies and bronchoalveolar lavage (BAL) cells after 6 hours of exposure.[82] IL-8 mRNA levels were as high in epithelium as in the BAL cells, and were induced 5-fold compared to cells obtained after control saline-exposure. IL-6 and TNF message levels were not increased above controls, and IL-1 increases were negligible when compared to levels in macrophages. These results suggest that epithelial cells are major producers of IL-8 in the airways, while contributing only a minor part of total IL-1 and no IL-6 after LPS exposure.

Cytokine Production by Airway Epithelial Cells in Response to Viral Infection

In BEAS-2B transformed human adenocarcinoma cell line, respiratory syncytial virus (RSV) infection caused increased expression of IL-8 mRNA within 4 hours of infection. Message levels for IL-6 and GM–CSF increased also, but only after 96 hours.[83] Interestingly enough, IL-1 was not found in BEAS-2B supernatants, although IL-1β mRNA was induced within 4 hours of infection. The pollutant gas, ozone, at noncytotoxic concentrations (0.5 ppm for 1 h) was found to induce IL-6 and IL-8 mRNA expression and protein secretion within 2 hours of exposure: mRNA levels peaked at 1–4 hours and returned to baseline levels by 8 hours.[83,84] When RSV infection of BEAS-2B cells was preceded by ozone exposure, additive effects of pollutant and virus on cytokine production were reported.[85] Freshly isolated nasal epithelial cells exposed to RSV *in vitro* showed only an increase in IL-8 mRNA and protein production, and did not produce IL-1, IL-6, or TNF during the first 24 hours of infection.

Cytokines in Airway Epithelium of Allergic/Asthmatic Individuals

Production of hematopoietic growth factors and inflammatory cytokines by airway epithelium has been of particular interest in allergic and asthmatic processes. These diseases are characterized by chronic inflammation, with an influx of monocytes, eosinophils, and neutrophilic granulocytes in the airway mucosa, and thus cytokines with effects on these cell types have been investigated in airway epithelium. Primary airway epithelial cell cultures from normal or allergic and/or asthmatic individuals were found to produce G–CSF, GM–CSF, IL-6, and IL-8.[86,87] Here, GM–CSF was found to be of primary importance, since, in addition to promoting monocyte and polymorphonuclear (PMN) leukocyte survival and differentiation, epithelial cell-conditioned medium promoted eosinophil survival, an effect abrogated by pretreatment with anti-GM–CSF antibody. Primary nasal epithelial cell cultures from nasal polyp tissue from allergic individuals produced four times more GM–CSF than control cultures, while there was no difference in production of IL-6 or G–CSF.[86] Marini *et al.*[87] used the PCR technique to demonstrate increased mRNA levels for GM–CSF in airway biopsies of asthmatic patients compared to normal controls. Thus, GM–CSF, together with cytokines such as IL-3 and IL-5, and the extracellular matrix component, fibronectin (also produced by airway epithelium), may interact to sustain the eosinophilic inflammatory activity in the airways.[88]

SUMMARY

Epithelial cells lining respiratory airways can participate in inflammation in a number of ways. They can act as target cells, responding to exposure to a variety of inflammatory mediators and cytokines by altering one or several of their functions, such as mucin secretion, ion transport, or ciliary beating. Aberrations in any of these functions can affect local inflammatory responses and compromise pulmonary defense. For example, oxidant stress can increase secretion of mucin and depress ciliary beating efficiency, thereby affecting the ability of the mucociliary system to clear potentially pathogenic microbial agents. Recent studies have indicated that airway epithelial cells also can act as "effector" cells, synthesizing and releasing cytokines, lipid mediators, and reactive oxygen species in response to a number of pathologically relevant stimuli, thereby contributing to inflammation. Many of these epithelial-derived substances can act locally, affecting both neighboring cells and tissues, or, via autocrine or paracrine mechanisms, affect structure and function of the epithelial cells themselves. Studies in our laboratories utilized cell cultures of both human and guinea pig tracheobronchial and nasal epithelial cells, and isolated human nasal epithelial cells, to investigate activity of respiratory epithelial cells *in vitro* as sources of cytokines and inflammatory mediators. Primary cultures of guinea pig and human tracheobronchial and nasal epithelial cells synthesize and secrete low levels of IL-6 and IL-8 constitutively. Production and release of these cytokines increases substantially after exposure to specific inflammatory stimuli, such as TNF or IL-1, and after viral infection.

REFERENCES

1. LE, J. & J. VILCEK. 1987. Tumor necrosis factor and interleukin 1: Cytokines with multiple overlapping biological activities. Lab. Invest. **56:** 234–248.

2. MING, W. J., L. BERSANI & A. MANTOVANI. 1987. Tumor necrosis factor is chemotactic for monocytes and polymorphonuclear leukocytes. J. Immunol. **138**: 1469–1474.
3. CAMUSSI, G., C. TETTA, F. BUSSOLINO & C. BAGLIONI. 1989. Tumor necrosis factor stimulates human neutrophils to release leukotriene B₄ and platelet activating factor. J. Biochem. **182**: 661–666.
4. CAMUSSI, G., F. BUSSOLINO, G. SALVIDIO & C. BAGLIONI. 1987. Tumor necrosis factor/cachectin stimulates peritoneal macrophages, polymorphonuclear neutrophils, and vascular endothelial cells to synthesize and release platelet activating factor. J. Exp. Med. **166**: 1390–1404.
5. PAGE, C. P. 1988. The role of platelet-activating factor in asthma. J. Allergy Clin. Immunol. **81**: 144–151.
6. BARNES, P. J. 1988. Platelet-activating factor and asthma. J. Allergy Clin. Immunol. **81**: 152–158.
7. MORLEY, J. 1988. Platelet activating factor and asthma. Agents Actions **19**: 100–108.
8. SALARI, H. & A. WONG. 1990. Generation of platelet activating factor (PAF) by a human epithelial cell line. Eur. J. Pharmacol. **175**: 253–259.
9. ADLER, K. B., N. J. AKLEY & W. C. GLASGOW. 1992. Platelet-activating factor provokes release of mucin-like glycoproteins from guinea pig respiratory epithelial cells via a lipoxygenase-dependent mechanism. Am. J. Respir. Cell Mol. Biol. **6**: 550–556.
10. ADLER, K. B., J. E. SCHWARZ, W. H. ANDERSON & A. F. WELTON. 1987. Platelet activating factor stimulates secretion of mucin by explants of rodent airways in organ culture. Exp. Lung Res. **13**: 25–43.
11. LARIVÉE, P., S. J. LEVINE, A. MARTINEZ, C. LOGUN & J. H. SHELHAMER. 1993. Protein kinase C zeta isozyme mediates the airway mucin secretory effect of platelet activating factor. Am. Rev. Respir. Dis. **147**: A934.
12. GOSWAMI, S. K., E. GOLLUB, J. Y. VANDERHOEK & Z. MAROM. 1993. 15-HETE (hydroxy eicosatetraenoic acid) enhances mucus like glycoprotein (MLGP) secretion from an epithelial cell line via protein kinase C (PKC). Am. Rev. Respir. Dis. **147**: A439.
13. CHOE, N.-H., N. J. AKLEY & K. B. ADLER. 1993. Unpublished data.
14. NISHIZUKA, Y. 1992. Intracellular signaling by hydrolysis of phospholipids and activation of protein kinase C. Science **258**: 607–614.
15. ONO, Y., T. FUJII, K. OGITA, U. KIKKAWA, K. IGARASHI & Y. NISHIZUKA. 1989. Protein kinase C zeta subspecies from rat brain: Its structure, expression, and properties. Proc. Natl. Acad. Sci. U.S.A. **86**: 3099–3103.
16. WAYS, D. K., P. P. COOK, C. WEBSTER & P. J. PARKER. 1992. Effect of phorbol esters on protein kinase C-zeta. J. Biol. Chem. **267**: 4799–4805.
17. NAKANISHI, H. & J. H. EXTON. 1992. Purification and characterization of the zeta isoform of protein kinase C from bovine kidney. J. Biol. Chem. **267**: 16347–16354.
18. LEVINE, S. J., C. LOGUN, P. LARIVÉE & J. H. SHELHAMER. 1993. TNF-a induces secretion of respiratory mucous glycoprotein from human airways *in vitro*. Am. Rev. Respir. Dis. **147**: A1011.
19. ———. 1993. IL-1β induces secretion of respiratory mucous glycoprotein from human airways *in vitro*. Am. Rev. Respir. Dis. **147**: A437.
20. SATO, M., T. SASAKI, S. SHIMURA, I. OHNO, Y. TANNO, H. SASAKI & T. TAKISHIMA. 1989. Regulatory effect of TNF on bioelectrical properties of canine tracheal epithelium. Am. Rev. Respir. Dis. **139**: A476.
21. ENDO, T., Y. UCHIDA, H. MATSUMOTO, N. SUZUKI, A. NOMURA, F. HIRATA & S. HASEGAWA. 1992. Regulation of endothelin-1 synthesis in cultured guinea pig airway epithelial cells by various cytokines. Biochem. Biophys. Res. Commun. **186**: 1594–1599.
22. TAMAOKI, J., T. KANEMURA, N. SAKAI, K. ISONO, K. KOBAYASHI & T. TAKIZAWA. 1991. Endothelin stimulates ciliary beat frequency and chloride secretion in canine cultured tracheal epithelium. Am. J. Respir. Cell Mol. Biol. **4**: 426–431.
23. NALLY, J. E., L. C. YOUNG, M. J. O. WAKELAM, N. C. THOMSON & J. C. MCGRATH. 1993. Endothelin-1 evokes IP₃ formation, but not protein kinase C activation in bovine and human bronchi. Am. Rev. Respir. Dis. **147**: A181.

24. NALLY, J. E., R. McCALL, L. C. YOUNG, M. J. O. WAKELAM & N. C. THOMSON. 1992. Mechanical and biochemical responses to endothelin-1 and endothelin-3 in bovine bronchial smooth muscle. Br. J. Pharmacol. **107:** 173P.

25. MAROM, Z., J. SHELHAMER, M. BERGER, M. FRANK & M. KALINER. 1985. Anaphylatoxin C3a enhances mucous glycoprotein release from human airways in vitro. J. Exp. Med. **161:** 657–668.

26. BALLARD, P. L., H. G. LILEY, L. W. GONZALES, M. W. ODOM, A. J. AMMANN, B. BENSON, R. T. WHITE & M. C. WILLIAMS. 1990. Interferon-gamma and synthesis of surfactant components by cultured human fetal lung. Am. J. Respir. Cell Mol. Biol. **2:** 137–143.

27. WISPÉ, J. R., J. C. CLARK, B. B. WARNER, D. FAJARDO, W. E. HULL, R. B. HOLTZMAN & J. A. WHITSETT. 1990. Tumor necrosis factor-alpha inhibits expression of pulmonary surfactant protein. J. Clin. Invest. **86:** 1954–1960.

28. WEGNER, C. D., R. H. GUNDEL, P. REILLY, N. HAYNES, L. G. LETTS & R. ROTHLEIN. 1990. Intercellular adhesion molecule-1 (ICAM-1) in the pathogenesis of asthma. Science **247:** 456–459.

29. TOSI, M. F., J. M. STARK, C. W. SMITH, A. HAMEDANI, D. C. GRUENERT & M. D. INFELD. 1992. Induction of ICAM-1 expression on human airway epithelial cells by inflammatory cytokines: Effects on neutrophil-epithelial cell adhesion. Am. J. Respir. Cell Mol. Biol. **7:** 214–221.

30. LOOK, D. C., S. R. RAPP, B. T. KELLER & M. J. HOLTZMAN. 1992. Selective induction of intracellular adhesion molecule-1 by interferon-gamma in human airway epithelial cells. Am. J. Physiol. **263:** L79–L87.

31. SUBAUSTE, M. C., B. S. BOCHNER & D. PROUD. 1993. Modulation of ICAM-1 expression on a human bronchial epithelial cell line (BEAS-2B) by cytokines. Am. Rev. Respir. Dis. **147:** A435.

32. SCHROTH, M. K. & D. M. SHASBY. 1992. Cytokine-mediated changes in PMN adherence to canine tracheal epithelial cells. Chest **101**(3, Suppl.): 39S–40S.

33. KOYAMA, S., S. I. RENNARD, L. CLASSEN & R. A. ROBBINS. 1991. Dibutyryl cAMP, prostaglandin E$_2$, and antioxidants protect cultured bovine bronchial epithelial cells from endotoxin. Am. J. Physiol. **261:** L126–L132.

34. STANDIFORD, T. J., S. L. KUNKEL, S. H. PHAN, B. J. ROLLINS & R. M. STRIETER. 1991. Alveolar macrophage-derived cytokines induce monocyte chemoattractant protein-1 expression from human pulmonary type II-like epithelial cells. J. Biol. Chem. **266:** 9912–9918.

35. VON ESSEN, S. G., S. I. RENNARD, D. O'NEILL, R. F. ERTL, R. A. ROBBINS, S. KOYAMA & I. RUBINSTEIN. 1992. Bronchial epithelial cells release neutrophil chemotactic activity in response to tachykinins. Am. J. Physiol. **263:** L226–L231.

36. MASUDA, T., M. YAMAYA, T. AIZAWA, G. TAMURA, S. SHIMURA, H. SASAKI, T. TAKISHIMA & K. SHIRATO. 1993. PAF induces eosinophil-penetration through human cultured epithelium in the presence of a protein kinase C activator. Am. Rev. Respir. Dis. **147:** A46.

37. SHEPPARD, D., D. S. COHEN, A. WANG & M. BUSK. 1992. Transforming growth factor β differentially regulates expression of integrin subunits in guinea pig airway epithelial cells. J. Biol. Chem. **267:** 17409–17414.

38. MAHESHWARI, R. K., V. P. KEDAR, H. C. COON & D. BHARTIYA. 1991. Regulation of laminin expression by interferon. J. Interferon Res. **11:** 75–80.

39. MAHESHWARI, R. K., V. P. KEDAR, D. BHARTIYA, H. C. COON & Y. H. KANG. 1990. Interferon enhances fibronectin expression in various cell lines. J. Biol. Regul. Homeost. Agents **4:** 117–124.

40. ITO, H., D. J. ROMBERGER, S. I. RENNARD & J. R. SPURZEM. 1993. TNF-a bronchial epithelial cell migration and attachment to fibronectin. Am. Rev. Respir. Dis. **147:** A46.

41. ADLER, K. B., V. L. KINNULA, N. J. AKLEY, J. LEE, L. A. COHN & J. D. CRAPO. 1992. Inflammatory mediators and the generation and release of reactive oxygen species by airway epithelium *in vitro*. Chest **101**(3, Suppl.): 53S–54S.

42. KINNULA, V. L., K. B. ADLER, N. J. AKLEY & J. D. CRAPO. 1992. Release of reactive

oxygen species by guinea pig tracheal epithelial cell in vitro. Am. J. Physiol. **262:** L708–L712.

43. LOPEZ, A., S. SHOJI, J. FUJITA, R. ROBBINS & S. RENNARD. 1988. Bronchoepithelial cells can release hydrogen peroxide in response to inflammatory stimuli. Am. Rev. Respir. Dis. **137:** A81.

44. ADLER, K. B., W. J. HOLDEN-STAUFFER & J. E. REPINE. 1990. Oxygen metabolites stimulate release of high-molecular-weight glycoconjugates by cell and organ cultures of rodent respiratory epithelium via an arachidonic acid-dependent mechanism. J. Clin. Invest. **85:** 75–85.

45. ADLER, K. B. & N. J. AKLEY. 1988. Oxygen radicals stimulate secretion of mucin by rodent airway epithelial cells in organotypic culture. *In* Oxy-Radicals in Molecular Biology and Pathology: 101–108.

46. WRIGHT, D., B. M. FISCHER, N. J. AKLEY & K. B. ADLER. Unpublished data.

47. HOTCHKISS, J. A. & J. R. HARKEMA. 1992. Endotoxin or cytokines attenuate ozone-induced DNA synthesis in rat nasal transitional epithelium. Toxicol. Appl. Pharmacol. **114:** 182–187.

48. VISNER, G. A., W. C. DOUGALL, J. M. WILSON, I. A. BURR & H. S. NICK. 1990. Regulation of manganese superoxide dismutase by lipopolysaccharide, interleukin-1, and tumor necrosis factor. J. Biol. Chem. **265:** 2856–2864.

49. MIYASHITA, A., J. G. HAY & R. G. CRYSTAL. 1993. Expression and regulation of secretory and cytosolic phospholipase A_2 in the human lung. Am. Rev. Respir. Dis. **147:** A664.

50. WU, T., M. LAWRENCE, C. LOGUN & J. SHELHAMER. 1993. Interferon-gamma (IFNg) induces the expression of cytosolic phospholipase A_2 in human tracheal epithelial cells. Am. Rev. Respir. Dis. **147:** A19.

51. ———. 1993. Interferon-gamma increases 15-HETE production in human tracheal epithelial cells: Involvement of cytosolic phospholipase A2 activation. Am. Rev. Respir. Dis. **147:** A437.

52. WU, T., P. LARIVÉE, C. LOGUN & J. H. SHELHAMER. 1993. The effect of interleukin-5 on arachidonate metabolism in human tracheal epithelial cells. Am. Rev. Respir. Dis. **147:** A1011.

53. TAMAOKI, J., K. TAKEYAMA, A. CHIYOTANI, F. YAMAUCHI & K. KONNO. 1993. Interleukin-1β inhibits airway smooth muscle contraction by releasing epithelium-derived relaxing factor. Am. Rev. Respir. Dis. **147:** A849.

54. PRIE, S., A. CADIEUX & P. SIROIS. 1990. Removal of guinea pig bronchial and tracheal epithelium potentiates the contractions to leukotrienes and histamine. Eicosanoids **3**(1): 29–37.

55. MUNAKATA, M., H. CHEN, H. UKITA, Y. MASAKI, Y. HOMMA & Y. KAWAKAMI. 1993. Effect of interleukin-2 (IL-2) and interferon gamma (IFN-r) on guinea-pig airway strips. Am. Rev. Respir. Dis. **147:** A1013.

56. ROTHMAN, B. L., A. W. DESPINS & D. L. KREUTZER. 1990. Cytokine regulation of C3 and C5 production by the human type II pneumocyte cell line, A549. J. Immunol. **145:** 592–598.

57. KHIRWADKAR, K., G. ZILOW, M. OPPERMANN, D. KABELITZ & K. ROTHER. 1993. Interleukin-4 augments production of the third complement component by the alveolar epithelial cell line A549. Int. Arch. Allergy Immunol. **100:** 35–41.

58. HARBECK, R. J., N. W. GEGEN, D. STRUHAR & R. MASON. 1988. Class II molecules on rat alveolar type II epithelial cells. Cell. Immunol. **111:** 139–147.

59. ROSSI, G. A., O. SACCO, B. BALBI, S. ODDERA, T. MATTIONI, G. CORTE, C. RAVAZZONI & L. ALLEGRA. 1990. Human ciliated bronchial epithelial cells: Expression of the HLA-DR antigens and of the HLA-DR alpha gene, modulation of the HLA-DR antigens by gamma-interferon and antigen-presenting function in the mixed leukocyte reaction. Am. J. Respir. Cell Mol. Biol. **3:** 431–439.

60. MOMBURG, F., N. KOCH, P. MOLLER, G. MOLDENHAUER & G. J. HAMMERLING. 1986. *In vivo* induction of H-2K/D antigen by recombinant interferon-g. Eur. J. Immunol. **16:** 551–557.

61. MEZZETTI, M., M. B. SOLOPERTO, A. FASOLI & S. MATTOLI. 1991. Human bronchial

epithelial cells modulate CD3 and mitogen-induced DNA synthesis in T cells but function poorly as antigen-presenting cells compared to pulmonary macrophages. J. Allergy Clin. Immunol. **87:** 930–938.

62. SPURZEM, J. R., O. SACCO, G. A. ROSSI, J. D. BECKMANN & S. I. RENNARD. 1992. Regulation of major histocompatibility complex class II gene expression on bovine bronchial epithelial cells. J. Lab. Clin. Med. **120:** 94–102.

63. JOHNSON, A. R., K. B. KOENIG & S. IDELL. 1993. TGF-β and TNF-a influence fibrin turnover in human tracheal epithelial cells in vitro. Am. Rev. Respir. Dis. **147:** A309.

64. MARSHALL, B. C., N. V. RAO, B. R. BROWN & J. R. HOIDAL. 1992. Cytokine modulation of plasminogen activator/plasminogen activator inhibitor expression by pulmonary epithelial cells. Chest **101**(3, Suppl.): 21S–22S.

65. MARSHALL, B. C., Q.-P. XU, N. V. RAO, B. R. BROWN & J. R. HOIDAL. 1992. Pulmonary epithelial cell urokinase-type plasminogen activator. Induction by interleukin-1β and tumor necrosis factor-a. J. Biol. Chem. **267:** 11462–11469.

66. GROSS, T. J., R. H. SIMON & R. G. SITRIN. 1990. Expression of urokinase-type plasminogen activator by rat pulmonary alveolar epithelial cells. Am. J. Respir. Cell Mol. Biol. **3:** 449–456.

67. HOWE, P. H., M. R. CUNNINGHAM & E. B. LEOF. 1990. Inhibition of mink lung epithelial cell proliferation by transforming growth factor-beta is coupled through a pertussis toxin-sensitive substrate. Biochem. J. **266:** 537–543.

68. KELLEY, J., L. BALDOR & M. ABSHER. 1992. Complex cytokine modulation of a continuous line of mink lung epithelial cells (Mv1Lu). Exp. Lung Res. **18:** 877.

69. ZABEL, P., C. KREIKER & M. SCHLAAK. 1990. [Initial results of a controlled study of small cell and squamous epithelial bronchial cancer: Polychemotherapy and interferons] (in German). Pneumologie **44**(Suppl 1): 586–587.

70. KELLEY, J. 1990. Cytokines in the lung. Am. Rev. Respir. Dis. **1141:** 765–788.

71. MATTOLI, S., S. MIANTE, F. CALABRO, M. MEZZETTI, A. FASOLI & L. ALLEGRA. 1990. Bronchial epithelial cells exposed to isocyanates potentiate activation and proliferation of T cells. Am. J. Physiol. **259:** L320–L327.

72. MATTOLI, S., F. COLOTTA, G. FINCATO, M. MEZZETTI, A. MANTOVANI, F. PATALANO & A. FASOLI. 1991. Time course of IL-1 and IL-6 synthesis and release in human bronchial epithelial cell cultures exposed to toluene diidocyanate. J. Cell. Physiol. **149:** 260–268.

73. TAKIZAWA, H., et al. 1993. Interleukin 6/B cell stimulatory factor II is expressed and released by normal and transformed human bronchial epithelial cells. Biochem. Biophys. Res. Commun. **187:** 596–602.

74. HENKE, D., R. BOUCHER & S. BECKER. 1993. Interleukin 6 metabolism by freshly isolated and cultured normal human and cystic fibrosis airway epithelium. Unpublished data.

75. NAKAMURA, H., K. YOSHIMURA, N. G. MCELVANEY & R. G. CRYSTAL. 1992. Neutrophil elastase in respiratory lining fluid of individuals with cystic fibrosis induces IL-8 gene expression in a human bronchial epithelial cell line. J. Clin. Invest. **89:** 1478–1484.

76. CHURCHILL, L., B. FRIEDMAN, R. P. SCHLEIMER & D. PROUD. 1992. Production of granulocyte macrophage colony stimulating factor by cultured human tracheal epithelial cells. Immunology **75:** 189–195.

77. BECKER, S., H. S. KOREN & D. HENKE. 1993. Interleukin-8 expression in normal nasal epithelium and its modulation by infection with respiratory syncytial virus and cytokines tumor necrosis factor, interleukin-1 and interleukin-6. Am. J. Respir. Cell. Mol. Biol. **8:** 20–27.

78. STANDIFORD, T. J., S. L. KUNKEL, M. A. BASHA, S. W. CHENSUE, J. P. LYNCH III, G. B. TOEWS, J. WESTWICK & R. M. STRIETER. 1990. Interleukin-8 gene expression by pulmonary epithelial cell line. A model for cytokine networks in the lung. J. Clin. Invest. **86:** 1945–1953.

79. NAKAMURA, H., K. YOSHIMURA, H. A. JAFFE & R. G. CRYSTAL. 1991. Interleukin-8 gene expression in human bronchial epithelial cells. J. Biol. Chem. **266:** 19611–19617.

80. CROMWELL, O., Q. HAMID, C. J. CORRIGAN, J. BARKANS, Q. MENG, P. D. COLLINS

& A. B. KAY. 1992. Expression and generation of interleukin-8, IL-6 and granulocyte-macrophage colony-stimulating factor by bronchial epithelial cells and enhancement by IL-1beta and tumor necrosis factor. Immunology **77:** 330–337.

81. SNYERS, L. & J. CONTENT. 1992. Enhancement of IL-6 receptor beta chain (gp 130) expression by IL-6, IL-1 and TNF in human epithelial cells. Biochem. Biophys. Res. Commun. **185:** 902–908.

82. QUAY, J. S., S. BECKER, H. S. KOREN, W. A. CLAPP & D. A. SCHWARTZ. 1993. Comparison of cytokine (IL-1, sIL-1RA, IL-6 and TNF) expression in human bronchial epithelium and in alveolar macrophages exposed to endotoxin-contaminated grain dust. Am. Rev. Respir. Dis. **147:** A19.

83. NOAH, T. & S. BECKER. 1993. Respiratory syncytial virus-induced cytokine production by a human bronchial epithelial cell line. Am. J. Physiol. In press.

84. DEVLIN, R. B., K. P. McKINNON, T. NOAH, S. BECKER & H. S. KOREN. 1993. Cytokine and fibronectin production by human alveolar macrophages and airway epithelial cells exposed to ozone *in vitro*. Am. J. Physiol. In press.

85. SOUKUP, J., K. P. McKINNON, T. NOAH, R. B. DEVLIN & S. BECKER. 1993. Ozone exposure before virus infection of human airway epithelial cells results in decreased virus production and increased cytokine release. Submitted for publication in Am. J. Physiol.

86. OHNISHI, M., J. RUHNO, J. BIENENSTOCK, J. DOLOVICH & J. DENBURG. 1989. Hematopoietic growth factor production by cultured cells of human nasal polyp epithelial scrapings: Kinetics, cell source, and relationship to clinical status. J. Allergy Clin. Immunol. **83:** 1091–1100.

87. MARINI, M., E. VITTORI, J. HOLLEMBORG & S. MATTOLI. 1992. Expression of potent inflammatory cytokines, granulocyte-macrophage colony stimulating factor, and interleukin-6 and interleukin-8, in bronchial epithelial cells of patients with asthma. J. Allergy Clin. Immunol. **89:** 1001–1009.

88. ANWAR, A. R. F., R. MOQBEL, G. M. WALSH, A. B. KAY & A. J. WARDLAW. 1993. Adhesion to fibronectin prolongs eosinophil survival. J. Exp. Med. **177:** 839–843.

Chemical Mediators and Adhesion Molecules Involved in Eosinophil Accumulation *In Vivo*[a]

V. B. WEG AND T. J. WILLIAMS

Department of Applied Pharmacology
National Heart & Lung Institute
Dovehouse Street
London SW3 6LY, United Kingdom

INTRODUCTION

Eosinophil accumulation in tissues is a prominent feature of local host defence reactions to helminth parasites, and these cells are equipped to adhere to and kill such organisms. For an unknown reason, eosinophils also accumulate in high numbers in the lungs of asthmatics, and the number of cells present correlates with the degree of lung dysfunction in terms of bronchial hyperreactivity to spasmogens.[1,2] A causal relationship has been suggested by the observation that inhibition of eosinophil accumulation in a monkey model of allergic asthma reduces bronchial hyperreactivity in parallel.[3] Thus, in asthmatics an inappropriate reaction appears to be triggered in which eosinophils are targeted on lung tissue, inducing cell damage notably in the epithelial cells lining the conducting airways. These observations have raised considerable interest in the mechanisms underlying eosinophil accumulation in inflammatory reactions, and particularly in cell–cell signaling by soluble mediators and the adhesion processes involved.

The mechanisms involved in eosinophil accumulation are complex, as with all leukocyte types. This situation is compounded by the fact that several chemically different mediators can serve the same function; the complexity probably reflecting the evolutionary pressures to limit chemical subversion by parasites.

CHEMICAL MEDIATORS

Detection of a potentially injurious stimulus triggers the local release of chemical mediators essential to orchestrate the accumulation of eosinophils in the affected tissue. At least three types of signal are implicated. One type of signal (the "chemoattractant") regulates the local events involved in eosinophil accumulation from the microvascular bed (usually via venules). A second type of signal "primes" eosinophils in the circulation. A third type releases marginated eosinophils from bone-marrow sinusoids and stimulates eosinophilopoiesis. Experimental inhibition of the release or action of any of these can suppress eosinophil accumulation *in vivo*, which leads to some confusion in identifying the important endogenous

[a] This research was generously supported by the National Asthma Campaign, UK, and the Wellcome Trust, UK.

146

chemoattractants involved. Several different endogenous molecules have been shown to have chemoattractant activity for eosinophils. Many of these are not eosinophil-specific in their actions. Phases of selective eosinophil accumulation are prominent *in vivo,* however, suggesting that selective mediators are of particular interest. For a number of years the major *in vitro* system for detecting chemoattractants has been the Boyden chamber. This has been of enormous value in detecting such agents, but is clearly a poor analogue of the dynamic events occurring *in vivo* in terms of mechanisms. *In vivo* the chemoattractant has to induce the trapping of moving eosinophils on the endothelial surface followed by migration through endothelial junctions, and subsequently passage through the perivascular basement membrane and then through the tissue matrix. This process is dependent on upregulation of adhesion molecules on the leukocyte and/or on microvascular endothelial cells, followed by the attachment of these molecules to their complementary ligands (see sections on adhesion molecules).

The major chemical mediators implicated as eosinophil chemoattractants are outlined below.

Lipid Mediators

The phospholipid, platelet activating factor (PAF) induces chemotaxis in Boyden chambers[4] and induces the accumulation of eosinophils when administered to a skin window chamber in man.[5,6] Interestingly, eosinophil accumulation in human skin was only observed in atopic subjects, implying that the eosinophils are already primed in these individuals.[5,6] Accordingly, it has been shown that eosinophils from atopics are more sensitive to PAF in Boyden chambers.[7] Several other interactions have been observed, that is, the cytokines granulocyte-macrophage colony stimulating factor (GM–CSF), interleukin-3 (IL-3), IL-5 and the neuropeptides substance P and CGRP have all been shown to prime eosinophils to enhance chemotactic responses to PAF.[7,8] Several papers have described eosinophil accumulation induced by administration of exogenous PAF in animals.[9–12] In one of these studies in the rat there was evidence that PAF induced the synthesis of a secondary peptide mediator that was responsible for eosinophil accumulation.[12]

Leukotriene B_4, in addition to its potent effects on neutrophils,[13] is also chemotactic for eosinophils *in vitro.*[14] Intradermally injected LTB_4 is potent in inducing the accumulation of ^{111}In-eosinophils in the guinea-pig.[10] The eosinophil chemoattractant activity produced by challenged/sensitized guinea-pig lung fragments, formerly thought to reside in small peptides, was later identified as LTB_4 and a related arachidonate metabolite 8,15-di-HETE.[15] Further, aerosolized LTB_4 administered by inhalation to guinea pigs was shown to induce eosinophil accumulation[16] and a selective LTB_4 antagonist to inhibit eosinophil accumulation induced by antigen challenge of sensitized guinea pigs.[17] Other arachidonate metabolites have also been implicated as chemoattractants. Peptidoleukotrienes are better known for their potent spasmogenic effects on airway and vascular smooth muscle. However, one study showed the peptidoleukotrienes LTC_4 and LTD_4 inducing eosinophil accumulation in guinea-pig lungs, and a LTD_4 antagonist suppressing eosinophil accumulation in response to antigen challenge of sensitized guinea pigs.[18] Another study showed a potent eosinophil chemotactic agent generated on incubation of eosinophils with arachidonic acid.[19] This agent differed from other known arachidonic acid metabolites. Further, 20-hydroxy-LTB_4 and LTB_4 have been shown to induce eosinophil accumulation in skin window experiments in man.[20]

Peptide Mediators

The complement-derived peptide C5a is a potent chemoattractant for eosino-phils in Boyden chambers[21] and in skin.[10] However, the effect is nonselective, with C5a also exerting potent effects on neutrophils and other cell types.

More interest has focused on IL-5. This cytokine was originally discovered because of its potent activity on eosinophilopoiesis and eosinophil survival.[22,23] The report that human recombinant IL-5 was selectively chemotactic for human eosinophils in Boyden chambers led to the suggestion that this cytokine may be an important chemoattractant for eosinophils in allergic reactions *in vivo*.[24] In support of this, IL-5 mRNA has been shown to be elevated in bronchial biopsies from asthmatics and expression correlates with the infiltration of secreting eosinophils.[25] Further, it has been shown that a neutralizing antibody against IL-5 suppresses eosinophil accumulation in the lungs of challenged/sensitized guinea pigs[26-28] and in the peritoneal cavities of challenged/sensitized mice.[29] In contrast, recombinant human IL-5 was shown not to induce eosinophil accumulation in guinea-pig skin *in vivo*.[30] These observations can be reconciled if IL-5 is generated locally in tissues, but has the major function of stimulating the bone marrow and priming eosinophils. In support of this IL-5 has been demonstrated in the circulation of allergic asthmatics[31] and has a marked priming effect on eosinophils to other agents such as PAF.[32-34] Interestingly, only cells from normal subjects exhibited this effect; eosinophils from asthmatics appearing to be already primed.[33] Although not specific for eosinophils, GM–CSF and IL-3 are similarly elevated in the circulation of allergic asthmatics, and these agents may also have a priming function on eosinophils.[35] Some evidence suggests that other cytokines, IL-1 and tumor necrosis factor (TNF),[36] may play a role in eosinophil accumulation, perhaps because of their action in inducing adhesion molecule expression on the endothelium, or alternatively they may be intermediates in triggering the release of eosinophil chemoattrac-tants. IL-4 may also have a role *in vivo* by stimulating the upregulation of endothelial cell VCAM-1, as described in the following section on adhesion molecules.

The discovery of IL-8 and related chemotactic cytokines (chemokines) has stimulated renewed interest in uncovering selective leukocyte chemoattractants. The chemokine family is divided into two branches (C-X-C and C-C) according to the relative position of the *N*-terminal two cysteines.[37,38] Members of the C-X-C branch of the family are predominantly potent neutrophil chemoattractants. How-ever, normal human eosinophils primed with GM–CSF or IL-3 do exhibit chemo-tactic responses to IL-8,[39] and human IL-8 induces the accumulation of eosinophils in guinea-pig skin,[30] although this is not a potent effect.

The potential importance of the C-C branch of the chemokine family as eosino-phil chemoattractant was revealed by studies on platelets. Initially it was shown that platelets could be stimulated to release an eosinophil chemoattractant.[20,40] Subsequently the important observation was made that platelet-derived regulated and normal T-lymphocyte expressed and secreted (RANTES), formerly recog-nized as a mononuclear cell stimulus, was also a potent eosinophil chemotactic agent *in vitro*.[40] This was confirmed by other groups that observed eosinophil activation in addition,[41,42] and the further observation was made that another member of the same branch, macrophage inflammatory protein-1α (MIP-1α), also stimulated eosinophils *in vitro*.[41] Little information is available concerning the *in vivo* activity of these molecules. Recently it has been shown that human RANTES induces eosinophil accumulation when injected intradermally in the dog;[43] how-ever, human RANTES and MIP-1α were inactive when tested in guinea-pig skin.[44]

The potential importance of this family has been further highlighted by recent experiments in our laboratory.[44,45] These experiments were designed to detect eosinophil chemoattractants generated *in vivo* in allergic reactions using an *in vivo* bioassay to measure relevant activity. Sensitized guinea pigs were challenged with aerosolized ovalbumin and bronchoalveolar lavage (BAL) fluid collected at intervals up to 24 hours postchallenge. BAL fluid was then injected intradermally into unsensitized assay guinea pigs injected intravenously with ^{111}In-labeled eosinophils. Radioactivity was measured in excised skin punch samples after a defined accumulation period. Activity was maximal in 3- to 6-hour BAL fluid samples. Pooled BAL samples were purified by a series of HPLC steps, using the skin system to test fractions throughout. Microsequencing revealed a novel 73 amino acid C-C chemokine, "eotaxin," showing low homology with human RANTES and MIP-1α, and approximately 50% homology with human MCP-1, MCP-2 and MCP-3. Eotaxin is highly potent in inducing eosinophil accumulation in the skin and lung,[45] but has no significant effect on neutrophil accumulation.[44] Interestingly, eotaxin stimulates both guinea-pig and human eosinophils *in vitro*.[44,45]

In addition to these agents, several partially characterized chemoattractants have been described[46–48] that may represent new molecules. On chemical identification these factors may prove to correspond to molecules discussed earlier, or they may represent new molecular structures.

ADHESION MOLECULES

Assays of leukocyte adhesion *in vitro* to gelatinized tissue culture plates or to cultured human umbilical vein endothelial cells (HUVEC) have been used to investigate the role of adhesion molecules and their ligands in the process of eosinophil attachment. Investigations of the interaction between purified human eosinophils and HUVEC showed that treatment of endothelial cells with IL-1, TNFα, and lipopolysaccharide (LPS) led to a time- and dose-dependent increase in adhesiveness for unstimulated eosinophils.[49] In addition, a variety of mediators, such as N-formyl-methionyl-leucyl-phenylalanine (FMLP), PAF, and TNF, directly activate eosinophils for enhanced adhesiveness to both unstimulated HUVEC and gelatinized plates.[49,50] In these studies, increased adhesion of stimulated eosinophils was inhibited by monoclonal antibodies (mAb) directed against the common β_1-subunit of the leukocyte integrin family (CD11/CD18). These observations were further extended with the demonstration that eosinophil expression of the α-chains of the CD11/CD18 integrins was comparable to that of neutrophils.[51] IL-5 and IL-3 have also been shown to enhance eosinophil, but not neutrophil, adherence reactions *in vitro*, by a mechanism dependent, at least in part, on the CD11/CD18 family of adhesion molecules.[52] The existence of mediators that cause selective hyperadherence of eosinophils may partly explain the preferential accumulation of this cell type at sites of allergic inflammation.

Cultured endothelial cells stimulated with IL-1, TNF, or LPS can express a variety of molecules that may play a role in eosinophil adhesion. As with the neutrophil, eosinophil adherence to cytokine-stimulated endothelial cells has been shown to be inhibited by mAbs against ICAM-1 and E-selectin.[53–55] More recently, it was shown that eosinophils can adhere via E-selectin or ICAM-1 expressed in isolation by COS cells transfected with cDNA for these molecules; adhesion via E-selectin or ICAM-1 did not depend on the activation of eosinophils by pretreatment with inflammatory mediators.[56] Thus, eosinophil adhesion to cultured endothelial cells has many functional and molecular characteristics similar to those of neutrophil–endothelial cell interactions. In contrast to neutrophils, however, eosinophils and lymphocytes, can emigrate in patients with leukocyte adhesion deficiency (LAD) syndrome where leukocyte CD18 is deficient. This indicates that eosinophils can use mechanisms both dependent and independent of the binding of CD18 with ICAM-1 in order to adhere to vascular endothelial cells and migrate into tissues.[57]

Recent studies have demonstrated the existence of a novel eosinophil–endothelial cell adhesion pathway, independent of the β_2 integrins CD11/CD18, and involving the β_1 integrin, very late activation antigen-4 (VLA-4) (CD49d/CD29) and its ligand, VCAM-1, which is expressed by cytokine-stimulated cultured endothelial cells.[55,58,59] Within the β_1 integrin family, VLA-4 is atypical since it participates in both cell–extravascular matrix[60] and cell–cell adhesive interactions.[61] Human eosinophils, but not neutrophils, have been shown to express VLA-4 constitutively and to adhere to COS cells transfected with VCAM-1 in an $\alpha_4\beta_1$-dependent manner.[59] VLA-4 expression is not increased on hypodense eosinophils or normodense eosinophils stimulated with PAF.[59] Furthermore, eosinophil, but not neutrophil adhesion to HUVEC stimulated by IL-1,[58,59] TNFα,[58,59] and LPS[58] was significantly inhibited by anti-VLA-4 or anti-VCAM-1 mAbs. It has also been demonstrated that eosinophils can use the VLA-4 adhesion pathway independent of its activation status,[59] unlike eosinophil CD11/CD18.[52] This may offer an initial step for the selective binding of unstimulated eosinophils to activated endothelial cells via the VLA-4/VCAM-1 pathway. This process could be promoted by cytokines, such as IL-4, which has been shown to up-regulate VCAM-1 specifically, without causing the expression of E-selectin.[62,63] These findings suggest that eosinophil expression of VLA-4 and adherence to VCAM-1 may enable eosinophils, in contrast to neutrophils, to be preferentially localized in tissue sites of allergic reactions.

Relatively few studies have so far addressed the potential role of adhesion molecules in eosinophil accumulation *in vivo*. In order to investigate whether ICAM-1 and E-selectin are expressed *in vivo* during late phase allergic responses in the skin, human skin biopsies were examined 6 hours after antigen or saline challenge.[53] At this time an eosinophil infiltrate, and to a lesser extent neutrophils and mononuclear cells, were present at those sites injected with antigen. Both E-selectin and ICAM-1 were up-regulated in antigen-challenged sites, suggesting that these molecules may be involved in leukocyte recruitment *in vivo*. In an Ascaris-challenge primate model an anti-ICAM-1 antibody-inhibited lung eosinophil accumulation and also reduced bronchial hyperreactivity.[3] More recently, increased ICAM-1 and VCAM-1 expression in human allergic airway disease has been demonstrated.[64] However, these authors were unable to establish any relationship between the up-regulation of these molecules and the number of eosinophils and T-cells present in the tissue. It is generally believed that eosinophils, like neutrophils, undergo an initial tethering phase to venular endothelial cells *in vivo* that is induced by a selectin–carbohydrate interaction. This is then thought to be followed by firm attachment and emigration in which β-integrins are important. A possible role for L-selectin in eosinophil accumulation *in vivo* has also been suggested.[65] L-Selectin expression was measured on eosinophils in peripheral blood and bronchoalveolar lavage fluid 4 hours after allergen challenge of asthmatic patients. It was observed that blood eosinophils expressed L-selectin and the extravasation of eosinophils into the lung after allergen challenge caused down-modulation of this molecule.

P-Selectin expression on endothelial cells may also be involved in tethering. Mediators such as histamine, thrombin, and LTC_4 have been shown to cause a rapid exocytosis of *P*-selectin,[66] but the importance of this *in vivo* is not known.

Recently, using an *in vivo* test system, we investigated the role of VLA-4 in eosinophil accumulation in allergic and nonallergic inflammatory reactions.[67] Eosinophil infiltration and edema formation were measured as the local accumulation of intravenously injected ^{111}In-labeled eosinophils and ^{125}I-human serum albumin. The inflammatory reactions investigated were a passive cutaneous anaphylaxis (PCA) reaction and responses elicited by intradermal soluble inflammatory mediators (PAF, LTB_4, and C5a des Arg), arachidonic acid, and zymosan particles. The *in vitro* pretreatment of ^{111}In-eosinophils with the anti-VLA-4 monoclonal antibody HP1/2, which cross-reacts with guinea-pig eosinophils, effectively suppressed eosinophil accumulation in all the inflammatory reactions investigated. Furthermore, intravenous mAb HP1/2, while suppressing stimulus-induced eosinophil accumulation, had no significant effect on edema formation. These findings indicate a dissociation between the inflammatory events of eosinophil accumulation and plasma protein leakage. In this study, while demonstrating an important role for VLA-4 in eosinophil accumulation, the possible ligands with which VLA-4 may be interacting were not identified. A possible candidate is VCAM-1, which may be basally expressed on venular endothelial cells *in vivo*. In addition, since an *in vivo* test period of 2 hours was used, an increase in the expression of VCAM-1 may have been induced; however, the maximal rate of influx was over the first 30 minutes. Time-course experiments with cytokine-activated cultured endothelial cells have shown that significant levels of VCAM-1 can be detected as early as 1 to 2 hours, though expression peaks after 6 to 10 hours of cytokine treatment.[68,69] It is possible that induction of VCAM-1 is faster on venular endothelial cells *in vivo* to account for the rapid appearance of eosinophils. In addition to cytokines such as IL-1 and IL-4, chemoattractants that induce eosinophil accumulation, such as LTB_4 and C5a, may also have a role in up-regulating VCAM-1 expression *in vivo*, although this remains to be established.

While several studies have investigated the interaction of VLA-4 and VCAM-1 with respect to leukocyte–endothelial cell adhesion, very few have addressed the involvement of this adhesion pathway in the process of transendothelial cell migration. In this respect it is interesting to note that blocking VLA-4, but not VCAM-1, was found to suppress transendothelial migration of T-cells across cultured endothelial cells activated with IL-1.[70] These *in vitro* results suggest VLA-4 can interact with a different ligand to VCAM-1 during leukocyte transendothelial migration. Although the ligands with which VLA-4 is interacting *in vivo* are yet to be determined, our results strongly indicate a role for VLA-4 in the process of eosinophil accumulation *in vivo*. An alternative pathway shared with neutrophils is via CD11/CD18 as monoclonal antibodies directed against CD18 also effectively suppress eosinophil accumulation *in vivo*.[71]

CONCLUSION

Because of their prominence in asthma there has been an explosion of interest in mechanisms underlying eosinophil accumulation *in vivo*. Intensive research has resulted in exciting new findings, revealing potent endogenous eosinophil chemoattractant molecules and selective adhesion mechanisms. These findings provide the opportunity for the development of selective therapeutic agents able to block eosinophil accumulation in man. It is generally thought that this would not unduly compromise host defence, but it would provide the ultimate test of the relationship between eosinophil accumulation and lung dysfunction in asthma.

REFERENCES

1. BOUSQUET, J., et al. 1990. Eosinophilic inflammation in asthma. New Eng. J. Med. **323:** 1033–1039.
2. BRADLEY, B. L., et al. 1991. Eosinophils, T-lymphocytes, mast cells, neutrophils, and macrophages in bronchial biopsy specimens from atopic subjects with asthma: Comparison with biopsy specimens from atopic subjects without asthma and normal control subjects and relationship to bronchial hyperresponsiveness. J. Allergy Clin. Immunol. **88:** 661–674.
3. WEGNER, C. D., et al. 1990. Intercellular adhesion molecule-1 (ICAM-1) in the pathogenesis of asthma. Science **247:** 456–459.
4. WARDLAW, A. J., R. MOQBEL, O. CROMWELL & A. B. KAY. 1986. Platelet-activating factor. A potent chemotactic and chemokinetic factor for human eosinophils. J. Clin. Invest. **78:** 1701–1706.
5. HENOCQ, E. & B. B. VARGAFTIG. 1986. Accumulation of eosinophils in response to intracutaneous Paf-acether and allergens in man. Lancet **i:** 1378–1379.
6. ———. 1988. Skin eosinophilia in atopic patients. J. Allergy Clin. Immunol. **81:** 691–695.
7. WARRINGA, R. A. J., et al. 1992. In vivo priming of platelet-activating factor-induced eosinophil chemotaxis in allergic asthmatic individuals. Blood **79:** 1836–1841.
8. NUMAO, T. & D. K. AGRAWAL. 1992. Neuropeptides modulate human eosinophil chemotaxis. J. Immunol. **149:** 3309–3315.
9. SANJAR, S., et al. 1990. Eosinophil accumulation in pulmonary airways of guinea-pigs induced by exposure to an aerosol of platelet-activating factor: Effect of anti-asthma drugs. Br. J. Pharmacol. **99:** 267–272.
10. FACCIOLI, L. H., et al. 1991. The accumulation of ^{111}In-eosinophils induced by inflammatory mediators in vivo. Immunology **73:** 222–227.
11. WEGNER, C. D., C. C. CLARKE, C. A. TORCELLINI, L. G. LETTS & R. H. GUNDEL. 1992. Effects of single and multiple inhalations of platelet-activating factor on airway cell composition and responsiveness in monkeys. Clin. Exp. Allergy **22:** 51–57.
12. SILVA, P. M. R., et al. 1991. Generation of an eosinophilotactic activity in the pleural cavity of platelet-activating factor-acether-injected rats. J. Pharmacol. Exp. Ther. **257:** 1039–1044.
13. FORD-HUTCHINSON, A. W., M. A. BRAY, M. V. DOIG, M. E. SHIPLEY & M. J. H. SMITH. 1980. Leukotriene B, a potent chemokinetic and aggregating substance released from polymorphonuclear leukocytes. Nature **286:** 264–265.
14. NAGY, L., T. H. LEE, E. J. GOETZL, W. C. PICKETT & A. B. KAY. 1982. Complement receptor enhancement and chemotaxis of human neutrophils and eosinophils by leukotrienes and other lipoxygenase products. Clin. Exp. Immunol. **47:** 541–547.
15. SEHMI, R., O. CROMWELL, G. W. TAYLOR & A. B. KAY. 1991. Identification of guinea pig eosinophil chemotactic factor of anaphylaxis as leukotriene B_4 and 8(S)-Dihydroxy-5,9,11,13(Z,E,Z,E)-Eicosatetraenoic acid. J. Immunol. **147:** 2276–2283.
16. SILBAUGH, S. A., et al. 1987. Effects of leukotriene B_4 inhalation. Airway sensitization and lung granulocyte infiltration in the guinea pig. Am. Rev. Respir. Dis. **136:** 930–934.
17. RICHARDS, I. M., et al. 1989. Effect of the selective leukotriene B_4 antagonist U-75302 on antigen-induced bronchopulmonary eosinophilia in sensitized guinea pigs. Am. Rev. Respir. Dis. **140:** 1712–1716.
18. FOSTER, A. & C. C. CHAN. 1991. Peptide leukotriene involvement in pulmonary eosinophil migration upon antigen challenge in the actively sensitized guinea pig. Int. Arch. Allergy Appl. Immunol. **96:** 279–284.
19. MORITA, E., J.-M. SCHRODER & E. CHRISTOPHERS. 1990. Identification of a novel

and highly potent eosinophil chemotactic lipid in human eosinophils treated with arachidonic acid. J. Immunol. **144:** 1893–1900.

20. BRUIJNZEEL, P., E. STORZ, E. VAN DER DONK & C. BRUIJNZEEL-KOMEN. 1993. Skin eosinophilia in patients with allergic asthma, patients with nonallergic asthma, and healthy controls. J. Allergy Clin. Immunol. **91:** 634–642.

21. KAY, A. B., H. S. SHIN & K. F. AUSTEN. 1973. Selective attraction of eosinophils and synergism between eosinophil chemotactic factor of anaphylaxis (ECF-A) and a fragment cleaved from the fifth component of complement (C5a). Immunology **24:** 969–976.

22. LOPEZ, A. F., et al. 1986. Murine eosinophil differentiation factor. An eosinophil-specific colony-stimulating factor with activity for human cells. J. Exp. Med. **163:** 1085–1099.

23. CLUTTERBUCK, E. J. & C. J. SANDERSON. 1988. Human eosinophil hematopoiesis studied in vitro by means of murine eosinophil differentiation factor (IL-5): Production of functionally active eosinophils from normal human bone marrow. Blood **71:** 646–651.

24. WANG, J. M., et al. 1989. Recombinant human interleukin 5 is a selective eosinophil chemoattractant. Eur. J. Immunol. **19:** 701–705.

25. HAMID, Q., et al. 1991. Interleukin-5 in the pathogenesis of asthma. J. Clin. Invest. **87:** 1541–1546.

26. GULBENKIAN, A. R., et al. 1992. Interleukin-5 modulates eosinophil accumulation in allergic guinea pig lung. Am. Rev. Respir. Dis. **146:** 263–265.

27. CHAND, N., et al. 1992. Anti-IL-5 monoclonal antibody inhibits allergic late phase bronchial eosinophilia in guinea pigs: A therapeutic approach. Eur. J. Pharm. **211:** 121–123.

28. VAN OOSTERHOUT, A. J. M., et al. 1993. Effect of anti-IL-5 and IL-5 on airway hyperreactivity and eosinophils in guinea pigs. Am. Rev. Respir. Dis. **147:** 548–552.

29. KANEKO, M., Y. HITOSHI, K. TAKATSU & S. MATSUMOTO. 1991. Role of interleukin-5 in local accumulation of eosinophils in mouse allergic peritonitis. Int. Arch. Allergy Appl. Immunol. **96:** 41–45.

30. COLLINS, P. D., et al. 1993. Eosinophil accumulation induced by human interleukin-8 in the guinea-pig in vivo. Immunology **79:** 312–318.

31. WALKER, C., J.-C. VIRCHOW, P. L. B. BRUIJNZEEL & K. BLASER. 1991. T cell subsets and their soluble products regulate eosinophilia in allergic and nonallergic asthma. J. Immunol. **146:** 1829–1835.

32. COEFFIER, E., D. JOSEPH & B. B. VARGAFTIG. 1991. Activation of guinea pig eosinophils by human recombinant IL-5. Selective priming to platelet-activating factor-acether and interference of its antagonists. J. Immunol. **147:** 2595–2602.

33. SEHMI, R., et al. 1992. Interleukin-5 selectively enhances the chemotactic response of eosinophils obtained from normal but not eosinophilic subjects. Blood **79:** 2952–2959.

34. PRETOLANI, M., M. J. LEFORT & B. B. VARGAFTIG. 1993. Inhibition by nedocromil sodium of recombinant human interleukin-5-induced lung hyperresponsiveness to platelet-activating factor in actively sensitized human guinea pigs. J. Allergy Clin. Immunol. **91:** 809–816.

35. LOPEZ, A. F., et al. 1986. Recombinant human granulocyte-macrophage colony-stimulating factor stimulates in vitro mature human neutrophil and eosinophil function, surface receptor expression, and survival. J. Clin. Invest. **78:** 1220–1228.

36. WATSON, M. L., D. SMITH, A. D. BOURNE, R. C. THOMPSON & J. WESTWICK. 1993. Cytokines contribute to airway dysfunction in antigen-challenged guinea pigs: Inhibition of airway hyperreactivity, pulmonary eosinophil accumulation and tumor necrosis factor generation by pretreatment with an interleukin-1 receptor antagonist. Am. J. Respir. Cell Mol. Biol. **8:** 365–369.

37. OPPENHEIM, J. J., C. O. C. ZACHARIAE, N. MUKAIDA & K. MATSUSHIMA. 1991. Properties of the novel proinflammatory supergene "intercrine" cytokine family. Ann. Rev. Immunol. **9:** 617–648.

38. SCHALL, T. J. 1991. Biology of the RANTES/SIS cytokine family. Cytokine **3:** 165–183.

39. WARRINGA, R. A. J., L. KOENDERMAN, P. T. M. KOK, J. KREUKNIET & P. L. B. BRUIJNZEEL. 1991. Modulation and induction of eosinophil chemotaxis by granulocyte-macrophage colony-stimulating factor and interleukin-3. Blood **77:** 2694–2700.

40. KAMEYOSHI, Y., A. DORSCHNER, A. I. MALLET, E. CHRISTOPHERS & J.-M. SCHRODER.
     1992. Cytokine RANTES released by thrombin-stimulated platelets is a potent at-
     tractant for human eosinophils. J. Exp. Med. **176:** 587–592.
41. ROT, A., *et al.* 1992. RANTES and macrophage inflammatory protein 1α induce the
     migration and activation of normal human eosinophil granulocytes. J. Exp. Med.
     176: 1489–1495.
42. ALAM, R., *et al.* 1993. RANTES is a chemotactic and activating factor for human
     eosinophils. J. Immunol. **150:** 3442–3447.
43. MEURER, R., *et al.* 1993. Formation of eosinophilic and monocytic intradermal inflam-
     matory sites in the dog by injection of human RANTES but not human monocyte
     chemoattractant protein 1, human macrophage inflammatory protein 1α, or human
     interleukin 8. J. Exp. Med. **178:** 1913–1921.
44. JOSE, P. J., *et al.* 1994. Eotaxin: A potent eosinophil chemoattractant cytokine detected
     in a guinea-pig model of allergic airways inflammation. J. Exp. Med. **179:** 881–887.
45. GRIFFITHS-JOHNSON, D. A., P. D. COLLINS, A. G. ROSSI, P. J. JOSE & T. J. WILLIAMS.
     1993. The chemokine, eotaxin, activates guinea-pig eosinophils in vitro, and causes
     their accumulation into the lung in vivo. Biochem. Biophys. Res. Commun. **197:**
     1167–1172.
46. THORNE, K. J. I., *et al.* 1989. Production of eosinophil-activating factor (EAF) by
     peripheral blood mononuclear cells from asthma patients. Int. Arch. Allergy Appl.
     Immunol. **90:** 345–351.
47. MAZZA, G., K. J. I. THORNE, B. A. RICHARDSON & A. E. BUTTERWORTH. 1913. The
     presence of eosinophil-activating mediators in sera from individuals with Schistosoma
     mansoni infections. Eur. J. Immunol. **21:** 901–905.
48. DENNIS, V. A., T. R. KLEI & M. R. CHAPMAN. 1993. Generation and partial character-
     ization of an eosinophil chemotactic cytokine produced by sensitized equine mononu-
     clear cells stimulated with Strongylus vulgaris antigen. Vet. Immunol. Immunopa-
     thol. **37:** 135–149.
49. LAMAS, A. M., C. M. MULRONEY & R. P. SCHLEIMER. 1988. Studies on the adhesive
     interaction between purified human eosinophils and cultured vascular endothelial
     cells. J. Immunol. **140:** 1500–1505.
50. KIMANI, G., M. G. TONNESEN & P. M. HENSON. 1988. Stimulation of eosinophil
     adherence to human vascular endothelial cells in vitro by platelet-activating factor.
     J. Immunol. **140:** 3161–3166.
51. HARTNELL, A., R. MOQBEL, G. M. WALSH, B. BRADLEY & A. B. KAY. 1990. Fc-
     gamma and CD11/CD18 receptor expression on normal density and low density
     human eosinophils. Immunology **69:** 264–270.
52. WALSH, G. M., *et al.* 1990. IL-5 enhances the in vitro adhesion of human eosinophils,
     but not neutrophils, in a leucocyte integrin (CD11/18)-dependent manner. Immunol-
     ogy **71:** 258–265.
53. KYAN-AUNG, U., D. O. HASKARD, R. N. POSTON, M. H. THORNHILL & T. H. LEE.
     1991. Endothelial leukocyte adhesion molecule-1 and intercellular adhesion
     molecule-1 mediate the adhesion of eosinophils to endothelial cells in vitro and are
     expressed by endothelium in allergic cutaneous inflammation in vivo. J. Immunol.
     146: 521–528.
54. BOCHNER, B. S., *et al.* 1991. Adhesion of human basophils, eosinophils, and neutrophils
     to interleukin 1-activated human vascular endothelial cells: Contributions of endothe-
     lial cell adhesion molecules. J. Exp. Med. **173:** 1553–1556.
55. WELLER, P. F., T. H. RAND, S. E. GOELZ, G. CHI-ROSSO & R. R. LOBB. 1991. Human
     eosinophil adherence to vascular endothelium mediated by binding to vascular cell
     adhesion molecule 1 and endothelial leukocyte adhesion molecule 1. Proc. Natl.
     Acad. Sci. U.S.A. **88:** 7430–7433.
56. WALSH, G. M., A. J. WARDLAW & A. B. KAY. 1993. Eosinophil accumulation, secretion
     and activation. *In* Immunopharmacology of Eosinophils, H. Smith and R. M. Cook,
     Eds.: 73–89. Academic Press. London.
57. ANDERSON, D. C., *et al.* 1985. The severe and moderate phenotypes of heritable Mac-1,
     LFA-1 deficiency: Their quantitative definition and relation to leukocyte dysfunction
     and clinical features. J. Infect. Dis. **152:** 668–689.

58. Dobrina, A., *et al.* 1991. Mechanisms of eosinophil adherence to cultured vascular endothelial cells. Eosinophils bind to the cytokine-induced endothelial ligand vascular cell adhesion molecule-1 via the very late activation antigen-4 integrin receptor. J. Clin. Invest. **88:** 20–26.
59. Walsh, G. M., J.-J. Mermod, A. Hartnell, A. B. Kay & A. J. Wardlaw. 1991. Human eosinophil, but not neutrophil, adherence to IL-1 stimulated human umbilical vascular endothelial cells is $\alpha_4\beta_1$ (very late antigen-4) dependent. J. Immunol. **146:** 3419–3423.
60. Wayner, E. A., A. Garcia-Pardo, J. Lotvall, J. A. McDonald & W. G. Carter. 1989. Identification and characterisation of the lymphocyte adhesion receptor for an alternative cell attachment domain in plasma fibronectin. J. Cell Biol. **109:** 1321–1330.
61. Elices, M. J., *et al.* 1990. VCAM-1 on activated endothelium interacts with the leukocyte integrin VLA-4 at a site distinct from the VLA-4/fibronectin binding site. Cell **60:** 577–584.
62. Masinovsky, B., D. Urdal & W. M. Gallatin. 1990. IL-4 acts synergistically with IL-1β to promote lymphocyte adhesion to microvascular endothelium by induction of vascular cell adhesion molecule-1. J. Immunol. **145:** 2886–2895.
63. Thornhill, M. H. & D. O. Haskard. 1990. IL-4 regulates endothelial cell activation by IL-1, tumor necrosis factor, or IFN-gammal. J. Immunol. **145:** 865–872.
64. Montefort, S., *et al.* 1992. The expression of leukocyte-endothelial adhesion molecules is increased in perennial allergic rhinitis. Am. J. Respir. Cell Mol. Biol. **7:** 393–398.
65. Mengelers, H. J. J., *et al.* 1993. Down regulation of L-selectin expression on eosinophils recovered from bronchoalveolar lavage fluid after allergen provocation. Clin. Exp. Allergy **23:** 196–204.
66. McEver, R. P., *et al.* 1989. GMP-140, a platelet α-granule membrane protein, is also synthesized by vascular endothelial cells and is localized in Weibel-Palade bodies. J. Clin. Invest. **84:** 92–99.
67. Weg, V. B., T. J. Williams, R. R. Lobb & S. Nourshargh. 1993. A monoclonal antibody recognising very late activation antigen-4 (VLA-4) inhibits eosinophil accumulation in vivo. J. Exp. Med. **177:** 561–566.
68. Osborn, L., *et al.* 1989. Direct expression cloning of vascular cell adhesion molecule 1, a cytokine-induced endothelial protein that binds to lymphocytes. Cell **59:** 1203–1211.
69. Rice, G. E., J. M. Munro & M. P. Bevilacqua. 1990. Inducible cell adhesion molecule 110 (INCAM-110) is an endothelial receptor for lymphocytes: A CD11/CD18-independent adhesion mechanism. J. Exp. Med. **171:** 1369–1374.
70. Oppenheimer-Marks, N., L. S. Davis, D. T. Bogue, J. Ramberg & P. E. Lipsky. 1991. Differential utilization of ICAM-1 and VCAM-1 during the adhesion and transendothelial migration of human T lymphocytes. J. Immunol. **147:** 2913–2921.
71. Teixeira, M. M., *et al.* 1994. Role of CD18 in the accumulation of eosinophils and neutrophils and local oedema formation in inflammatory reactions in guinea pig skin. Br. J. Pharmacol. **111:** 811–818.

Transendothelial Migration of Eosinophils: Unanswered Questions[a]

RENÉ MOSER

Department of Internal Medicine/Hematology
University Hospital
A-Hof 143
CH-8091 Zurich, Switzerland

INTRODUCTION

In the course of allergic inflammation increased numbers of eosinophils are circulating in the peripheral blood from which they infiltrate the perivascular tissue. Such accumulation precedes penetration of the vessel wall. The key role of the endothelial cell lining in the initiation and timely control of this process is meanwhile coming on age.[1] Governed by induced expression of endothelial adhesion molecules leukocytes are recruited from the circulation.[2] Immobilized at the luminal surface of "inflamed" endothelium, transendothelial migration proceeds as an inevitable step controlled by proinflammatory cytokines such as interleukin-1β (IL-1β) and tumor necrosis factor-α (TNF-α).[3] Only recently, this research has been extended to minor leukocyte populations such as the eosinophils. Lamas *et al.* first described the ability of eosinophils to interact in a neutrophil-like fashion with IL-1-activated umbilical vein endothelial cells in culture.[4] Recently, we demonstrated that further transendothelial migration depends on *in vitro* or *in vivo* priming of eosinophils.[5] Taken together, these reports allow the assumption that IL-1 and TNF also have the capacity to initiate the endothelial-dependent extravasation of eosinophils. This work, however, does not explain the preferential accumulation of eosinophils in allergic diseases. Thus, alternative mechanisms were predicted, leading to selective recruitment of eosinophils. IL-5, specifically chemotactic for eosinophils, was proposed as the causative agent of tissue eosinophilia, despite the fact that the low sensitivity casts doubt on its physiological importance. Regarding selective localization, it has been demonstrated that IL-5 activates eosinophils, but not neutrophils, allowing them to adhere to endothelial cells (EC) in culture.[6] At the endothelial level, IL-4 promotes the selective adherence of eosinophils,[7] inevitably leading to transendothelial migration.[8] This selective pathway of transendothelial migration also depended on eosinophil priming.[8] In mice, intradermal injection of IL-4-induced local accumulation of eosinophils, and intraperitoneal application resulted in marked peritoneal eosinophilia.[9]

Thus, whether eosinophil recruitment takes place in a selective or nonselective way may be decided at the endothelial level. There, the pattern of endothelial adhesion molecules determines the recognition of leukocytes.[2] Once recruited at the luminal site of the vessel wall, a dynamic interplay is going on by sequential engagement of specific adhesion ligand pairs.[10]

[a] The author's studies were supported by Swiss National Foundation Grants 32-09532.88 and 32-31405.91.

ENDOTHELIAL-DEPENDENT ADHERENCE OF EOSINOPHILS

Eosinophils adhere together with neutrophils to activated EC. IL-1 and TNF are known to provoke the nonselective eosinophil recruitment.[4] These cytokines significantly induce endothelial leukocyte adhesion molecule-1 (ELAM-1) and enhance constitutively expressed intercellular adhesion molecule-1 (ICAM-1), which interacts with the β_2-integrins LFA-1 (CD11a/CD18) and Mac-1 (CD11b/CD18).[11–13] Correspondingly, adherence of eosinophils and neutrophils depends on CD11/CD18 and involves ELAM-1.[4] Additionally, IL-1 and TNF also induced expression of vascular cell adhesion molecule-1 (VCAM-1), which binds to very late antigen-4 (VLA-4), a member of the β_1-integrin family.[14] VLA-4 is expressed on eosinophils, but not on neutrophils.[15] The partial inhibition of eosinophil adher-

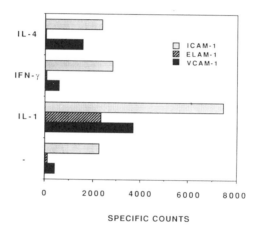

FIGURE 1. Endothelial expression of adhesion molecules in response to preincubation with cytokines. EC-monolayers in 24-well plates were preincubated for 16 h with culture medium alone ($-$), culture medium containing IL-1 (IL-1; 5 U/ml), interferon-γ (IFN-γ; 100 U/ml), or IL-4 (IL-4; 10 U/ml). Endothelial ICAM-1, ELAM-1, and VCAM-1 were detected by the monoclonal antibodies 84H10, BBIG-E6, and BBIG-V1, respectively. Specific binding was determined by J^{125}-goat antimouse IgG antibodies. Data represent mean of triple determinations of one of three congruent experiments (SD $<$ 10 percent).

ence by the mAb against VLA-4 (HP2/1) indicates a functional role of the VLA-4/VCAM-1 ligand pair in nonselective eosinophil adherence.[15]

Regarding IL-4-stimulated endothelial monolayers, induction of VCAM-1 was predominant even though it was far below the level induced by IL-1. ICAM-1 generally remained at the basic level, and ELAM-1 was not induced by IL-4 (FIG. 1). It is interesting in this regard that IL-4, along with IL-1 or TNF, inhibits expression of ELAM-1 and ICAM-1.[16] Thus, the pattern of adhesion molecules expressed by IL-4 exactly explains the recently observed selective adherence of eosinophils.[7,8] Based on the restricted expression of VLA-4 on eosinophils, selective eosinophil adherence was significantly inhibited by the mAb HP2/1 directed against VLA-4, but also included CD11/CD18.[7] With respect to ICAM-1 as counterpart of CD11/CD18, these results allow two interpretations: either CD11/CD18 is capable of binding to constitutively expressed ICAM-1, or conversion of ICAM-1 into its active form does not necessarily include increased expression. Taken together, the principle of selective adherence depends, on the one hand, on the selective expression of VLA-4 on eosinophils. To the other hand, the rationale of the selective eosinophil recruitment by IL-4 is that ELAM-1 induction is restricted to IL-1 and TNF.

ENDOTHELIAL-DEPENDENT TRANSMIGRATION: COMPARISON OF TWO *IN VITRO* MODELS

Since the fate of the adhering granulocytes that reach the extravascular compartment crucially depends on subsequent endothelial-dependent transmigration (ETM), this final step may additionally modify selectivity. Therefore, special emphasis was given in our group to the characterization of ETM using two different *in vitro* systems. On the one hand, HUVEC were grown on microporous membranes, separating the upper and lower compartments of modified Boyden-chambers. This monolayer-on-filter system allowed us to count eosinophils having passed the endothelial layer and slipped through the pores of the carrier material. Ideally, the assay served to compare ETM with transendothelial chemotaxis and to study the vectorial properties of ETM.[17] The inherent problem of the monolayer-on-filter method is the obligatory contact of the traveling leukocytes with the microporous membrane. For neutrophils, such interference may initiate immobilization by spreading followed by respiratory burst activation and enzyme release.[18] On the other hand, we have introduced an *in vitro* bilayer model consisting of HUVEC cultured on an extracellular matrix of human fibroblasts. This model avoids any contact of transmigrating leukocytes with tissue culture plastic and allows further processing for light and electron microscopy.[3,19]

Comparison of both *in vitro* systems surprisingly resulted in divergent data uncovering new aspects of the functional organization of ETM. With regard to the monolayer-on-filter system, eosinophils and neutrophils transmigrated in marked numbers across the IL-1 and TNF-activated endothelial monolayers[5,17,19] (TABLE

TABLE 1. Endothelial-dependent Adherence and Transendothelial Migration of Neutrophils and Eosinophils

Pretreatment of Endothelial Cells[a]	Adherence	Transendothelial Migration	
	Monolayers on 24-Well Plates	Bilayer Vascular Constructs	Monolayer-on-Filter System
		Neutrophils	
IL-1	+++	+++	+++
TNF	+++	+++	+++
IL-4	−	−	−
		Eosinophils	
IL-1	+++	− (+)	+++
TNF	+++	− (+)	+++
IL-4	++	+++	−

Note: Comparison of two different *in vitro* systems of transmigration.

[a] The endothelial monolayers in the different assay systems were preincubated for 16 h with IL-1 (5 U/ml), TNF (10 ng/ml), and IL-4 (10 U/ml) prior to coincubation with granulocytes for 2 h.

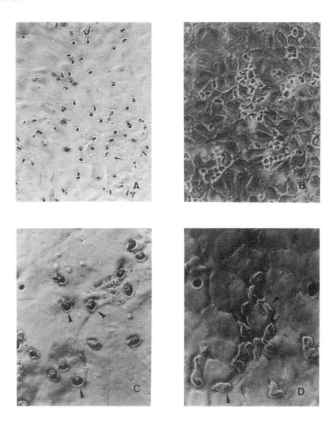

FIGURE 2. Phase contrast and Nomarski contrast micrographs demonstrating eosinophils interacting with cytokine-activated EC from human umbilical veins in culture. The mono-layers were preincubated, either with IL-1 (5 U/ml; **A, C**) or IL-4 (10 U/ml; **B, D**) for 16 h. Eosinophil primed for 24 h with 10 pM of IL-3 and granulocyte macrophage colony-stimulating factor were coincubated for 30 min with activated EC. Adhering eosinophils were randomly distributed on IL-1-preincubated monolayers (**A**), whereas IL-4-activation led to a patchy adherence (**B**; magnification 67.2 ×). On IL-1-activated EC, the majority of eosinophils were round shaped and adhered in a sticky fashion (**C**). Close association to the intercellular region and tight attachment of strongly polarized eosinophils resulted from endothelial pretreatment with IL-4 (**D**; magnification 168 ×).

1). Regarding the expression of ICAM-1, ELAM-1, and VCAM-1 by IL-1-activated EC (FIG. 1), this form of eosinophil transmigration strongly depended upon CD11/CD18, but unexpectedly did not involve the VLA-4 epitope recognized by the mAb HP2/1.[5] These data allow the suggestion that VCAM-1, despite playing a role in IL-1-provoked adherence,[15] is obviously not involved in successive ETM. Morphologically, the interacting eosinophils were randomly distributed on the EC monolayer and predominantly adhered in a sticky fashion (FIG. 2A, C) clearly distinct from the interaction initiated by IL-4. Thus, the question arises why these eosinophils transmigrate across IL-1-activated EC monolayers on microporous filters while they do not on bilayer vascular constructs[8] (TABLE 1). Concerning this difference, we hypothesize that for eosinophils the IL-1- and TNF-provoked interactions are restricted to adherence, and transmigration occurs secondarily by transendothelial chemotaxis. ETM of neutrophils seems to involve chemotaxis to transendothelial gradients of endothelium-derived IL-8 and platelet-activating factor (PAF).[20] Additionally, it has been shown that ELAM-1 induces polarization of neutrophils, upregulation of β_2-integrins, and to possess chemotactic activity for neutrophils.[21] Fluorocytometric experiments in our laboratory revealed that ELAM-1, IL-8, and PAF contribute to the increased regulation of neutrophil CD11/CD18 during the IL-1-provoked interaction (unpublished observation). These experiments are in progress for eosinophils. However, these arguments do not explain why eosinophils do not transmigrate on bilayer vascular constructs. The development of endothelial tight junctions in our bilayer vascular model[19] might inhibit eosinophil penetration and free diffusion of endothelial chemotactic mediators.

IL-4-treated bilayer vascular constructs, however, initiated marked eosinophil transmigration[8] (TABLE 1). Interestingly, IL-4-provoked ETM did not run in the monolayer-on-filter system (TABLE 1). Interference with the microporous filter seems to stop traveling eosinophils, pointing to an increase in stickiness due to the contact with IL-4-activated EC. Compared to the random distribution of eosinophils interacting with IL-1-activated EC, IL-4 pretreatment resulted in a patchy adherence pattern of (FIG. 2B). The eosinophils were polarized and tightly attached at the intercellular region of EC (FIG. 2D). Moreover, they closely resembled neutrophils in contact with IL-1-stimulated endothelium.[17] From video microscopic observations we conclude that the previously described flat polarized shape resulted from the fast movement of these granulocytes. With reference to Dierich et al.,[22] such surface-attached movement was called *haptotaxis*.[17]

CONCLUDING REMARKS

Adherence of eosinophils is selectively induced by IL-4-activated EC. Such adherence is inevitably linked to ETM, representing a potent pathway for selective eosinophil recruitment. Using only bilayer vascular constructs, we demonstrated that it is predominantly IL-1 and TNF that initiate ETM of neutrophils, whereas IL-4 exclusively promotes ETM of eosinophils. However, the monolayer-on-filter assay, which is a more artificial system, provokes the IL-1-induced transmigration of neutrophils and eosinophils. The causative mechanism and the *in vivo* relevance of this difference remain to be determined. Finally, these diverging data call special attention to the importance of more physiological *in vitro* systems.

REFERENCES

1. LAWRENCE, B. W. & T. A. SPRINGER. 1991. Leukocytes roll on a selectin at physiologic flow rates: Distinction from a prerequisite for adhesion through integrins. Cell **65:** 859–873.
2. SPRINGER, T. A. 1990. Adhesion receptors of the immune system. Nature **346:** 425–434.
3. MOSER, R., B. SCHLEIFFENBAUM, P. GROSCURTH & J. FEHR. 1989. Interleukin 1

and tumor necrosis factor stimulate human vascular endothelial cells to promote transendothelial neutrophil passage. J. Clin. Invest. **83:** 444–455.

4. LAMAS, A. M., C. M. MULRONEY & R. P. SCHLEIMER. 1988. Studies on the adhesive interaction between purified human eosinophils and cultured vascular endothelial cells. J. Immunol. **140:** 1500–1505.

5. MOSER, R., J. FEHR, L. OLGIATI & P. L. B. BRUIJNZEEL. 1992. Migration of primed human eosinophils across cytokine-activated endothelial cell monolayers. Blood **79:** 30–38.

6. WALSH, G. M., A. HARTNELL, A. J. WARDLAW, K. KURIHARA, C. J. SANDERSON & A. B. KAY. 1990. IL-5 enhances the in vitro adhesion of human eosinophils, but not neutrophils, in a leucocyte integrin (CD11/18)-dependent manner. Immunology **71:** 258–265.

7. SCHLEIMER, R. P., S. A. STERBINSKY, J. KAISER, C. A. BICKEL, D. A. KLUNK, K. TOMIOKA, W. NEWMAN, F. W. LUSCINSKAS, M. A. GIMBRONE, JR., B. W. MCINTIRE & B. S. BOCHNER. 1992. IL-4 induces adherence of human eosinophils and basophils but not of neutrophils to endothelium. Association with expression of VCAM-1. J. Immunol. **148:** 1086–1092.

8. MOSER, R., J. FEHR & P. L. B. BRUIJNZEEL. 1992. Interleukin-4 controls the selective endothelium-driven extravasation of eosinophils from allergic individuals. J. Immunol. **149:** 1432–1438.

9. MOSER, R., P. GROSCURTH, J. CARBALLIDO, P. L. B. BRUIJNZEEL, K. BLASER, C. H. HEUSSER & J. FEHR. 1993. Interleukin-4 induces tissue eosinophilia in mice: Correlation with its in vitro capacity to stimulate the endothelial cell-dependent selective transmigration of human eosinophils. J. Lab. Clin. Med. **122:** 567–575.

10. BUTCHER, E. C. 1991. Leucocyte-endothelial cell recognition: Three (or more) steps to specificity and diversity. Cell **67:** 1033–1036.

11. MARLIN, S. D. & T. A. SPRINGER. 1987. Purified intercellular adhesion molecule-1 (ICAM-1) is a ligand for lymphocyte function associated antigen 1 (LFA-1). Cell **51:** 813–819.

12. DIAMOND, M. S., D. E. STAUNTON, A. R. DEFOUGEROLLES, S. A. STACKER, J. GARCIA-AGUILAR, M. L. HIBBS & T. A. SPRINGER. 1990. ICAM-1 (CD54): A counter-receptor for Mac-1 (CD11b/CD18). J. Cell Biol. **111:** 3129–3139.

13. DIAMOND, M. S., D. E. STAUNTON, S. D. MARLIN & T. A. SPRINGER. 1991. Binding of the integrin Mac-1 (CD11b/CD18) to the third immunoglobulin-like domain of ICAM-1 (CD54) and its regulation by glycosylation. Cell **65:** 961–971.

14. ELICES, M. J., L. OSBORN, Y. TAKADA, C. CROUSE, S. LUHOWSKYJ, M. E. HEMLER & R. R. LOBB. 1990. VCAM-1 on activated endothelium interacts with the leukocyte integrin VLA-4 at a site distinct from the VLA-4/fibronectin binding site. Cell **60:** 577–584.

15. WELLER, P. F., T. H. RAND, S. E. GOELZ, G. CHI-ROSSO & R. R. LOBB. 1991. Human eosinophil adherence to vascular endothelium mediated by binding to vascular cell adhesion molecule 1 and endothelial leukocyte adhesion molecule 1. Proc. Natl. Acad. Sci. U.S.A. **88:** 7430–7433.

16. THORNHILL, M. H. & D. O. HASKARD. 1990. IL-4 regulates endothelial cell activation by IL-1, tumor necrosis factor, or IFN-gamma. J. Immunol. **145:** 865–872.

17. MOSER, R., B. SCHLEIFFENBAUM, P. GROSCURTH & J. FEHR. 1989. Interleukin 1 and tumor necrosis factor stimulate human vascular endothelial cells to promote transendothelial neutrophil passage. J. Clin. Invest. **83:** 444–455.

18. FEHR, J., R. MOSER, D. LEPPERT & P. GROSCURTH. 1985. Antiadhesive properties of biological surfaces are protective against stimulated granulocytes. J. Clin. Invest. **76:** 535–542.

19. MOSER, R., P. GROSCURTH & J. FEHR. 1990. Promotion of transendothelial neutrophil passage by human thrombin. J. Cell. Sci. **96:** 737–744.

20. KUIJPERS, T. W., B. C. HAKKERT, M. H. L. HART & D. ROOS. 1992. Neutrophil migration across monolayers of cytokine-prestimulated endothelial cells: A role for platelet-activating factor and IL-8. J. Cell Biol. **117:** 565–572.

21. LO, S. K., S. LEE, R. A. RAMOS, R. LOBB, M. ROSA, G. CHI-ROSSO & S. D. WRIGHT.

1991. Endothelial-leukocyte adhesion molecule 1 stimulates the adhesive activity of leukocyte integrin CR3 (CD11b/CD18, Mac-1, $\alpha_m\beta_2$) on human neutrophils. J. Exp. Med. **173:** 1493–1500.

22. DIERICH, M. P., D. WILHELMI & G. TILL. 1977. Essential role of surface-bound chemoattractant in leukocyte migration. Nature **270:** 351–352.

Increased Expression of ELAM-1, ICAM-1, and VCAM-1 on Bronchial Biopsies from Allergic Asthmatic Patients[a]

P. GOSSET,[a] I. TILLIE-LEBLOND,[a] A. JANIN,[b]
C. H. MARQUETTE,[c] M. C. COPIN,[b] B. WALLAERT,[a]
AND A. B. TONNEL[a]

[a]INSERM-CJF 90.96
Institut Pasteur
BP 245
59019-Lille
France

[b]Service d'Anatomie et de Cytologie Pathologique
Hospital Calmette
CHR
Lille, France

[c]Departement de Pneumologie
Hospital Calmette
CHR
Lille, France

INTRODUCTION

The eosinophil, T-lymphocyte, and monocyte infiltrate in bronchial mucosa are mainly involved in asthma; they also play an important role in allergic chronic inflammation.[1,2] The mechanism by which these cells are recruited in asthma is not clearly defined.

The adhesion of these inflammatory cells to endothelium is mediated by interaction of adhesion molecules expressed by endothelial cells with their counterpart ligands present onto leucocytes. Studies in *in vitro* models indicated that intercellular adhesion molecule-1 (ICAM-1) (belonging to the superfamily of immunoglobulins) is implicated on adhesion of leucocytes on endothelial and epithelial cells via their cell-surface LFA-1.[3-5] The E-selectin (endothelial leucocyte adhesion molecule-1, ELAM-1), which belongs to the selectin family, is mainly implicated in the subacute influx of neutrophils during an inflammatory response.[6] Its ligand on leucocytes is the sialyl-lewis X oligosaccharide. The vascular cell adhesion molecule-1 (VCAM-1) (belonging to the superfamily of immunoglobulins) is involved in adhesion of eosinophils,[7,8] monocytes, and T lymphocytes[9] via their cell-surface integrin VLA-4. ELAM-1 and VCAM-1 are only expressed on activated endothelial cells.

Moreover, in a monkey model of allergic asthma, Wegner *et al.* have shown that ICAM-1 was implicated in the induction of antigen-induced airway inflammation and hyperresponsiveness.[10,11] The infusion of anti-ICAM-1 antibody attenu-

[a] This work was supported by CHRU de Lille (93-02).

ated eosinophil infiltration and bronchial hyperreactivity in this monkey model. Gundel *et al.* demonstrated in the same model the implication of ELAM-1 in the late phase bronchoconstriction observed after a single allergen inhalation.[12]

In human allergic disease, three studies demonstrated the implication of adhesion molecules in leucocyte influx. The first study showed that in late allergic cutaneous reaction endothelium expressed ICAM-1 and ELAM-1 with greater intensities in allergen-challenge biopsies (6 h after) compared with saline-challenge skin; this event being contemporaneous with eosinophil and neutrophil influx.[13] The second one described a marked increase of ICAM-1 expression on epithelial cells of conjunctiva after an allergen challenge, with a concomitant local inflammatory cell infiltrate.[14] The third one concerned the perennial allergic rhinitis.[15] Montefort *et al.* have shown an increased expression of ICAM-1 and VCAM-1 on endothelial cells compared with healthy volunteers, the ICAM-1 expression being correlated with the LFA-1 positive cells. The neutrophil count was correlated with the number of LFA-1 positive cells and the ELAM-1 expression. These data demonstrated an increased regulation of the expression of adhesion molecules in allergic disease and suggested their role in the recruitment of leucocytes.

In contrast, Montefort *et al.* showed no difference between the ICAM-1 and ELAM-1 expression in the bronchial mucosa of allergic asthmatics compared with normals.[16] However, a significant mucosal eosinophilia was apparent in the asthmatics but not in the biopsies from normals. This surprising result led us to develop a study concerning the involvement of adhesion molecules (including VCAM-1, which has not been evaluated) in the leucocyte infiltrate observed in bronchial biopsy from asthmatics. Correlations were measured between the clinical severity of asthma, the inflammatory infiltrate, and the level of adhesion molecule expression on endothelial and epithelial cells in bronchial mucosa. In addition, the results obtained in allergic asthma were compared with those of nonallergic asthma and of controls.

MATERIALS AND METHODS

Patients

Two groups of patients with asthma, based on the definition of the American Thoracic Society, were selected:

1. The group of allergic asthma sufferers included 17 patients (11 males and 6 females) with a mean age of 39.7, and who ranged in age from 18 to 69 years old. Seven were not treated with corticosteroid, 6 were treated with inhaled corticosteroid (1500 mg/day), and 4 with oral corticosteroid (40 mg/day of prednisolone) and with inhaled corticosteroid (1500 mg/day). All were allergic as judged by positive skin responses to common allergens (*Dermatophagoïdes pteronyssimus* or *farinae* and cat dander) and specific IgE against the relevant allergen. All the patients had airways that responded hyperreactively to inhaled metacholine or/and a completely reversible airway obstruction.

2. The group of nonallergic asthma patients included 18 (7 males and 11 females), with a mean age of 48, and an age range of 18 to 68 years old. One was not treated with corticosteroid, 12 were treated by inhaled corticosteroid (1500 mg/day), and 5 with oral corticosteroid (40 mg/day of prednisolone) and inhaled corticosteroid (1500 mg/day). All were nonallergic as judged by negative skin responses to common allergens (*Dermatophagoïdes ptero-*

nyssimus or *farinae,* mixed grass pollen, and cat dander) and none had occupationnal asthma. All had airways that responded hyperreactively to inhaled metacholine or/and a completely reversible airway obstruction. All patients with asthma were nonsmokers.

The control population included 12 patients (12 males), with a mean age of 56, and an age range of 41 to 84 years old, who had a fiberoptic bronchoscopy for a lung cancer depistage. None had a history of asthma or atopy. Skin tests were negative to common allergens (*Dermatophagoïdes pteronyssimus* or *farinae,* mixed grass pollen, and cat dander). All of them were smokers.

In the three groups, none had experienced respiratory infection within six weeks before investigations. FEV-1 was measured before the fiberoptic bronchoscopy and expressed as the percentage of the theorical value.

Clinical Evaluation

In order to evaluate the severity of the disease, the AAS score was defined for each patient at the time of fiberoptic bronchoscopy. Moreover, the treatment by inhaled or oral corticosteroids was evaluated and defined using the following score: 0 = no corticosteroid; 1 = inhaled corticosteroid (1500 mg/day); 2 = corticosteroid by inhalation (1500 mg/day); and per os (40 mg/day of prednisolone).

Fiberoptic Bronchoscopy

Endobronchial mucosal biopsies were obtained during a fiberoptic bronchoscopy. The FEV-1 (best of three attempts) was measured before the fiberoptic bronchoscopy and expressed as the percentage of the theoric value as a safety precaution, and the investigations were done only for values of more than 70 percent. Bronchoscopy was carried out according to the guidelines outlined by the American Thoracic Society.[17] The asthmatics were also given 5 mg of preservative-free salbutamol via an inspiron nebulizer. Fiberoptic bronchoscopy was performed with Olympus FT20 bronchoscope (Olympus Optical Co., Tokyo, Japan). The larynx and upper airways were anesthetized with xylocaïne 2 percent spray. The oxygen saturation was monitored with a digital oximeter. Four endobronchial mucosal biopsies were taken between the carena and the right lower lobes using alligator forceps.

Sample Processing

The biopsies were fixed in 4 percent paraformaldehyde in cacodylate buffer for 8 hours at 20°C, dehydrated in a series of ethanol dilution, and embedded in paraffin. For each patient, paraffin sections were stained with May-Grunwald-Giemsa (MGG) for specific counts of inflammatory cells. The slides were examined by two investigators who specialized in pathological data. On the MGG stained sections, the quantitative studies performed were expressed with a scale defined as 0 = none; 1 = from 1 to 10 cells/mm^2; 2 = from 10 to 50 cells/mm^2; 3 = more than 50 cells/mm^2.

Immunohistochemistry

The following paraffin-embedded sections were processed with monoclonal mouse antihuman ICAM-1 (clone 84H10, Immunotech, Luminy, France), ELAM-1 and VCAM-1 antibody (clone BBIG-E6 and BBIG-V1, British Bio-Technology, Oxford, UK). The antibodies were diluted at 1/200, 1/50, and 1/200, respectively. The incubation times were 18 h, 48 h, and 18 h, respectively. Nonspecific binding was measured by adding a nonrelevant mouse monoclonal antibody at the same concentration during 48 h. Subsequently, rabbit antibody biotinyled against mouse IgG was added and amplified by a streptavidin-peroxydase complex (both from DAKO). Sections were counterstained with haematoxylin. On immunohistochemical sections, the cells stained positively with the antibody were counted in the epithelium and endothelium by two observers, and the results were expressed as a percentage of positive cells.

Statistical Analysis

The statistical analysis was performed by using the Man Whitney U-test. The Spearman test was used to calculate the correlation.

RESULTS

Clinical Evaluation

These data are summarized in TABLE 1. The severity of asthma was appreciated with the AAS score; the mean score was not significantly different between the patients with allergic asthma and those with nonallergic asthma, although it was higher in the last group.

Concerning the corticosteroid treatment, in the group of allergic or nonallergic patients, respectively, 7 and 1 had no corticosteroid, 6 and 12 had inhaled cortico-

TABLE 1. Clinical Characteristics and Bronchial Mucosal Cellular Infiltrate in Biopsies from Patients with Asthma and from Controls

	n	AAS Score	FEV-1 (%)	Treatment[b]	Cellular Infiltrate[a]		
					MNC[c]	Eosinophil	Total
Control population	12	0	86.8 ± 4	0	0.9 ± 0.3	0.3 ± 0.3	1.1 ± 0.5
Allergic asthma	17	2.6 ± 0.2	83 ± 3.8	0.8 ± 0.2	1.3 ± 0.2	1.1 ± 0.3^d	2.4 ± 0.3^d
Nonallergic asthma	18	3.2 ± 0.2	84.8 ± 2.8	1.2 ± 1	1.5 ± 0.3	0.56 ± 0.2	2.1 ± 0.4^d

[a] Cellular infiltrate (0–3): 0 = none; 1 = from 1 to 10 cells/mm^2; 2 = from 10 to 50 cells/mm^2; 3 = more than 50 cells/mm^2. Total means the sum of lymphocyte and eosinophil infiltrate.

[b] Treatment by corticotherapy (0–3): 0 = absence; 1 = inhaled corticotherapy; 2 = inhaled and per os treatments.

[c] MNC = mononuclear cells.

[d] $p < 0.05$ compared with the results of the control population.

steroid, and 4 and 5 had inhaled an oral corticosteroid. No patient in the control population was treated with corticosteroids.

These results showed that patients with nonallergic asthma had a more severe disease and received corticosteroids more frequently compared with allergic asthmatics.

Pathological Data

The thickness of the basement membrane was increased in 15/17 patients with allergic disease, in 17/18 patients with nonallergic disease, and in 2/12 patients in the control population.

The measurement of cell infiltrate showed that no neutrophil migrated in the bronchial mucosa of patients with asthma. In contrast, an eosinophil and a mononuclear cell (essentially composed of lymphocytes) infiltrate was detected for some patients. The mean score of lymphocyte and eosinophil infiltrate was higher in the patients with allergic asthma compared with the control population (respectively, $p = NS$ and $p < 0.05$) (TABLE 1). In the patients with nonallergic asthma, lymphocyte and eosinophil infiltrate was not significantly different from that of the control population, although it was higher in the asthmatic patients. As shown, the eosinophil infiltrate was less frequent in the nonallergic asthmatic patients (5/18, 26%) than in the group of allergic asthma (9/17, 53%), but the difference is not significant.

The score of leucocyte infiltrate was significantly higher in both groups of asthmatic patients compared with the control population ($p < 0.05$ in both cases) (TABLE 1). These data showed that the bronchial mucosa from asthmatic patients contained a greater number of inflammatory cells than those from the control population.

Adhesion Molecule Expression on Bronchial Mucosa

Adhesion Molecule Expression on Epithelial Cells

The mean results for all patients are shown in TABLE 2. Only ICAM-1 was overexpressed on the epithelial cells from asthmatic patients. Compared with the

TABLE 2. Mean Results of Immunohistochemical Study with Anti-ICAM-1, Anti-ELAM-1, and Anti-VCAM-1 Antibodies on Biopsies from Patients with Asthma or from Controls

	Epithelial Cell			Endothelial Cell		
	ICAM-1	ELAM-1	VCAM-1	ICAM-1	ELAM-1	VCAM-1
Control population	9.6 ± 2.7	2.6 ± 0.8	3.5 ± 1	11.2 ± 4.1	7.3 ± 2.6	6.8 ± 2
Allergic asthma	28 ± 5.3^b	3 ± 0.7	5.6 ± 1.4	35.6 ± 5^b	17.4 ± 4.8^a	12.8 ± 3.6^a
Nonallergic asthma	14.1 ± 5.2	3.7 ± 1.1	1.6 ± 0.7	15.3 ± 3.6	7.4 ± 2.9	5.1 ± 2.1

Note: Results are expressed in percentages of positive cells (mean ± SEM).
[a] $p < 0.05$ compared with the results of control population.
[b] $p < 0.01$ compared with the results of control population.

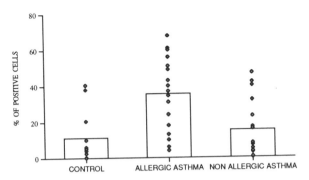

FIGURE 1. Individual results of ICAM-1 expression on endothelium of bronchial mucosa from patients with allergic or nonallergic asthma and from control subjects. Results are expressed in % of positive cells. The columns represent the mean of these individual results in each group.

control population, there was a significantly increased expression of ICAM-1 on epithelium from allergic asthmatics (respectively, $9.6 \pm 2.7\%$ and $28 \pm 5.3\%$ positive epithelial cells, $p < 0.01$). There was no significant difference in the ICAM-1 expression on epithelial cells obtained from the control population compared with results in the nonallergic asthmatic patients (mean of positive cells = $14.1 \pm 5.2\%$).

Evaluation of the relationship between ICAM-1 expression and the clinical or pathological data revealed no correlation between the expression of ICAM-1 on epithelial cells from patients with allergic asthma and the infiltrate or the severity of asthma.

No significant increase of VCAM-1 or ELAM-1 expression was identified on epithelial cells in the asthmatics compared with the control population. Indeed, in bronchial epithelial cells, only the ICAM-1 expression was described.

ICAM-1, ELAM-1, and VCAM-1 on Endothelial Cells

An increased expression of ICAM-1, ELAM-1, and VCAM-1 on bronchial mucosal endothelium from allergic asthmatics was identified when compared with the control population (TABLE 2). Concerning the ICAM-1, $35.6 \pm 5\%$ endothelial cells were stained with the specific antibody compared with $11.2 \pm 4.1\%$ in the control population ($p < 0.01$, FIG. 1). Although ELAM-1 and VCAM-1 expression was also significantly increased in allergic patients compared with the control population ($p < 0.05$), the percentage of positive cells was lower than that obtained with the anti-ICAM-1 antibody ($p = $ NS).

Evaluation of the relationship between these data and the clinical or pathological data showed that the ICAM-1 and ELAM-1 expression on endothelium in patients with allergic asthma was correlated with the eosinophil and the total cell infiltrate (TABLE 3). Moreover, although ICAM-1 was significantly overexpressed on endothelium from allergic asthmatics compared with the ELAM-1 and VCAM-1, a significant relationship was observed between the expression of the three molecules on endothelium. No other significant correlation was observed in this group.

TABLE 3. Correlation between Biological Parameters and the Immunohistochemical Study in the Patients with Allergic Asthma

r p Value	ICAM-1 Endothelium	ELAM-1 Endothelium	VCAM-1 Endothelium	Eosinophil Infiltrate	Total Infiltrate
ICAM-1 epithelium	**0.53** **0.03**	0.17 0.53	0.22 0.4	0.38 0.11	0.35 0.14
ICAM-1 endothelium		**0.63** **0.007**	**0.5** **0.04**	**0.69** **0.003**	**0.56** **0.02**
ELAM-1 endothelium			**0.61** **0.01**	**0.6** **0.01**	**0.48** **0.05**
VCAM-1 endothelium				0.45 0.08	0.36 0.13
Eosinophil infiltrate					**0.84** **0.0001**

In patients with nonallergic asthma, no significant difference was observed between adhesion molecule expression in the bronchial biopsy from these patients compared with the control population (TABLE 2). Although the eosinophil infiltrate was less frequent in this group than in allergic patients, the endothelium of the few patients presenting an eosinophil infiltrate or important mononuclear cells (6/18) expressed high levels of adhesion molecules. Moreover, this association was confirmed by the correlation of ICAM-1 expression on endothelium with the total cell infiltrate ($r = 0.52$, $p = 0.02$).

DISCUSSION

In Allergic Asthma

In this study we demonstrated that ICAM-1 and, at a lower level, ELAM-1 and VCAM-1 were overexpressed on endothelium from patients with allergic asthma. Moreover, an increased expression of ICAM-1 on epithelium was also shown in this group. ICAM-1 mediates the adhesion of most of the leucocytes,[3-5] ELAM-1 expression is mainly associated with neutrophil migration,[6] and VCAM-1 is implicated in adherence of lymphocyte, monocyte, and eosinophil.[7-9] ICAM-1 and VCAM-1 expression on bronchial mucosa endothelium might mediate the eosinophil adherence and then allow their migration, as seen in the patients with allergic asthma and suggested by the correlation of ICAM-1 expression with eosinophil infiltrate. Then, mediated by ICAM-1 expression detected on these cells, eosinophil present in the mucosa might reach the lumen by adherence on the epithelium. No relationship has been observed between mononuclear cell infiltrate and the adhesion molecule expression, suggesting that they do not participate in this process. However, we do not evaluate the infiltrate of lymphocyte subpopulation and of monocyte separately; thus, we cannot draw a conclusion about the role of these adhesion molecules in this process. In order to do so it would be necessary to identify these subpopulations.

The fact that ICAM-1 was present at a higher level required discussion. Among the three adhesion molecules studied *in vitro*, ICAM-1 is the one in which the expression on endothelial cells is the highest. Moreover, its expression persists for 3 to 4 days as VCAM-1 expression induced by IL-4, whereas that of ELAM-1 does not exceed 24 hours.[18,19] Some allergic patients (particularly those with a low AAS score) included in this study did not develop a bronchospastic reaction during the day before the bronchoscopy. This delay and the highest intensity of ICAM-1 expression might explain the preferential detection of ICAM-1 on bronchial endothelium. Nevertheless, an increase of ELAM-1 and VCAM-1 expression was found in the majority of allergic patients, suggesting that in some cases, the transient expression of these adhesion molecules could be sustained by a chronic inflammatory reaction. Such an inflammatory reaction induces the release of cytokines potentially involved in the expression of adhesion molecules. Moreover, the correlations observed between the expression of the three adhesion molecules on endothelium from allergic subjects suggest that their induction is triggered by one or a group of related mediators. Two cytokines [interleukin-1β (IL-1β) and TNF] are able to induce the expression of the three adhesion molecules on endothelial cells.[18-20] The presence of both cytokines in bronchoalveolar lavage from symptomatic asthmatics have been shown previously.[21] These data suggest that TNF and IL-1β might induce the adhesion molecule expression detected in allergic asthmatic patients.

In Nonallergic Asthma

No significant difference was noted between the expression of adhesion molecules in bronchial mucosa and nonallergic asthmatics compared with the control population. Nevertheless, for the patients with an eosinophil infiltrate, an increased expression of adhesion molecules was detected, suggesting that these molecules could play a role in these cases. The fact that no significant differences were observed in the expression of the adhesion molecules could be attributed to different hypotheses: (1) patients with nonallergic asthma were more treated with corticosteroids. This could explain the less important inflammatory infiltrate found in this group. In the same way, the glucocorticoids in vitro repress the expression of ICAM-1 molecules in human monocytic and bronchial epithelial cells.[22] Similarly, steroids in vitro decrease the ELAM-1 and ICAM-1 on endothelial cells,[23] suggesting a mechanism by which corticosteroids suppress inflammation. In this way, the lower level of the expression of adhesion molecules in this group could be explained by the inhibiting activity of corticosteroids. (2) The mechanisms and the cells involved in inflammation in nonallergic asthma could be different from those found in allergic asthma. T-cell activation is much more strongly associated with nonallergic asthma. T-cell mediators, such as soluble IL-2 receptor of IFN-γ, increase in the sera of patients with acute attacks of asthma.[24] The development of an autoimmune process has also been evoked: a relationship has been shown between the clinical severity of asthma and the T- and B-cell autoreactivity against an endothelial cell antigen.[25] These data and the detection of IFN-γ that are not found in allergic asthma, suggest the involvement of a different subpopulation of T-cell (perhaps of TH1) in nonallergic asthma, whereas TH2 cells are implicated in allergic asthma. However, since we cannot withdraw corticosteroid treatment in the patients with nonallergic asthma, analysis of the mechanisms regulating inflammatory reaction in these patients seems difficult.

This study and previous reports[10-12] suggest that drugs that counteract inflammatory cytokines, such as TNF and IL-1β, and/or adhesion molecule expression on endothelial cells might be useful in the therapeutic management of allergic asthma.

REFERENCES

1. BOUSQUET, J., *et al.* 1990. New Eng. J. Med. **323:** 1033–1039.
2. DJUKANOVIC, R., *et al.* 1990. Quantitation of mast cells and eosinophils in the bronchial mucosa of symptomatic atopic asthmatics and healthy controls using immunohisto- chemistry. Am. Rev. Respir. Dis. **142:** 863–871.
3. DUSTIN, M., R. ROTHLEIN, A. K. BHAN C. A. DINARELLO & T. A. SPRINGER. 1986. Induction by IL-1 and IFN-γ, tissue distribution, biochemistry and function of a natural adherence molecule (ICAM-1). J. Immunol. **137:** 245–254.
4. SMITH, C. W., S. D. MARLIN, R. ROTHLEIN, C. TOMAN & D. C. ANDERSON. 1989. Co-operative interactions of LFA-1 and Mac-1 with ICAM-1 in facilitating adherence and transendothelial migration of human neutrophils *in vitro*. J. Clin. Invest. **83:** 2008–2013.
5. DUSTIN, M., K. H. SINGER, D. T. TUCK & T. A. SPRINGER. 1988. Adhesion of T- lymphoblasts to epidermal keratinocytes is regulated by IFN-γ and is mediated by ICAM-1. J. Exp. Med. **167:** 1323–1340.
6. BEVILACQUA, M., S. STENGILIN, M. H. GIMBRONE & B. SEED. 1989. ELAM-1: An inducible receptor for neutrophils related to complement regulatory proteins and lectins. Science **243:** 1160–1164.
7. BOCHNER, B. S., *et al.* 1991. Adhesion of human basophils, eosinophils and neutrophils to interleukin-1 actived human vascular endothelial cells: Contributions of endothelial cell adhesion molecules. J. Exp. Med. **173:** 1553–1556.
8. WALSH, G. M., J. J. MERMOD, A. HARTNELL, A. B. KAY & A. J. WARDLAW. 1991. Human eosinophil but not neutrophil adherence to IL-1 stimulated human umbilical vascular endothelial cells is $\alpha_4\beta_4$ (VLA-4) dependent. J. Immunol. **146:** 3419–3423.
9. OSBORN, L., *et al.* 1989. Direct expression cloning of vascular cell adhesion molecule 1, a cytokine-induced endothelial protein that binds to lymphocytes. Cell **59:** 1203–1211.
10. WEGNER, C. D., *et al.* 1990. ICAM-1 in the pathogenesis of asthma. Science **247:** 416–418.
11. WEGNER, C. D., *et al.* 1991. Inhaled anti-ICAM-1 reduces antigen-induced airway hyperresponsiveness in monkeys. Am. Rev. Respir. Dis. **143:** A418.
12. GUNDEL, R. H., *et al.* 1991. ELAM-1 mediates antigen-induced acute airway inflamma- tion and late-phase obstruction in monkeys. J. Clin. Invest. **88:** 1407–1411.
13. KYAN-AUNG, U., D. O. HASKARD, R. N. POSTON, M. H. TORNHILL & T. H. LEE. 1991. ELAM-1 and ICAM-1 mediate the adhesion of eosinophils to endothelial cells *in vitro* and are expressed by endothelium in allergic cutaneous inflammation *in vivo*. J. Immunol. **146:** 521–528.
14. CIPRANDI, G., *et al.* 1993. Allergic subjects express ICAM-1 (CD 54) on epithelial cells of conjunctiva after allergen challenge. J. Allergy. Clin. Immunol. **91:** 783–792.
15. MONTEFORT, S., *et al.* 1992. The expression of leukocyte-endothelial adhesion mole- cules is increased in perennial allergic rhinitis. Am. J. Respir. Cell. Mol. Biol. **7:** 393–398.
16. MONTEFORT, S., *et al.* 1992. Intercellular adhesion molecule-1 (ICAM-1) and endothe- lial leucocyte adhesion molecule-1 (ELAM-1) expression in the bronchial mucosa of normal and asthmatic subjects. Eur. Respir. J. **5:** 815–823.
17. SUMMARY AND RECOMMENDATIONS OF A WORKSHOP ON THE INVESTIGATIVE USE OF FIBEROPTIC BRONCHOSCOPY AND BRONCHOALVEOLAR LAVAGE IN ASTHMATICS. 1985. Am. Rev. Respir. Dis. **132:** 180–182.
18. POBER, J. S., *et al.* 1986. Two distinct monokines, interleukin 1 and tumour necrosis factor, each independently induce the biosynthesis and transient expression of the same antigen on the surface of cultured human vascular endothelial cells. J. Immunol. **136:** 1680–1687.
19. WELLICOME, S. M., *et al.* 1990. A monoclonal antibody that detects a novel antigen on endothelial cells that is induced by TNF, IL-1 or lipopolysaccharide. J. Immunol. **144:** 2558–2565.
20. ROTHLEIN, R., *et al.* 1988. Induction of ICAM-1 on primary and continuous cell lines by pro-inflammatory cytokines. J. Immunol. **141:** 1665–1669.

21. BROIDE, D. H., *et al*. 1992. Cytokines in symptomatic asthma airways. J. Allergy Clin. Immunol. **89:** 958–967.
22. VAN DE STOLPE, A., E. CALDENHOVEN, J. A. M. RAAIJMAKERS, P. T. VAN DER SAAG & L. KOEDERMAN. 1993. Glucocorticoid-mediated repression of ICAM-1 expression in human monocytic and bronchial epithelial cell line. Am. J. Respir. Cell Mol. Biol. **8:** 340–347.
23. CRONSTEIN, B. N., F. C. KIMMEL, R. I. LEVINE, F. MARTINIUK & G. WEISSMANN. 1992. A mechanism for the antiinflammatory effect of corticosteroid: The glucocorticoid receptor regulates leukocyte adhesion to endothelial cells and expression of ELAM-1 and ICAM-1. Proc. Natl. Acad. Sci. U.S.A. **89:** 9991–9995.
24. CORRIGAN, C. J. & A. B. KAY. 1990. CD4 T-lymphocyte activation in acute severe asthma. Relationship to disease severity and atopic status. Am. Rev. Respir. Dis. **141:** 970–977.
25. LASSALLE, PH., *et al*. 1993. T and B cell immune response to a 55-kDa endothelial cell-derived antigen in severe asthma. Eur. J. Immunol. **23:** 796–803.

Endotoxin-Induced Neutrophil Adherence to Endothelium: Relationship to CD11b/CD18 and L-Selectin Expression and Matrix Disruption

ADAM FINN,[a] STEPHEN STROBEL,[b]
MICHAEL LEVIN,[c] AND NIGEL KLEIN[c]

[a]Department of Paediatrics
University of Sheffield
Children's Hospital
Sheffield S10 2TH, England

[b]Division of Cell and Molecular Biology
Institute of Child Health
30 Guilford Street
London WC1N 1EH, England

[c] Department of Paediatrics
St. Mary's Hospital Medical School
South Wharf Road
London W2 1NY, England

INTRODUCTION

Increased microvascular permeability during the acute inflammatory response and its association with leukocyte adhesion and accumulation was first described over a century ago.[1] It is now appreciated that inflammatory modification of the endothelium may contribute significantly to the pathophysiology of diseases, such as severe infection with gram-negative bacteria, and that endotoxin may mediate this vascular injury through its effects on cells and inflammatory mediators.[2] Under such conditions, neutrophils, adherent to the endothelium, may release proteolytic enzymes, cationic proteins, and reactive oxygen intermediates, resulting in cellular and extracellular damage.[3]

Two important molecular species associated physically and functionally with vascular endothelial cells are the sulphated glycosaminoglycans[4] and fibronectin (FN).[5] Located on the endothelial cell surface and in the pericellular matrix, they are particularly vulnerable to enzymatic degradation and may therefore be a sensitive marker of experimental endothelial injury.[6,7] The sulphated glycosaminoglycans are important in regulating vascular permeability to plasma proteins,[8] maintaining endothelial cell thromboresistance,[9] modulating cellular traffic across the vascular wall, and binding important macromolecules.[10,11] The most prominent endothelial-associated sulphated glycosaminoglycan, heparan sulphate (HS), also binds specifically to other extracellular matrix proteins including FN, laminin, and collagen.[4] Together they help to maintain the physical integrity of the vascular endothelium. Fibronectin, synthesized by endothelial cells, is involved in cell motility, wound healing, tissue repair, and leukocyte adhesion.[12,13] Endothelial cells bind to FN through specific attachment sites, including the RGD (Arg-Gly-Asp) sequence, important in integrin-mediated cell adhesion.[14] Recent evidence also suggests that proteolytic cleavage of FN is a potent stimulus of neutrophil activation.[15,16] By inducing the release of proteolytic enzymes,[17] enhancing the respiratory burst,[18] and increasing neutrophil adherence,[19] FN degradation may be an important component of the pathophysiological cascade seen in overwhelming sepsis. Modulation of the glycosaminoglycans-FN matrix in response to inflammatory mediators and cells would therefore be expected to compromise significantly the homeostatic functions of vascular endothelial cells.

A conceptual model of the processes of leukocyte adhesion to endothelium, first described by Cohnheim,[1] has now emerged, which requires at least three sequential events.[20,21] The first stage involves transition of the leukocyte from the circulating state, moving at speeds of around 1000 μm/s with erythrocytes along the center of the lumen of the capillary or venule, to a rolling state, tumbling along the wall of the vessel at much slower speeds of around 30 μm/s. This rolling appears to involve a family of adhesion molecules designated the selectins, members of which are expressed by leukocytes and endothelial cells. The second stage is an essential activation step, made possible by rolling, which is mediated by chemotactic agents released from, or attached to the endothelial surface. This activation enables the third stage of firm adhesion and transendothelial migration to occur by promoting the function of integrin adhesion molecules on the leukocyte surface. Rolling involves L-selectin expressed on the neutrophil.[22] Subsequent transmigration of the neutrophil to the extravascular space includes adherence via the leukocyte (β_2) integrins CD11a/CD18 and CD11b/CD18.[23] Circulating, unstimulated neutrophils express high levels of surface L-selectin and low levels of CD11b/CD18; the reverse is true of those that have migrated through the endothelium.[24,25] This, and the fact that several neutrophil chemoattractants induce the shedding of L-selectin and the rapid mobilization of CD11b/CD18 from intracellular stores onto the cell surface,[22,25] suggests that these changes may be important regulatory steps in the transition between margination and transmigration. CD11b/CD18 binds endothelial intercellular adhesion molecule (ICAM)1[23] and fibrinogen[26] and may adhere to other proteins of the endothelial extracellular matrix, since it binds iC3b through an Arg-Gly-Asp (RGD) sequence,[27] one shared by many extracellular matrix proteins.[14] Adhesion via CD11b/CD18 has been shown to promote neutrophil release of both reactive oxygen intermediates[28] and proteolytic enzymes.[29] However, the association between the quantitative expression of these adhesion molecules and endothelial injury is currently unclear.

In this study, we measured L-selectin and CD11b/CD18 expression and adhesion of neutrophils purified from peripheral blood when added to monolayers of cultured human umbilical vein endothelial cells and correlated these values to disruption of HS and FN extracellular matrices as assessed immunohistochemically.[6,7] We used lipopolysaccharide (LPS) and the tripeptide secretagogue f-Met-Leu-Phe to modulate cellular activation.

METHODS

Endothelial Cell Culture

Second passage human umbilical vein endothelial cells were cultured on gelatinized 13-mm glass coverslips in 24 well plates as previously described.[30] Cells

TABLE 1. Experimental Conditions Used

A	B	C	D	E	F
HUVEC only	HUVEC	HUVEC LPS	HUVEC LPS	HUVEC LPS 4 h pre	HUVEC LPS 4 h pre
	PMN	PMN	PMN	PMN	PMN
			fMLP		fMLP

Note: HUVEC = Human umbilical vein endothelial cells; PMN = polymorphonuclear leukocytes (1.25×10^5 cells/well); LPS = lipopolysaccharide (endotoxin) (1 μg/ml); fMLP = formyl methionine leucine phenylalanine (1 μM); 4 h pre = added 4 hours prior to addition of neutrophils.

were verified as endothelial by their characteristic morphology, the presence of Von Willibrand factor, and prostacyclin production.

Preparation of Neutrophils

Venous blood from adult donors was collected into 3.8% trisodium citrate and neutrophils separated by centrifugation on mono-poly resolving medium (Flow Laboratories, High Wycombe, England) according to the manufacturer's instructions. Morphological assessment of neutrophil purity and viability were estimated to be >93% and >95%, respectively.

Incubation of Neutrophils with Endothelial Cells

In each experiment three identical rows of six wells of cultured human umbilical vein endothelial cells (HUVEC) were treated as shown in TABLE 1. In addition, samples of neutrophils were held as suspensions in culture medium and stimulated with LPS and formyl methionine leucine phenylalanine (fMLP) (both from Sigma, London, UK) identically to wells B, C, and D to assess changes in the absence of endothelial cells. Fifteen minutes after the addition of neutrophils to HUVECs, saturating concentrations of fluorochrome-conjugated antibodies to CD11b (44, Cymbus, Southampton, UK) and L-selectin (TQ1, Coulter Electronics, Hialeah, FL USA) were added to two rows of wells and to the neutrophil suspensions. After a further 15 minutes the supernatants (nonadherent cells) from the same rows were removed by aspiration using a Pasteur pipette. Adherent cells were then removed by treatment with 10-mM ethylenediaminetetraacetic acid (EDTA) for one minute at 37°C and similarly aspirated. Nonadherent cells and control suspensions were also EDTA treated. All samples were added to an equal volume of fixative (2% formaldehyde, 2 g/l glucose in phosphate-buffered saline (PBS) and held at 4°C until flow cytometry.

Staining for Endothelial Fibronectin and Heparan Sulphate

The monolayers from the third row were fixed in cold (−20°C) methanol for 10 minutes. Cells were stained with a mouse monoclonal antibody to the cell attachment domain of FN (Boehringer, Mannheim, Germany), detected with fluorescein-isothiocynate (FITC) labeled goat antimouse IgG (TAGO, TCS, Botolph Claydon, UK), washed and stained for HS with cationic gold as previously described.[31] Semiquantitative analysis of FN and HS integrity was assessed by scoring the presence or absence of staining in 10 high power microscopic fields. If the fibrillar pattern of staining was seen in eight or more fields, the coverslip was given a score of 3; 5–7 fields scored 2; 2–4 fields scored 1; and staining in 1 field or less scored 0.

Flow Cytometry

A Becton-Dickinson FACScan™ was used. On forward and orthogonal light scatter 2-dimensional dot plots, neutrophils and EDTA-treated endothelial cells were clearly distinguishable. Cell concentrations in each sample were assessed by acquisition over a fixed period of 10 seconds and adhesion quantified by subtraction of the number of adherent and nonadherent cells in the control (A-HUVEC only) from those in the sample under study. The mode fluorescence was computed on the appropriate color fluorescence detector histogram for the gated granulocyte population, corresponding to the average level of expression of L-selectin or CD11b/CD18 on the cells' surface. Addition of anti-CD11b and anti-L-selectin monoclonal antibodies prior to addition of neutrophils did not reduce neutrophil-induced changes to endothelial HS and FN, nor change the adherence of the neutrophils to endothelium as compared to wells in which the antibodies were added 15 minutes after the neutrophils. Incubation of endothelial cells with LPS and fMLP at the same concentrations and for the same time periods in the absence of neutrophils consistently failed to produce any change in HS and FN staining.

Statistics

The effects of endotoxin stimulation of endothelium on adherence and adhesion molecule expression were compared by one-way analysis of variance and t tests modified by the Bonferroni method. Differences were considered significant if $p \leq 0.05$. Values in the text are expressed as mean $\pm 2 \times$ SEM.

Endothelial staining was performed in five experiments under identical conditions, in three of which neutrophil adhesion, CD11b/CD18, and L-selectin expression were measured.

RESULTS

Fibronectin and Heparan Sulphate Morphology

Changes in the HS and FN matrices are shown in FIGURE 1. The corresponding experimental conditions are shown in detail in TABLE 1. In the absence of neutrophils (A), HUVEC monolayers were extensively covered in colocalizing fibrillar networks of FN and HS as shown previously.[31] The conditions used resulted in a progressively more marked loss of HS varying from little or no change when neutrophils were added with LPS (B) to complete dissolution of the matrix when endothelial cells were preincubated with LPS and neutrophils added with fMLP (F), with intermediate levels of damage in between as shown. Changes in FN

Endothelial matrix integrity

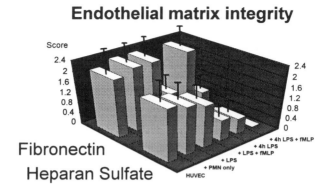

FIGURE 1. Integrity of endothelial cell heparan sulphate and fibronectin extracellular matrices following exposure to neutrophils under the conditions shown (see also TABLE 1). Values are mean score ± 2 SEM of 5 experiments. Note that disruption of the 2 matrices, which colocalize, can be dissociated.

staining follow a different pattern. Addition of fMLP with the neutrophils (D) resulted in numerous discrete areas of matched FN and HS loss throughout much of the monolayer. Phase contrast microscopy revealed a positive correlation between the presence of neutrophils and extracellular matrix destruction (data not shown). The predominant feature of HUVEC monolayers stimulated with LPS prior to incubation with neutrophils (E), was a marked disparity between HS and FN staining. Dissolution of the charged network of HS was almost complete in the face of an FN matrix that was predominantly intact. In marked contrast to this, addition of fMLP (F) induced an almost complete destruction of both HS and FN fibrillar matrices. In spite of these changes, the endothelial monolayer remained intact under these experimental conditions, as previously shown.[7,31]

Neutrophil Adhesion

FIGURE 2 shows that, as expected, the numbers of nonadherent and adherent neutrophils showed an approximately reciprocal relationship. Prior stimulation of HUVEC with LPS for 4 hours (E) resulted in a marked increase in neutrophil adherence (as indicated by a marked fall in numbers of nonadherent cells and a rise in numbers of adherent cells). By contrast, addition of LPS with the neutrophils (C) did not produce these changes. Analysis of these two sets of results (C vs. E) showed a significant effect of endothelial cell preincubation with LPS on adhesion ($n = 6$, $p = 0.02$). The pattern of changes in adherence (FIG. 2) was notable for its similarity to that observed for HS staining (FIG. 1), but no such association was observed between adherence and loss of FN.

Neutrophil Adhesion Molecule Expression

CD11b/CD18 expression rose markedly under all experimental conditions relative to unstimulated cells (FIG. 3 shows these data from one experiment). No

Neutrophil adhesion

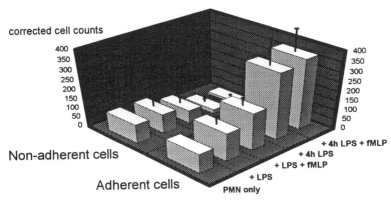

FIGURE 2. Adhesion of neutrophils to endothelial cells under the conditions shown (see also TABLE 1) as reflected by numbers of adherent and nonadherent cells harvested. Values are mean ± 2 SEM of 3 experiments. Note how the rise in adhesion mirrors the fall in HS integrity seen in FIGURE 1.

consistent difference was evident between nonadherent cells, adherent cells, and those in suspension. Endothelial preincubation with LPS did not result in significant change in CD11b/CD18 expression by either adherent or nonadherent cells. FIGURE 4 shows equivalent data for L-selectin expression. While conditions that produced a rise in CD11b/CD18 expression tended to cause a loss of L-selectin

Neutrophil CD11b/CD18 expression

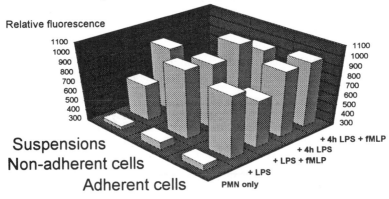

FIGURE 3. Expression of CD11b/CD18 by adherent and nonadherent neutrophils as well as control cells held in suspension under the conditions shown (see also TABLE 1). Values are taken from a single representative experiment. Note that CD11b/CD18 is raised under all stimulated conditions and neither correlates with matrix disruption nor even the adherent state of the cells.

Neutrophil L-selectin expression

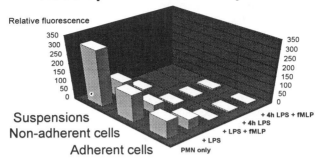

FIGURE 4. Expression of L-selectin by adherent and nonadherent neutrophils as well as control cells held in suspension under the conditions shown (see also TABLE 1). Values are taken from a single representative experiment. Note that L-selectin is entirely lost following exposure to fMLP or endothelium preincubated with LPS. Expression also falls on exposure to endothelium without stimuli—conditions that do not alter CD11b/CD18 expression.

expression, the relationship between the two parameters was not entirely reciprocal. Comparison of neutrophils held in suspension with those exposed to unstimulated HUVEC (B) showed a significant drop in L-selectin expression in both adherent (range 67–78%, $n = 3$, $p < 0.01$) and nonadherent (range 52–78%, $n = 3$, $p < 0.01$) cells. Neutrophils added with LPS to HUVEC (C) showed a further loss of L-selectin, leaving some residual expression in both adherent and nonadherent cells; in HUVEC, prestimulated with LPS, there was no residual expression discernible relative to negative controls. The addition of fMLP always induced complete L-selectin loss (D & F). Percentage differences between neutrophil L-selectin expression in cells added to HUVEC without or with prior stimulation with LPS (C vs. E) showed a significant difference only in nonadherent neutrophils ($n = 3$, $p = 0.01$).

DISCUSSION

Disruption of the HS matrix was observed in this study under conditions where little endothelial activation had had time to occur. The degree of this disruption appeared to correlate with neutrophil adhesion, suggesting the mechanisms involved in the two processes may be interrelated in this model.

Neutrophil expression of CD11b/CD18 was not quantitatively related to neutrophil adherence or to the reduction in HS. Elevated CD11b/CD18 expression was observed both under conditions that did not increase adherence (C) and when the overall level of adhesion was increased (E) and no difference in CD11b/CD18 expression was observed between nonadherent and strongly adherent cells in the same well. These findings support previous work suggesting that upregulation of CD11b/CD18 alone is insufficient to induce adherence,[32] which in as much as it is CD11b/CD18-mediated is likely to depend on further functional changes in the adhesion molecule. Additionally, CD11a/CD18[33,34] and members of the β_1 integrin family[35] have been shown to contribute to neutrophil adhesion to endothelial cells and the extracellular matrix, including fibronectin.

Reduction in neutrophil surface L-selectin expression was induced with unstimulated endothelium, conditions that did not alter CD11b/CD18 expression. LPS directly induced similar degrees of L-selectin loss from neutrophils in suspension. Exposure to LPS-prestimulated endothelium or fMLP induced complete loss of L-selectin from both adherent and nonadherent cells. In this model, therefore, adhesion is inversely related to L-selectin expression. Since our model measures adhesion under static conditions, this is consistent with reports of a role for L-selectin in inducing margination under conditions of flow.[22] It also demonstrates that L-selectin loss can occur in the absence of CD11b/CD18 upregulation, indicating that despite the frequent appearance of synchronous changes in these two adhesion molecules,[25] they can be independently regulated.

Conditions that produced maximal neutrophil adhesion to endothelium, maximal expression of CD11b/CD18, and loss of neutrophil L-selectin are those that also resulted in the greatest degree of damage to the endothelial extracellular matrix. However, our results also demonstrated that such changes in neutrophil adhesion molecule expression were not always related to neutrophil adhesion and extracellular matrix destruction. This suggests that although these molecular changes may be necessary to facilitate endothelial injury, they do not alone determine or indicate the extent of endothelial damage as assessed in this model. It can be inferred from our results that modulation of endothelial cells by LPS may be critical in inducing the generalized reduction of HS staining following the addition of neutrophils. These results highlight the importance of the endothelium in regulating leukocyte adhesion and leukocyte-induced endothelial injury.

SUMMARY

The injury to vascular endothelium seen in severe bacterial infection may be mediated by neutrophil-derived enzymes. Neutrophil adhesion to endothelium, a prerequisite for this process, is mediated sequentially by the leukocyte adhesion molecules L-selectin and the β_2 integrins, including CD11b/CD18. We have explored the relationship between expression of these molecules, neutrophil adherence, endothelial activation, and consequent endothelial injury, as assessed *in vitro* by changes to HS and FN matrices that colocalize. Endothelial prestimulation with LPS (endotoxin) caused an increase in adherence and an inversely proportional disruption in the HS matrix; disruption of the FN matrix only occurred on the further addition of fMLP. Although maximal changes in these matrices were associated with elevation of neutrophil CD11b/CD18 and reduction in L-selectin expression, these changes did not determine either the nature or extent of endothelial damage. CD11b/CD18 expression was similar in both adherent and nonadherent neutrophils, while L-selectin was shed in association with adherence in the absence of other stimuli. These changes in expression were thus independently regulated. This model may provide further insights into the interrelationship between neutrophil adhesion and activation and endothelial damage in infection with gram-negative bacteria.

REFERENCES

1. COHNHEIM, J. 1889. Lectures on General Pathology (Transl. from the second German edition). The New Sydenham Society. London, UK.

2. GLAUSER, M. P., G. ZANETTI, J. D. BAUMGARTNER & J. COHEN. 1991. Septic shock: Pathogenesis. Lancet **338:** 732–736.

3. HENSON, P. M. & R. B. JOHNSTON, JR. 1987. Tissue injury in inflammation. Oxidants, proteinases, and cationic proteins. J. Clin. Invest. **79:** 669–674.

4. KJELLEN, L. & U. LINDAHL. 1991. Proteoglycans: Structures and interactions. Annu. Rev. Biochem. **60:** 443–475.

5. RUOSLAHTI, E. 1988. Fibronectin and its receptors. Annu. Rev. Biochem. **57:** 375–413.

6. FORSYTH, K. & R. J. LEVINSKY. 1990. Fibronectin degradation; An in vitro model of neutrophil mediated endothelial cell damage. J. Pathol. **161:** 313–319.

7. KLEIN, N. J., G. I. SHENNAN, R. S. HEYDERMAN & M. LEVIN. 1992. Alteration in glycosaminoglycan metabolism and surface charge on human umbilical vein endothelial cells induced by cytokines, endotoxin and neutrophils. J. Cell Sci. **102:** 821–833.

8. LINDAHL, U. & M. HOOK. 1978. Glcosaminoglycans and their binding to biological macromolecules. Annu. Rev. Biochem. **23:** 1730–1737.

9. MARCUM, J. A. & R. D. ROSENBERG. 1984. Anticoagulantly active heparin-like molecules from vascular tissue. Biochemistry **23:** 1730–1737.

10. GALLAGHER, J. T., M. LYON & W. P. STEWARD. 1986. Structure and function of heparan sulphate proteoglycans. Biochem. J. **236:** 313–325.

11. SAKSELA, O. & D. B. RIFKIN. 1990. Release of basic fibroblast growth factor-heparan sulfate complexes from endothelial cells by plasminogen activator-mediated proteolytic activity. J. Cell. Biol. **110:** 767–775.

12. ANON. 1989. Fibronectins and vitronectin. Lancet **1:** 474–476.

13. MONBOISSE, J. C., R. GARNOTEL, A. RANDOUX, J. DUFER & J. P. BOREL. 1991. Adhesion of human neutrophils to and activation by type-I collagen involving a beta 2 integrin. J. Leukoc. Biol. **50:** 373–380.

14. RUOSLAHTI, E. & M. D. PIERSCHBACHER. 1986. Arg-Gly-Asp: A versatile cell recognition signal. Cell **44:** 517–518.

15. WACHTFOGEL, Y. T., W. ABRAMS, U. KUCICH, G. WEINBAUM, M. SCHAPIRA & R. W. COLMAN. 1988. Fibronectin degradation products containing the cytoadhesive tetrapeptide stimulate human neutrophil degranulation. J. Clin. Invest. **81:** 1310–1316.

16. ODEKON, L. E., M. B. FREWIN, P. DEL VECCHIO, T. M. SABA & P. W. GUDEWICZ. 1991. Fibronectin fragments released from phorbol ester-stimulated pulmonary artery endothelial cell monolayers promote neutrophil chemotaxis. Immunology **74:** 114–120.

17. DAUDI, I., P. W. GUDEWICZ, T. M. SABA, E. CHO & P. VINCENT. 1991. Proteolysis of gelatin-bound fibronectin by activated leukocytes: A role for leukocyte elastase. J. Leukoc. Biol. **50:** 331–340.

18. SUD'INA, G. F., A. V. TATARINTSEV, A. A. KOSHKIN, S. V. ZAITSEV, N. A. FEDOROV & S. D. VARFOLOMEEV. 1991. The role of adhesive interactions and extracellular matrix fibronectin from human polymorphonuclear leukocytes in the respiratory burst. Biochim. Biophys. Acta. **1091:** 257–260.

19. VERCELLOTTI, G. M., J. MCCARTHY, L. T. FURCHT, H. S. JACOB & C. F. MOLDOW. 1983. Inflamed fibronectin: An altered fibronectin enhances neutrophil adhesion. Blood **62:** 1063–1069.

20. BUTCHER, E. C. 1991. Leukocyte-endothelial cell recognition: Three (or more) steps to specificity and diversity. Cell **67:** 1033–1036.

21. POBER, J. S. & R. S. COTRAN. 1990. The role of endothelial cells in inflammation. Transplantation **50:** 537–544.

22. SMITH, C. W., et al., 1991. Chemotactic factors regulate lectin adhesion molecule 1 (LECAM-1)-dependent neutrophil adhesion to cytokine-stimulated endothelial cells in vitro. J. Clin. Invest. **87:** 609–618.

23. SMITH, C. W., S. D. MARLIN, R. ROTHLEIN, C. TOMAN & D. C. ANDERSON. 1989. Cooperative interactions of LFA-1 and Mac-1 with intercellular adhesion molecule-1 in facilitating adherence and transendothelial migration of human neutrophils in vitro. J. Clin. Invest. **83:** 2008–2017.

24. HUBER, A. R., S. L. KUNKEL, R. F. TODD III & S. J. WEISS. 1991. Regulation of transendothelial neutrophil migration by endogenous interleukin-8. Science **254:** 99–102.

25. KISHIMOTO, T. K., M. A. JUTILA, E. L. BERG & E. C. BUTCHER. 1989. Neutrophil Mac-1 and MEL-14 adhesion proteins inversely regulated by chemotactic factors. Science 245: 1238–1241.

26. WRIGHT, S. D., J. I. WEITZ, A. J. HUANG, S. M. LEVIN, S. C. SILVERSTEIN & J. D. LOIKE. 1988. Complement receptor type three (CD11b/CD18) of human polymorpho-nuclear leukocytes recognizes fibrinogen. Proc. Natl. Acad. Sci. U.S.A. 85: 7734–7738.

27. WRIGHT, S. D., P. A. REDDY, M. T. JONG & B. W. ERICKSON. 1987. C3bi receptor (complement receptor type 3) recognizes a region of complement protein C3 contain-ing the sequence Arg-Gly-Asp. Proc. Natl. Acad. Sci. U.S.A. 84: 1965–1968.

28. SHAPPELL, S. B., C. TOMAN, D. C. ANDERSON, A. A. TAYLOR, M. L. ENTMAN & C. W. SMITH. 1990. Mac-1 (CD11b/CD18) mediates adherence-dependent hydrogen peroxide production by human and canine neutrophils. J. Immunol. 144: 2702–2711.

29. RICHTER, J., J. NG SIKORSKI, I. OLSSON & T. ANDERSSON. 1990. Tumor necrosis factor-induced degranulation in adherent human neutrophils is dependent on CD11b/CD18-integrin-triggered oscillations of cytosolic free Ca2+. Proc. Natl. Acad. Sci. U.S.A. 87: 9472–9476.

30. JAFFE, E. A., N. L. NACHMAN, C. G. BECKER & C. R. MINICK. 1973. Culture of human endothelial cells derived from umbilical veins. J. Clin. Invest. 52: 2745–2764.

31. KLEIN, N. J., G. I. SHENNAN, R. S. HEYDERMAN & M. LEVIN. 1992. Detection of glycosaminoglycans on the surface of human umbilical vein endothelial cells using gold conjugated poly-1-lysine with silver enhancement. Histochem. J. In press.

32. VEDDER, N. B. & J. M. HARLAN. 1988. Increased surface expression of CD11b/CD18 (Mac-1) is not required for stimulated neutrophil adherence to cultured endothelium. J. Clin. Invest. 81: 676–682.

33. LO, S. K., G. A. VAN SEVENTER, S. M. LEVIN & S. D. WRIGHT. 1989. Two leukocyte receptors (CD11a/CD18 and CD11b/CD18) mediate transient adhesion to endothe-lium by binding to different ligands. J. Immunol. 143: 3325–3329.

34. TONNESEN, M. G., D. C. ANDERSON, T. A. SPRINGER, A. KNEDLER, N. AVDI & P. M. HENSON. 1989. Adherence of neutrophils to cultured human microvascular endothelial cells. Stimulation by chemotactic peptides and lipid mediators and depen-dence upon the Mac-1, LFA-1, p150,95 glycoprotein family. J. Clin. Invest. 83: 637–646.

35. BOHNSACK, J. F. & X. ZHOU. 1992. Divalent cation substitution reveals CD18- and very lage antigen-dependent pathways that mediate human neutrophil adherence to fibronectin. J. Immunol. 149: 1340–1347.

Role of Macrophage-derived Cytokines in Coal Workers' Pneumoconiosis[a]

D. VANHEE, P. GOSSET, B. WALLAERT, AND
A. B. TONNEL[b]

*Pathologie Immunoallergique Respiratoire
et Cellules Inflammatoires
INSERM-CJF 90.96
Institut Pasteur
BP 245
59019 Lille, France*

INTRODUCTION

Coal workers' pneumoconiosis (CWP) represents, with asbestosis, one of the most widespread occupational diseases caused by the inhalation of inorganic dust particles.[1] However, its pathophysiological mechanism, although extensively studied, is incompletely understood. As in other chronic interstitial lung diseases, many of the alterations in the lung structure and function are believed to be a consequence of the accumulation and activation of inflammatory cells in the lower respiratory tract.[2,3] Among cells present in airways, current concepts in the pathogenesis of pneumoconiosis suggest that alveolar macrophages play a cental role because of their capacity to release mediators potentially implicated in the induction of the initial inflammatory alveolitis then in the development of a subsequent extensive fibrosis.[4-6]

ALVEOLAR MACROPHAGE ACTIVATION AND CYTOKINE PRODUCTION AFTER *IN VITRO* EXPOSURE TO MINERAL PARTICLES

In response to inorganic dust particles, alveolar macrophages (AM) are known to secrete reactive oxygen radicals and eicosanoids. Generation of free radicals from the freshly fractured silica dust is thought to play a role in silica injury;[7] various active oxygen species are also involved in asbestos toxicity.[8] Moreover other inflammatory cells, like polymorphonuclear phagocytes, locally recruited after AM activation are also able to produce toxic oxydant species and to amplify structural alterations of the lung. AMs are also apt to release a large panel of cytokines and fibroblast growth or inhibitory factors when cultured in the presence of mineral particles.[9] So several studies have evaluated the biological properties of different kinds of mineral compounds, including pure silica, asbestos, coal mine dust, or inert particles such as titanium oxide.

It has been shown that silica was able to trigger the secretion of tumor necrosis factor alpha (TNF),[10] interleukin-1 (IL-1),[11] or interleukin-6 (IL-6)[12] at levels higher than those observed after inert mineral exposure like titanium oxide.[13] Moreover

[a] This work was supported by Grant 72-80-0318 from the Commission of European Communities.

[b] To whom correspondence should be addressed.

TABLE 1. Secretion of Human Alveolar Macrophage-derived Cytokines after 24 h of *in vitro* Mineral Dust Exposure

	Conditions of Culture				
Monokines	Medium	TiO_2 (1 mg/ml)	TiO_2 + Silica (1 + 0.03 mg/ml)	Silica (0.03 mg/ml)	Coal dust (1 mg/ml)
TNF (pg/ml)	284 ± 139	330 ± 138	423 ± 209	488 ± 395	3526 ± 3509[a]
IL-1β (pg/ml)	149 ± 81	196 ± 80	195 ± 147	169 ± 95	274 ± 220[b]
IL-6 (U/ml)	61 ± 35	72 ± 34	67 ± 39	60 ± 36	224 ± 74[a]

Note: All values are mean ± SEM.
[a] $P < 0.01$ when compared to TiO_2 exposed AM (Wilcoxon test).
[b] P = NS.

this cytokine production appears to be influenced by the mineral particles in a density- and time-dependent manner. Moreover, Dubois *et al.*[14] demonstrated that alveolar macrophages incubated in the presence of asbestos or silica produced both leukotriene B4 (LTB4) and TNF, and that endogenous lipoxygenase metabolites as well as exogenous LTB4 could act *in vitro* to amplify TNF production. In addition, it has been suggested that IL-1 and IL-6 secretions were triggered by endogenous TNF,[15] which allowed precisely the activation cascade leading to the production of monokines.

However, the respective roles of silica and other compounds present in coal mine dust has to be discussed. So, Gosset *et al.*[12] investigated the effects of *in vitro* exposure to coal dust and to its silica content on TNF, IL-1, and IL-6 production by normal human AM. As shown in TABLE 1, coal dust triggered significant release of TNF and IL-6 compared to titanium oxide (TiO_2), which was used as a biologically inert control dust. In contrast no modification of IL-1β concentration could be evidenced in AM exposed to coal dust, although an increased expression of specific mRNA expression was detected. This discrepancy between IL-1β mRNA expression and the absence of monokine secretion was previously observed with alveolar macrophages retrieved from allergic asthmatic patients and stimulated by an IgE-dependent mechanism. Under these conditions, AM released a specific IL-1 inhibitory factor, potentially IL-1RA,[16] which was also detected in supernatants from AM exposed to coal dust. Moreover, in regard to the respective potentiality of silica (α-quartz, 30 μg/ml, which is the concentration of silica present in 1 mg of the coal dust used in this study) and coal mine dust (1 mg/ml) to stimulate alveolar macrophages, the comparison of the level of monokines (TNF, IL-1, IL-6) secretion demonstrated a higher biological reactivity for the complex mineral dust. So it appeared that the cytokine secretion was induced by other mineral compounds or a complex interaction of substances and was not exclusively related to the simple presence of silica.

Besides the secretion of proinflammatory cytokines, numerous works also describe the presence in supernatants of AMs exposed to mineral particles, of factors susceptible to modify fibroblast proliferation and collagen deposition.[17,18] Both compact and fibrous particles induce fibronectin secretion.[19] Asbestos-exposed alveolar macrophages were able to secrete large amounts of platelet-derived growth factor (PDGF),[20,21] which is considered a competence factor for fibroblast proliferation.[22]

Alveolar macrophages might also act as a regulating cell. Mohr *et al.*[23] described an enhanced release of prostaglandin E2, prostaglandin D2, and thromboxane B2 from alveolar macrophages exposed to silica particles. In the case of PGE2, this prostanoid is able to modulate fibroblast or macrophage functions elicited by TNF: TNF stimulate PGE2 release which, in turn, suppressed TNF synthesis in an autocrine manner. Thus PGE2 or LTB4[14,23] could represent two important regulatory molecules in the pulmonary response to inorganic particle exposure.

Indeed all these publications reported effects related to *in vitro* treatment of cells with mineral particles. These publications explain the mechanisms that trigger and regulate the alveolar macrophage activation after mineral dust exposure. In contrast they do not give information about the respective roles of these different AM-derived mediators in the development of inflammatory and fibrotic processes *in vivo*.

CYTOKINE PRODUCTION AND ITS ROLE IN EXPERIMENTAL PNEUMOCONIOSIS

Several recent experimental studies have produced data arguing in favor of the implication of cytokines in experimental models of pneumoconiosis. The role of TNF in fibrosis development has been clearly documented in an animal model of silicosis.[24] After intratracheal instillation of silica, a marked increase in the level of lung TNF mRNA was observed, which persisted up to the seventieth day. More interestingly, silica-induced collagen production, measured as the total lung hydroxyproline content, was significantly reduced after anti-TNF antibody treatment.[24] The role of IL-1RA has also been discussed: the treatment of silica-exposed mice by IL-1RA prevented the development of fibrotic lesions.[25] It is possible that IL-1RA, which is spontaneously produced by AM in a physiological situation,[12,16] may protect against the development of fibrosis.

In another animal model of mineral dust exposure, the production of chemotactic factor for inflammatory cells has been identified. Recently, Driscoll *et al.*[26] described the production of chemokines—that is, macrophage inflammatory protein 1 and 2 (MIP-1, MIP-2)—by alveolar macrophages but also by fibroblasts or epithelial cells in rats exposed to silica. On the basis of their biological properties, both these chemokines might be responsible, at least in part, for the recruitment of inflammatory cells after particle deposition.

CYTOKINE AND ALVEOLAR MACROPHAGE ACTIVATION IN COAL WORKERS' PNEUMOCONIOSIS

To determine the *in vivo* pertinency of these *in vitro* observations, studies have been made on coal workers exposed to an occupational inorganic dust, in order to identify the precise involvement of cytokines and various profibrotic factors. In some studies, alveolar macrophages, recovered from bronchoalveolar lavage of patients exposed to mineral dust and from unexposed controls,[27] were tested for their spontaneous ability to secrete these different factors. In both silicosis and asbestosis, an increased release of TNF, IL-1 by alveolar macrophage was observed in patients when compared to controls. Moreover, when patients with coal workers' pneumoconiosis were divided according to the degree of severity into two groups called simple pneumoconiosis (SP) and progressive massive fibrosis (PMF), an increased secretion of inflammatory cytokines in PMF was observed when compared to SP and controls.[28] In a model of chronic beryllium disease, Bost et al.[29] also reported an increased incidence of TNF and IL-6 mRNA by alveolar macrophages.

In our laboratory, we recently confirmed the relationship between the levels of TNF and IL-6 production in AM supernatants, the detection by in situ hybridization of signals for the mRNA encoding for both these monokines, and the presence of particles in macrophages recovered by BAL from coal miners and also from lung fragments obtained from patients with pneumoconiosis and requiring lobectomy or pneumonectomy for lung cancer.[30] The percentage of BAL cells expressing TNF and IL-6 was significantly higher in patients with PMF (TNF: 55% ± 6; IL-6: 46% ± 12.8) than in those with SP (TNF: 34% ± 11.6; IL-6: 26% ± 10.2) or controls (TNF: 15% ± 5.5; IL-6: 13.3% ± 6). Furthermore, for the two groups of patients, mRNA expression was associated with the presence of coal dust in the cells. In lung tissue, hybridization signals for TNF and IL-6 were detected in mononuclear phagocytes; IL-6 mRNA was also detected in other cell-type like endothelial cells. This study shows evidence of an endothelial cell activation in the lung of pneumoconiotic patients and confirms the probable involvement of TNF and IL-6 in the pathophysiology of coal workers' pneumoconiosis.

Besides TNF, IL-1, and IL-6, other cytokines, such as platelet-derived growth factor (PDGF), insulin-like growth factor-1 (IGF-1), or transforming growth factor-β (TGFβ),[31-33] are known to activate or stimulate fibroblast growth directly or by induction of growth factors potentially active in fibroblast proliferation.

The development of fibrosis, namely of the fibroblast proliferation, needs the interaction of two signals: a competence signal and a progression signal.[34] In this regard, alveolar macrophages expressed both types of activities by their capacities to release PDGF, a competence factor, and IGF-1, a progression factor, in response to mineral dust. For example, Rom et al.[35] demonstrated that alveolar macrophages spontaneously released significant amounts of an alveolar-macrophage-derived growth factor (AMDGF), later identified as IGF-1. Moreover additional works described the production of fibronectin, which is known to be a chemotactic factor for fibroblast and to prime or facilitate fibroblast proliferation.[36,37]

Another cytokine, TGFβ, appears to play an important, though controversial, role in lung fibrosis.[38,39] The role of this cytokine is not definitively established, but it is thought to act as a mediator that regulates chemotaxis and proliferation of fibroblast, as well as the propagation of the inflammatory reaction.

We recently investigated the capacity of AMs recovered from 28 coal workers (19 simple pneumoconiosis and 9 progressive massive fibrosis) and 8 control subjects to release factors possibly implicated in fibroblast proliferation: PDGF, IGF-1, and TGFβ. As shown in TABLE 2, levels of PDGF and IGF-1 concentrations were increased in AMs from PMF compared to SP or controls. The assay of the TGFβ used in this study detected only the active form, comparisons of the values observed before or after acidification[40] of AM-conditioned media led to the demonstration that only the latent form of TGFβ was significantly secreted in AM supernatants. In contrast to PDGF and IGF-1, TGFβ concentration showed the opposite profile in the three groups. The level of TGFβ concentration was increased in acidified AM supernatants from SP in comparison to PMF or controls (FIG. 2). In the second step, the effects of the conditioned media were tested for their ability to induce the growth of a human lung fibroblast cell line (MRC5) in a low concentration of fetal calf serum (1%). The role of TGFβ in this model was indirectly increased by the addition to the MRC5 culture of anti-TGFβ antibodies. As expected, acidified AM supernatants from patients with PMF, but also from

TABLE 2. Secretion of PDGF, IGF-1, and TGFβ by Alveolar Macrophages from Pneumoconiotic Patients with Simple Pneumoconiosis (SP) or Progressive Massive Fibrosis (PMF), and from Control Subjects

Cytokines	Subjects		
	Controls ($n = 8$)	SP ($n = 19$)	PMF ($n = 9$)
PDGF (fmol/ml)	1.64 ± 0.57	3.40 ± 1.71	5.24 ± 2.58[a]
IGF-1 (ng/ml)	23.86 ± 5.19	23.16 ± 2.84	44.49 ± 8.17[a]
TGFβ (pg/ml)	48.88 ± 10.51	**168.20 ± 17.54**[a]	72.93 ± 7.10

Note: All values are mean ± SEM. Supernatants were obtained from a 3-h culture of 3×10^6 AMs.

[a] $P < 0.01$ when compared to the other groups.

five patients with idiopathic pulmonary fibrosis (IPF), were able to promote proliferation of fibroblasts. Neutralization of TGFβ was without effect. In contrast, AMs from patients with SP-induced inhibition of ³H-thymidine incorporation and fibroblast growth was restored after neutralization of TGFβ by the specific antibodies (FIG. 1).

Although additional experiments are needed, it seems possible to hypothesize that TGFβ, present in the alveolar macrophage supernatants, was responsible for the inhibition of fibroblast proliferation, providing evidence that activation of latent TGFβ occurs *in vivo* in an acidic environment or by proteasic cleavage (plasmin or cathepsin D).[41] Indeed TGFβ has recently been described as a potent inhibitor of fibroblast growth.[42-44] Evidence suggests that this effect was dose related and due to modulation of the expression of the PDGF receptor.[45,46] At low concentrations TGFβ would induce the production of PDGF, which promotes fibroblast growth; at higher concentrations, as was observed in SP, TGFβ would down-regulate the PDGF receptor expression that blocks the autocrine PDGF

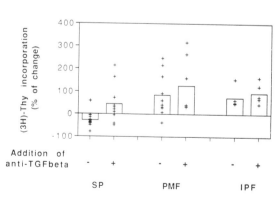

FIGURE 1. Proliferation of a human lung fibroblast cell line (MRC5) induced by AM supernatants from patients with coal workers' pneumoconiosis (SP or PMF), patients with idiopathic pulmonary fibrosis (IPF), or control subjects. Supernatants were obtained from a 3-h culture of 3×10^6 AMs in 2 ml. Before the assay, supernatants were "activated" by acid treatment to release the active form of TGFβ. Results are expressed as the % of change of ³H-thymidine incorporation between patients and the mean incorporation obtained with a pool of control subjects (1253 cpm ± 115).

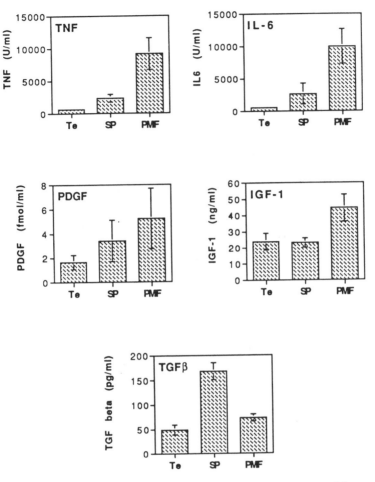

FIGURE 2. Profiles of cytokine secretion by alveolar macrophages recovered from patients with coal workers' pneumoconiosis (SP, $n = 10$; or PMF, $n = 6$) or control subjects ($n = 6$). The same profile was observed for the first 4 cytokines (TNF, IL-6, PDGF, IGF-1). By contrast an opposite profile for the secretion of TGFβ was obtained from AM recovered from patient with SP. Supernatants were obtained from a 3-h culture of 3×10^6 AMs in 2 ml. All values are mean ± SEM.

loop, or possibly inhibits directly fibroblast proliferation. Another way TGFβ acts is related to its anti-inflammatory properties: indeed, TGFβ could act at different points in the development of the inflammatory reaction. Gamble et al.[47–49] demonstrated that TGFβ could inhibit endothelial cell adhesiveness to leukocytes via inhibition of the cellular adhesion molecule E-selectin. Moreover, the importance of TGFβ was also substantiated by results observed in TGFβ-deficient mice that spontaneously developed a multifocal inflammatory disease from cellular infiltration.[50] In support of this hypothesis Dubois et al.[51] showed that TGFβ is a potent inhibitor of IL-1 receptor expression. TGFβ also induces monocyte production of IL-1RA,[52,53] a molecule that is known for its ability to prevent the development of silica-induced pulmonary fibrosis in mice.[25]

Even though some other studies supported the theory of profibrotic action of TGFβ,[38,39] Denholm *et al.*[54] showed that TGFβ increased in the lungs of animals treated with bleomycin, and postulated that TGFβ mediated the bleomycin-induced fibrosis. Nevertheless, other cytokines, such as PDGF, may also influence the pulmonary fibrotic lesions.[22,55]

These data obtained from *in vitro* experiments strengthen our *in vivo* observations. Other recent observations could support our hypothesis. For example, Moreland *et al.*[56] recently described a significantly higher concentration of TGFβ in normal lungs compared to fibrotic scleroderma lungs. On the other hand, Yamauchi *et al.*[57] discussed the possible action of TGFβ to stabilize the lung structure and the behavior of cell populations present in the normal lung. So if at the present time the exact role of TGFβ in the development of fibrosis, and more precisely of pulmonary fibrosis, remains a matter of debate, results observed after *in vitro* or *in vivo* exposure to silica or mineral dust appear, in this clinical situation, to support the idea that TGFβ acts as a protection.

CONCLUSION

Alveolar macrophages are present in exagerated numbers in the lower respiratory tracts of patients with coal workers' pneumoconiosis. In these patients, these cells produce exagerated amounts of a large panel of mediators and of cytokines. While the load of inhaled particles is often similar in mining workers, quantitative and qualitative differences in the release of macrophage mediators might represent an interesting explanation for differences observed in patients.[4] Some coal miners, through a different profile of cytokine production, might develop, despite a similar exposure, a more severe form of pneumoconiosis with enhanced alterations of pulmonary lesions and increased pulmonary function test impairment. So evaluation of the cytokine profile, and particularly of TGFβ, could open new insights into the understanding of pneumoconiosis, but also probably of other interstitial pulmonary disorders.

REFERENCES

1. DAVIS, J. M. G., *et al.*, 1983. Variations in the histological patterns of the lesions of coal workers' pneumoconiosis in Britain and their relationship to lung dust content. Am. Rev. Respir. Dis. **128:** 118–124.
2. ROM, W. N., P. B. BITTERMAN, S. I. RENNARD, A. CANTIN & R. G. CRYSTAL. 1987. Characterization of the lower respiratory tract inflammation of nonsmoking subjects with interstitial lung disease associated with chronic inhalation of inorganic dusts. Am. Rev. Respir. Dis. **136:** 1429–1434.
3. DRISCOLL, K. E., R. C. LINDENSCHMIDT, J. K. MAURER, J. M. HIGGINS & G. RIDDER. 1990. Pulmonary response to silica or titanium dioxide: Inflammatory cells, alveolar macrophage-derived cytokines, and histopathology. Am. J. Respir. Cell. Mol. Biol. **2:** 381–390.
4. ROM, W. N. 1991. Relationship of inflammatory cell cytokines to disease severity in individuals with occupational inorganic dust exposure. Am. J. Ind. Med. **19:** 15–27.
5. WARHEIT, D. B., *et al.* 1986. Pulmonary macrophage accumulation and asbestos-induced lesions at the site of fiber deposition. Am. Rev. Respir. Dis. **134:** 128–133.

6. ROM, W. N., B. BITTERMAN, S. RENNARD & R. G. CRYSTAL. 1984. Alveolar mediated fibroblast proliferation in the pneumoconiosis. Am. Rev. Respir. Dis. 119: 160.

7. VALLYATHAN, V., X. SHI, N. S. DALAL, W. IRR & V. CASTRANOVA. 1988. Generation of free radicals from freshly fractured silica dust: Potential role in acute silica-induced lung injury. Am. Rev. Respir. Dis. 138: 1213–1219.

8. MOSSMAN, B. T., et al. 1987. Implication of active oxygen species as a second messenger of asbestos toxicity. Drug Chem. Toxicol. 10: 157–180.

9. DRISCOLL, K. E., J. M. HIGGINS, M. J. LAYTART & L. L. CROSBY. 1990. Differential effects of mineral dust on the in vitro activation of alveolar macrophage eicosanoid and cytokine release. Toxicol. In vitro 4: 284–288.

10. BORM, P. J. A., N. PAMEN, J. J. M. ENGELEN & W. A. BUURMAN. 1988. Spontaneous and stimulated release of Tumor Necrosis Factor α (TNF) from blood monocytes of miners with coal worker pneumoconiosis. Am. Rev. Respir. Dis. 138: 1589–1594.

11. SCHMIDT, J. A., C. N. OLIVER, J. L. LEPE-ZUNIGA, I. GREEN & I. GREY. 1984. Silica-stimulated monocytes release fibroblast proliferation factors identical to Interleukin-1: Potential role for Interleukin-1 in the pathogenesis of silicosis. J. Clin. Invest. 73: 1462–1472.

12. GOSSET, P., et al. 1991. Production of Tumor Necrosis Factor alpha and Interleukin-6 by human alveolar macrophages exposed to in vitro coal mine dust. Am. J. Respir. Cell. Mol. Biol. 5: 431–436.

13. LINDERSCHMIDT, R. C., et al. 1990. The comparison of a fibrogenic and two nonfibrogenic dusts by bronchoalveolar lavage. Toxicol. Appl. Pharmacol. 102: 268–281.

14. DUBOIS, C. M., E. BISSONNETTE & M. ROLA-PLESZCZYNSKI. 1989. Asbestos fibers and silica particles stimulates rat alveolar macrophages to release tumor necrosis factor. Am. Rev. Respir. Dis. 139: 1257–1264.

15. SHERON, N., J. N. LAU, J. HOFMANN, R. WILLIAMS & G. J. M. ALEXANDER. 1990. Dose-dependent increase in plasma interleukin-6 after recombinant tumor necrosis factor infusion in humans. Clin. Exp. Immunol. 82: 427–432.

16. GOSSET, P., et al. 1988. Production of an interleukin-1 inhibitory factor by human alveolar macrophages from normal and allergic asthmatic patients. Am. Rev. Respir. Dis. 138: 40–46.

17. GRITTER, H. L., I. Y. R. ADAMSON & G. M. KING. 1986. Modulation of fibroblast activity by normal and silica exposed alveolar macrophages. J. Pathol. 148: 263–271.

18. BROWN, G. P., M. MONICK & G. W. HUNNINGHAKE. 1988. Fibroblast proliferation induced by silica-exposed human alveolar macrophages. Am. Rev. Respir. Dis. 138: 85–89.

19. DAVIES, P., G. ERGODU, R. J. HILL & J. H. EDWARD. 1985. Secretion of fibronectin by dust induced alveolar macrophages. In In vitro Effects of Mineral Dusts, E. G. Beck and J. Bignon, Eds. 63: 353–358. NATO A.S.I. Series. Springer-Verlag. Berlin/Heidelberg.

20. SCHAPIRA, R. M., A. OSORNIO-VARGAS & A. R. BRODY. 1991. Inorganic particles induce secretion of a macrophage homologue of platelet-derived growth factor in a density and time dependent manner in vitro. Exp. Lung Res. 17: 1011–1024.

21. BAUMAN, M. D., et al. 1990. Secretion of a platelet-derived growth factor homologue by rat alveolar macrophages exposed to particulates in vitro. Eur. J. Cell Biol. 51: 327–334.

22. MARINELLI, W. A., V. A. POLUNOVSKI, K. R. HARMON & P. B. BITTERMAN. 1991. Role of platelet-derived growth factor in pulmonary fibrosis. Am. J. Respir. Cell Mol. Biol. 5: 503–504.

23. MOHR, C., G. S. DAVIS, C. GRAEBNER, D. R. HEMENWAY & D. GEMSA. 1992. Enhanced release of prostaglandin E2 from macrophages of rats silicosis. Am. J. Respir. Cell Mol. Biol. 6: 390–396.

24. PIGUET, P. F., M. A. COLLART, G. E. GRAU, A. P. SAPPINO & P. VASSALLI. 1990. Requirement of tumor necrosis factor for the development of silica-induced pulmonary fibrosis. Nature 344: 245–247.

25. PIGUET, P. F., C. VESIN, G. E. GRAU & R. C. THOMPSON. 1993. Interleukin-1 receptor antagonist (IL-1ra) prevents or cures pulmonary fibrosis elicited by bleomycin or silica. Cytokine 5: 57–61.

26. DRISCOLL, K. E., *et al.* 1993. Macrophage inflammatory proteins 1 and 2: Expression by rat alveolar macrophages, fibroblasts, and epithelial cells in rat lung after mineral dust exposure. Am. J. Respir. Cell Mol. Biol. **8:** 311–318.
27. VOISIN, C., *et al.* 1983. Le lavage broncho-alvéolaire dans la pneumoconiose des mineurs de charbon. Aspects cytologiques. Rev. Fr. Mal. Respir. **11:** 455–466.
28. LASSALLE, P., *et al.* 1990. Abnormal secretion of Interleukin-1 and Tumor Necrosis Factor alpha by alveolar macrophages in coal worker pneumoconiosis: Comparison between simple pneumoconiosis and progressive massive fibrosis. Exp. Lung. Res. **16:** 73–80.
29. BOST, T., L. NEWMAN & D. RICHES. 1993. Increased TNF-alpha and IL-6 mRNA expression by alveolar macrophages in chronic beryllium disease. Chest **103:** 138.
30. VANHEE, D., *et al.* 1993. Secretion and mRNA expression of TNFα and IL-6 in alveolar macrophages and in the lung of pneumoconiotic patients. Am. Rev. Respir. Dis. In press.
31. SUGARMAN, B. J., *et al.* 1985. Recombinant human tumor necrosis factor-a: Effects on proliferation of normal and transformed cells *in vitro.* Science **230:** 943–945.
32. VILCEK, J., *et al.* 1986. Fibroblast growth enhancing activity of tumor necrosis factor and its relationship to other polypeptide growth factors. J. Exp. Med. **163:** 632–643.
33. FLYNN, R. M. & M. A. PALLADINO. 1991. TNF and TGF-β: The opposite sides of the avenue? *In* Tumor Necrosis Factors: The Molecules and Their Emerging Role in Medicine, B. Beutler, Ed.: 131–144. Raven Press. New York.
34. PLEDGER, W. J., C. D. STILES, H. N. ANTONIADES & C. D. SCHER. 1978. An ordered sequence of events is required before BALB/c-3T3 cells become committed to DNA synthesis. Proc. Natl. Acad. Sci. U.S.A. **75:** 2839–2843.
35. ROM, W. N., *et al.* 1988. Alveolar macrophages release an insulin-like growth factor 1-type molecule. J. Clin. Invest. **82:** 1685–1693.
36. WALLAERT, B., *et al.* 1990. Superoxide anion generation by alveolar inflammatory cells in simple pneumoconiosis and in progressive massive fibrosis of nonsmoking coal workers. Am. Rev. Respir. Dis. **141:** 120–133.
37. BITTERMAN, P. B., S. I. RENNARD, S. ADELBERG & R. G. CRYSTAL. 1983. Role of fibronectin as a growth factor for fibroblasts. J. Cell Biol. **97:** 1925–1932.
38. KOVACS, E. J. 1991. Fibrogenic cytokines: The role of immune mediators in the development of scar tissue. Immunol. Today **12:** 17–23.
39. WAHL, S. M., N. MCCARTNEY-FRANCIS & S. E. MERGENHAGEN. 1989. Inflammatory and immunomodulatory role of TGFβ. Immunol. Today **10:** 258–261.
40. ASSOIAN, R. K., *et al.* 1987. Expression and secretion of type beta transforming growth factor by activated human macrophage. Proc. Natl. Acad. Sci. U.S.A. **84:** 6020–6024.
41. LYONS, R. M., J. KESKI-OJA & H. L. LOSES. 1988. Proteolytic activation of latent transforming growth factor-β from fibroblast-conditioned medium. J. Cell Biol. **106:** 1659–1665.
42. PAULSSON, Y., M. P. BECKMANN, B. WESTERMARK & C. H. HELDIN. 1988. Density-dependent inhibition of cell growth by transforming growth factor $\beta 1$ in normal human fibroblasts. Growth Factors **1:** 19.
43. MOSES, H. L., E. Y. YANG & J. A. PIETEMPOL. 1990. TGFb stimulation and inhibition of cell proliferation: New mechanistic insights. Cell **63:** 245–247.
44. OSORNIO-VARGAS, A., *et al.* Early-passage rat lung fibroblats do not migrate *in vitro* to transforming growth factor β. Am. J. Respir. Cell Mol. Biol. **8:** 468–471.
45. BATTEGAY, E. J., E. W. RAINES, R. A. SEIFERT, D. F. BOWEN-POPE & R. ROSS. 1990. TGFb induces bimodal proliferation of connective tissue cells via complex control of autocrine PDGF loop. Cell **63:** 515–524.
46. ANZANO, M. A., A. B. ROBERTS & M. B. SPORN. 1986. Anchorage-independent growth of primary rat embryo cells is induced by platelet-derived growth factor and inhbited by type-beta transforming growth factor. J. Cell Physiol. **126:** 312–318.
47. GAMBLE, J. R., Y. KHEW-GOODALL & M. A. VADAS. 1993. Transforming growth factor β inhibits E-Selectin expression on human endothelial cells. J. Immunol. **150:** 4494–4503.
48. GAMBLE, J. R. & M. A. VADAS. 1988. Endothelial cell adhesiveness for blood neutrophils is inhibited by transforming growth factor β. Science **242:** 97.

49. ———. 1991. Endothelial cell adhesiveness for human T lymphocytes is inhibited by TGFβ. J. Immunol. **146:** 1149.
50. SHULL, M., *et al.* 1992. Targeted disruption of the mouse transforming growth factor β1 gene results in multi-focal inflammatory disease. Nature **359:** 693.
51. DUBOIS, C. M., *et al.* 1990. Transforming growth factor β is a potent inhibitor of interleukin 1 (IL-1) receptor expression: Proposed mechanism of inhibition of IL-1 action. J. Exp. Med. **172:** 737–744.
52. WAHL, S. M., G. L. COSTA, M. CORCORAN, L. M. WAHL & A. E. BERGER. 1993. Transforming growth factor β mediates IL-1-dependent induction of IL-1 receptor antagonist. J. Immunol. **150:** 3553–3560.
53. TURNER, M., *et al.* 1991. Induction of the interleukin 1 receptor antagonist protein by transforming growth factor β. Eur. J. Immunol. **21:** 1635.
54. DENHOLM, E. M. & S. M. ROLLINS. 1993. Expression and secretion of transforming growth factor β by bleomycin-stimulated rat alveolar macrophages. Am. J. Physiol. **264:** L36–L42.
55. VIGNAUD, J. M., *et al.* 1991. Presence of platelet-derived growth factor in normal and fibrotic lung is specifically associated with interstitial macrophages, while both interstitial macrophages and epithelial cells express the c-sis proto-oncogene. Am. J. Respir. Cell Mol. Biol. **5:** 531–538.
56. MORELAND, L. W., K. T. GOLDSMITH, W. J. RUSSELL, K. R. YOUNG & R. I. GARVER. 1992. Transforming growth factor β within fibrotic scleroderma lungs. Am. J. Med. **93:** 628–636.
57. YAMAUCHI, K., *et al.* 1988. High levels of transforming growth factor β are present in epithelial lining fluid of the normal lower respiratory tract. Am. Rev. Respir. Dis. **137:** 1360–1363.

Control of Lung Fibroblast Proliferation by Macrophage-derived Platelet-derived Growth Factor

ARNOLD R. BRODY

Department of Pathology
Tulane University Medical Center
1430 Tulane Avenue
New Orleans, Louisiana 70112

INTRODUCTION

A key feature of interstitial fibrogenic lung disease is an increase in the population of fibroblasts that synthesize and secrete extracellular matrix components of the "scarring" process.[1] The biology, biochemistry, and molecular characteristics of this cell type have been studied extensively over the past decades.[2-4] If we knew the basic mechanisms through which these cells were stimulated to divide and produce connective tissue, it would be more likely that a therapeutic intervention could be developed where none now exists for interstitial pulmonary fibrosis (IPF).

There are a number of strategies that could be employed to halt the development of IPF. For example, investigators have partially blocked lung fibrosis by treating animals with antioxidants.[5,6] Presumably, this blocks some cellular injury at the alveolar level and clearly ameliorates the disease process.[5,6] Another approach has been to develop antibodies that might block the biological activities of factors known to cause cell proliferation or matrix production.[7,8] Both of these strategies offer exciting new possibilities for controlling fibrosis and have added to our understanding of the disease process. There is, however, a great deal we do not know about the mechanisms of disease and much must be learned before IPF can actually be prevented or cured by practical modalities.

One of the major obstacles to firmly establishing a mechanism of fibrogenesis is the huge array of inflammatory mediators, cytokines, and growth factors that are known to affect fibroblast biology.[9] For example, prostaglandin E2 reduces fibroblast proliferation, while platelet-derived growth factor dramatically enhances this activity, and both are produced by lung macrophages as well as the fibroblasts themselves. How do we sort out which of the agents is doing what and which ones actually are significant *in vivo*? It is clear that no individual or group of investigators can even attempt to answer these questions by studying a morass of antagonistic molecules. One must carefully choose a single agent or a small interactive group of factors upon which to focus a series of experiments. We have been studying platelet-derived growth factor (PDGF) because it is the most potent known stimulator of fibroblast proliferation;[10] it is produced by a number of lung cell types;[10-12] and increased expression of the mRNA coding for the PDGF protein as well as PDGF secretion are upregulated by fibrogenic agents *in vitro* and *in vivo*. Following is a review of some findings that support our working hypothesis that PDGF is the predominant mitogen mediating fibroblast growth during the development of IPF.

In 1974, PDGF originally was found in serum as the major growth factor for mesenchymal cells.[10] Synthesized by megakaryocytes, PDGF is stored in the alpha granules of blood platelets until released at sites of tissue injury.[10] PDGF thus aids in healing of wounds and general tissue repair. In 1985, investigators from Russell Ross's laboratory discovered that human lung macrophages synthesize and secrete PDGF.[13] In 1988, we found that rat macrophages produce a similar molecule that is neutralized by a polyclonal antibody to human PDGF.[14] Other normal cell types such as endothelium,[15] smooth muscle,[16] fibroblasts,[17] and recently, lung epithelium[18] have been shown to secrete the same molecule. Thus, it is clear that PDGF is produced by a number of cell types and that it is a potent mitogen and chemotactic factor for mesenchymal cells.[10,19] However, its function in normal development, and particularly in tissue repair, is not clear. There are several good models that suggest that PDGF plays a major role in wound healing[20] and the pathogenesis of atherosclerosis.[21] There are no data that tell us whether or not PDGF is at all significant in any lung disease. However, given its biological potential and known role in other fibrogenic processes,[20,21] it is reasonable to speculate (as several investigators have[22]) that PDGF can play a central role in the development of interstitial pulmonary fibrosis.

RESULTS AND DISCUSSION

In Vitro: *Macrophage and Fibroblast-Derived PDGF*

Our approach has been to study the two cell types considered by many to be the main effector and target cells in fibrogenic disease, that is, the macrophage and fibroblast. As previously noted, lung macrophages from humans and animals produce PDGF, but it was not known if these cells released all three isoforms of the growth factor and if the isoforms were biologically active on the target cells. Bonner et al.[23] showed that alveolar macrophages from rats indeed secrete the two peptide chains that form the three possible combinations of the PDGF molecules, that is, the A- and B-chain monomers of PDGF combine to form the AA, AB, and BB isoforms.[10,23] The rat macrophages produced predominantly BB isoforms (~50%), which proved to be the most potent mitogen of the three for early passage lung fibroblasts.[23] The AA isoform exhibited little mitogenic activity because these fibroblasts possess few alpha (α)-type receptors, which bind the A-chain peptide.[24] It was fascinating to learn that the mRNA coding for this receptor type was upregulated by treating the fibroblasts with inorganic particles (see below for further discussion). Also, treatment with asbestos fibers caused the macrophages to consistently produce increased amounts of PDGF in a concentration-dependent fashion.[25]

Bonner et al.[26] also demonstrated that the PDGF isoforms were released by lung macrophages *in vitro* along with a high molecular weight-binding protein, which proved to be alpha-2 macroglobulin (α-2M). This finding solved an apparent paradox, that is, a significant component of the PDGF-like mitogenic activity in serum and macrophage-conditioned medium was blocked by α-2M. In addition, in the presence of the binding protein, little PDGF could be detected by standard immunoassay techniques.[20] Since PDGF is acid stable, treatment of macrophage-conditioned medium with 1 M acetic acid released the growth factor from its binding protein. Only then could the full mitogenic and chemotactic potential of the macrophage-derived (MD) PDGF be demonstrated.[26–28] Interestingly enough, when the binding protein was altered by treatment with an amine, to induce the receptor-recognized ("fast") form, the α-2M increased the mitogenic activity of the MD-PDGF.[29] While a number of growth factors, including transforming growth factor beta and fibroblast growth factor, bind to α-2M, PDGF exhibits a specific binding site that can be competed for only by the isoforms of PDGF itself.[30]

As is discussed below, inhaled fibrogenic asbestos fibers are actively translocated to the lung interstitium where they are taken up by interstitial macrophages and fibroblasts.[31] Therefore, we carried out a series of studies to establish whether or not these cells release PDGF after treatment *in vitro*. Interstitial macrophages separated from rat lung tissue by enzymatic digestion produced the same form of PDGF molecules as alveolar macrophages.[32] This PDGF also had to be separated from the α-2M binding protein before it could be quantified by an enzyme immunoassay.[32] The information on fibroblast-derived PDGF is less clear, although there is no doubt that these cells from both humans and animals produce PDGF.[33] Our experiments suggest that the A-chain is predominant, and asbestos induces increased secretion of the peptide.[33] Most interesting was the finding that asbestos treatment of rapidly dividing fibroblasts caused cytotoxicity and loss of cells from the culture surface. When the cells were treated while in a quiescent phase, however, they began to divide again, resulting in a significant increase in cell number. This apparently is due to an autocrine effect caused by the fibroblasts' own PDGF.[33] The added growth can be blocked essentially 100 percent by an antibody to PDGF, but nonimmune IgG had no effect. This could be a significant finding in understanding interstitial fibrosis if this event takes place *in vivo*. The autocrine effect appears to take place through binding of the A-chain PDGF to the α-receptor subunit. We recently have shown that this receptor type is increased *in vitro* after the fibroblasts are treated with asbestos fibers.[24] This treatment causes upregulation of the mRNA, which codes for the α-receptor, and the number of high-affinity membrane receptors for the A-chain thus increases about 40 percent.[24] This probably is a critical event in the autocrine loop described earlier, but further work will be necessary to establish the mechanism of this effect on receptor mRNA and whether or not such an event occurs *in vivo* in the interstitium of exposed animals and humans.

Finally, we have used the relatively new technology of *in situ* hybridization to learn if the genes coding for the A- and B-chains of PDGF express message in lung macrophages. Using nonisotopically labeled 40-mer oligonucleotides, it was clear that rat lung macrophages expressed both chains of PDGF (Fig. 1), as expected, since all three isoform proteins have been identified.[23] More important was to establish that treatment with asbestos fibers caused increased percentages of cells to express message, again correlating with what we found by immunoassay for the protein. FIGURE 1 shows that asbestos-treated macrophages exhibit clear expression of the mRNA for the B-chain of PDGF. Preliminary quantitative data have shown that asbestos treatment induces 3- to 5-fold increases in the percentages of macrophages expressing the A-chain message. The B-chain message also was increased, but the findings were not sufficiently consistent to reach statistical significance in every experiment. Further experiments are ongoing to establish the concentration and time-dependent effect of fibers and the specificity of the response to other respirable agents.

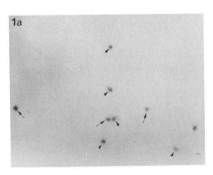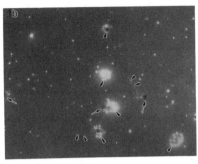

FIGURE 1. *In situ* hybridization using an oligonucleotide probe for the A-chain of PDGF was carried out on these rat lung macrophages treated with chrysotile asbestos fibers. Cells with *arrows* have not hybridized. *Arrowheads* identify the labeled cells and *double arrowheads* show asbestos fibers. **(a)** *Bright-field image* shows the cells adherent to the glass substrate. **(b)** *Dark-field image* of the same field seen in **(a)** demonstrates the bright silver grains that have bound to the macrophages expressing mRNA for the PDGF A-chain. Most, but not all, of the macrophages in this field exhibited hybridization. Treatment of the cells *in vitro* caused up to 5-fold increases in percentages of hybridized cells compared to untreated controls.

In Vivo: *Identification of PDGF mRNA Expression*

In vitro experiments are useful for exploring the biochemistry and biological potential of the various factors released by cells. For any of the findings made *in vitro* to be useful in understanding the mechanisms of a disease process, however, the appropriate experiments must be carried out *in vivo*. We have initiated a series of studies designed to determine whether or not the genes that code for various growth factors are expressing messenger (m)RNA at specific postexposure times and in the cell types that are participating in the development of lesions. At the time of this writing, we have preliminary results from a single experiment in which rats were exposed to chrysotile asbestos fibers for three hours/day for three consecutive days. We know from our previous studies using immunohistochemistry and electron microscopy that this exposure induces a progressive fibrogenic lesion at alveolar duct bifunctions and along the alveolar duct walls.[34–36] The fibrosis persists at these sites for at least six months (unpublished observations), and within the lesions there are clear increases in interstitial fibronectin content, smooth muscle actin, and strong antibody staining of transforming growth factor beta in the macrophages that accumulate at the developing lesions.[37,38]

Two weeks after the exposure described earlier, *in situ* hybridization of the mRNA for PDGF A- and B-chains demonstrated striking localization in macrophages, as well as in epithelial and mesenchymal cells associated with developing lesions (FIG. 2). The silver-amplified label on specific oligonucleotide probes could be readily visualized in dark-field microscopy (FIG. 2). Tissues from unexposed rats exhibited little labeling, and control tissues treated with a random sequence oligonucleotide showed no labeling.

Little is known about the role any of the growth factors may play in the development of interstitial lung disease. We postulate that if growth factors are indeed involved in the pathogenesis, it should be possible to predict the anatomic

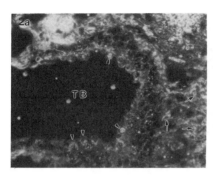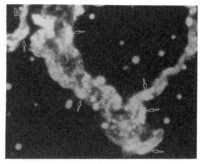

FIGURE 2. Lung tissue from animals exposed to chrysotile asbestos for three days and sacrificed two weeks later. **(a)** *Dark-field image* showing clear hybridization of the probe for the PDGF A-chain in many epithelial cells (*arrowheads*) lining the end of this terminal bronchide (TB) where it opens to an alveolar duct. Interstitial cells (*arrows*) also are labeled. **(b)** *Dark-field image* of alveolar duct walls demonstrating a number of cells (*arrows*) hybridized with a probe for the B-chain.

compartment and temporal sequence in which the specific messenger RNAs will be expressed. To carry out such studies, it is essential to know where the initial lesions develop, the pathogenetic sequence of events, and the cell types involved. Inasmuch as we have established these parameters in our animal model of asbestosis,[34-38] it now is possible to test the postulate; and the findings with *in situ* hybridization at two weeks postexposure (FIG. 2) lend support to the overall concept. Experiments are ongoing to ask whether or not the mRNAs for the PDGF isoforms and for other growth factors (such as TGFB, TGFα, FGF, TNF) are expressed in developing lesions and if the site and time of expression can be predicted.

CONCLUSIONS

A major challenge in today's pathobiological experiments is to establish whether or not any of the multitude of growth factors and cytokines produced by lung cells actually are playing a mechanistic role in a disease process. There are a number of lung diseases in which the cytokines could be involved, including asthma, fibrosis, and neoplasia. We have chosen to focus on two of the factors, TGFB and PDGF. In ongoing experiments we are asking if and when and in which cells expression of the appropriate mRNAs is upregulated after exposure to a known fibrogenic agent, in this case, asbestos.[34] Preliminary findings support our hypothesis that the PDGF isoforms play a major role in maintaining asbestos-induced fibrogenic lesions in the alveolar interstitium (FIG. 2). If this mesenchymal cell growth factor were not participating in the pathogenetic process, one would expect expression of the mRNA coding for the specific protein to remain at control levels and not be concentrated at sites of macrophage accumulation and cell proliferation. Further studies using combinations of techniques *in vitro* and *in vivo* will be necessary to determine if any of the potent cytokines and growth factors are mediating interstitial lung disease.

ACKNOWLEDGMENTS

The author is grateful to his colleagues and students whose data form the majority of this review. He particularly thanks James C. Bonner, Joseph A. Lasky, and Lynn Blalock.

REFERENCES

1. CROUCH, E. 1990. Pathobiology of pulmonary fibrosis. Am. J. Physiol. **259:** L159–L170.
2. ADLER, K. B., R. B. LOW, K. O. LESLIE, J. MITCHELL & J. N. EVANS. 1989. Contractile cells in normal and fibrotic lung. Lab. Invest. **60:** 473–485.
3. GOLDSTEIN, R. H. & A. FINE. 1986. Fibrotic reactions in the lung: Activation of the lung fibroblast. Exp. Lung Res. **11:** 245–260.
4. PHAN, S. H., J. VARANI & D. SMITH. 1985. Rat lung fibroblast collagen metabolism in bleomycin-induced pulmonary fibrosis. J. Clin. Invest. **72:** 241–247.
5. MOSSMAN, B. T., et al. 1990. Inhibition of lung injury, inflammation, and interstitial pulmonary fibrosis by polyethyleneglycol conjugated catalase in a rapid inhalation model of asbestosis. Am. Rev. Respir. Dis. **141:** 1266–1271.
6. WANG, Q., D. M. HYDE & S. N. GIRI. 1992. Abatement of bleomycin induced increases in vascular permeability, inflammatory cell infiltration, and fibrotic lesions in hamster lungs by combined treatment with taurine and niacin. Lab. Invest. **67:** 234–242.
7. PIGUET, P. F., M. A. COLLART, G. E. GRAU, A. P. SAPPINO & P. VASSALLI. 1990. Requirement of tumor necrosis factor for development of silica-induced pulmonary fibrosis. Nature **344:** 245–248.
8. GIRI, S. N., D. M. HYDE & M. A. HOLLINGER. 1993. Treatment with antitransforming growth factor-β antibody reduces the bleomycin-induced increases in lung collagen accumulation in mice. Am. Rev. Respir. Dis. **147:** A757.
9. NATHAN, C. 1987. Secretory products of macrophages. J. Clin. Invest. **79:** 319–327.
10. ROSS, R., E. W. RAINES & D. F. BOWEN-POPE. 1986. The biology of platelet-derived growth factor. Cell **46:** 155–166.
11. KELLY, J. 1990. Cytokines of the lung. Am. Rev. Respir. Dis. **141:** 765–788.
12. ANTONIADES, H. N., et al. 1990. PDGF in idiopathic pulmonary fibrosis. J. Clin. Invest. **86:** 1055–1062.
13. SHIMOKADO, K., et al. 1985. A significant part of macrophage-derived growth factor consists of at least two forms of PDGF. Cell **43:** 277–285.
14. KUMAR, R. K., R. A. BENNETT & A. R. BRODY. 1988. A homologue of platelet-derived growth factor produced by alveolar macrophages. Fed. Am. Soc. Exp. Biol. J. **2:** 2272–2277.
15. DiCORLETO, P. E. & D. F. BOWEN-POPE. 1983. Cultured endothelial cells produce a PDGF-like protein. Proc. Natl. Acad. Sci. U.S.A. **80:** 1919–1925.
16. MAJESKY, M. W., E. P. BENDITT & S. M. SCHWARTZ. 1988. Expression and developmental control of platelet-derived growth factor A-chain and B-chain/Sis genes in rat aortic smooth muscle cells. Proc. Natl. Acad. Sci. U.S.A. **85:** 1524–1528.
17. FABISIAK, J. P., M. ABSHER, J. N. EVANS & J. KELLEY. 1992. Spontaneous production of PDGF A-chain homodimer by rat lung fibroblasts in vitro. Am. J. Physiol. L185–L193.
18. FINKELSTEIN, J. N. & C. KRAMER. 1993. Alveolar epithelial proliferation and production of growth factors and cytokines in pulmonary fibrosis. Am. Rev. Respir. Dis. **147:** A153.
19. WESTERMARK, B. & C.-H. HELDIN. 1989. Platelet-derived growth factor: Structural and functional aspects. J. Intern. Med. **225:** 55–67.
20. GREENHALGH, D. G., K. H. SPRUGEL, M. J. MURRAY & R. ROSS. 1990. PDGF and FGF stimulate wound healing in the genetically diabetic mouse. Am. J. Pathol. **136:** 1235–1246.

21. Ross, R., *et al.* 1990. Localization of PGDFβ protein in macrophages in all phases of atherogenesis. Science **248:** 1009–1012.
22. Hertz, M. I., *et al.* 1992. Obliterative bronchiolitis after lung transplantation: A fibroproliferative disorder associated with platelet-derived growth factor. Proc. Natl. Acad. Sci. U.S.A. **89:** 10385–10389.
23. Bonner, J. C., A. Osornio-Vargas, A. Badgett & A. F. Brody. 1991. Differential proliferation of rat lung fibroblasts induced by the PDGF, AA, AB, and BB isoforms secreted by rat alveolar macrophages. Am. J. Respir. Cell Mol. Biol. **5:** 539–547.
24. Bonner, J. C., A. L. Goodell, P. G. Coin & A. R. Brody. 1993. Chrysotile asbestos upregulates gene expression and production of alpha-receptors for platelet-derived growth factor (PDGF-AA) on rat lung fibroblasts. J. Clin. Invest. **92:** 425–430.
25. Schapira, R. M., A. R. Osornio-Vargas & A. R. Brody. 1991. Inorganic particles induce secretion of a macrophage homologue of platelet-derived growth factor in a density and time-dependent manner *in vitro*. Exp. Lung Res. **17:** 1011–1024.
26. Bonner, J. C., M. Hoffman & A. R. Brody. 1989. Alpha-macroglobulin secreted by alveolar macrophages serves as a binding protein for a macrophage-derived homologue of platelet-derived growth factor. Am. J. Respir. Cell Mol. Biol. **1:** 171–179.
27. Bonner, J. C. & A. R. Brody. 1992. Cytokine binding proteins. *In* Lung Biology in Health and Disease, J. Kelley, Ed.: 459–490. Dekker. New York.
28. Osornio-Vargas, A. R., J. C. Bonner, A. Badgett & A. R. Brody. 1990. Rat alveolar macrophage-derived platelet-derived growth factor is chemotactic for rat lung fibroblasts. Am. J. Respir. Cell Mol. Biol. **3:** 595–602.
29. Bonner, J. C., A. Badgett, A. R. Osornio-Vargas, K. Hoffman & A. R. Brody. 1990. PDGF-stimulated fibroblast proliferation is enhanced synergistically by receptor-recognized α2-macroglobulin. J. Cell Physiol. **145:** 1–8.
30. Bonner, J. C., A. L. Goodell, J. A. Lasky & M. R. Hoffman. 1992. Reversible binding of platelet-derived growth factor-AA, -AB, and -BB isoforms to a similar site on the "slow" and "fast" conformations of alpha-2 macroglobulin. J. Biol. Chem. **267:** 12837–12844.
31. Brody, A. R. & L. H. Hill. 1982. Interstitial accumulation of inhaled chrysotile asbestos fibers and consequent formation of microcalcifications. Am. J. Pathol. **109:** 107–114.
32. Bauman, M. D., *et al.* 1990. Secretion of platelet-derived growth factor homologue by rat alveolar macrophages exposed to particulates in vitro. Eur. J. Cell Biol. **51:** 327–334.
33. Lasky, J. A., *et al.* 1994. Chrysotile asbestos stimulates gene expression and secretion of PDGF-AA by rat lung fibroblasts *in vitro*: Evidence for an autocrine loop. Am. J. Resp. Cell Mol. Biol. In Press.
34. Brody, A. R. 1992. Asbestos exposure as a model of inflammation inducing interstitial pulmonary fibrosis. *In* Inflammation: Basic Principles and Clinical Correlates: 1033–1049. Raven Press. New York.
35. McGavran, P. D., C. J. Butterick & A. R. Brody. 1990. Tritiated thymidine incorporation and the development of an interstitial lesion in the bronchiolar-alveolar regions of normal and complement deficient mice after inhalation of chrysotile asbestos. J. Environ. Pathol. Toxicol. Oncol. **6:** 377–388.
36. Chang, L. Y., L. H. Overby, A. R. Brody & J. D. Crapo. 1988. Progressive lung cell reactions and extracellular matrix production after a brief exposure to asbestos. Am. J. Pathol. **131:** 156–170.
37. Warheit, D. B., L. H. Hill, G. George & A. R. Brody. 1986. Time course of chemotactic factor generation and the corresponding macrophage response to asbestos inhalation. Am. Rev. Respir. Dis. **134:** 128–133.
38. Perdue, T. D. & A. R. Brody. 1994. Distribution of TGF-beta 1, fibronectin and smooth muscle actin in asbestos induced pulmonary fibrosis in rats. J. Histochem. Cytochem. In press.

The Role of Alveolar Macrophages in Regulation of Lung Inflammation

T. THEPEN,[a] G. KRAAL,[b] AND P. G. HOLT[c]

[a]Department of Dermatoallergology
University Hospital Utrecht
Heidelberglaan 100
3584 CX Utrecht
The Netherlands

[b]Department of Cellbiology
Vrije Universiteit
vd Boechorststraat 7
1081 BT, Amsterdam
The Netherlands

[c]The Western Australian Research
Institute for Child Health
GPO Box D184
Perth, Western Australia, 6001

INTRODUCTION

In air-breathing animals the respiratory system is the principal organ for gas exchange. The respiratory system can be subdivided in an upper and a lower respiratory tract, the former being considered the conductive part, while the latter can be referred to as the respiratory part where the actual gas exchange takes place. In order to perform this vital function the lungs have a large surface area where the internal environment is exposed to external air.

Together with oxygen, airborne antigenic material present in ambient air, enters the lungs. These incoming antigens make contact with the respiratory epithelium from the nasal cavity to the most distal part, the air-filled alveoli. Considering the large surface area and the volume of air inspired on a daily base, the low prevalence of inflammation under normal circumstances is remarkable. This indicates tight control and restriction of the response to potentially pathogenic antigens.

To respond adequately to pathogenic antigens the respiratory system is equipped with an elaborate immune system. This system comprises lymph nodes draining the respiratory system via afferent lymphatics, lymphoid structures associated with the mucosal epithelium [mucosa-associated lymphoid tissue (MALT)], and immunocompetent cells in the respiratory epithelium, lung parenchyma, and alveolar space.

IMMUNOCOMPETENT CELLS IN THE RESPIRATORY EPITHELIUM AND LUNG PARENCHYMA

T Cells in the Respiratory System

Intraepithelial lymphocytes are predominantly T cells and occur as single cells in airway epithelium, underlying mucosa, in the alveolar septal walls, and on the epithelial surface. Experiments in which lung digests were used have demonstrated a large population of T cells in lung parenchyma of rats, which is comparable in size to the peripheral blood T cell pool.[1,2] These T cells can be found in lung tissue sections as randomly distributed single cells in the alveolar septal wall.

Lung T cells show a higher $CD8^+/CD4^+$ ratio and contain more blasts than peripheral blood T cells, which indicates some selectivity in retaining T cells in the lungs.[3] In addition to this, Nelson *et al.* showed functional suppression of the majority of $CD4^+$ and in particular $CD8^+$ T cells, during their temporary arrest in the vascular bed of the lungs. When the proliferative capacity of lung T cells in rat and human was compared to that of T cells derived from peripheral blood or the spleen, a marked reduction was found.[3,4] These results indicate that T cells, during their sequestration in the lungs, are subjected to down-regulation, restricting their functional capacity.

Dendritic Cells in Respiratory Tract

Recently, the presence of dendritic cells (DC) in the respiratory tract has been demonstrated by several authors.[2,5–10] Dendritic cells are present in tracheal epithelium and also in lung parenchyma. Interestingly, DCs in the respiratory epithelium form a dense network bearing a great resemblance to the Langerhans' cell network in skin.[9,11] The pulmonary DCs have been shown to possess an antigen-presenting capability.[6,10] It has been demonstrated, that endogenous macrophage populations suppress the antigen presentation of these DCs.[7,8] Therefore DCs are at present considered to be the principal antigen-presenting cell in the respiratory tract. In addition to this it has been shown that in broncho alveolar lavage in humans, a subpopulation can be identified that exhibit "dendritic" characteristics.[12] These cells were identified by staining with a set of monoclonal antibodies that discriminate between macrophages and DCs,[13] and were strong stimulators in mixed lymphocyte reactions. This stimulatory effect of the putative DCs was suppressed by alveolar macrophages (AM) in broncho-alveolar lavage characterized as "suppressor macrophages" by the same set of monoclonal antibodies.

ALVEOLAR MACROPHAGES

Probably the most frequently examined cell type in the respiratory tract is the AM, probably because they are easily accessible in broncho-alveolar lavage.[14–17] The AM is situated at the air–tissue interface in the alveoli and alveolar ducts, and are the first cell type to encounter inhaled foreign material.

In Vitro *Immunoregulatory Functioning of Alveolar Macrophages*

Many *in vitro* studies examined the role of AMs in pulmonary immunity, and in particular their capacity to support T- and B-cell activation. Though interspecies differences were observed, these studies consistently indicate that AMs are inefficient in providing accessory cell activity *in vitro* compared to macrophages derived from other sources or monocytes.[18] In fact, AMs have been demonstrated to be efficient suppressors of T-cell activation and in antibody production by B cells, measured by a plaque-forming cell assay.[18,19] A reservation should be made regarding the AM : T-cell ratio. At a high AM : T-cell ratio AMs are strongly suppressive, whereas at a low AM : T-cell ratio some stimulatory effect is present. This can be explained by either the balance of suppressive versus stimulatory factors produced by the AM itself, indicating a "dilution" of suppressive factors and the remainder of the activity of the stimulatory factors at low AM : T-cell ratios, or by the presence of a strong stimulatory signal from DCs in AM preparation, which is abrogated by the suppressive signal from AMs at high AM : T-cell ratios.[18] In summary it can be concluded from the previously mentioned *in vitro* data that AMs function poorly as accessory cells and that their general action is suppressive. At this point, their exact *in vivo* role and their mode of action remains to be established.

In Vivo *Elimination of Alveolar Macrophages*

Recently a technique was developed to selectively eliminate AMs from the lungs of experimental animals *in vivo*, by the use of the cytotoxic drug dichloromethylene diphosphanate (Cl$_2$MDP) encapsulated in liposomes.[20] After intratracheal administration of these liposomes they are avidly phagocytosed by AMs, which causes accumulation of the drug in AM. The AMs are subsequently selectively killed without damage to the surrounding tissue or causing any change in cell populations in the lungs.[21,22] Both in rats and mice a single intratracheal injection of Cl$_2$MDP liposomes leads to the rapid depletion of AMs, reducing the AM population to a nadir of approximately 10 percent after 24 to 48 hours. The AM population remains at this very low level for at least one week, while no influx of inflammatory cells is observed and the remaining population is >95 percent AM.

The use of this method creates an AM-depleted animal model that enables the study of the *in vivo* role of AM in the regulation of the pulmonary immune response and the control of inflammation in the lungs by AMs.

Effect of In Vivo *Alveolar Macrophage Depletion on Pulmonary Immune Response*

When antigen is delivered in normal animals as a bolus via the intratracheal route, virtually no response is elicited. When the same amount of antigen is identically administered to animals that were previously depleted of their AM population, a drastic increase in response is found. Large amounts of specific antibody-forming cells (AFCs) were found in draining lymph nodes and in lung parenchyma. This is in contrast to the normal controls, where only a very few AFCs were present in the draining lymph nodes and not in the lung parenchyma. The response was not only dramatically increased, but was also longer lasting then in the control animals.[21] This effect, however, was only observed when T-cell-dependent antigens were used, either particulate or soluble. Administration of T-cell-independent antigens, either soluble, particulate, Type-1, or Type-2, did not result in an increase in the pulmonary response.[23] These data strongly suggest regulation of AM at the level of pulmonary T cells under normal circumstances.

This hypothesis was confirmed in a set of experiments in which the functioning of lung T cells derived from normal untouched controls or animals that were AM depleted prior to T-cell isolation was studied. Lung T cells have a suppressed phenotype, making it unlikely that they could respond to inhaled antigens under normal steady conditions.[3] A marked increase in proliferative capacity, however, was observed when T cells were isolated from the lungs of AM-depleted animals. The proliferative capacity of these lung T cells reached values normal for splenic T cells, showing that the suppression was abolished, enabling them to respond to stimulation. This effect of AM elimination was restricted to the lung, since splenic T cells showed no change in proliferative capacity.[24] These results demonstrate that AMs down regulate T-cell functioning in lungs, thereby preventing T-cell activation and subsequent pulmonary inflammation.

The normal baseline response to repeated inhalation of aeroallergens is the induction of immunological tolerance. This takes place in the upper respiratory tract and protects the body upon ensuing contact with that allergen by shutting down immune responses, especially IgE responses, against that allergen. When the effect of AM depletion on the induction of protective tolerance was studied, no difference was observed between normal and AM-depleted animals, demonstrating that AMs do not play a role in this process.[23]

When this protective tolerance is not induced, but the animals are instead primed for an allergen, the effect of *in vivo* AM depletion on the pulmonary immune response was found to be even more drastic.[23,25] In these experiments animals were intraperitoneally primed for ovalbumin (OVA) with a very low dose, known to form immunological memory, but not eliciting an immune response. When thus treated normal control animals were subsequently challenged with an aerosol of OVA, a low immune response was observed as could be expected. However, when OVA presensitized, AM-depleted animals were challenged with aerosolized OVA, a strong immune response was found. In particular the IgE response was strongly increased, demonstrated by the presence of large numbers of anti-OVA IgE-secreting AFCs in draining lymph nodes and more importantly in lung parenchyma. Not only was the OVA-specific IgE response increased, but many IgE-producing AFCs of other specificity were found, again in draining lymph nodes and even more strongly in lung parenchyma, indicating a strong "bystander" IgE response in the AM-depleted animals. In the identically treated, but not AM-depleted animals, the lung parenchyma was completely devoid of any IgE-producing AFC. Similar results were observed at the level of IgE mRNA, a strong increase in IgE mRNA production in draining lymph nodes, trachea, and lung parenchyma. In addition to this a large influx of T cells was found in the AM-depleted animals that by far exceeded that of control animals. This stresses the importance of AM in not just down regulation of pulmonary immune responses by the suppression of T cells present in the lungs, but also by controlling the influx of T cells into the lungs. Moreover, these data show that AMs *in vivo* play an important role in determining the outcome of the response in presensitized animals, namely the prevention of unwanted IgE responses in the respiratory tract and especially in the lower respiratory tract.[25]

Dendritic cells can be found throughout the respiratory tract and, especially in the lungs, these cells are in close proximity to AM.[26] *In vitro* experiments indicate that AMs may have a suppressive effect on the presentation of antigens by pulmonary DCs to T cells. We have shown that, in analogy to Langerhans' cells in the skin,[27] the capacity of lung DCs to present antigens to both naive and primed T cells increases the culture remains overnight in an appropriate medium.[26] This *in vitro* maturation could be abrogated by coculturing the DCs with AMs across a semipermeable membrane, indicating that the role of AMs in preventing antigen presentation by DCs in the lung is by the secretion of soluble mediators. The inhibitory effect of AMs on antigen presentation by

DCs could be blocked by adding the nitric oxide synthetase inhibitor mono-methyl-arginine (MMA) to the overnight culture, strongly suggesting that nitric oxide plays a direct role in this inhibition. Addition of TNF-a to the overnight culture can partly mimic the AM suppression, and synergy with AM suppression was observed.

That this inhibitory effect of AMs on the antigen-presenting cell function of DCs also holds true for the *in vivo* situation was shown in a set of experiments in which the antigen-presenting capacity of the DCs was compared with that of DCs isolated from the lungs in AM-depleted and normal animals. Depletion of AMs resulted in a rapid upregulation of the antigen-presenting function of freshly isolated pulmonary DCs, comparable to that achieved by overnight culturing of pulmonary DCs isolated in normal animals. This is in contrast to freshly isolated pulmonary DCs from normal animals which, as mentioned before, show a low antigen-presenting capacity. This indicates that under normal circumstances AMs *in vivo* prohibit the presentation of antigens by pulmonary DCs, and thereby limit pulmonary inflammation.[26]

It has been shown previously that AMs may play a role in particle transportation from alveolar space to draining lymph nodes.[28] No information was available, however, as to where AMs migrate in draining lymph nodes. We examined the translocation of a fluorescent particulate antigen to the draining lymph node.[29] In addition to this we studied the capability of AMs to migrate from alveoli to the draining lymph node. These experiments show that liposomes intratracheally instilled as a model particulate antigen, translocate to the paracortical T-cell area of the draining lymph node. Besides this, also intratracheally injected, fluorescent-labeled AMs migrated to the same area in the lymph node. Subsequent double labeling studies, using red-labeled liposomes phagocytized by green-labeled AM, demonstrated that AMs were capable of migrating to the paracortical area of the draining lymph node with the phagocytized antigen. This specific migration to the paracortical T-cell area is a striking phenomenon, since macrophages normally migrate to the subcapsular sinus and medulla of draining lymph nodes.[30] The migration pattern of macrophages appears to be determined by microenvironmental conditions at the site of origin. The draining lymph node is not a determining factor, since both localization patterns can be demonstrated in the same paratracheal lymph nodes, which drains both the lower respiratory tract and the peritoneal cavity. Intratracheal instillation of either AMs or PMs resulted in the localization in the paracortical T-cell area in paratracheal lymph nodes, whereas intraperitoneal injection of AMs or PMs resulted in the localization in the subcapsular sinus and medulla of this lymph node.[29] The paracortical T-cell area of the lymph nodes contains cells of the DC lineage, interdigitating cells. Dendritic cells are also present in the respiratory epithelium and it is assumed that pulmonary DCs migrate to the paracortical T-cell area in the draining lymph nodes, where they appear as interdigitating cells and participate in initiating immune responses. As has been demonstrated in the aforementioned experiments, AMs play a down-regulating role in the respiratory tract, preventing antigen presentation by DCs and suppressing T-cell reactivity in the lung *in vivo*. In addition we showed that AMs play a key role in limiting IgE responses in lung parenchyma and draining lymph nodes. The migration of AMs into precisely that area of the lymph node where antigen presentation by DCs to T cells occurs could imply that in the paracortical T-cell area the AMs together with antigen provides a down-regulating, immuno-regulating signal, besides the positive signal of the migrated DCs, thus preventing or limiting the immune response in the draining lymph node.

CONCLUSIONS

The *in situ* depletion of PAM from the lungs of experimental animals, using intratracheal administration of Cl_2MDP incorporated in liposomes, provides a good animal model with which to study the *in vivo* role of PAMs in controlling pulmonary immune responses.

The data here presented demonstrate the importance of PAMs in maintaining homeostasis in the lower respiratory tract. Besides their capacity to clear antigens deposited on the epithelial surface of the lung, they prevent activation of the elaborate immune system present in lung tissue and draining lymph nodes. This activation is achieved by preventing the presentation of allergen by DCs to T cells in the lungs by down regulation of the antigen presentation of DCs. In addition to this they prevent the activation of T cells by limiting their proliferative capacity. Furthermore, they control T-cell infiltration in the lungs after contact with an aeroallergen. In these ways they prevent sensitization to allergens in the lower respiratory tract.

They are, however, not involved in the induction of protective tolerance, which is the normal baseline response upon contact with a nonpathogenic aeroallergen via the respiratory mucosa, and is induced in the upper respiratory tract.

Instead of just providing blanket suppression by preventing T-cell activation in the lungs, the PAMs are also involved in the regulation of both allergen-specific and nonspecific secondary IgE responses. So under normal circumstances PAMs limit the induction of IgE responses in the lungs.

This regulatory role might not be limited to lung tissue, but can extend to the draining lymph nodes, since AMs were shown to migrate from alveolar space into the paracortical T-cell area of these lymph nodes. This location, where there is close contact between interdigitating cells and T cells, is especially important for the initiation of immune responses, and AMs might perform an immunoregulatory function after migration to this area with antigen sampled from the alveolar surface.

The observation that PAMs are capable of down regulation of the immune responses, even when protective tolerance has not been induced, suggests an important role for PAMs in atopic disease and lung inflammation. Aberrant functioning of PAMs in sensitized individuals, which have a T-helper response against allergen instead of having acquired a protective tolerance, can lead to vigorous, ongoing allergen-specific and nonspecific IgE responses. These raised IgE levels can subsequently lead to atopic disease by the activation of mast cells and facilitated IgE-mediated antigen presentation by DCs in the respiratory tract and other tissues, such as skin, causing T-cell infiltration, activation, and inflammatory responses.

REFERENCES

1. HOLT, P. G., A. DEGEBRODT, C. O'LEARY, K. KRSKA & T. M. PLOZZA. 1985. Clin. Exp. Immunol. **62:** 586–594.
2. HOLT, P. G. & M. A. SCHON-HEGRAD. 1987. Immunology **62:** 349–356.
3. NELSON, S., D. STRICKLAND & P. G. HOLT. 1990. Immunology **69:** 476–481.
4. HOLT, P. G., *et al.* 1988. Immunology **64:** 649–654.
5. HOLT, P. G., *et al.* 1985. Immunology **54:** 139.
6. SERTL, K., *et al.* 1986. J. Exp. Med. **163:** 436–451.
7. HOLT, P. G., M. A. SCHON-HEGRAD & J. OLIVER. 1988. J. Exp. Med. **167:** 262–274.
8. ROCHESTER, C. L., E. M. GOODELL, J. K. STOLTENBERG & W. BOWERS. 1988. Am. Rev. Respir. Dis. **138:** 121–128.

9. HOLT, P. G., M. A. SCHON-HEGRAD, M. J. PHILLIPS & P. G. MCMENAMIN. 1989. Clin. Exp. Allergy **19:** 597–601.
10. POLLARD, A. M. & M. F. LIPSCOMB. 1990. J. Exp. Med. **172:** 159–167.
11. ROWDEN, G. 1981. CRC Crit. Rev. Immunol. **3:** 95–180.
12. SPITERI, M. A. & L. W. POULTER. 1991. Clin. Exp. Immunol. **83:** 157–162.
13. POULTER, L. W., D. A. CAMPBELL, C. MUNRO & G. JANOSSY. 1986. Scand. J. Immunol. **24:** 351.
14. BOWDEN, D. H. 1984. Environ. Health Perspect. **55:** 327–341.
15. HERSCOWITZ, H. B. 1985. Ann. Allergy **55:** 634–648.
16. BRAIN, J. D. 1988. Am. Rev. Respir. Dis. **137:** 507–509.
17. SIBILLE, Y. & H. Y. REYNOLDS. 1990. Am. Rev. Respir. Dis. **141:** 471–501.
18. HOLT, P. G. 1986. Clin. Exp. Immunol. **63:** 261–270.
19. MURPHY, M. A. & H. B. HERSCOWITCH. 1984. J. Leuk. Biol. **35:** 39–54.
20. VAN ROOIJEN, N. 1989. J. Immunol. Method. **124:** 1–6.
21. THEPEN, T., N. VAN ROOIJEN & G. KRAAL. 1989. J. Exp. Med. **170:** 499–509.
22. THEPEN, T., C. MCMENAMIN, J. OLIVER, G. KRAAL & P. G. HOLT. 1991. Eur. J. Immunol. **21:** 2845–2850.
23. THEPEN, T., K. HOEBEN, J. BREVE & G. KRAAL. 1992. Immunology **76:** 60–64.
24. STRICKLAND, D. H., T. THEPEN, U. R. KEES, G. KRAAL & P. G. HOLT. 1993. Immunology. In press.
25. THEPEN, T., C. MCMENAMIN, B. GIRN, G. KRAAL & P. G. HOLT. 1992. Clin. Exp. Allergy **22:** 1107–1114.
26. HOLT, P. G., et al. 1993. J. Exp. Med. **177:** 397–407.
27. SCHULER, G. & R. M. STEINMAN. 1985. J. Exp. Med. **161:** 526–532.
28. HARMSEN, A. G., B. A. MUGGENBURG, M. B. SNIPES & D. E. BICE. 1985. Science **230:** 1277–1280.
29. THEPEN, T., E. CLAASSEN, K. HOEBEN, J. BREVE & G. KRAAL. 1993. Submitted for publication in.
30. ROSEN, H. & S. GORDON. 1990. Eur. J. Immunol. **20:** 1251–1258.

Asbestos-induced Nitric Oxide Production: Synergistic Effect with Interferon-γ

GEORGE THOMAS,[a] TASUKE ANDO,[b] KIRAN VERMA,[b]
AND ELLIOTT KAGAN[b]

[a]Department of Physiology and Biophysics
Georgetown University Medical Center
Washington, District of Columbia 20007

[b]Department of Pathology
Georgetown University Medical Center
Washington, District of Columbia 20007

INTRODUCTION

Asbestos is a generic name for a group of naturally occurring, hydrated, fibrous silicates that have an aspect ratio of 3 : 1 or greater. There are two major mineralogic categories of asbestos minerals: amphiboles and serpentines. Inhalation of asbestos fibers can cause a variety of clinical disorders afflicting the lungs and serous membranes. These diseases include both fibrotic reactions (asbestosis, parietal pleural plaques, and visceral pleural fibrosis) and malignant lesions (diffuse malignant mesothelioma and bronchogenic carcinoma).[1,2] Studies of asbestos workers and of asbestos-exposed rodents have shown that alveolar macrophages (AMs) are recruited to the sites of deposition of inhaled asbestos fibers.[3,4] There is evidence that asbestos fibers can induce the release of a diverse array of inflammatory mediators from AMs, including cytokine growth factors, chemoattractants, and arachidonic acid metabolites.[3,4] Several studies also have demonstrated that the *in vitro* phagocytic uptake of asbestos fibers can generate a variety of oxygen-derived free radicals, such as the superoxide anion (O_2^{*-}), hydrogen peroxide, and the hydroxyl radical (OH*).[3-5] Furthermore, *in vitro* asbestos exposure can induce lipid peroxidation and chemiluminescence in rodent AMs.[6] It also has been reported that scavengers of oxygen free radicals, such as superoxide dismutase (SOD) and catalase, may ameliorate the injurious effects of asbestos exposure.[7,8] These studies, which are predicated on O_2^{*-}-driven Fenton–Haber–Weiss (i.e., iron-catalyzed) reactions that generate the OH* radical,[9] suggest that reactive oxygen species may have an important role in the pathobiology of asbestos-related disease.

Recently, a great deal of attention has been focused on another type of free radical, namely nitric oxide (NO*).[9,10] Nitric oxide is a labile molecule that is synthesized by the enzyme, NO* synthase. It has important biological properties, being a potent vasodilator as well as an inhibitor of platelet aggregation and smooth muscle proliferation.[11] There is considerable evidence that many cells (including endothelial cells, smooth muscle cells, neutrophils, and macrophages) are capable of generating NO* or a nitric oxidelike molecule.[9,10] A recent study also has shown that NO* can be synthesized by rat AMs.[12] Recent reports suggest that, in addition to its beneficial effects, NO* may be involved in several pathologic reactions such as inflammation and immune complex-mediated cell injury.[13,14] It has been

207

suggested that many of these effects are mediated by the generation of secondary radicals as a consequence of the interaction of O_2^{*-} and NO^*, which yields the peroxynitrite anion ($ONOO^-$). The latter, when protonated, can undergo homolytic cleavage, generating OH^* and NO_2^* radicals that, in turn, can produce oxidation of tissue sulfhydryl groups.[13]

Given the pivotal role of the alveolar macrophage in asbestos-mediated pulmonary injury, the present study was undertaken to determine whether *in vitro* asbestos exposure might stimulate the production of NO^* in rat AMs. In this regard, the effects of two mineralogically dissimilar commercial types of asbestos were compared: crocidolite (an amphibole) and chrysotile (a serpentine). The possible interaction of O_2^{*-} and NO^* was studied with the addition of SOD to macrophage cultures in some experiments. Several cytokines such as interferon-γ, interleukin-1β (IL-1β), and tumor necrosis factor-α (TNF-α) are known to induce the expression of NO^* synthase in cells.[9,15] This could have importance in the context of asbestos-induced injury, since bronchoalveolar lavage lymphocytes from asbestos workers are known to secrete increased amounts of interferon-γ.[16,17] Accordingly, we also have investigated whether the effect of asbestos exposure on NO^* production might be modulated by interferon-γ.

MATERIALS AND METHODS

Alveolar Macrophage Cultures

The AMs were harvested by bronchoalveolar lavage from Sprague-Dawley rats. The AMs were suspended in RPMI medium containing 10 percent fetal bovine serum and allowed to attach for 2 h in 24-well culture plates. Thereafter, the AMs were cultured, in the presence or absence of NIEHS crocidolite or NIEHS chrysotile asbestos fibers (2.5–10 μg/ml), at 37°C in a humidified environment containing 5 percent CO_2 for 48 h. In some experiments, the AMs were cultured in the presence of recombinant rat interferon-γ (250–500 IU/ml). In other experiments, the NO^* synthase inhibitor, N^G-monomethyl-L-arginine acetate (L-NMMA,

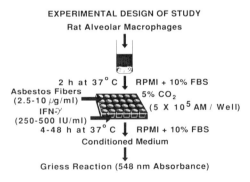

EXPERIMENTAL DESIGN OF STUDY

Rat Alveolar Macrophages

2 h at 37°C | RPMI + 10% FBS

Asbestos Fibers
(2.5-10 μg/ml) — 5% CO_2

IFN-γ
(250-500 IU/ml) (5 X 10^5 AM / Well)

4-48 h at 37°C | RPMI + 10% FBS

Conditioned Medium

Griess Reaction (548 nm Absorbance)

FIGURE 1. Schematic diagram illustrating the experimental protocol for the studies.

500 μg/ml) was added to the cultures. In another set of experiments, the AMs were cultured in the presence of SOD (150 U/ml).

The experimental protocol is schematically represented in FIGURE 1.

Nitric Oxide Assay

Nitric oxide formation was determined by measuring its oxidation product, nitrite (NO_2^-), by the Griess reaction.[18] Absorbance was measured at 548 nm. A functional bioassay for endothelial cell-derived relaxing factor (EDRF) -like activity also was used to determine the presence of NO* activity in macrophage culture supernatants.[10] For this purpose, EDRF-like activity was evaluated on deendothelialized rat aortic rings that were precontracted with the α adrenergic agonist, phenylephrine.

RESULTS

When rat AMs were cultured in the presence of crocidolite asbestos fibers, there was a progressive, time-dependent increase in NO* production (measured as NO_2^-), which was maximal in 48-h cultures. Significantly greater NO_2^- production was noted in supernatants from crocidolite-containing cultures than in those from control cultures devoid of added asbestos fibers ($p < 0.001$). Furthermore, exposure of AM for 48 h to crocidolite, at doses ranging from 2.5 to 10 μg/ml, increased NO_2^- production in a concentration-dependent manner (TABLE 1).

TABLE 2 compares the effects of chrysotile and crocidolite asbestos fibers on

TABLE 1. Effect of Crocidolite Fibers on NO* Production by Rat Alveolar Macrophages in 48-h Cultures

Concentration of Crocidolite (μg/ml)	NO_2^- Production (nmol/5 × 10⁵ AM)
0	0.92 ± 0.13
2.5	1.57 ± 0.13^a
5.0	2.92 ± 0.33^b
10.0	4.58 ± 0.23^b

^{a} $p < 0.005$ compared with control cultures devoid of asbestos.
^{b} $p < 0.001$ compared with control cultures devoid of asbestos.

TABLE 2. Effects of Asbestos Fibers (10 μg/ml) and Interferon-γ (250 IU/ml) on NO* Production by Rat Alveolar Macrophages in 48-h Cultures

Test Category	Without Interferon-γ NO_2^- Production (nmol/5 × 10⁵ AM)	With Interferon-γ
Control	1.16 ± 0.58	20.28 ± 2.01
Crocidolite	2.87 ± 0.66^a	30.09 ± 1.87^b
Chrysotile	4.30 ± 0.90^b	26.10 ± 4.96

^{a} $p < 0.05$ compared with control cultures devoid of asbestos.
^{b} $p < 0.001$ compared with control cultures devoid of asbestos.

TABLE 3. Effect of L-NMMA (500 μg/ml) on NO* Production by Rat Alveolar Macrophages in 48-h Cultures Stimulated with Interferon-γ (250 IU/ml)

Test Category	With L-NMMA	Without L-NMMA
	NO_2^- Production (nmol/5 $\times$ 10^5 AM)	
Control	14.56 ± 3.81	20.28 ± 2.01
Crocidolite	15.59 ± 1.55	30.09 ± 1.87
Chrysotile	13.82 ± 3.61	26.10 ± 4.96

TABLE 4. Effect of SOD (150 U/ml) on NO* Production by Rat Alveolar Macrophages in 48-h Cultures

Test Category	Without SOD	With SOD
	NO_2^- Production (nmol/5 $\times$ 10^5 AM)	
Control	1.5 ± 1.00	3.82 ± 0.19
Crocidolite	2.43 ± 1.05	10.75 ± 2.07[a]
Chrysotile	2.8 ± 0.80	7.36 ± 0.30[a]

[a] $p < 0.001$ compared with similar cultures devoid of added SOD.

NO* production by rat AMs at 48 h. It is apparent that both commercial types of asbestos significantly increased the generation of NO_2^- in culture supernatants. As was anticipated, the addition of interferon-γ (250–500 IU/ml) to control cultures markedly augmented the production of NO*. As shown in TABLE 2, however, the effects of interferon-γ and both types of asbestos (250 IU/ml) were synergistic with respect to NO* production by AMs.

In TABLE 3 it can be seen that the NO* synthase inhibitor, L-NMMA, attenuated the increase in NO* production elicited by chrysotile and crocidolite in the presence of cultures containing interferon-γ (250 IU/ml). This confirms that the NO_2^- detectable in the culture supernatants was a measure of NO* production by the AMs. By contrast, the addition of SOD to the macrophage cultures significantly enhanced the production of NO* (TABLE 4). Although the effect of SOD was noted both in control and in asbestos-containing cultures, significantly greater amounts of NO_2^- were evident in the asbestos-exposed culture supernatants. This observation provides indirect evidence that both types of asbestos induced the formation of O_2^{*-} anion by AMs. Moreover, since the stability of NO* is enhanced by O_2^{*-} and since the addition of SOD significantly increased the amount of NO_2^- in asbestos-containing cultures, our findings indicate that asbestos exposure is likely to induce the formation of $ONOO^-$ anion within rat AMs.

DISCUSSION

Previous studies have shown that rodent macrophages exposed to cytokines (interferon-γ, TNF-α, and IL-1β) can generate NO*, due to activation of the inducible form of the enzyme, NO* synthase.[9,15] In the present study we have shown that amphibole (crocidolite) as well as serpentine (chrysotile) asbestos exposure also stimulated the production of NO* by rat AMs. Furthermore, the addition of recombinant rat interferon-γ greatly enhanced NO* synthesis by AMs. The formation of NO* in macrophage culture supernatants was confirmed by the detection of an augmented EDRF-like effect of supernatants from asbestos-exposed AMs on precontracted, deendothelialized rat aorta preparations (data not shown). Furthermore, NO_2^- production was markedly reduced by the addition of the NO* synthase inhibitor, L-NMMA, to the macrophage cultures. This study has not addressed the issue of whether the asbestos-related effect is mediated directly via activation of inducible NO* synthase. It is conceivable, however, that asbestos may exert its action indirectly via the induction of cytokine synthesis by AMs.[1,3,4] Whatever mechanism is involved, to our knowledge, this is the first demonstration that asbestos exposure stimulates the generation of NO* by AMs.

Superoxide anion interacts with NO*, to generate the highly toxic $ONOO^-$ anion.[13] Peroxynitrite mediates the oxidation of both nonprotein and protein sulfhydryl moieties. In addition, the decomposition of the protonated form of $ONOO^-$ generates another potentially harmful oxidant, the OH* free radical.[13] Our observations have shown that asbestos-exposed rat AMs generated increased quantities of both NO* and O_2^{*-}. This therefore represents a novel mechanism of asbestos-mediated injury that is distinct from iron-catalyzed Fenton reactions.[9] It is possible that some of the toxic effects of asbestos published previously may be mediated by the generation of secondary radicals generated from the interaction of NO* and O_2^{*-}. This might also explain the reported beneficial effect of SOD on asbestos-induced cytotoxicity.[7,8] Finally, it should be noted that some NO* metabolites (NO_2^*, N_2O_3, and N_2O_4) are potent N-nitrosating agents and can generate potentially carcinogenic nitrosamines.[9]

SUMMARY

This study has shown, for the first time, that *in vitro* exposure of rat AMs to either crocidolite (amphibole) or chrysotile (serpentine) asbestos fibers induces the synthesis not only of the O_2^{*-} anion, but also of the nitrogen radical, NO*. Furthermore, this asbestos-related effect is enhanced in the presence of interferon-γ. NO* has been implicated in several pathologic reactions, such as inflammation and immune complex-mediated cell injury. Additionally, NO* may interact with secondary amines to generate nitrosamines, which are potent carcinogens. Our findings could represent a novel type of asbestos-mediated injury, and we propose that the injurious effects of asbestos might be mediated via the interaction of NO* with O_2^{*-}, with the generation of $ONOO^-$ and other potent toxic free radicals.

REFERENCES

1. KAGAN, E. 1985. Ann. Allergy **54:** 464–473.
2. MOSSMAN, B. T. & J. B. L. GEE. 1989. New Eng. J. Med. **320:** 1721–1730.
3. KAGAN, E. 1988. J. Thorac. Imag. 3(4): 1–9.
4. ROM, W. N., W. D. TRAVIS & A. R. BRODY. 1991. Am. Rev. Respir. Dis. **143:** 408–422.
5. SHULL, S., M. MANOHAR, J. P. MARSH, Y. M. W. JANSSEN & B. T. MOSSMAN. 1992. *In* Free Radical Mechanisms of Tissue Injury, M. T. Moslen and C. V. Smith, Eds.: 153–162. CRC Press. Boca Raton, Fla.
6. GULUMIAN, M., F. SARDIANOS, T. KILROE-SMITH & G. OCKERSE. 1985. Biochem. J. **225:** 259–263.
7. MOSSMAN, B. T., J. P. MARSH & M. A. SHATOS. 1986. Lab. Invest. **54:** 204–212.
8. MOSSMAN, B. T., *et al.* 1990. Am. Rev. Respir. Dis. **141:** 1266–1261.
9. GRISHAM, M. B. 1992. Reactive Metabolites of Oxygen and Nitrogen in Biology and Medicine. Landes. Austin, Tex.

10. NATHAN, C. 1992. Fed. Am. Soc. Exp. Biol. J. **6:** 3051–3064.
11. ROEDIGER, W. E. W., M. J. LAWSON, S. H. NANCE & B. C. RADCLIFFE. 1986. Digestion **35:** 199–204.
12. JORENS, P. G., F. J. VAN OVERVELD, H. BULT, P. A. VERMEIRE & A. G. HERMAN. 1991. Eur. J. Pharmacol. **200:** 205–209.
13. BECKMAN, J. S., T. W. BECKMAN, J. CHEN, P. A. MARSHALL & B. A. FREEMAN. 1990. Proc. Natl. Acad. Sci. U.S.A. **87:** 1620–1624.
14. MULLIGAN, M. S., J. M. HEVEL, M. A. MARLETTA & P. A. WARD. 1991. Proc. Natl. Acad. Sci. U.S.A. **88:** 6338–6342.
15. MONCADA, S., R. M. J. PALMER & E. A. HIGGS. 1991. J. Pharmacol. Exp. Theory **43:** 109–142.
16. ROBINSON, B. W. S., A. H. ROSE, A. HAYES & A. W. MUSK. 1988. Am. Rev. Respir. Dis. **138:** 278–283.
17. ROM, W. N. & W. D. TRAVIS. 1992. Chest **101:** 779–786.
18. ARCHER, A. 1993. Fed. Am. Soc. Exp. Biol. J. **7:** 349–360.

Involvement of Both Cyclooxygenase and Lipoxygenase Pathways in Platelet-activating Factor-induced Interleukin-6 Production by Alveolar Macrophages[a]

MARYSE THIVIERGE AND
MAREK ROLA-PLESZCZYNSKI

Immunology Division
Faculty of Medicine
University of Sherbrooke
3001, North 12th Avenue
Sherbrooke, Québec, Canada J1H 5N4

INTRODUCTION

The alveolar macrophages (AM) are among the essential immune cells of the lung, and they participate in the modulation of the inflammatory response by the production of a variety of factors. Among them are various cytokines, including platelet-derived growth factor,[1] transforming growth factor-α and -β,[2] tumor necrosis factor (TNF),[3,4] interleukin (IL)-1,[5] IL-6,[6] and IL-8,[7] and a variety of lipid mediators, such as the arachidonic acid metabolites prostaglandins (PGs),[8] and leukotrienes (LTs),[9] and the phospholipid platelet-activating factor (PAF).[10] These cytokines and metabolites may be involved in the pathogenesis of either acute or chronic pulmonary inflammation via autocrine or paracrine activation of other macrophages, neutrophils, fibroblasts, epithelial cells, or endothelial cells.

In the last few years, it has become increasingly apparent that the metabolism of PAF and that of arachidonic acid are interrelated in a number of inflammatory cells. The release of arachidonic acid and the production of eicosanoids is an early event in the activation of macrophages by many types of inflammatory stimuli. Eicosanoids have been considered to be responsible for some actions of PAF, and have been found to modulate the effects of PAF itself.[11,12] Hence, previous studies from our laboratory and others have examined the regulatory potential of endogenous leukotrienes in PAF-induced augmentation of TNF-α or IL-6 production by macrophages.[13,14] While both PAF and LTB$_4$ can stimulate IL-6 and TNF gene expression, PGE$_2$ has been shown to stimulate the former[15] and inhibit the latter.[16-18] Furthermore, it was recently demonstrated that PGs and LTs are produced by macrophages upon stimulation with PAF.[19,20] It was therefore of interest to determine whether PGE$_2$ was involved in the modulation of macrophage-derived IL-6 and TNF-α production induced by PAF.

In this report, we present evidence that, in addition to 5-lipoxygenase (5-LOX), the cyclooxygenase (COX) pathway could also be implicated in the modulation of IL-6 and TNF-α release by PAF-stimulated AM and that the production of

[a] This work was supported by the Medical Research Council of Canada and the Fonds de Recherche en Santé du Québec.

these cytokines is differently regulated by COX and 5-LOX metabolites in response to PAF.

MATERIALS AND METHODS

Reagents

PAF (hexadecyl-PAF, Bachem, Torrance, Calif.) was dissolved in ethanol and resuspended in RPMI 1640 medium containing bovine serum albumin (0.25%). LTB$_4$ and MK 886 were a generous gift from Dr. A. Ford-Hutchinson (Merck-Frosst, Pointe-Claire, Canada) and were resuspended in methanol and ethanol, respectively, and further diluted in RPMI 1640 medium. Muramyl dipeptide (MDP: N-acetylmuramyl-L-alanyl-D-isoglutamine) was obtained from Behring Diagnostics (La Jolla, Calif.). PGE$_2$, dBcAMP, dBcGMP, indomethacin and aspirin were from Sigma (St-Louis, Mo.). Ibuprofen was from the Upjohn Company (Don Mills, Ont. Canada).

Alveolar Macrophage Preparation

Male Wistar rats weighing 200 to 250 g were purchased from Charles River Canada Inc. (St-Constant, QC, Canada). Rat AMs were obtained by bronchoalveolar lavage. Ketamine hydrochloride-anesthetized rats were exsanguinated, the thoracic cavity opened, and the trachea was canulated. The lungs were lavaged with a total volume of 60-ml phosphate-buffered saline (PBS) in 10-ml aliquots. After recovery, the bronchoalveolar cells were centrifuged, washed twice in PBS, and resuspended in RPMI 1640 medium supplemented with 5% FBS. Cells were counted in a hemocytometer chamber and viability was determined by Trypan blue exclusion. The cells (>98% AMs, determined by nonspecific esterase and Wright-Giemsa staining) were incubated overnight at 1×10^6 cells/ml in RPMI 1640 supplemented with 5% FBS in polystyrene tubes.

Supernatant Production

Following adherence, AMs were washed once, and fresh serum-free medium was added to the adherent cells with or without MDP (1 μg/ml) and further treated with the appropriate stimuli. After 18 hours of culture or less, the AM-containing tubes were centrifuged at $400 \times g$ for 10 min and the cell-free supernatants were harvested and stored at $-80°C$ until used in the IL-6 or TNF-α bioassay. Control cultures contained corresponding vehicle only and were otherwise treated as experimental cultures. Final concentration of ethanol or methanol were <0.08% and had no effect by themselves in the experiments.

Interleukin-6 and TNF-α Bioassay

Bioactivity of IL-6 was assayed using the IL-6-sensitive B9 hybridoma cell line as described previously,[14] according to the method of Aarden et al.[21] TNF-α

activity was measured essentially as described elsewhere[22] on actinomycin D-treated L-929 cells as target cells.

PGE₂ and LTB₄ Assays

Alveolar macrophages (1×10^6 cells/ml) were incubated in RPMI medium in the presence or absence of PAF, LTB_4, cyclooxygenase, or lipoxygenase inhibitors either alone or in combination. Supernatants were collected and assayed for PGE_2 or LTB_4 content using a commercial enzyme-linked immunoassay (Cayman Chemical, Ann Arbor, Mich.). PGE_2 and LTB_4 values are expressed as pg/1×10^6 cells.

Statistical Analysis

Data were analyzed for statistical significance using the analysis of variance (Anova, Scheffé test, for multiple comparisons). Differences were considered significant at $p < 0.05$.

RESULTS

Enhanced Production of IL-6 and TNF-α by PAF-stimulated AMs

Alveolar macrophages stimulated with the macrophage activator MDP (1 μg/ml) were cultured overnight with graded concentrations of PAF (10^{-14} to 10^{-7} M). As shown in FIGURE 1, PAF at 10^{-10} M induced a two- to fivefold increase in

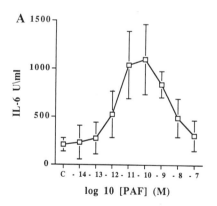 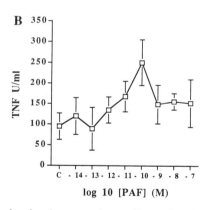

FIGURE 1. Effect of PAF on cytokine production by alveolar macrophages. Macrophages (10^6/ml) stimulated with MDP (1 μg/ml) were cultured in the absence (vehicle control: C) or presence of graded concentrations of PAF for 18 hours. Cell-free supernatants were then analyzed for IL-6 (**A**) or TNF-α (**B**) bioactivity. Data are mean ± SE of six and five experiments, respectively. Statistically significant effects were noted for PAF concentrations of 10^{-11}–10^{-9} M ($p < 0.01$) in (**A**), and 10^{-10} M ($p < 0.01$) in (**B**).

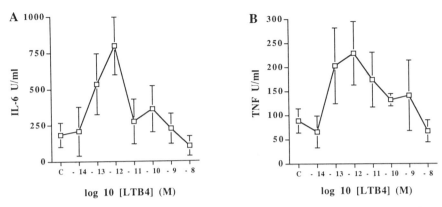

FIGURE 2. Effect of graded concentrations of LTB_4 on IL-6 (**A**) and TNF-α (**B**) production. Data represent mean $\pm$ SE of five experiments. Statistically significant effects were noted for LTB_4 concentrations of 10^{-13} M ($p < 0.05$) and 10^{-12} M ($p < 0.01$) in (**A**), and 10^{-13}–10^{-12} M ($p < 0.05$) in (**B**).

TNF-α and IL-6 production, respectively, by MDP-stimulated AMs. In parallel experiments we assessed whether LTB_4 could reproduce and mimic the effect of PAF on the release of TNF-α and IL-6. Under the same culture conditions, our data indicated that exogenous LTB_4 could enhance TNF-α and IL-6 production by two- to fourfold, respectively (FIG. 2). Picomolar concentrations were sufficient to induce significant augmentation of release of these cytokines.

PGE₂ and LTB₄ Production by PAF-stimulated AMs

Release of arachidonic acid and production of arachidonate metabolites in response to PAF have been reported in various cells, including guinea pig alveolar

TABLE 1. LTB_4 and PGE_2 Production by Alveolar Macrophages Stimulated with PAF or LTB_4[a]

	LTB_4[b]	PGE_2
C	240	100
PAF	440	200
LTB_4	—	220
INDO	380	45
INDO + PAF	500	13
MK 886	64	70
MK + PAF	76	130

[a] Data are from an experiment representative of three experiments, in which 1×10^6 AM/ml stimulated with MDP (1 μg/ml) were preincubated or not with COX inhibitor indomethacin (10^{-6} M) or 5 LOX inhibitor MK 886 (2×10^{-6} M) then cultured for 18 h with or without PAF (10^{-10} M) or LTB_4 (10^{-12} M).

[b] LTB_4 and PGE_2 expressed as pg/ml were detected by EIA as described in the section titled "Materials and Methods."

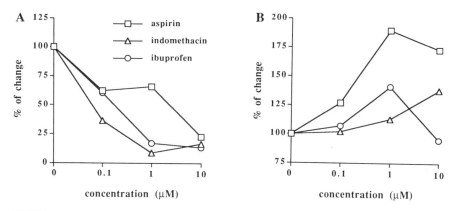

FIGURE 3. Effect of cyclooxygenase inhibition on PAF-induced IL-7 **(A)** and TNF-α **(B)** production. Macrophages were preincubated 30 min with graded concentrations of aspirin, indomethacin, or ibuprofen and further incubated 18 hours in the presence of MDP and PAF (10^{-10} M). Data are mean of five and six experiments, respectively.

macrophages,[23] rat Kupffer cells,[24] and the mouse macrophagelike cell line P388D$_1$.[20] We investigated the effect of PAF directly on PGE$_2$ and LTB$_4$ production by AMs. As shown in TABLE 1, treatment of AMs with PAF at 10^{-10} M enhanced by twofold their PGE$_2$ and LTB$_4$ production. As could be expected, inhibition of COX or 5-LOX by inhibitors of these pathways abrogated the augmentation induced by PAF.

Effect of COX and 5-LOX Inhibitors on PAF-stimulated IL-6 and TNF-α Production

Previous findings have shown a regulatory potential of endogenous leukotrienes in PAF-induced augmentation of TNF-α or IL-6 production by macrophages.[13,14] Since PAF could enhance LTB$_4$ as well as PGE$_2$ secretion by AMs, we assessed whether in this system endogenous COX metabolites could also be implicated in the mechanism of PAF action. For these experiments, AMs were preincubated 30 min at 37°C with the different inhibitors of COX pathway and further incubated 18 hours in the presence of MDP and PAF, at concentrations known to enhance IL-6 and TNF-α production. Data shown in FIGURE 3 indicate that indomethacin, aspirin, and ibuprofen reduced PAF-stimulated IL-6 production while they potentiated PAF-induced TNF-α production. These effects were concentration dependent.

On the other hand, we had already reported that LTB$_4$ could stimulate IL-6 and TNF-α production by AM.[13,14] Surprisingly, we observed that LTB$_4$ could also enhance by twofold their PGE$_2$ production (as illustrated in TABLE 1). Therefore we investigated whether indomethacin could affect the LTB$_4$-induced release of IL-6 and TNF-α. As shown in FIGURE 4, pretreatment of AMs with this inhibitor effectively blocked the LTB$_4$-induced IL-6 production while it further augmented its effect on TNF-α production.

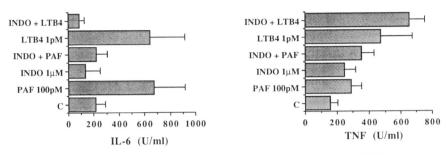

FIGURE 4. Effect of cyclooxygenase inhibition on LTB$_4$-induced IL-6 and TNF-α production. Macrophages were preincubated or not 30 min with indomethacin, then stimulated 18 hours with LTB$_4$ or PAF. Data represent mean $\pm$ SE of three experiments.

Effect of PGE$_2$ and dBcAMP on the Release of IL-6 and TNF-α

It is known that PGE$_2$ produced by activated macrophages may participate in the autoregulation of cytokine production by stimulation of adenylate cyclase and the induction of cyclic AMP-dependent signal pathways. FIGURE 5 shows the effects of PGE$_2$ and of the cell-permeable cAMP analogue, dibutyryl cAMP (dBcAMP), on IL-6 and TNF-α release by AMs. Treatment of AMs with exogenous PGE$_2$ or dBcAMP resulted in five- to tenfold enhancement in IL-6 production while it concomitantly inhibited TNF-α production. In parallel, increasing levels of intracellular cGMP by dBcGMP had no effect on either cytokine release.

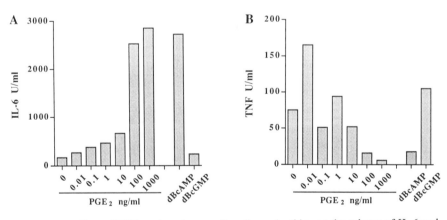

FIGURE 5. Effect of PGE$_2$ and analogues of cyclic nucleotides on the release of IL-6 and TNF-α. Macrophages were stimulated 18 hours with graded concentrations of PGE$_2$ or dBcAMP (10^{-4} M) or with dBcGMP (10^{-4} M). Cell-free supernatants were then analyzed for their content in IL-6 **(A)** or TNF-α **(B)**. Data are mean of three experiments.

DISCUSSION

We have previously shown that PAF induces IL-6 and TNF-α production by AMs. These effects are stereospecific, and endogenous 5-LOX metabolites can act as secondary mediators in the underlying mechanism of action.[13,14] The present study provides evidence for the possible involvement of both COX and 5-LOX pathways in the mechanism by which PAF could modulate release of these cytokines. Furthermore, our data indicate a differential regulation of IL-6 and TNF-α production by COX and 5-LOX metabolites in response to PAF, and suggest that PAF induces both positive and negative feedback mechanisms in its interactions with macrophages and their cytokine networks.

The 5-LOX metabolites of arachidonic acid, and in particular LTB$_4$, have been recognized as powerful activators of several phagocyte functions and modulators of cytokine production. Recently, we reported that LTB$_4$ could stimulate IL-6 production by human monocytes by both transcriptional and posttranscriptional mechanisms.[25] Furthermore, we also observed that exogenous and endogenous LTB$_4$ can up-regulate TNF-α as well as IL-6 production.[13,14]

Our results are in accordance with observations by other investigators concerning the participation of lipoxygenase metabolites in some mononuclear cell functions. Hence, it has been observed that lipoxygenase inhibitors suppress thioglycolate-elicited mouse peritoneal macrophage release of IL-1[26] and TNF-α,[27] inhibit mouse peritoneal macrophage release of FGF,[28] prevent human peripheral blood mononuclear cell release of leukocyte pyrogen,[29] block TPA-induced increases in TNF-α mRNA levels in HL-60 cells,[18] and inhibit both LTB$_4$ and NAP/IL-8 release.[30]

On the other hand, we observed that inhibition of the COX pathway abrogated the PAF- and LTB$_4$-induced augmentation of IL-6 production, but further enhanced PAF-stimulated TNF-α production. Less information is available on the effects of endogenous cyclooxygenase metabolites on regulation of cytokines, although certain studies have demonstrated effects of COX inhibition on augmentation of TNF-α production.[31,32] COX metabolites such as PGE$_2$ have been shown to inhibit TNF-α production, presumably by augmenting cAMP levels in the cells.[16,17] The inhibitory effect of PGE$_2$ upon TNF-α production has been well documented. This inhibition occurs predominantly if not totally at the level of mRNA production.[18,33] It has been reported, however, that low concentrations of PGE$_2$ could augment TNF-α production in rat peritoneal macrophages, presumably by stimulating cGMP accumulation.[34] Our data also show augmented TNF-α production by AMs at 0.01 ng/ml PGE$_2$.

On the other hand, it is possible that the induction by PGE$_2$ of macrophage IL-6 synthesis involves cAMP, since cAMP-responsive DNA elements have been functionally implicated in IL-6 gene expression.[35] Similar observations on a differential regulation of TNF-α and IL-6 have been reported with phosphodiesterase inhibitor studies and in LPS-stimulated human monocytes.[36–38] PGE$_2$ and other agents that increase intracellular cAMP levels reduced TNF-α production, while IL-6 production was increased.

An interesting finding in this investigation was the observation of PGE$_2$ production by AM in response to LTB$_4$ stimulation. Such a potential regulatory role of endogenous and exogenous 5-LOX metabolites on the COX pathway has been suggested in some studies. For instance, leukotrienes C4 and D4 have been shown to induce the release of PGE$_2$, 6-keto PGF$_{1\alpha}$, and TXB$_2$ release from rat peritoneal macrophages.[39,40] Further studies will be required to clarify the complex signaling process involved in macrophage activation by PAF and to identify the putative link between 5-LOX and COX metabolites. These results may reflect the underlying complexities of a system in which multiple, convergent pathways can be involved in the modulation of cytokine production and where interactions between them can occur in sequential steps during the biosynthetic process. However, we speculate that the ability of PAF to induce concomitant production of endogenous 5-LOX and COX metabolites may be important, even crucial, in modulating the effects of PAF in several cell systems.

Differential modulation of TNF-α and IL-6 production and secretion by AMs would permit the fine tuning of the response to inflammatory stimuli. It is interesting to observe that a single stimulus such as PAF, which promotes the expression of inflammatory cytokines, simultaneously initiates the production of eicosanoids, which, directly or indirectly, can autoregulate cytokine synthesis in a selective fashion. Such differential autocrine modulation could play an important role in the regulation of the production of cytokines participating in immune and inflammatory responses. PAF could induce both positive and negative feedback mechanisms in its interaction with macrophages. Since cellular sources of PAF and stimuli for its production are present in many inflammatory reactions, these observations might have relevance in PAF-mediated events in the lung.

REFERENCES

1. MORNEX, J. F., et al. 1986. Spontaneous expression of the c-sis gene and release of platelet-derived growth factorlike molecule by human alveolar macrophages. J. Clin. Invest. **78:** 61–66.
2. DERYNCK, R., et al. 1985. Human transforming growth factor-beta complementary sequence and expression in normal cells. Nature **316:** 701–707.
3. BEUTLER, B., et al. 1985. Identity of tumor necrosis factor and macrophage-secreted factor cachectin. Nature **316:** 552–556.
4. STRIETER, R. M., D. G. REMICK, J. P. LYNCH, R. N. SPENGLER & S. L. KUNKEL. 1989. Interleukin-2 induced tumor necrosis factor-alpha (TNF-α) gene expression in human alveolar macrophages and blood monocytes. Am. Rev. Respir. Dis. **139:** 335–342.
5. KORETZKY, G. A., et al. 1983. Spontaneous production of interleukin-1 by human alveolar macrophages. Clin. Immunol. Immunopathol. **29:** 443–450.
6. HORII, Y., et al. 1988. Regulation of BSF-2/IL-6 production by human mononuclear cells: Macrophage-dependent synthesis of BSF-2/IL-6 by T cells. J. Immunol. **141:** 1529–1535.
7. STRIETER, R. M., et al. 1990. Human alveolar macrophage gene expression of interleukin-8 by tumor necrosis factor-α, lipopolysaccharide, and interleukin-1β. Am. J. Respir. Cell. Mol. Biol. **2:** 321–326.
8. STENSON, W. F. & C. W. PARKER. 1980. Prostaglandins, macrophages and immunity. J. Immunol. **125:** 1–5.
9. GOLDYNE, M. E., G. F. BURRISH, P. POUBELLE & P. BORGEAT. 1984. Arachidonic acid metabolism among human mononuclear leukocytes: Lipoxygenase-related pathways. J. Biol. Chem. **259:** 8815–8819.
10. ALBERT, D. H. & F. SNYDER. 1983. Biosynthesis of 1-alkyl-2-acetyl-sn-glycero-3-phosphocholine (platelet-activating factor) from 1-alkyl-2-acyl-sn-glycero-3-phosphocholine by rat alveolar macrophages. J. Biol. Chem. **258:** 97–102.
11. CAMUSSI, G., C. TETTA & C. BAGLIONI. 1990. The role of platelet-activating factor in inflammation. Clin. Immunol. Immunopathol. **57:** 331–338.

12. PEPLOW, P. V. & D. P. MIKHAILIDIS. 1990. Platelet-activating factor (PAF) and its relation to prostaglandins, leukotrienes and other aspects of arachidonate metabolism. Prostagl. Leuk. Essent. Fatty Acids **41:** 71–76.

13. DUBOIS, C., E. BISSONNETTE & M. ROLA-PLESZCZYNSKI. 1989. Platelet-activating factor (PAF) stimulates tumor necrosis factor production by alveolar macrophages: Prevention by PAF receptor antagonists and lipoxygenase inhibitors. J. Immunol. **143:** 964–971.

14. THIVIERGE, M. & M. ROLA-PLESZCZYNSKI. 1992. Platelet-activating factor (PAF) enhances interleukin-6 production by alveolar macrophages. J. Allergy Clin. Immunol. **90:** 796–802.

15. ZHANG, Y., J. X. LIN & J. VILCEK. 1988. Synthesis of interleukin 6 (interferon-$\beta2$/B cell stimulatory factor 2) in human fibroblasts is triggered by an increase in intracellular cyclic AMP. J. Biol. Chem. **263:** 6177–6182.

16. KUNKEL, S. L., et al. 1988. Prostaglandin E_2 regulates macrophage-derived tumor necrosis factor gene expression. J. Biol. Chem. **263:** 5380–5384.

17. RENZ, H., et al. 1988. Release of tumor necrosis factor-α from macrophages. Enhancement and suppression are dose-dependently regulated by prostaglandin E_2 and cyclic nucleotides. J. Immunol. **141:** 2388–2393.

18. HORIGUCHI, J., et al. 1989. Role of arachidonic acid metabolism in transcriptional induction of tumor necrosis factor gene expression by phorbol ester. Mol. Cell Biol. **9:** 252–258.

19. LISTER, M. D., K. B. GLASER, R. J. ULEVITCH & E. A. DENNIS. 1989. Inhibition studies on the membrane-associated phospholipase A2 *in vitro* and prostaglandin E_2 production *in vivo* of the macrophage-like P388D_1 cell. J. Biol. Chem. **264:** 8520–8528.

20. GLASER, K. B., R. ASMIS & E. A. DENNIS. 1990. Bacterial lipopolysaccharide priming of P388D_1 macrophage-like cells for enhanced arachidonic acid metabolism. J. Biol. Chem. **265:** 8658–8664.

21. AARDEN, L. A., E. R. DE GROOT, O. L. SCHAAP & P. M. LANSDORP. 1987. Production of hybridoma growth factor by human monocytes. Eur. J. Immunol. **17:** 1411–1416.

22. POUBELLE, P. E., et al. 1991. Platelet-activating factor (PAF-acether) enhances the concomitant production of tumor necrosis factor-alpha and interleukin-1 by subsets of human monocytes. Immunology **72:** 181–187.

23. KADIRI, C., et al. 1990. Mechanism of N-formyl-methionyl-leucyl-phenylalanine- and platelet-activating factor-induced arachidonic acid release in guinea pig alveolar macrophages: Involvement of a GTP-binding protein and role of protein kinase A and protein kinase C. Mol. Pharmacol. **38:** 418–425.

24. CHAO, W., H. LIU, D. J. HANAHAN & M. S. OLSON. 1990. Regulation of platelet-activating factor receptor and PAF receptor-mediated arachidonic acid release by protein kinase C activation in rat Kupffer cells. Arch. Biochem. Biophys. **282:** 188–197.

25. ROLA-PLESZCZYNSKI, M. & J. STANKOVA. 1992. Leukotriene B_4 enhances interleukin-6 (IL-6) production and IL-6 messenger RNA accumulation in human monocytes *in vitro:* Transcriptional and post-transcriptional mechanisms. Blood **80:** 1004–1011.

26. BRANDWEIN, S. R. 1986. Regulation of interleukin-1 production by mouse peritoneal macrophages. Effects of arachidonic acid metabolites, cyclic nucleotides, and interferons. J. Biol. Chem. **261:** 8624–8632.

27. SCHADE, U. F., M. ERNST, M. REINKE & D. T. WOLTER. 1989. Lipoxygenase inhibitors suppress formation of tumor necrosis factor *in vitro* and *in vivo*. Biochem. Biophys. Res. Commun. **159:** 748–754.

28. PHAN, S. H., B. M. MCGARRY, K. M. LOEFFLER & S. L. KUNKEL. 1987. Regulation of macrophage-derived fibroblast growth factor release by arachidonate metabolites. J. Leuk. Biol. **42:** 106–113.

29. DINARELLO, C. A., I. BISHAI, L. J. ROSENWASSER & F. COCEANI. 1984. The influence of lipoxygenase inhibitors on the *in vitro* production of human leukocyte pyrogen and lymphocyte activating factor (interleukin-1). Int. J. Immunopharmacol. **6:** 43.

30. RANKIN, J. A. & P. HARRIS. 1993. The effect of inhibition of leukotriene B_4 release

on lipopolysaccharide-induced production of neutrophil attractant/activation protein-1 (interleukin-8) by human alveolar macrophages. Prostaglandins **45:** 77–84.

31. ENDRES, S., *et al.* 1989. *In vitro* production of IL-1β, IL-1α, TNF and IL-2 in healthy subjects: Distribution, effect of cyclooxygenase inhibition, and evidence of independent gene regulation. Eur. J. Immunol. **19:** 2327–2333.

32. ENDRES, S., *et al.* 1989. The effect of supplementation with n-3 polyunsaturated fatty acids on the synthesis of interleukin-1 and tumor necrosis factor by mononuclear cells. New Eng. J. Med. **320:** 265–271.

33. TANNENBAUM, C. S. & T. A. HAMILTON. 1989. Lipopolysaccharide-induced gene expression in murine peritoneal macrophages is selectively suppressed by agents that elevate intracellular cAMP. J. Immunol. **142:** 1274–1280.

34. GONG, J.-H., H. RENZ, H. SPRENGER, M. NAIN & D. GEMSA. 1990. Enhancement of tumor necrosis factor-α gene expression by low doses of prostaglandin E_2 and cyclic GMP. Immunobiology **182:** 44–55.

35. RAY, A., P. SASSONE-CORSI & P. B. SEGHAL. 1989. A multiple cytokine- and second messenger-responsive element in the enhancer of the human IL-6 gene: Similarities with c-fos gene regulation. Mol. Cell Biol. **9:** 5537.

36. ZABEL, P., D. T. WOLTER, M. M. SCHÖNHARTING & U. F. SCHADE. 1989. Oxpentifylline in endotoxaemie. Lancet **II:** 1474–1477.

37. WAAGE, A., M. SORENSEN & B. STORDAL. 1990. Differential effect of oxpentifylline on tumour necrosis factor and interleukin-6 production. Lancet **II:** 543.

38. BAILLY, S., B. FERRUA, M. FAY & M. A. GOUGEROT-POCIDALO. 1990. Differential regulation of IL-6, IL-1α, IL-1β and TNF-α production in LPS-stimulated human monocytes: Role of cyclic AMP. Cytokine **2:** 205–210.

39. FEUERSTEIN, N., M. FOEGH & P. W. RAMWELL. 1981. Leukotrienes C_4 and D_4 induce prostaglandin and thromboxane release from rat peritoneal macrophages. Br. J. Pharmacol. **72:** 389–391.

40. SCHENKELAARS, E.-J. & I. L. BONTA. 1983. Effect of leukotriene C_4 on the release of secretory products by elicited populations of rat peritoneal macrophages. Eur. J. Pharmacol. **86:** 477–480.

Eosinophils, Cytokines, and Allergic Inflammation

REDWAN MOQBEL

Department of Allergy and Clinical Immunology
National Heart and Lung Institute
Dovehouse Street
London, England SW3 6LY

INTRODUCTION

Eosinophils are prominent inflammatory cells associated with allergic disease and inflammatory responses against metazoan helminthic parasites.[1,2] This association has been most extensively characterized in relation to asthma where large numbers of eosinophils and their granule products are found in and around the airways in asthma deaths.[2] An inverse correlation between the degree of bronchial hyperreactivity and peripheral blood eosinophilia has been observed in subjects who exhibited dual response following antigen challenge.[3] Furthermore, using more invasive methods such as fiberoptic bronchoscopy, an increase in the number of activated eosinophils present in the airways was shown to correlate with asthma severity.[4] Despite the close association between eosinophils and the pathogenesis of allergic disease and asthma, the evidence for a cause and effect relationship remains largely circumstantial.

Eosinophils are nondividing, granule-containing cells that arise principally in the bone marrow.[5] They are 8 μm in diameter and their granules avidly take up acidic dyes such as eosin. In laboratory animals, parasite-induced eosinophilia has been shown to be dependent on T lymphocytes.[6] This effect was shown to be mediated by soluble factors released from sensitized lymphocytes.[7] Recent advances in human eosinophil research have indicated that eosinophil infiltration into the tissue in allergic-type responses and asthma may be regulated by a complex series of events that involve immunological and inflammatory mechanisms including T cells and cytokines.[8,9]

EOSINOPHIL MEDIATORS

Granule-derived Proteins

Eosinophils are granulocytic inflammatory leukocytes that contain specialized and unique granules that avidly take up acidic dyes due to their cationic nature.[5,10] A number of preformed biologically active mediators are stored within the eosinophil granules. It is now thought that these granule-derived products, which have potent cytotoxic properties against bronchial epithelial cells and pneumocytes, may be largely responsible for the damage associated with eosinophil infiltration into the bronchial mucosa in asthma.[10] Each granule is comprised of a rectangular or square crystalline-like core that is surrounded by a less electron dense matrix.[11,12] The core of the granule contains mainly major basic protein (MBP), while the matrix contains three other eosinophil basic proteins, eosinophil cationic protein

223

(ECP), eosinophil peroxidase (EPO), and eosinophil-derived neurotoxin (EDN).[5,10] In addition, mature eosinophils contain small granules that contain acid phosphatase and aryl sulphatase.[13]

Membrane-derived Mediators

Eosinophils are a rich source of the sulphidopeptide leukotriene LTC_4 (5S-hydroxy-6R,S-glutathionyl-7,9,-$trans$-11,14-cis-eicosatetraenoic acid).[14,15] Stimulation with the calcium ionophore A-23187, generates up to 40 ng/10^6 cells of LTC_4 from normal density eosinophils, while light-density eosinophils elaborate 70 ng/10^6 cells. Eosinophils produce negligible amounts (6 ng/10^6 cells) of LTB_4 (5S-12R-dihydroxy-6,14-cis-8,10-$trans$-eicosatetraenoic acid) compared with up to 200 ng/10^6 cells from neutrophils. LTC_4 generation by human eosinophils was also observed after stimulation with both opsonized zymosan and via an FcγRII-dependent mechanism using Sepharose beads coated with IgG.[16] Release was maximal at 45 minutes, greater in hypodense eosinophils than normal density eosinophils and enhanced by fMLP. Eosinophils can also generate substantial quantities of 15-HETE via the 15-lipoxygenase pathway.

Eosinophils generate large amounts of PAF after both stimulation with calcium ionophore-, zymosan-, and IgG-coated Sepharose beads.[17–20] PAF (1-0-alkyl-2-acetyl-sn-glycerol-3-phosphatidycholine) is a potent phospholipid mediator which causes leukocyte activation. For instance, eosinophils elaborated 25 ng/10^6 cells of PAF after stimulation with calcium ionophore and up to 2 ng/10^6 cells after IgG stimulation. Much of the PAF remained cell associated, possibly acting as an intracellular messenger, or alternatively binding to PAF receptors on eosinophils, thus acting as an autocrine agent. Interestingly, stimulation of eosinophils with fMLP did not augment PAF release, and hypodense eosinophils from patients with a marked eosinophilia released less PAF than normal eosinophils. ^{3}H.PAF added to hypodense eosinophils was much more rapidly incorporated into the phospholipid pool than ^{3}H.PAF with normal density cells.[19] This suggests that hypodense eosinophils were metabolizing the exogeneous PAF at a greater rate than the normodense cells and may explain why stimulation with fMLP did not result in an increased amount of PAF generation. As with leukotriene synthesis, eosinophil-derived release of PAF was maximal at 45 minutes. Eosinophils also generate mediators of the cyclooxygenase pathway, including PGE_1 and PGE_2, and thromboxane B_2.

Eosinophil-derived Cytokines

A number of recent studies have demonstrated the capacity of the human eosinophil to synthesize and elaborate a number of cytokines. Human eosinophils have already been shown to express messenger RNA (mRNA) for, and release a number of important proinflammatory cytokines, including TGFα, TGFβ_1, granulocyte/macrophage–colony-stimulating factor (GM–CSF), IL-3, IL-5, IL-6, IL-8, and IL-1α[21–28] (see TABLE 1). mRNA for both GM–CSF and IL-6 were shown to be translated and the mature proteins detected using immunocytochemical staining techniques.[23,26] In addition, picogram amounts of GM–CSF, IL-3, and IL-6 were measured in supernatants of stimulated eosinophils.[24,26] Studies have demonstrated that the production of IL-3 and GM–CSF by eosinophils may be important in prolonging the survival of these cells, possibly by a putative autocrine

TABLE 1. Cytokines Synthesized by and Released from Human Eosinophils

Cytokine	Reference
Transforming growth factor α	21
Transforming growth factor β	22
Granulocyte/macrophage colony-stimulating factor	23, 24
Interleukin-1α	28
Interleukin-3	24
Interleukin-5	25
Interleukin-6	26
Interleukin-8	27

loop.[24,29] Observations on eosinophil cytokine release have been mainly studied *in vitro*, but have, with most cytokines, been confirmed *in vivo*.[21,22,25,30,31] The physiological triggers for eosinophil cytokine generation are, however, not fully clear. The recognition of the capacity of the eosinophil to synthesize and release these cytokines has introduced a new dimension toward understanding the potential of the eosinophil as an effector cell in allergic inflammation. However, the full capacity of the eosinophil to elaborate cytokines, the precise microenvironment requirements for such synthesis, and the intracellular pattern of production and storage are yet to be fully investigated.

EOSINOPHIL DIFFERENTIATION

Peripheral blood and tissue eosinophils are derived in hemopoiesis from CD34$^+$ myeloid progenitors found in the bone marrow. The factors that influence the proliferation and the differentiation of the eosinophil lineage are cytokine growth factors of which IL-3, granulocyte/macrophage–colony-stimulating factor (GM–CSF), and IL-5 are important in promoting eosinophil differentiation.[32,33] It is now well recognized that IL-5 is the key cytokine in terminal differentiation of eosinophils from committed precursors. The obligatory role of IL-5 in the differentiation of the eosinophil has been confirmed by elegant studies on transgenic mice in which the expression of the gene for IL-5 developed marked eosinophilia and contain increasing numbers of eosinophil precursors in their bone marrow.[34,35] Interestingly, eosinophil differentiation in this transgenic model appeared to be completely independent of IL-3 and GM–CSF, suggesting that IL-5 alone was sufficient to generate an eosinophilia from stem cell precursors. This was in contrast with *in vitro* eosinopoiesis studies using cultures of eosinophil progenitors from either bone marrow or cord blood mononuclear cells where IL-3 and GM–CSF appeared to be necessary at least at a proximal (early) stage of proliferation and lineage commitment, and where IL-5 played a critical role only at a distal (terminal) stage of differentiation.[32,33] These discrepant observations highlight the need for a more precise delineation of the factors, both autocrine and paracrine, involved in the growth proliferation and differentiation of eosinophils from myeloid precursor cells.

EOSINOPHIL HETEROGENEITY

Peripheral blood eosinophils from normal individuals are dense cells that separate out from other leukocytes in the lower bands of Percoll or Metrizamide discontinuous density gradients. A proportion of eosinophils from individuals with a raised eosinophil count are of lower density than eosinophils from normal subjects.[36] The mechanism for this heterogeneity is not clear. Hypodense eosinophils appear vacuolated and contain smaller sized granules although of equal numbers to normal-density eosinophils. They also have a greater cell volume than normodense eosinophils.[37] The presence of low-density (or hypodense) eosinophils appears to be a nonspecific phenomenon that occurs in any eosinophilic condition, including allergic disease.[38] It is generally thought that hypodense eosinophils are more activated. They show elevated oxygen consumption,[39] increased cytotoxicity toward helminthic targets,[40] and release more LTC_4 after physiological stimulation.[16] Activation of eosinophils *in vitro* with inflammatory mediators, such as platelet activating factor (PAF), as well as long-term culture with cytokines, was also associated with a decrease in eosinophil density.[41-43] In contrast, there was no difference in receptor expression between normal and hypodense eosinophils.[44] Normal-density eosinophils from patients with an eosinophilia have enhanced function compared with eosinophils from normal individuals. It is possible, therefore, that the association between hypodensity and activation is coincidental with the less dense cells being more immature.

EOSINOPHIL TISSUE ACCUMULATION

The mechanisms involved in the selective recruitment of eosinophils in allergic reaction remains speculative. Among these mechanisms are chemotaxis, selective adhesion of eosinophils to both vascular endothelial cells and extracellular matrix proteins, *in situ* differentiation of committed precursors, and prolonged survival. It now appears that many of these mechanisms may be controlled at the level of the T-cell response to antigens and the subsequent release of cytokines, which in turn regulate the activity of eosinophils.[8] There is now ample evidence demonstrating the presence of mRNA encoding for the IL-3, IL-4, IL-5, and GM–CSF gene cluster family in allergen-induced cutaneous late-phase reaction (LPR) in atopic subjects where an association between the degree of eosinophilic inflammation and cytokine expression has been observed.[45] IL-5 mRNA was also expressed in bronchial biopsies from symptomatic, but not asymptomatic, atopic asthmatics, and this was again correlated with eosinophil activation.[46] Similar findings have been described in nasal LPR in atopic individuals.[47,48] The profile of cytokine release in these allergen-induced inflammatory responses appears to be akin to the pattern observed in the murine Th2-type; that is, IL-4 and IL-5.[45,49,50] In contrast, in the classic delayed-type hypersensitivity (DTH) reaction observed 24 hours after tuberculin injection, a Th1-type cytokine mRNA profile (i.e., IL-2 and IFNγ) was predominant in nonatopic individuals.[51] Thus, IL-5 released by sensitized Th2-type T-cells as a consequence of their stimulation with specific allergen may be related to the development for the eosinophilia during allergic disease.

Eosinophil Chemotaxis

While cytokines are important in growth and differentiation of eosinophils from precursors, they may also influence the locomotory function of the ma-

TABLE 2. Functional Activity of Cytokines and Chemokines on Human Eosinophils

	Chemotaxis	Adhesion	Survival Factor	Cytotoxicity	Mediator Release
IL-2	+ +	?	?	?	?
IL-3	weak[a]	+[b]	+ +[b]	+ +[b]	+ +[b]
IL-5	weak[a]	+ + +	+ +	+ +	+ +
IL-8	weak[a]	?	?	?	?
GM–CSF	weak	+ +[b]	+ + +	+ +	+ +
RANTES	+ + +	?	?	?	?
IFNγ	—	?	+ +	+ +	—
MIP-1α	+ +	?	?	?	?
LCF[c]	+ +	?	?	?	?

[a] Primes for enhanced response.
[b] Not selective for eosinophils.
[c] Lymphocyte chemotactic factor.

ture eosinophil, which may in turn contribute to the accumulation of these cells within the inflammatory tissue foci. IL-3, IL-5, and GM–CSF are all weakly chemotactic for eosinophils (TABLE 2). However, IL-5 has been shown to prime eosinophils for better chemotactic response to other chemotactic mediators such as PAF, LTB_4, or IL-8.[52,53] IL-5 also has a stronger chemotactic activity for resting (normal density) eosinophils than activated (low density obtained from eosinophilic patients).[52] These *in vitro* migratory responses can be down-regulated by antiallergic, H_1 histamine antagonists such as cetirizine,[54] an agent that also inhibits chemotactic factor-induced cell activation, including adhesion, cytotoxic effector function, and mediator release.[55] Regulated and normal T-lymphocyte expressed and secreted (RANTES), a member of the IL-8 family of chemokines, has been shown to be a potent eosinophilotactic factor.[56]

Adhesion

In health, eosinophils reside mainly in the tissues; however, the mechanism of their tissue localization is not yet fully understood. The initial step in tissue accumulation is adherence to postvenular endothelium, which occurs following interaction between receptors on the surface of inflammatory cells and their ligands on the endothelial cell surface. An increasingly complex array of receptors is involved in this process.[57,58] These receptors are grouped into a number of gene superfamilies that include the integrin superfamily, the immunoglobulin superfamily, and another gene family termed the Selectins, the members of which are characterized by a lectin binding domain. It is becoming clear that adhesion and transmigration of leukocytes involve a number of carefully regulated steps. First, the Selectins are involved in the initial anchoring of the inflammatory cells to the venular endothelium. This has been shown to occur under flow conditions that mimic those in the venular endothelium where immunoglobulin family receptor/integrin interactions are inactive. Once anchored, the leukocytes roll until they become activated by a chemoattractant stimulus that induces a change in the integrin receptor on the leukocyte surface, which allows it to bind to the relevant ligand and rapidly induces flattening and transmigration.

In vitro assays of leukocyte adhesion to cultured human umbilical vein endothelial cells (HUVEC) have clarified the role of the individual receptors and their ligands in adhesion. Eosinophil adhesion to unstimulated HUVEC is upregulated by inflammatory mediators, including PAF.[59] This increase in adhesion appears to be mediated primarily through CR3 (Mac-1).[60] IL-5 also upregulates eosinophil, but not neutrophil, adhesion to unstimulated endothelium, offering a selective pathway of eosinophil adhesion.[61] Both stimulated and unstimulated eosinophils have increased adherence to IL-1-stimulated HUVEC compared with resting HUVEC. This adhesion is inhibited by monoclonal antibodies against ICAM-1 and ELAM-1 on the endothelium and by antibodies against LFA-1 and Mac-1 on the eosinophil.[62] To this extent the mechanism of eosinophil adhesion is very similar to that described for neutrophils.

A number of adhesion pathways have been defined that could potentially mediate the transmigration of eosinophils through the vascular endothelium. Particular interest is focused on the specific accumulation of eosinophils in allergic-type response, which may be due to the selective adhesion of eosinophils to vascular endothelium via receptors that are expressed on eosinophils. Recent studies by our group and others have described an eosinophil adhesion pathway that is not available for neutrophils, namely VLA-4 (constitutively expressed on eosinophils and lymphocytes, but not on neutrophils), which binds to its ligand VCAM-1 on vascular endothelium.[63-65] IL-4 is a key cytokine in the immunological induction of IgE synthesis[66] and has no known direct effect on human eosinophils. Interestingly, this cytokine was shown to enhance selective VLA-4-mediated eosinophil adhesion to vascular endothelial cells by increasing the expression of endothelial VCAM-1 receptors.[67] These findings have important implications in allergic asthma where preferential accumulation of eosinophils is a feature of atopic (IgE-dependent) inflammatory conditions.

Once the eosinophils adhere to vascular endothelium, they begin the process of extravasation (diapedesis) by which they emerge out of the capillaries and traverse the adjacent connective tissue *en route* to the focus of the inflammatory response.

Prolonged Survival

An alternative mechanism for eosinophil accumulation in tissues is prolonged survival. Like neutrophils, eosinophils are end-stage cells that, in culture, rapidly undergo cell death. However, eosinophil-active cytokines, such as IL-3, IL-5, and GM–CSF prolong eosinophil survival in culture for up to two weeks.[41,68,69] They also enhance eosinophil functions such as cytotoxicity for metazoan targets and mediator release.[70] Activated eosinophils can also generate a number of cytokines *in vitro*.[23,24] Extracellular matrix proteins have been shown to modulate eosinophil response to physiological soluble stimuli.[71] Research from our laboratory has demonstrated that eosinophils can adhere specifically to fibronectin,[72] an abundant extracellular matrix protein, and that VLA-4, a known receptor for fibronectin,[73] was involved in mediating eosinophil/fibronectin interactions.[72] Moreover, eosinophil adhesion to fibronectin resulted in short-term priming of eosinophils for enhanced leukotriene C_4 (LTC_4) release.[72] When eosinophil survival was measured by trypan blue exclusion, a significant enhancement of survival with fibronectin was observed as compared with both BSA-coated and uncoated wells.[29] Fibronectin-induced eosinophil survival was comparable to that obtained with exogenous IL-3 or GM–CSF and was inhibitable by antibodies against fibronectin, VLA-4, IL-3, and GM–CSF.[29] Supernatants from fibronectin-, but not BSA-coated wells, contained picogram amounts of IL-3 and GM–CSF, and eosinophils cultured on fibronectin for 24 hours expressed mRNA for GM–CSF as determined by *in situ* hybridization.[29] Therefore, fibronectin has the potential of acting as an important eosinophil survival factor, at least in culture, by triggering autocrine generation of cytokines by eosinophils. Since neutrophils lack VLA-4, this observation may provide a partial explanation for the preferential accumulation of eosinophils at sites of allergic inflammation, as well as the predominantly tissue localization of eosinophils in healthy individuals.

COLOCALIZATION OF mRNA TO EOSINOPHILS IN NASAL INFLAMMATORY REACTION

IL-5 is known to be a product of activated T cells.[74] However, recent studies have suggested that other cell types, such as mast cells[75] and eosinophils[25,30] are also capable of synthesizing IL-5. It is therefore important to determine the precise cellular source of this cytokine in allergic reactions. In a recent study,[31] nasal biopsies from allergen-induced late phase reactions, in subjects with allergic rhinitis, were used to determine the source of IL-5 transcripts among infiltrating T cells, mast cells, and eosinophils. The phenotype of interleukin-5 (IL-5) mRNA+ cells in the nasal mucosa was determined by simultaneous detection methods for cell phenotype by immunocytochemistry (APAAP) and IL-5 mRNA by *in situ* hybridization, using a Digoxigenin-labeled IL-5 riboprobe. This was conducted on serial nasal biopsy sections obtained from six atopic rhinitic patients, pre- and 24-hour postlocal allergen-challenge. For immunocytochemistry, monoclonal antibodies against T cells (CD3), mast cells (antitryptase), and eosinophil major basic protein (anti-MBP, BMK-13) were used to identify cell phenotypes. *In situ* hybridization was performed using nitroblue tetrazolium (NBT) and *X*-phosphate-5-bromo-4-chloro-3-indoly phosphate (BCIP), which served as chromogens to detect hybridized IL-5 mRNA. While the majority of IL-5 mRNA-positive cells were CD3+ (>80%), a percentage of MBP+ eosinophils were also IL-5 mRNA+ (>5%); the remainder were tryptase+ mast cells (>11%). Only few IL-5 mRNA+ cells were observed in prechallenged nasal biopsies, all of which were colocalized to CD3+ cells. These results suggested that CD3+ cells are the main source of IL-5 transcripts in allergen-induced late phase nasal reactions, but that subpopulations of both eosinophils and mast cells had the capacity to synthesize IL-5.[31]

CONCLUSIONS

While the mechanism of eosinophilia in association with allergic disease is not yet fully understood, it seems likely to be controlled at the level of the T-cell response to antigen and the subsequent elaboration of cytokines that exert both direct and indirect effect on these inflammatory cells. The profile of cytokines generated in allergic reactions, such as the allergen-induced late phase response (LPR) in the skin, nose, and lung, appears to conform to a Th2 profile since mRNA expression of IL-4 and IL-5, but not IFNγ or IL-2, was detected in tissue sections by *in situ* hybridization.[45–47] The release of IL-5 by Th2-type T-cells following stimulation with allergen may therefore be responsible for the eosinophilia of allergic disease. Thus a complex network of T cells, eosinophils, and other inflammatory cells and their cytokine products participate in a cascade of events that lead to specific accumulation of eosinophils in sites of allergic inflammation and asthma. Tissue damage, a feature of these disease conditions, may be the consequence of the activation and exocytosis of these infitrating cytotoxic cells and the release of their highly basic protein products. A more adequate understanding of the regulatory role of T cells and their cytokines, as well as a better appreciation of the full capacity of eosinophils and other inflammatory cells to synthesize and release their own range of cytokines should aid in the search for a more precise target for therapy aimed at inhibiting the selective accumulation of eosinophils in allergy and asthma.

REFERENCES

1. KAY, A. B., *et al.* 1985. Leucocyte activation initiated by IgE dependent mechanisms in relation to helminthic parasitic disease and clinical models of asthma. Int. Arch. Allergy Clin. Immunol. **77:** 69–72.
2. WARDLAW, A. J. & R. MOQBEL. 1992. The eosinophil in allergic and helminth related inflammatory responses. *In* Allergy and Immunity to Helminths, R. Moqbel, Ed: 154–186. Taylor & Francis. London.
3. DURHAM, S. R. & A. B. KAY. 1985. Eosinophils, bronchial hyperreactivity and late-phase asthmatic reactions. Clin. Allergy **15:** 411–418.
4. AZZAWI, M., *et al.* 1990. Identification of activated T lymphocytes and eosinophils in bronchial biopsies in stable atopic asthma. Am. Rev. Respir. Dis. **142:** 1407–1413.
5. SPRY, C. J. F. 1988. Eosinophils. A Comprehensive Review and Guide to the Scientific and Medical Literature: 484 pp. Oxford Univ. Press. Oxford.
6. BASTEN, A. & P. B. BEESON. 1970. Mechanism of eosinophilia. II. Role of the lymphocyte. J. Exp. Med. **131:** 1288–1305.
7. COLLEY, D. 1980. Lymphokine-related eosinophil responses. Lymphokine Res. **1:** 133–155.
8. CORRIGAN, C. J. & A. B. KAY. 1992. T cells and eosinophils in the pathogenesis of asthma. Immunol. Today **13:** 501–507.
9. KAY, A. B. 1991. Asthma and inflammation. J. Allergy Clin. Immunol. **87:** 893–910.
10. GLEICH, G. J. & C. R. ADOLPHSON. 1986. The eosinophil leucocyte. Ann. Rev. Immunol. **39:** 177–253.
11. BESSIS, M. & H. THIERY. 1961. Electron microscopy of human white blood cells and their stem cells. Int. Rev. Cytol. **12:** 199–241.
12. MILLER, F., E. DE HARVEN & G. E. PALDE. 1966. The structure of eosinophil leukocyte granules in rodents and man. J. Cell. Biol. **31:** 349–362.
13. PARMLEY, R. T. & S. S. SPICER. 1974. Cytochemical ultrastructural identification of a small type granule in human late eosinophils. Lab. Invest. **30:** 557–567.
14. WELLER, P. F., *et al.* 1983. Generation and metabolism of 5-lipoxygenase pathway leukotrienes by human eosinophils: Predominant production of leukotriene C_4. Proc. Natl. Acad. Sci. U.S.A. **80:** 7625–7630.
15. SHAW, R. J., O. CROMWELL & A. B. KAY. 1984. Preferential generation of leukotriene C_4 by human eosinophils. Clin. Exp. Immunol. **56:** 716–722.
16. SHAW, R. J., *et al.* 1985. Activated human eosinophils generate SRS-A leukotrienes following physiological (IgG-dependant) stimulation. Nature **316:** 150–152.
17. HENDERSON, W. R., J. B. HARLEY & A. S. FAUCI. 1984. Arachadonic acid metabolism in normal and hypereosinophilic syndrome human eosinophils: Generation leukotrienes B_4, C_4, D_4 and 15-lipoxygenase products. J. Immunol. **124:** 1383–1388.
18. LEE, T., D. J. HANAHAN, B. MALONE, L. L. RODDY & S. I. WASSERMAN. 1984. Increased biosynthesis of platelet activating factor in activated human eosinophils. J. Biol. Chem. **259:** 5526–5530.

19. CROMWELL, O., *et al*. 1990. IgG-dependent generation of platelet activating factor by normal and low density eosinophils. J. Immunol. **145:** 3862–3868.
20. BURKE, L. A., *et al*. 1990. Comparison of the generation of platelet-activating factor and leukotriene C_4 in human eosinophils stimulated by unopsonized zymosan and by the calcium ionophore A23187: The effects of nedocromil sodium. J. Allergy Clin. Immunol. **85:** 26–35.
21. WONG, D. T. W., *et al*. 1990. Human eosinophils express transforming growth factor α. J. Exp. Med. **172:** 673–681.
22. WONG, D. T. W., *et al*. 1991. Eosinophils from patients with blood eosinophilia express transforming factor β_1. Blood **78:** 2702–2707.
23. MOQBEL, R., *et al*. 1991. Expression of mRNA and immunoreactivity for the granulo-cyte/macrophage-colony stimulating factor (GM-CSF) in activated human eosinophils. J. Exp. Med. **174:** 749–752.
24. KITA, H., *et al*. 1991. GM-CSF and interleukin 3 release from human peripheral blood eosinophils and neutrophils. J. Exp. Med. **174:** 743–748.
25. DESREUMAUX, P., *et al*. 1992. Interleukin-5 mRNA expression by eosinophils in the intestinal mucosa of patients with coeliac disease. J. Exp. Med. **175:** 293–296.
26. HAMID, Q., *et al*. 1992. Human eosinophils synthesize and secrete interleukin-6, *in vitro*. Blood **80:** 1496–1501.
27. BRAUN, R. K., *et al*. 1993. Human peripheral blood eosinophils produce and release interleukin-8 on stimulation with calcium ionophore. Eur. J. Immunol. **23:** 956–960.
28. WELLER, P. F., *et al*. 1993. Accessory cell function of human eosinophils: HLA-DR-dependent, MHC-restricted antigen presentation and interleukin-1α formation. J. Immunol. **150:** 2554–2562.
29. ANWAR, A. R. E., R. MOQBEL, G. M. WALSH, A. B. KAY & A. J. WARDLAW. 1993. Adhesion to fibronectin prolongs eosinophil survival. J. Exp. Med. **177:** 839–843.
30. BROIDE, H., M. PAINE & G. FIRESTEIN. 1992. Eosinophils express interleukin 5 and granulocyte macrophage-colony-stimulating factor mRNA at sites of allergic inflammation. J. Clin. Invest. **90:** 1414–1424.
31. SUN YING, *et al*. 1993. T cells are the principal source of interleukin-5 mRNA in allergen-induced allergic rhinitis. Am. J. Respir. Cell Mol. Biol. **9:** 356–360.
32. SAITO, H., *et al*. 1988. Selective differentiation and proliferation of haematopoietic cells induced by recombinant human interleukins. Proc. Natl. Acad. Sci. U.S.A. **85:** 2288–2292.
33. CLUTTERBUCK, E. J., E. M. A. HIRST & C. J. SANDERSON. 1988. Human interleukin 5 (IL-5) regulates the production of eosinophils in human bone marrow cultures: Comparison and interaction with IL-1, IL-3, IL-6 and GM-CSF. Blood **73:** 1504–1511.
34. DENT, L. A., M. STRATH, A. L. MELLOR & C. J. SANDERSON. 1990. Eosinophilia in transgenic mice expressing interleukin 5. J. Exp. Med. **172:** 1425–1431.
35. TOMINAGA, A., *et al*. 1991. Transgenic mice expressing a B cell growth and differentiation factor gene (interleukin 5) develop eosinophilia and auto-antibody production. J. Exp. Med. **173:** 429–437.
36. BASS, D. A., *et al*. 1980. Comparison of human eosinophils from normals and patients with eosinophilia. J. Clin. Invest. **66:** 1265–1273.
37. CAULFIELD, J. P., *et al*. 1990. A morphometric study of normodense and hypodense human eosinophils that are derived *in vivo* and *in vitro*. Am. J. Pathol. **137:** 27–41.
38. FUKUDA, T., *et al*. 1985. Increased numbers of hypodense eosinophils in the blood of patients with bronchial asthma. Am. Rev. Respir. Dis. **132:** 981–985.
39. WINQVIST, I., T. OLOFFSON, I. OLSSON, A. M. PERSSON & T. HALLBERG. 1982. Altered density, metabolism and surface receptors of eosinophils in eosinophilia. Immunology **47:** 531–539.
40. PRIN, L., M. CAPRON, A. B. TONNEL, O. BLENTRY & A. CAPRON. 1983. Heterogeneity of human peripheral blood eosinophils: Variability in cell density and cytotoxic ability in relation to the level and origin of hypereosinophilia. Int. Arch. Allergy Appl. Immunol. **72:** 336–346.
41. ROTHENBURG, M. E., *et al*. 1987. Eosinophils co-cultured with endothelial cells have increased survival and functional properties. Science **237:** 645–647.

42. OWEN, W. F., *et al.* 1987. Regulation of human eosinophil viability, density and function by granulocyte/macrophage colony-stimulating factor in the presence of 3T3 fibroblasts. J. Exp. Med. **166:** 129–141.

43. FUKUDA, T. & S. MAKINO. 1989. Eosinophil heterogeneity. *In* Eosinophils in Asthma, Chap. 7, J. Morley and I. Colditz, Eds.: 125–137. Academic Press. London.

44. HARTNELL, A., R. MOQBEL, G. M. WALSH, B. BRADLEY & A. B. KAY. 1990. Fcγ and CD11/CD18 receptor expression on normal density and low density human eosinophils. Immunology **69:** 264–270.

45. KAY, A. B., *et al.* 1991. Messenger RNA expression of the cytokine gene cluster, IL-3, IL-4, IL-5 and GM-CSF in allergen-induced late-phase cutaneous reactions in atopic subjects. J. Exp. Med. **173:** 775–778.

46. HAMID, Q., *et al.* 1991. Expression of mRNA for interleukin-5 in mucosal bronchial biopsies from asthma. J. Clin. Invest. **87:** 1541–1546.

47. WIERENGA, E. A., *et al.* 1990. Evidence for compartmentalization of functional subsets of CD4+ T lymphocytes in atopic patients. J. Immunol. **144:** 4651–4656.

48. DURHAM, S. R., *et al.* 1992. Cytokine messenger RNA expression for IL-3, IL-4, IL-5 and granulocyte/macrophage-colony-stimulating factor in the nasal mucosa after local allergen provocation: Relationship to tissue eosinophilia. J. Immunol. **148:** 2390–2394.

49. ROBINSON, D. S., *et al.* 1991. Evidence for a predominant Th2-type bronchoalveolar lavage T lymphocyte population in atopic asthma. New Eng. J. Med. **326:** 298–304.

50. ROMAGNANI, S. Human Th1 and Th2: Doubt no more. Immunol. Today, **12:** 256–257.

51. TSICOPOULOS A., *et al.* 1992. Preferential mRNA expression of Th1-type cells (IFN-gamma+, IL-2+) in classical delayed-type (tuberculin) hypersensitivity reactions in human skin. J. Immunol. **148:** 2058–2061.

52. SEHMI, R., *et al.* 1992. Interleukin-5 (IL-5) selectively enhances the chemotactic response of eosinophils obtained from normal, but not eosinophilic subjects. Blood **79:** 2952–2959.

53. SEHMI, R., O. CROMWELL, A. J. WARDLAW, R. MOQBEL & A. B. KAY. 1993. Interleukin-8 is a chemoattractant for eosinophils from patients with an eosinophilia but not from normal subjects. Clin. Exp. Allergy **23.** In press.

54. SEHMI, R., *et al.* 1993. Modulation of human eosinophil chemotaxis and adhesion by anti-allergic drugs, *in vitro*. Paediatr. Allergy Immunol. **4**(Suppl. 4): 13–18.

55. WALSH, G. M., R. MOQBEL, A. HARTNELL & A. B. KAY. 1991. The effects of Cetirizine on human eosinophil and neutrophil activation, *in vitro*. Int. Arch. Allergy Appl. Immunol. **95:** 158–162.

56. KAMEYOSHI, Y., A. DORSCHNER, A. I. MALLET, E. CHRISTOPHERS & J.-M. SCHRODER. 1992. Cytokine RANTES-released by thrombin-stimulated platelets is a potent attractant for human eosinophils. J. Exp. Med. **176:** 587–592.

57. SPRINGER, T. A. 1990. Adhesion receptors of the immune system. Nature **346:** 425–434.

58. WARDLAW, A. J. 1990. Leucocyte adhesion to endothelium. Clin. Exp. Allergy **20:** 619–626.

59. KIMANI, G., M. G. TONNESEN & P. M. HENSON. 1988. Stimulation of eosinophil adherence to human vascular endothelial cells *in vitro* by platelet activating factor. J. Immunol. **140:** 3161–3166.

60. LAMAS, A. M., C. M. MULRONEY & R. P. SCHLEIMER. 1988. Studies of the adhesive interaction between purified human eosinophils and cultured vascular endothelial cells. J. Immunol. **140:** 1500–1505.

61. WALSH, G. M., *et al.* 1990. IL-5 enhances the *in vitro* adhesion of human eosinophils, but not neutrophils, in a leucocyte integrin (CD11/18)-dependent manner. Immunology **71:** 258–265.

62. KYAN-AUNG, U., D. O. HASKARD, R. N. POSTON, M. H. THORNHILL & T. H. LEE. 1991. Endothelial leukocyte adhesion molecule-1 and intercellular adhesion molecule-1 mediate adhesion of eosinophils to endothelial cells *in vitro* and are expressed by endothelium in allergic cutaneous inflammation *in vivo*. J. Immunol. **146:** 521–528.

63. WALSH, G. M., A. HARTNELL, J.-J. MERMOD, A. B. KAY & A. J. WARDLAW. 1991. Human eosinophil, but nor neutrophil, adherence to IL-1 stimulated HUVEC is α4β1 (VLA-4) dependent. J. Immunol. **146:** 3419–3423.

64. BOCHNER, B. S., *et al.* 1991. Adhesion of human basophils, eosinophils and neutrophils to interleukin-1-activated human vascular endothelial cells: Contribution of endothelial cell adhesion molecules. J. Exp. Med. **173:** 1553–1556.

65. WELLER, P. F., T. H. RAND, E. J. GOETZL, G. CHI-ROSSO & R. R. LOBB. 1991. Human eosinophil adherence to vascular endothelium mediated by binding to vascular cell adhesion molecule-1 and endothelial cell adhesion molecule-1. Proc. Natl. Acad. Sci. U.S.A. **88:** 7430–7433.

66. DEL PRETE, G., *et al.* 1988. IL-4 is an essential co-factor for the IgE synthesis induced *in vitro* by human T cell clones and their supernatants. J. Immunol. **144:** 4193–4198.

67. SCHLEIMER, R. P., *et al.* 1992. IL-4 induces adherence of human eosinophils and basophils but not neutrophils to endothelium. Association with expression of VCAM-1. J. Immunol. **148:** 1086–1092.

68. ROTHENBURG, M. E., *et al.* 1988. Human eosinophils have prolonged survival, enhanced functional properties and become hypodense when exposed to human interleukin 3. J. Clin. Invest. **81:** 1986–1992.

69. SILBERSTEIN, D. S., K. F. AUSTEN & W. F. OWEN. 1989. Hemopoietins for eosinophils. Glycoprotein hormones that regulate the development of inflammation in eosinophilia-associated disease. Haemat./Oncol. Clinics North Am. **3:** 511–532.

70. SILBERSTEIN, D. S. & J. R. DAVID. 1987. The regulation of human eosinophil function by cytokines. Immunol. Today **8:** 380–385.

71. DRI, P., R. CRAMER, R. SPESSOTTO, M. ROMANO & P. PATRIARCA. 1991. Eosinophil activation on biological surfaces. Production of O_2 in response to physiologic soluble stimuli is differentially modulated by extracellular matrix components and endothelial cells. J. Immunol. **147:** 613–620.

72. ANWAR, A. R. E., G. M. WALSH, O. CROMWELL, A. B. KAY & A. J. WARDLAW. Adhesion to fibronectin primes eosinophils via $\alpha4\beta1$ (VLA-4). Immunology. In press.

73. MOULD, A. P., *et al.* 1990. Affinity chromatic isolation of the melanoma adhesion receptor for the III CS region of fibronectin and its identification as the integrin $\alpha4\beta1$. J. Biol. Chem. **265:** 4020–4028.

74. YOKOTA, T., *et al.* 1987. Isolation and characterization of lymphokine cDNA clones encoding mouse and human IgA-enhancing factor and eosinophil colony-stimulating factor activities: Relationship to interleukin-5. Proc. Natl. Acad. Sci. U.S.A. **84:** 7388–7392.

75. PLAUT, M., *et al.* 1989. Mast cell lines produce lymphokines in response to cross-linkage of $Fc_\varepsilon RI$ or calcium ionophore. Nature **339:** 64–67.

Human Granulocytes Express Functional IgE-Binding Molecules, Mac-2/εBP

MARIE-JOSÉ TRUONG,[a] FU-TONG LIU,[b]
AND MONIQUE CAPRON[a]

[a]Centre d'Immunologie et de Biologie Parasitaire
Unité Mixte INSERM U 167–CNRS 624,
Institut Pasteur
Lille, France

[b]Allergy Research Section
Department of Molecular and Experimental Medicine
Research Institute of Scripps Clinic
La Jolla, California 92037

INTRODUCTION

Inflammatory reactions generally involve a vast array of mediators and a variety of effector cells, such as mast cells, macrophages, eosinophils, platelets, and neutrophils. Among them, eosinophils and neutrophils accumulate at inflammatory sites, especially during the late phase of the asthmatic reaction. These two types of granulocytes can be distinguished by several important features, such as the expression of receptors for IgE. Indeed, neutrophils represent the only leukocyte population that does not seem to express conventional Fc receptors for IgE, neither FcεRI, like basophils or mast cells,[1] nor FcεRII, like macrophages, eosinophils, or platelets.[2] Besides these IgE Fc receptors, other molecules present the ability to bind both IgE and selective carbohydrates. They belong to S-type lectins (thiol-dependent) with a specific β-galactoside recognition domain.[3] Members of the family include Mac-2, a murine macrophage cell surface protein that was originally identified from thioglycollate-elicited peritoneal macrophages.[4] The nucleotide sequence of Mac-2 cDNA is identical to that of carbohydrate-binding protein (CBP35), a galactose-specific lectin found in fibroblasts[5] and highly homologous to that of rat IgE-binding protein (εBP), described in rat basophilic leukemia cell line (RBL).[6] They are endogenous soluble lectins and can be detected on the cell surface, in the cytoplasm, and the nucleus of various cell types, specifically after activation.[7,8] One feature of εBP molecules is their restricted recognition by specific glycoforms of IgE. The majority of myeloma IgE proteins, as well as polyclonal IgE, from patients are able to bind to εBP only after desialylation.[9] The precise functions of these lectins are still unknown; however, εBP has been recently proposed as a cell adhesion protein.[9] The purpose of the present study was to investigate whether human eosinophils and neutrophils can express IgE-binding molecules of this lectin family.

DETECTION OF mRNA ENCODING MAC-2/εBP

The expression of IgE-binding molecules, such as Mac-2/εBP, by purified eosinophils and neutrophils was first analyzed by Northern blot with the Mac-2

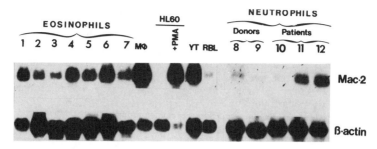

FIGURE 1. Northern blot analysis of RNA of eosinophils from 7 HE patients, various cell lines (promyelocytic HL60, NK-like YT, rat basophilic RBL cell lines) and neutrophils from normal donors or patients with various diseases. Total RNA were extracted by using the guanidine thiocyanate/CsCl gradient method.[28] HL60 were induced or not toward the macrophage phenotype (+PMA).[7] The blots were subsequently hybridized with ^{32}P-labeled Mac-2[7] and β-actin probes. Washes were carried out in $1 \times$ SSC, 0.05% SDS at 55°C.

cDNA (Fig. 1). All eosinophil preparations (lanes 1 to 7) and neutrophils from normal donors (lanes 8 and 9) or patients with various diseases (lanes 10 to 12) expressed the 1.2-kb mRNA corresponding to Mac-2/hεBP. The level of expression varied according to the eosinophil populations from hypereosinophilic (HE) patients. Neutrophils purified from some patients (lanes 11 and 12) appeared to express higher amounts of Mac-2/εBP mRNA than neutrophils purified from other patients or from normal donors. As controls, the analysis of RNA from alveolar macrophages (Mϕ) and from several cell lines (HL60, NK-like (YT), and RBL) also revealed the presence of the 1.2-kb mRNA. The β-actin mRNA was used as a monitor of the amount of RNA loaded onto each gel. In contrast to neutrophils, only eosinophils from HE patients have been analyzed. No apparent difference in mRNA expression was detected between hypodense eosinophils, previously defined as "activated" eosinophils, and normodense eosinophils (data not shown). However, it would have been interesting to compare the level expression of Mac-2 by eosinophils from HE patients and from normal subjects, or by eosinophils differentiated *in vitro* from cord blood cell precursors. Findings obtained with neutrophils seem in agreement with the variable levels of S-type lectin expression during cell differentiation and maturation, such as in HL60 differentiated to macrophages[1] or in different mast cell lines.[9] The variations in Mac-2 mRNA denoted in patients suggest that, in some diseases, neutrophils could be in different stages of maturation, leading therefore to higher expression of Mac-2 mRNA. In contrast, the negative results obtained by Northern blot with the CD23 probe confirmed that neutrophils did not express CD23 mRNA.[10]

SURFACE EXPRESSION OF MAC-2 AND IgE-BINDING SITES ON HUMAN GRANULOCYTES

The detection of Mac-2/εBP mRNA by Northern blot led us to investigate their surface expression on eosinophils from different HE patients and on neutrophils from normal donors or patients, by flow cytometry (TABLE 1). Among eosinophils that bound IgE, two groups of eosinophil donors have been described: eosinophils from group I both expressed Mac-2 molecules (mean: 18.8 ± 3.3) and bound IgE (mean: 26.4 ± 9.7); whereas, eosinophils from group II did not express Mac-2 molecules (mean: 3.1 ± 1.7) on the surface, although they bound IgE (mean: 33.8 ± 14.1). Interestingly, patient eosinophils expressing variable surface Mac-2/εBP protein levels, possessed a relatively comparable Mac-2/εBP mRNA content. Similar observations of variable cell surface εBP levels, with comparable total εBP mRNA, have been recently reported for several mast cell lines.[9] Our results suggest that expression of Mac-2/εBP on a cell surface can be differentially regulated according to the patients. The mechanism of surface expression has still to be established. The role of various cytokines, known to influence eosinophil differentiation and survival, as well as expression of membrane markers, should be highlighted.

No striking difference was observed in the expression of Mac-2 molecules by neutrophils from normal donors or from patients. However, neutrophils bound significantly less IgE–BL than IgE–PS. Since Mac-2/εBP lectins have the capacity to bind to restricted IgE glycoforms, we investigated whether the difference observed in IgE binding was in relation with the degree of glycosylation of the IgE myeloma protein. Experiments were performed with the same myeloma IgE proteins previously desialylated by treatment with neuraminidase (TABLE 2). A significant increase of IgE binding was observed both for IgE–PS and for IgE–BL, but more pronounced for the latter. In contrast, neuraminidase treatment did not affect the binding of serum IgA to neutrophils, which occurs through the myeloid FcαR.[11] It was concluded that similarly to eosinophils and other inflammatory cells, neutrophils can also bind IgE, but with some variability according to the myeloma IgE tested. Our results suggest that IgE binding to neutrophils involved surface Mac-2/εBP and not transmembrane CD23. In contrast to eosinophils,

TABLE 1. Flow Cytometry Analysis of Surface Expression of Mac-2 and IgE-binding Molecules by Human Granulocytes

Source of Granulocytes[a]	Percentage of Positive Cells[b]		
	Mac-2	IgE–PS	IgE–BL
Eosinophils from HE patients			
Group I	18.6 ± 3.3	26.4 ± 9.7	21.2 ± 11.12
Group II	3.1 ± 1.7	33.8 ± 14.1	24.6 ± 12.6
Neutrophils			
Patients	40.1 ± 4.7	40.1 ± 5.9	9.7 ± 3.6
Normal donors	54.6 ± 5.6	27.9 ± 8.0	13.8 ± 4.2

[a] Eosinophils were purified from HE patients ($n = 9$, group I; $n = 10$, group II) upon metrizamide gradients.[25] Neutrophils were purified from venous blood of patients with various diseases ($n = 16$) or from normal donors ($n = 10$) by the same technique or by centrifugation through a cushion of Ficoll according to Boyum's method.[26] The degree of purity ranged between 82 and 99 percent, and the morphologic integrity of cell populations was estimated after staining of centrifugated preparation with Giemsa.

[b] Granulocytes were incubated with anti-Mac-2 hybridoma supernatant (dilution 1/10)[27] or 50-μg/ml myeloma IgE (IgE–PS, donated by H. L. Spiegelberg, San Diego, Calif.; or IgE–BL, Bernett Laboratories, Buena Park, Calif.), prior to staining with the corresponding FITC-labeled anti-Ig antibodies (1:40 final dilution; Fab2′, Cappel Laboratories, Cochranville, Pa.). The percentage of positive cells was obtained after subtraction of the nonspecific binding with the control antibody or medium (mean ± SEM).

TABLE 2. Binding of Neuraminidase-treated Ig to Neutrophils

Treatment of Ig	Percentage of Positive Cells[a]		
	IgE–PS	IgE–BL	IgA
None	58.7 ± 8.1	16.8 ± 2.1	47.3 ± 7.9
Neuraminidase[b]	79.5 ± 4.4	55.7 ± 5.1	50.1 ± 8.5
Heat-inactivated[c] neuraminidase	60.7 ± 5.9	22.5 ± 4.0	52.7 ± 11.6

[a] Neutrophils were incubated with 50-μg/ml IgE–PS, IgE–BL, or serum IgA (Sigma Chemical Co, St-Louis, Mo.) and stained with the corresponding FITC-labeled anti-Ig (mean of 4 to 11 experiments ± SEM).

[b] The various Ig have been treated with neuraminidase (0.03 U/ml) for 90 min. at 37°C before incubation with neutrophils.

[c] Neuraminidase (*Clostridium perfringens* type, 0.5 U/mg of protein, Sigma Chemical Co.) was heat-inactivated for 1 hour at 56°C before incubation with Ig.

which express both CD23[12] and Mac-2/εBP, neutrophils seem to express only molecules of the S-type lectin family, with the IgE recognition capacity modulated by sialylation of IgE oligosaccharides.

CHARACTERIZATION OF IMMUNOREACTIVE MAC-2 MOLECULES IN GRANULOCYTE EXTRACTS

In parallel to the Northern blot analysis, the characterization of Mac-2 molecules was performed by immunoblotting with two types of antibodies: anti-Mac-2 (FIG. 2, lane b) and anti-εBP (FIG. 2, lane c) antibodies. These two immunoprobes

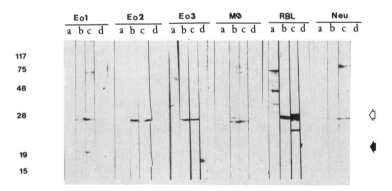

FIGURE 2. Western blot analysis of Mac-2 and εBP immune reactive proteins. Protein blots from eosinophil, alveolar macrophage, RBL, or neutrophil extracts were probed with anti-Mac-2 hybridoma supernatant (dilution 1/40, **lane b**) and by anti-εBP antisera (dilution 1/300, **lane c**),[9] and further detected by the addition of antirat or antirabbit antibodies conjugated with horseradish peroxidase, respectively. In controls, protein blots were incubated with normal rat serum **(lane a)** or normal rabbit serum **(lane d)**. The Mr is indicated in kD. The *white arrow* indicates the 29 kD and the *black arrow* indicates the 20 kD molecule.

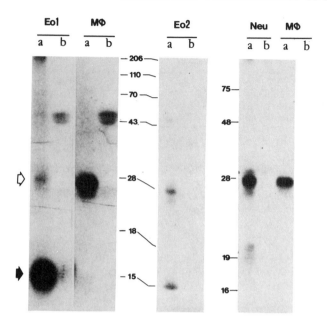

FIGURE 3. Immunoprecipitation of [125]iodine-labeled lysates of eosinophils from patients of both groups defined in TABLE 1 (Eo1, Eo2), neutrophils (Neu), and alveolar macrophages (Mø). Results obtained with anti-Mac-2 hybridoma supernatant were shown in **lane a** and with normal rat serum control in **lane b**. These antibodies were bound to protein G-sepharose (Pharmacia Biotech, St-Quentin Yvelines, France). The Mr is indicated in kD. The *white arrow* indicates the 29-kD molecule and the *black arrow* indicates the 15-kD molecule.

revealed the same protein pattern: a molecule at the expected molecular weight of 29 kD in both the group of eosinophils (Eo1 from group I; Eo2 and Eo3 from group II) and neutrophil (Neu) extracts. An additional molecule at approximately 20 kD was found only in eosinophil extracts. As control, RBL cell lines and alveolar macrophage extracts also showed the presence of the 29-kD molecule, but no additional molecule at 20 kD. Immunoprecipitation with anti-Mac-2 antibodies confirmed the presence of 29- and 20-kD in granulocyte extracts (FIG. 3). Surprisingly, an additional molecule at 15 kD, absent in Western blotting, was detected in eosinophil extracts (FIG. 3, lane a). The 45-kD band, also detected with the control serum, was nonspecific. The failure to detect surface Mac-2 in eosinophils from group II patients [Mac-2(−), IgE-R(+)], which are positive by Northern blot and by immunoprecipitation, can be explained by the fact that Mac-2/εBP proteins are predominantly found as cytosolic molecules.[7,8]

In order to demonstrate that both anti-εBP and anti-Mac-2 antibodies recognized the same molecule in eosinophils and neutrophils, immunoprecipitation by anti-εBP antibodies of cell extracts previously treated with anti-Mac-2 antibodies was performed (FIG. 4). The 29-kD and also the 20-kD molecules were immunoprecipitated from granulocyte extracts (FIG. 4, lane a), but not from those pretreated

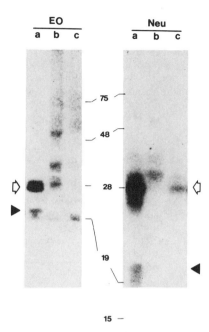

FIGURE 4. Immunoprecipitation of [125]iodine-labeled lysates of granulocytes performed with anti-εBP **(lane a)** or with normal rabbit serum **(lane b)**, bound to protein A-sepharose (Pharmacia Biotech, St-Quentin Yvelines, France); inhibition of immunoprecipitation with anti-εBP by anti-Mac-2 antibodies **(lane c)**. The Mr is indicated in kD. The *white arrow* indicates the 29-kD molecule, and the *black arrowhead* indicates the 20-kD molecule.

with anti-Mac-2 antibodies (FIG. 4, lane c). Additional molecules at 20 kD and 15 kD detected in granulocytes could correspond to degradation products of the 29-kD protein. Interestingly, various molecules at 14–16 kD located in eosinophil granules have been recently shown to exhibit sequence homology with εBP, such as the CLC protein,[13] and with the FcεRII/CD23, such as MBP.[14] Alternatively, the 15-kD molecule might correspond to another member of the β-galactoside lectin family previously found around Mr 14–16 kD.[15]

INVOLVEMENT OF MAC-2/εBP MOLECULES IN EOSINOPHIL FUNCTION

Mac-2/εBP and IgE-binding to Eosinophils

Mac-2/εBP molecules have been shown to bind several IgE glycoforms.[8] In order to investigate whether Mac-2/εBP expressed by eosinophils could be involved in IgE binding, experiments of inhibition of radiolabeled IgE binding were performed. As shown in FIGURE 5, anti-Mac-2 mAb significantly inhibited, in a dose-dependent manner, the binding of ^{125}I–IgE to human eosinophils. A similar level of inhibition was observed with unlabeled IgE and with the highest concentration of anti-Mac-2 supernatant. In contrast, no significant inhibition was detected with the control mAb used at the same concentrations (FIG. 5). Since Mac-2 has been described as a β-galactoside-binding lectin, detected by SDS–PAGE using either SDS or lactose elution but not in glucose-eluted samples, competition experiments with several carbohydrates have been performed. Only galactose and lactose, at 100 mM, induced the same level of inhibition as unlabeled IgE or anti-Mac-2 mAb. Glucose also inhibited but at a lower level the binding of ^{125}I–IgE to eosinophils.

Mac-2/εBP and IgE-dependent Eosinophil-mediated Cytotoxicity

Eosinophils and macrophages play an important role among inflammatory cells involved in the allergic reaction. Eosinophils have been reported as being able to present phagocytic properties facilitating ingestion of IgG or IgE immune complexes.[16] Lectin-mediated phagocytosis has been shown for activated macrophages in relation with secreted Mac-2 molecules.[4] It has also been suggested that Mac-2 protein present in macrophages play an important role in acute and chronic inflammation. The function of Mac-2 molecules was investigated in a cytotoxicity assay involving eosinophils and polyclonal IgE antibodies. Hypodense eosinophils were incubated together with IgE-containing immune serum from patients with schistosomiasis and various concentrations of purified anti-Mac-2 mAb or anti-Mac-2 hybridoma supernatant, in the presence of schistosomula targets. Results illustrated in FIGURE 6 clearly showed a highly significant and dose-dependent inhibition of eosinophil-mediated cytotoxicity in the presence of anti-Mac-2 mAb, by comparison to control supernatant, rat IgG or to medium. It has been shown that the receptor for IgE, FcεRII/CD23, was implicated in the IgE-dependent cytotoxicity mediated by eosinophils.[12] The involvement of the two groups of IgE binding molecules (CD23, C-type lectin and Mac-2/εBP, S-type lectin) in the cytotoxic function of eosinophils suggests an important role in the recognition of

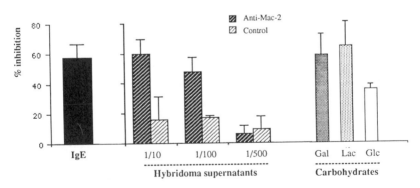

FIGURE 5. Inhibition of radiolabeled IgE-binding to eosinophils by unlabeled IgE (1-mg/ml final concentration) or various dilutions (1/10 to 1/500) of anti-Mac-2 and control hybridoma supernatants and various carbohydrates (galactose, lactose, and glucose) at 100-mM final concentration. The percentage of inhibition of binding was calculated after incubation with 10-μg/ml ^{125}I–IgE together with the antibodies or carbohydrates, for 90 min at +4°C (competition protocol) (mean of 3 to 6 experiments ± SEM).

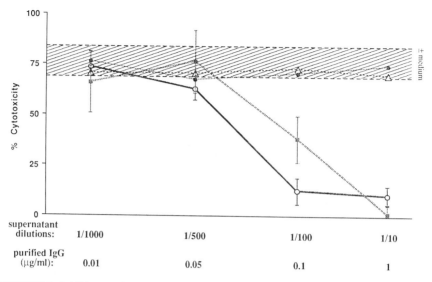

FIGURE 6. Inhibitory effect of anti-Mac-2 mAb on eosinophil-dependent cytotoxicity. The various antibodies [anti-Mac-2 —○— and control My43 hybridoma supernatant[24] (kindly donated by Dr. Chen, Hanover, N.H.) —△— or purified fraction Mab 3/38 (Boehringer Mannheim, Germany) —■— and control rat IgG —●—] were incubated directly at different concentrations to purified eosinophils, IgE-containing immune serum (1 : 32 final dilution), and *S. mansoni* schistosomula targets at a ratio of 5000 effector cells to one target. The percentage of dead larvae was estimated microscopically after 24 hours at 37°C and compared to positive control wells in the presence of medium (mean of 6 experiments ±SEM).

IgE proteins by CRD domains of the two types of lectin. In addition to the role of Mac-2/εBP in IgE binding to eosinophils, the inhibition by anti-Mac-2 mAb of eosinophil adhesion to parasite targets also suggests the function of such molecules as cell adhesion proteins, and should be explored in other adhesive properties of eosinophils.

INVOLVEMENT OF MAC-2/εBP MOLECULES IN NEUTROPHIL ACTIVATION

Neutrophil Activation by Myeloma or Polyclonal IgE

The function of IgE-binding molecules expressed on neutrophil surface has been investigated in an experimental assay measuring the respiratory burst by chemiluminescence (CL) induced by incubation of neutrophils with 10 µg/ml of IgE myeloma protein or serum IgA and then with the corresponding anti-Ig antibodies. As shown in FIGURE 7A, only myeloma IgE–PS, but not IgE–BL, induced a CL level close to that induced by serum IgA, as positive control.[11] It has been noticed that the magnitude order of IgE–PS- and IgA-dependent respira-

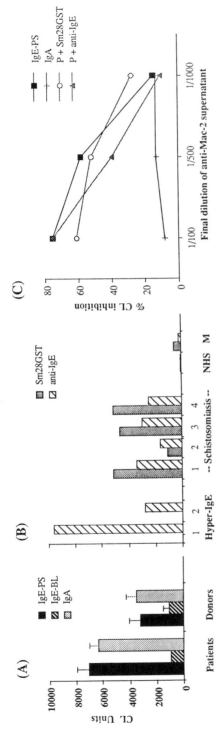

FIGURE 7. Role of Mac-2/εBP in IgE-dependent activation of neutrophils from individual donors measured by chemiluminescence (CL) procedure in the presence of luminol (250 μg/ml). **(A)** CL of neutrophils purified from patients with various diseases and from normal donors by incubation with 10-μg/ml myeloma IgE (IgE–PS and IgE–BL) or serum IgA, and 25-μg/ml anti-IgE or anti-IgA antibodies. **(B)** Normal donors' neutrophil CL induced by anti-IgE or Sm28GST Ag[29] with sera from two patients with hyper-IgE syndrome (numbers 1 and 2), which contained 8000 IU/ml IgE or sera from four different patients with schistosomiasis (numbers 1, 2, 3, and 4) (kindly donated by Dr. P. Desreumaux, Centre Hospitalier St. Louis, Senegal). Normal human serum (NHS), medium alone (M) represented the controls. **(C)** Dose-effect of anti-Mac-2 supernatant on myeloma IgE–PS- and IgA-dependent CL, on pool P (sera from three patients with schistosomiasis numbers 1, 3, and 4) -dependent activation induced by Sm28GST or anti-IgE on normal donors' neutrophils. Light emission of CL was monitored after 15–30 min of incubation at 37°C using a photometer (Nucleotimetre 107; Interbio CLV, Villeurbanne, France) and was expressed in mM (100 CL U = 1 mV). The evaluation of CL was calculated by comparison to results obtained with control used at the same concentrations.

tory burst was significantly higher for neutrophils from patients than from normal donors.

In addition to myeloma IgE, polyclonal IgE, with or without antibody specificity, could also induce neutrophil activation. Neutrophils were incubated either with the serum from patients with hyper-IgE syndrome or from schistosomiasis infected patients (FIG. 7B). The former sera, previously shown to bind to sepharose-linked hεBP,[17] induced a respiratory burst in the presence of anti-IgE antibodies; this burst varied with neutrophil donors and with patient sera. In the case of schistosomiasis patient sera, the incubation with specific antigen Sm28GST as well as with anti-IgE antibodies also induced a significant respiratory burst (FIG. 7B). No chemiluminescence was produced when only serum, antigen Sm28GST, or anti-IgE alone were added to the neutrophils. These results indicate that after cross-linking with antigen or anti-IgE, specific IgE antibodies can induce a respiratory burst in neutrophils.

Role of Mac-2/εBP in IgE-dependent Neutrophil Activation

To identify the nature of the molecules involved in IgE-dependent activation of neutrophils, inhibition procedures with anti-Mac-2 hybridoma supernatant were performed (FIG. 7C). In the case of activation with myeloma IgE and anti-IgE antibodies, a dose-dependent inhibition of CL was observed with anti-Mac-2 hybridoma supernatant, by comparison with control supernatant. In contrast, anti-Mac-2 antibodies showed no significant effect on IgA-dependent activation.

The involvement of Mac-2 was also investigated in neutrophil activation induced by polyclonal IgE antibodies. According to the stimulus (Sm28GST or anti-IgE), a significant dose-dependent inhibition of neutrophil respiratory burst was obtained with anti-Mac-2 mAb (FIG. 7C).

CONCLUDING REMARKS

The expression by human eosinophils from HE patients of FcεRII/CD23 epitopes was recently reviewed.[12,18] However, the low level of membrane and mRNA expression of CD23 led us to suggest the existence of additional IgE binding proteins. In the present paper, we describe the capacity of eosinophils to express Mac-2/εBP molecules belonging to the S-type lectin family, defined as a cytosolic lectin with the ability to bind to carbohydrates on the cell surface and on extracellular molecules.[4,7] Not only eosinophils, but also neutrophils from patients with various diseases and from normal donors, have the capacity to express functional IgE-binding molecules such as Mac-2/εBP. Compared to eosinophils, Mac-2/εBP molecules seemed to be expressed on the surface of a larger majority of neutrophil donors, whereas Mac-2 was expressed on the surface of only half of HE patients. This might indicate a difference in the regulatory process of surface expression of these endogenous lectins on the two cell populations, a mechanism that still has to be explored.

It has been previously reported that the expression of S-type lectins appears to be linked to cell differentiation or maturation.[3] The Mac-2 mRNA was found in various cell lines, particularly in HL60 differentiated toward the macrophage phenotype,[7] and has been shown to increase during macrophage maturation.[19]

Similarly to Mac-2, the εBP mRNA was detected in a variety of tissues and different cell lines.[8] The εBP was found in few of the human lymphoma cell lines tested,[8] and its surface expression widely varies among different mast cell lines.[6] Mac-2 and εBP molecules were identical in nucleotide sequence and molecular weight levels. The results of immunoprecipitation by anti-εBP antibodies of cell extracts previously treated with anti-Mac-2 antibodies, which did not reveal the 29- and 20-kD molecules, confirmed the similarity between Mac-2 and εBP proteins.

The present paper demonstrates that not only transmembrane receptors, such as FcεRII/CD23, but also soluble Mac-2/εBP molecules expressed on the eosinophil surface might participate to their IgE-dependent effector function, such as IgE-dependent cytotoxicity against parasite larvae. It has previously been stated that FcεRII/CD23 epitopes were also implicated in the release of cytotoxic mediators, in the presence of IgE antibodies.[12,18] FcεRII plays an important role in the regulation of IgE antibody response and presents significant sequence homology with a class of animal lectins.[20] However, in the case of C-type (calcium dependent binding) lectins, IgE binding to FcεRII is pH-dependent, but independent of the carbohydrate structure of IgE.[21,22] In contrast to FcεRII/CD23, which binds to the protein moiety of IgE,[21] Mac-2 and εBP bind to IgE in a carbohydrate-dependent manner and show heterogeneity in the binding of various IgE glycoforms.[8,17] The functional relationships between these two families of molecules, both exhibiting a lectin domain and expressed on a variety of cell populations, have still to be explored.

Interactions between mouse neutrophils and IgE antibodies in cytotoxicity assays have been previously reported; however, no attempt at characterization of IgE-binding molecules potentially expressed by neutrophils was made at this time.[23] We demonstrated here that neutrophils seemed to express only Mac-2, but not CD23. Our results indicate that not only restricted glycoforms of myeloma IgE proteins but also polyclonal IgE antibodies could induce neutrophil activation in an antigen-specific manner. These findings suggest that in addition to FcεR-bearing cell populations, neutrophils might participate to IgE-dependent reactions. It remains to be determined whether, in the case of other cell populations, such as eosinophils,[24] the IgE-dependent activation of neutrophils can induce the generation of mediators potentially involved in inflammatory reactions.

REFERENCES

1. METZGER, H. 1988. Molecular aspects of receptors and binding factors for IgE. Adv. Immunol. **43:** 277–312.
2. CAPRON, A., *et al.* 1986. From parasites to allergy: The second receptor for IgE (FcεR2). Immunol. Today **7**(1): 15–18.
3. DRICKAMER K. 1988. Two distinct classes of carbohydrate-recognition domains in animal lectins. J. Biol. Chem. **263**(20): 9557–9560.
4. CHERAYIL, B. J., S. J. WEINER & S. PILLAI. 1989. The Mac-2 antigen is a galactose-specific lectin that binds IgE. J. Exp. Med. **170**(6): 1959–1972.
5. JIA, S. & J. L. WANG. 1988. Carbohydrate binding protein 35. Complementary DNA sequence reveals homology with proteins of the heterogeneous nuclear RNP. J. Biol. Chem. **263**(13): 6009–6011.
6. ALBRANDT, K., N. K. ORIDA & F.-T. LIU. 1987. An IgE-binding protein with a distinctive sequence and homology with an IgG receptor. Proc. Natl. Acad. Sci. U.S.A. **84**(19): 6859–6863.
7. CHERAYIL, B. J., S. CHAITIVITZ, C. WONG & S. PILLAI. 1990. Molecular cloning of

a human macrophage lectin specific for galactose. Proc. Natl. Acad. Sci. U.S.A. **87**(18): 7324–7328.

8. ROBERTSON, M. W., K. ALBRANDT, D. KELLER & F. T. LIU. 1990. Human IgE-binding protein: A soluble lectin exhibiting a highly conserved interspecies sequence and differential recognition of IgE glycoforms. Biochemistry **29**(35): 8093–8100.

9. FRIGERI, L. G. & F.-T. LIU. 1992. Surface expression of functional IgE-binding protein, an endogenous lectin, on mast cells and macrophages. J. Immunol. **148**(3): 861–867.

10. TRUONG, M.-J., *et al.* 1993. Human neutrophils express immunoglobulin E (IgE)-binding proteins (Mac-2/εBP) of the S-type lectin family: Role in IgE-dependent activation. J. Exp. Med. **177**(1): 243–248.

11. STEWART, W. W. & M. A. KERR. 1990. The specificity of the human neutrophil IgA receptor (FcαR) determined by measurement of chemiluminescence induced by serum or secretory IgA1 or IgA2. Immunology **71**(3): 328–334.

12. CAPRON, M., *et al.* 1991. Heterogeneous expression of CD23 epitopes by eosinophils from patients. Relationships with IgE-mediated functions. Eur. J. Immunol. **21**(10): 2423–2429.

13. ACKERMAN, S. J., *et al.* 1993. Molecular cloning and characterization of human eosinophil Charcot-Leyden crystal protein (Lysophospholipase). Similarities to IgE-binding proteins and the S-type animal lectin superfamily. J. Immunol. **150**(2): 456–468.

14. PATTHY, L. 1989. Homology of cytotoxic protein of eosinophil leukocyte with IgE receptor FcεRII: The implications for its structure and function. Mol. Immunol. **136**(12): 1151–1154.

15. LEVI, G. & V. I. TEICHBERG. 1981. Isolation and physicochemical characterization of Electrolectin, a β-D-galactoside binding lectin from the electric organ of Electrophorus Electricus. J. Biol. Chem. **256**(11): 5735–5740.

16. FUJITA, Y., E. RUBINSTEIN, D. B. REISMAN & C. E. ARBESMAN. 1975. Antigen-antibody complexes in or on eosinophils in nasal secretions. Int. Arch. Allergy Appl. Immunol. **48**(5): 577–583.

17. ROBERTSON, M. W. & F.-T. LIU. 1991. Heterogeneous IgE glycoforms characterized by differential recognition of an endogenous lectin (IgE-binding protein). J. Immunol. **147**(9): 3024–3030.

18. GRANGETTE, C., *et al.* 1989. IgE receptor on human eosinophils (FcεRII): Comparison with B cell CD23 and association with an adhesion molecule. J. Immunol. **143**(11): 3580–3588.

19. LEENEN, P. J. M., A. M. A. C. JANSEN & W. VAN EWIJK. 1986. Murine macrophage cell lines can be ordered in a linear differentiation sequence. Differentiation **32**(2): 157–161.

20. IKUTA, K., *et al.* 1987. Human lymphocyte Fc receptor for IgE: Sequence homology of its cloned cDNA with animal lectins. Proc. Natl. Acad. Sci. U.S.A. **84**(2): 819–823.

21. VERCELLI, D., *et al.* 1989. The B cell binding site on human immunoglobulin E. Nature **338**(6217): 649–651.

22. RICHARDS, M. L. & D. H. KATZ. 1990. The binding of IgE to murine FcεRII is calcium-dependent but not inhibited by carbohydrate. J. Immunol. **144**(7): 2638–2646.

23. LOPEZ, A. F., M. STRATH & C. J. SANDERSON. 1983. Mouse immunoglobulin isotypes mediated cytotoxicity of target cells by eosinophils and neutrophils. Immunology **48**(3): 503–509.

24. CAPRON, M., *et al.* 1992. Eosinophil membrane receptors: Function of IgE and IgA binding molecules. *In* Eosinophils in Allergy and Inflammation. (Proceedings of the 1992 Conference on Eosinophils), G. J. Gleich, Ed. Dekker. New York. In press.

25. PRIN, L., M. CAPRON, A. B. TONNEL, O. BLETRY & A. CAPRON. 1983. Heterogeneity of human peripheral blood eosinophils. I. Variability in cell density and cytotoxic ability in relation to the level and the origin of hypereosinophilia. Int. Arch. Allergy Appl. Immunol. **72**(4): 336–346.

26. BOYUM, A. 1968. Isolation of mononuclear cells and granulocytes by combining centrifugation and sedimentation at 1 g. Scand. J. Clin. Lab. Invest. **21**(Suppl. 97): 77–80.

27. HO, M.-K. & T. A. SPRINGER. 1982. Mac-2, a novel 32,000 Mr mouse macrophage subpopulation-specific antigen defined by monoclonal antibodies. J. Immunol. **128**(3): 1221–1228.

28. CHIRGWIN, J. M., A. E. PRZYBYLA, J. MACDONALD & W. J. RUTTER. 1979. Isolation of biologically active ribonucleic acid from sources enriched in ribonuclease. Biochemistry **18**(2): 5294–5299.
29. BALLOUL, J. M., *et al.* 1987. Molecular cloning of a protective antigen against schistosomiasis. Nature **326**(6109): 149–151.

Cytokines–Eosinophil Interactions in Experimental Allergy

MARINA PRETOLANI[a] AND B. BORIS VARGAFTIG

Unité de Pharmacologie Cellulaire
Unité Associée Institut Pasteur/INSERM 285
Institut Pasteur
25, rue du Dr. Roux
75015, Paris, France

INTRODUCTION

Current theories concerning the mechanisms of allergic reactions highlight the role of non-histamine-dependent mechanisms, involving eosinophils, antigen-presenting cells, and lymphocytes. Accordingly, the established concept that allergy results from the production of specific IgE antibodies that bind to mast cells and trigger the release of bronchoconstrictor mediators following exposure to allergen has been superseded by a broader concept that considers asthma as "a chronic inflammatory disorder of the airways in which many cells play a role, including mast cells and eosinophils."[1] This formal recognition that the eosinophil is one of the effector cells, particularly involved in the chronic airways inflammation, followed the observation of an intense infiltration of eosinophils and mononuclear cells in the bronchial submucosa of asthmatic patients.[2] The analysis of bronchoalveolar lavage fluid (BALF) from asthmatics revealed that those infiltrating eosinophils were degranulated, as a consequence of their *in situ* activation.[3] Eosinophils release different cationic proteins,[4] such as major basic protein (MBP) and eosinophil peroxidase (EPO), which are stored in the core and matrix, respectively, of their large crystalloid-containing granules.[5] The role of the eosinophil-derived proteins in bronchial asthma may be linked to their ability to injure the respiratory epithelium,[6–8] resulting in the exposure of submucosal structures and sensory nerve endings to nonspecific bronchoconstrictor agents and/or stimulation of smooth muscle proliferation, two potential mechanisms for bronchopulmonary hyperreactivity. Recently, the administration of MBP has been shown to elicit bronchial hyperreactivity in different species,[9–12] further reinforcing the concept of a link between an altered airway function and eosinophil activation. However, the formal recognition that inhibition or antagonism of MBP, for instance, with specific antiserum, would suppress bronchial hyperreactivity in experimental models, is still missing. Circumstantially, heparin, which binds to cationic proteins, has been shown to inhibit bronchial hyperreactivity.[11,13]

ROLE OF EOSINOPHILS IN EXPERIMENTAL BRONCHIAL HYPERREACTIVITY

Models have been developed, particularly using the guinea pig, to investigate the mechanisms of the late-phase reaction and of the associated bronchial

---

[a] To whom correspondence should be addressed.

hyperreactivity. Other species, such as rats, rabbits, dogs, sheep, and monkeys have also been studied, but the guinea pig continues to be used, essentially because of the marked reactivity of its airways. Those models are based on the immunization and subsequent challenge with the specific allergen, on the exposure to irritants, or on the inoculation of virus.[14] A single inhalation of antigen by guinea pigs sensitized to ovalbumin by the subcutaneous route in the absence of adjuvant is reported to induce bronchial hyperreactivity to i.v. histamine and acetylcholine[15] within 24 hours, accompanied by eosinophil infiltration in the BALF. We failed to confirm these results, since in our recent experiments an intense BALF eosinophilia was not accompanied by bronchial hyperreactivity (see below). A careful examination of the literature shows that the models of allergic bronchial hyperreactivity are mostly based on the repeated exposures of the animals to the allergen.[16] In one report, allergen inhalation by guinea pigs sensitized by aerosol was followed by early- and late-phase bronchoconstriction with neutrophil and eosinophil infiltration in the BALF.[17] In view of its similarity with the human situation, this model seems relevant, particularly since the same authors showed more recently an increased proportion of hypodense eosinophils in the BALF from antigen-challenged animals, as compared to controls.[18] These results are consistent with the observation that the majority of the eosinophils of asthmatic patients are hypodense.[19] However, no evidence of bronchial hyperreactivity during the late-phase reaction following antigen challenge was reported in this model.

IS THE EOSINOPHIL INFILTRATION IN THE AIRWAYS ESSENTIAL FOR BRONCHIAL HYPERREACTIVITY?

While the pivotal role of the eosinophil in bronchial hyperreactivity is now generally accepted, it is clear that its presence in the airways is not sufficient to induce bronchial hyperreactivity. Gibson et al.[20] demonstrated that chronic eosinophilic bronchitis may occur without bronchial hyperreactivity, whereas the reverse, that is, bronchial hyperreactivity with no eosinophil infiltration, was shown by Lundgren et al.[21] A marked eosinophil recruitment into the airways was demonstrated in the BALF of guinea pigs sensitized by two different protocols, bronchial hyperreactivity being observed in only one of those groups,[22] suggesting that eosinophil infiltration per se does not modify airway reactivity. In fact, the intensity of activation of the airway eosinophils, rather than their numbers, may correlate with the severity of asthma and with the intensity of bronchial hyperreactivity.[23-25] Several investigators, including us,[26] have worked under the implicit hypothesis that airways inflammation is equivalent to the accumulation of cells in the BALF or in the lung parenchyma and bronchial submucosa. It is currently clear that the presence of eosinophils in the airways, even if recruited by the "natural" antigenic challenge, is not sufficient to induce bronchial hyperreactivity. An additional component, such as further activation and receptor expression on the eosinophil surface brought by secreted cytokines, or the active participation of other cell types, seems to be required. In addition, bronchial hyperreactivity may also be associated to other signs of airway inflammation, including the increase in vascular permeability and epithelium injury, and not only to the cellular infiltration in the airways. In a recent study,[27] we showed that eosinophil infiltration of the guinea-pig airways triggered by a single antigen provocation is not sufficient to increase the nonspecific bronchial reactivity to methacholine. However, the subsequent intratracheal instillation of leukotriene (LT)B$_4$, but not of platelet activating factor (PAF), leads to the activation of airway eosinophils, as assessed by increased levels of EPO and MBP in the BALF and by the development of bronchial hyperreactivity to methacholine (FIG. 1). These results further emphasize the absolute need of evaluating, together with the number of infiltrating eosinophils in allergic tissues, their activation status.

ROLE OF T-CELLS IN EXPERIMENTAL
BRONCHIAL HYPERREACTIVITY

Increasing evidence suggests that late-phase reactions, including eosinophilia and IgE production, are orchestrated by T-lymphocytes, particularly T helper cells of the Th2 subset. Following the specific recognition of the antigen, Th2 cells elaborate cytokines, such as IL-4, which favor the synthesis of IgE by B-lymphocytes, or IL-5, which accounts for the proliferation of eosinophils and for their differentiation from precursors, at a distance in the bone marrow or *in situ,* in the lung. Activated Th lymphocytes are present in the BALF, bronchial biopsies and peripheral blood from atopic subjects, their number correlating with that of circulating eosinophils.[29] More recently, the observation of increased numbers of cells expressing mRNA for IL-2, IL-3, IL-4, and IL-5, but not of interferon-γ, in BALF from asthmatics, suggests the presence of a Th2-like pattern of cytokine gene expression in allergic asthma.[30] Even though the presence of characterization of T-lymphocytes and of the genes expressing their derived cytokines is now well established in humans, the situation is not as clear in animals. Indeed, Frew et al.[31] described increased numbers of T cells with a CD8 negative phenotype in the lung parenchyma and bronchial submucosa of sensitized guinea pigs following exposure to antigen delivered by aerosol, leading to the hypothesis that CD4$^+$ cells predominate in the bronchial wall. Recently, using specific monoclonal antibodies, we demonstrated that guinea pigs actively sensitized to ovalbumin exhibit an increased number of CD4$^+$ lymphocytes infiltrating the bronchial mucosa, in the absence of augmented CD8$^+$.[32] The expansion of the CD4$^+$ subset parallels the development of nonspecific bronchial hyperresponsiveness, which we had demonstrated earlier, using isolated lungs obtained by guinea pigs sensitized by the same route.[33]

The characterization of lymphocyte subsets in the bronchial wall was described in the past in mice, a species in which most of the immunological tools have been developed so far. Curtis and Kaltreider[34] characterized by flow cytometry techniques the numbers and phenotypes of lymphocyte subpopulations recovered in the BALF from antigen-challenged mice, demonstrating that Th-cells predominate over suppressor T-cells and B-cells. However, the increment in those cells in the lung after antigen challenge did not correlate with changes in the lung function. Furthermore, the presence of T-cells at the site of antigen challenge is not proof that they participate in airway inflammation. This demonstration came, at least in part, from more recent studies showing that the increased contraction of isolated trachea from antigen-challenged Balb/c mice in response to carbachol is suppressed in athymic animals[35] and that the transfusion of nonimmunized mice with lymphoid cells purified from immunized donors, restored the *ex vivo* airway hyperreactivity.

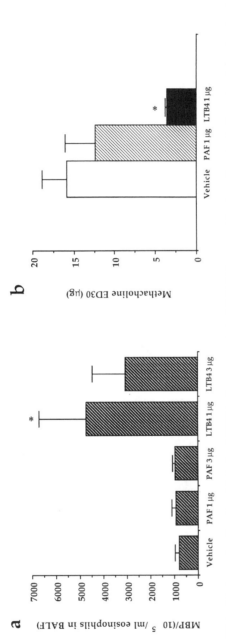

FIGURE 1. (a) Amounts of eosinophil-derived MBP in the supernatant of BALF from sensitized ovalbumin-challenged guinea pigs that have been treated intratracheally, 24 h after the challenge, with 100-μl saline solution containing 0.25% BSA (vehicle) or with 1, 3-μg PAF or LTB$_4$ 30 min prior to intravenous administrations of 1–64-μg methacholine. MBP was determined by specific ELISA, as described.[28] **(b)** Bronchial response to methacholine, expressed as the provocative dose capable of inducing a 30% increase in bronchial resistance to inflation (ED30), in ovalbumin-challenged guinea pigs treated intratracheally, 24 h after the challenge, with 100-μl saline solution containing 0.25% BSA (vehicle), or with 1-μg PAF or LTB$_4$. Guinea pigs were sensitized to ovalbumin (10 μg in 1-mg Al(OH)$_3$, injected subcutaneously). Fourteen days later they were challenged by aerosol with a 0.1% ovalbumin solution in sterile saline for 90 sec. Control animals were exposed to sterile saline. $p < 0.05$, as compared to vehicle-treated animals.

EVIDENCES FOR THE PARTICIPATION OF T-CELL-DERIVED CYTOKINES IN ANIMAL MODELS OF AIRWAY INFLAMMATION AND BRONCHIAL HYPERREACTIVITY

As indicated earlier, cytokines produced by Th lymphocytes in response to antigen stimulation may play a role in airway inflammation and in the consequent hyperresponsiveness. These cytokines include IL-3 and granulocyte-macrophage colony stimulating factor (GM–CSF), which share the ability to support the proliferation of granulocyte and macrophage precursors and IL-5, which selectively stimulates eosinophil differentiation. IL-5 is indeed unique in selectively acting on the eosinophil lineage and in enhancing the survival of mature eosinophils.[36] Furthermore, since those cytokines are capable of priming target cells for increased responses to stimuli by mechanisms involving the release of arachidonic acid metabolites, including LTC_4,[37] the link between the regulatory role of hematopoietic growth factors and lipid mediator appears likely. This led Coëffier et al.[38] to study the interaction between PAF and Th2-derived cytokines on isolated eosinophils and in vivo in the guinea pig. Preincubation of guinea-pig peritoneal eosinophils with recombinant human(rh)IL-5 increased significantly the migration, the superoxide anion production, and the calcium fluxes induced by PAF, but not by LTB_4.[38] The mechanism underlying this phenomenon has not been elucidated, but the recent findings showing that the incubation of a human eosinophilic cell line with IL-5 increased markedly the mRNA encoding for the PAF receptor[39] may be relevant to those findings.

Priming by rhIL-5 of the effects of PAF on purified guinea-pig eosinophils may extend to lung functions, since the intratracheal introduction of rhIL-5 into isolated lungs from actively sensitized guinea pigs triggered a marked time-dependent hyperresponsiveness to PAF.[40] The previous observation that actively sensitized and boosted guinea pigs exhibit an increased number of eosinophils in the BALF, as compared to nonimmunized animals,[41] and the evidences that IL-5 stimulates selectively mature eosinophils,[42] may explain the increased lung responses to PAF induced by this cytokine. On the basis of these results, it is suggested that repeated allergen exposures of asthmatic subjects is followed by the production of PAF and of IL-5 in the airways. The interaction between both mediators on the eosinophils leads to their activation, characterized by the release of arachidonate derivatives, free radicals, proteolytic enzymes, and cytotoxic basic proteins, as discussed earlier. Various cell types may produce PAF and IL-5 in the airways of asthmatic patients or of sensitized animals after antigen exposure, including mast cells, a recognized source for both PAF[43] and IL-5.[44]

Hyperresponsiveness to PAF induced by rhIL-5 applied to guinea-pig lungs enriched in eosinophils was inhibited by the antiallergic drug nedocromil sodium administered in vivo together with the antigenic provocation of the donor animal. Nedocromil sodium concomitantly suppressed rhIL-5-induced bronchopulmonary hyperresponsiveness to PAF and the increased numbers of eosinophils in the BALF induced by antigen challenge.[45] The observation that incubation with nedocromil sodium of normal-density human eosinophils inhibits IL-5, but not interferon-γ, induced increased survival,[46] leads to the hypothesis that this drug may interfere with the direct effects of IL-5 on the eosinophil. These results suggest that protection by nedocromil sodium against the late-phase reaction of asthma may derive from its ability to inhibit IL-5-induced up-regulation of the inflammatory activity of eosinophils. In recent experiments,[47] eosinophils purified from the BALF of antigen-challenged guinea pigs, exhibited a marked increase of migration induced by different stimuli, corroborating that they had been exposed continuously to priming factors generated in their environment. This eosinophil hyper-responsiveness was not reduced when the cells were collected from the nedocromil sodium-treated animals, even though their number was significantly decreased,[47] indicating that the reduction of the number of recruited inflammatory cells is the target of nedocromil sodium, but that the up-regulated eosinophil function is not modified. In contrast, pretreatment of sensitized animals with TRFK-5, a monoclonal antibody directed against IL-5, reduced both the infiltration of eosino-phils and their enhanced response, suggesting that endogenous secreted IL-5 accounts for *in vivo* priming of eosinophils recruited in the airways following antigen challenge.[47]

More recently, studies have correlated the concentrations of IL-5 in biological fluids with the number of T-cells and eosinophils in the BALF and in the serum from patients with allergic rhinitis[48] and bronchial asthma,[49] respectively. The segmental provocation of the airways of allergic patients with the specific antigen was followed by the generation of IL-5 activity. Most interestingly, the amount of IL-5 activity was proportional to the intensity of the late clinical response of the patients; little or no IL-5 activity was generated in patients who do not display late reactions. These results show that IL-5 is generated locally upon antigen provocation in humans as well, and suggest that this is not only involved in eosinophil recruitment but is also important for the bronchopulmonary late re-sponses. Interestingly enough, the concentrations of IL-5 significantly correlated with those of eosinophil secretion products, including cationic proteins and LTC_4,[48] suggesting once again a link between *in situ* eosinophil activation and the alteration of the lung functions.

Sanjar et al.[50] showed that the i.v. administration of IL-5 to guinea pigs is followed by a marked blood eosinophilia that peaks between 1 and 7 hours, depending on the route of administration, and persists for at least 24 hours. Also in the guniea pig, Iwama et al.[51] demonstrated that higher doses of murine IL-5 (mIL-5) instilled intratracheally elicited airway hyperresponsiveness to acetyl-choline. This phenomenon, however, could not be explained exclusively by the eosinophil recruitment into the airways induced by mIL-5, since its instillation is also followed by a marked increase in the total number of cells in the BALF, reflecting macrophage and neutrophil infiltration.[52] The role of IL-5 in antigen-induced eosinophil recruitment and bronchial hyperreactivity in the guinea pig has also been widely demonstrated.[40,51–55] Thus, treatment of the animals with an antibody directed against IL-5 was shown to inhibit the lung infiltration by eosinophils[53–55] and the subsequent bronchial hyperreactivity.[55] In parallel, the ability of systemic or airway administrations of human (h) or murine (m) IL-5 to induce airway eosinophilia and bronchial hyperreactivity in the guinea pig has been described.[40,51,52,55] However, the demonstration that IL-5 is effectively generated *in vivo* following antigenic stimulation and that this phenomenon may be a potential target for anti-inflammatory and antiallergic drugs, is still missing.

The ability of cytokines to modify the pulmonary function has also been de-scribed in rats. The systemic administration of rhIL-2, the major growth factor for T-lymphocytes, was shown to cause bronchial hyperreactivity to methacholine, accompanied by an augmented vascular leakage, by increased numbers of lympho-cytes, neutrophils, and eosinophils in the BALF and in the bronchial wall and by the detachment of the epithelium from the basement membrane.[56,57] The mecha-nisms of these effects have not been explained so far. One hypothesis involves the structural changes of the bronchial tree observed after the administration of IL-2. Indeed, the thickening of the bronchial wall secondary to edema formation and to the infiltration of inflammatory cells in the airways characterizes asthma and is claimed to be responsible for the development of nonspecific bronchial hyperreactivity.[58] On the other hand, the activation of T-lymphocytes by IL-2 is followed by the production of other cytokines acting on eosinophils, such as IL-5.[59] These cells may in turn release inflammatory lipid or granule-associated mediators that contribute to the alterations of the bronchial responsiveness.

The effect of cytokines other than those implicated with the regulation of the eosinophil functions has been investigated in experimental models of airway inflammation and bronchial hyperreactivity. Kips et al.[60] reported that an aerosol of tumor necrosis factor (TNF) induces bronchial hyperreactivity to 5-hydroxy-tryptamine (5-HT) in rats, associated with neutrophil infiltration into the BALF. Since the same authors had reported that the inhalation of endotoxin also induced bronchial hyperreactivity and neutrophil infiltration,[61] it was suggested that the release of TNF during endotoxic shock may account for the changes in the airway responsiveness observed. The situation in the guinea pig is different, and the intratracheal instillation of endotoxin was also followed by bronchopulmonary hyperreactivity and neutrophil infiltration in the airways, but both phenomena were dissociated, since neutrophil depletion failed to prevent hyperresponsiveness. In contrast, platelet depletion or inhibition of platelet function by prostacyclin removed endotoxin-induced bronchial hyperresponsiveness.[62] The generation of TNF in the BALF from antigen-challenged guinea pigs concomitantly with a marked bronchial hyperreactivity to histamine and cellular infiltration into the airways have been recently reported.[63] These phenomena were inhibited by the pretreatment of the animals with an aerosol of an IL-1 receptor antagonist, indicating that cytokines such as IL-1 and TNF contribute to the development of airway inflammation and the accompanying bronchial hyperreactivity following antigen administration.

STUDIES OF CYTOKINE NETWORKS IN THE MOUSE: A NEW APPROACH FOR FURTHER UNDERSTANDING THE MECHANISMS OF ALLERGIC EOSINOPHILIA

Cytokines such as rhIL-2, rhIL-3, rhIL-5, rhGM-CSF, and rhTNF may, to some extent, cross the species barrier. This is of particular interest for those groups working with guinea pigs, a species for which immunological tools have not been developed extensively. Nevertheless, firm conclusions will only be reached when adequate homologous tools will become available. For this reason, a mouse model, allowing immunological manipulations and cell transfer, is indispensable to unravel the molecular mechanisms of allergic reactions. Paradoxically, this model had not been developed before, probably because mice were reputed to respond poorly to bronchoconstrictor agents; this is certainly true for histamine, LTC_4, and antigen itself,[64] but less so for serotonin or cholinergic agents. Thus, the A/J mice strain has been described as being selectively hyperresponsive to methacholine, via M3 muscarinic receptors.[65,66] The genetic background of the susceptibility to passive cutaneous anaphylaxis mediated by allogeneic antibody in the mouse has been demonstrated,[67,68] but no such study seems to be available for bronchopulmonary responsiveness. Recently, Ewart et al.[69] claimed that hyper-responsiveness in those A/J mice is T-lymphocyte-dependent since it is suppressed by cyclosporine. We noted that a selection of hyper-IgE mice respond more intensively in terms of bronchoconstriction to methacholine or serotonin than other mice strains. However, those responses were not augmented by immunization and subsequent intranasal antigen provocation. Similarly, we demonstrated that the responsiveness to serotonin was not augmented in Swiss, Balb/C, and CBA mice made hypereosinophilic 24 hours after the intrapulmonary antigen instillation. Bronchial hyperreactivity was also not observed in "naturally" hypereosinophilic mice transgenic to IL-5[70] that show up to 40% eosinophils in blood, as compared to 1–3% in the CBA/J background animals.[71] As a consequence, it remains to be determined whether additional eosinophil activation will induce bronchial hyper-responsiveness, as is the case with the guinea pig, or if indeed intense eosinophilia and its bronchopulmonary counterpart cannot be linked in this animal species.

Pulmonary eosinophilia is obtained when C57Bl/6 mice are sensitized repeatedly with an *Ascaris suum* extract[72] and antigen-induced eosinophil infiltration into the mouse trachea is mediated by $CD4^+$ lymphocytes and IL-5, whereas $CD8^+$ seems not to be involved.[73] In this study, no increased eosinophil counts were detected in blood, whereas Lefort *et al.* (in preparation) noted a threefold increase in eosinophil counts in the mice circulation 24 hours after intranasal antigen challenge. Blood eosinophilia following the administration of IL-2 to mice was antagonized by a specific antibody directed against IL-5. Concomitantly, an enhancement of IL-5 mRNA expression in spleen cells of IL-2-treated mice was detected.[59] Similarly, another study demonstrated that the production of IL-5 by granuloma cells from mice infected with *Shistosoma mansoni* is enhanced by IL-2 and suppressed by the addition of an anti-IL-2 or an antibody directed against the IL-2 receptor.[74] Taken together, these results suggest that *in vivo* stimulation of T-lymphocytes of the Th2 subclass, which follows antigen exposures, leads directly to the generation of IL-5, but also of IL-2, which in turn is responsible for the production of IL-5.

CONCLUSIONS

Even though no comprehensive model for asthma using conventional laboratory animals is available, it is clear that many features of the disease can be reproduced. These features include acute antigen-induced bronchoconstriction in the guinea pig and in selected rats, which is due to the combined effects of different mediators and delayed effects, particularly bronchial hyperreactivity. The latter event, nevertheless, has not been shown to persist throughout the life span, as may occur in humans, but is rather an acute or subacute event, particularly in the guinea pig. In this respect, progress is needed.

The novelty of recent years is the demonstration that cytokines are not only involved in the proliferation/differentiation responses of haematopoietic and inflammatory cells but also as priming agents for acute migration and release[37,38] and for bronchopulmonary responses to unrelated, particularly lipid, mediators.[14,27,40] It remains to be demonstrated that indeed the descriptions can be completed with the analytical and therapeutical approaches. Immunohistochemistry and the search for gene expression on lungs from sensitized animals, particularly guinea pigs and mice, as well as the use of transgenic and knockout animals, and of specific anticytokine antibodies will be vital for the future trends in research on the mechanisms of allergy.

REFERENCES

1. INTERNATIONAL CONSENSUS REPORT ON DIAGNOSIS AND TREATMENT OF ASTHMA. 1992. Eur. Respir. J. **5:** 601–641.

2. DJUKANOVIC, R., *et al.* 1990. Mucosal inflammation in asthma. Am. Rev. Respir. Dis. **142:** 434–457.
3. METZGER, W. J., *et al.* 1987. Local allergen challenge and bronchoalveolar lavage of allergic asthmatic lungs: Description of the model and local airway inflammation. Am. Rev. Respir. Dis. **135:** 433–440.
4. GLEICH, G. J. 1990. The eosinophil and bronchial asthma: Current understanding. J. Allergy Clin. Immunol. **85:** 422–436.
5. EGESTEN, A., J. ALUMETS, C. VON-MECKLENBURG, M. PALMEGREN & I. OLSSON. 1986. Localization of eosinophil cationic protein, major basic protein and eosinophil peroxidase in human eosinophils by immunoelectron microscopic technique. J. Histochem. Cytochem. **34:** 1399–1404.
6. MOTOJIMA, S., E. FRIGAS, D. A. LOEGERING & G. J. GLEICH. 1989. Toxicity of eosinophil cationic proteins for guinea-pig tracheal epithelium in vitro. Am. Rev. Respir. Dis. **139:** 801–805.
7. GLEICH, G. J., E. FRIGAS, D. A. LOEGERING, D. L. WASSOM & D. STEINMULLER. 1979. Cytotoxic properties of the eosinophil major basic protein. J. Immunol. **123:** 2925–2927.
8. FRIGAS, E., D. A. LOEGERING & G. J. GLEICH. 1980. Cytotoxic effects of the guinea-pig major basic protein on tracheal epithelium. Lab. Invest. **42:** 35–43.
9. BROFMAN, J. D., *et al.* 1988. Epithelial augmentation of trachealis contraction caused by major basic protein of eosinophils. J. Appl. Physiol. **66:** 1867–1873.
10. GUNDEL, R. H., L. G. LETTS & G. J. GLEICH. 1991. Human eosinophil major basic protein induces airway constriction and airway hyperresponsiveness in primates. J. Clin. Invest. **87:** 1470–1473.
11. COYLE, A. J., S. J. ACKERMAN & C. G. IRVIN. 1993. Cationic proteins induce airway hyperresponsiveness dependent on charge interactions. Am. Rev. Respir. Dis. **147:** 896–900.
12. UCHIDA, D. A., *et al.* 1993. The effect of human eosinophil granule major basic protein on airway responsiveness in the rat *in vivo*. Am. Rev. Respir. Dis. **147:** 982–988.
13. SASAKI, M., C. M. HERD & C. P. PAGE. 1993. Effect of heparin and a low-molecular weight heparinoid on PAF-induced airway responses in neonatally immunized rabbits. Br. J. Pharmacol. **110:** 107–112.
14. PRETOLANI, M. & B. B. VARGAFTIG. 1992. From lung hypersensitivity to bronchial hyperreactivity. What can we learn from studies on animal models? Biochem. Pharmacol. **45:** 791–800.
15. COYLE, A. J., *et al.* 1988. The effect of the selective PAF antagonist BN 52021 on PAF- and antigen-induced bronchial hyperreactivity and eosinophil accumulation. Eur. J. Pharmacol. **148:** 51–58.
16. BOICHOT, E., *et al.* 1991. Bronchial hyperresponsiveness and cellular infiltration in lung from aerosol-sensitized and antigen-exposed guinea-pigs. Clin. Exp. Allergy **21:** 67–76.
17. HUTSON, P. A., M. K. CHURCH, T. P. CLAY, P. MILLER & S. T. HOLGATE. 1988. Early and late phase bronchoconstriction after allergen challenge of nonanesthetized guinea-pigs. I. The association of disordered airway physiology to leukocyte infiltration. Am. Rev. Respir. Dis. **137:** 548–557.
18. RIMMER, S. J., *et al.* 1992. Density profile of bronchoalveolar lavage eosinophils in the guinea-pig model of allergen-induced late-phase allergic responses. Am. J. Respir. Cell. Mol. Biol. **6:** 340–348.
19. KLOPROGGE, E., A. J. DE LEEUW, G. R. DE MONCHY & H. F. KAUFFMAN. 1989. Hypodense eosinophilic granulocytes in normal individual and patients with asthma: Generation of hypodense cell populations in vitro. J. Allergy Clin. Immunol. **83:** 393–400.
20. GIBSON, P. G., J. DENBURG, J. DOLOVICH, E. H. RAMSDALE & F. E. HARGREAVE. 1989. Chronic cough: Eosinophilic bronchitis without asthma. Lancet **i:** 1346–1348.
21. LUNDGREN, R., M. SODERBERG, P. HORSTEDT & R. STENLING. 1988. Morphological studies of bronchial mucosal biopsies from asthmatics before and after ten years of treatment with inhaled steroids. Eur. Respir. J. **1:** 883–889.

22. SANJAR, S., S. AOKI, A. KRISTERSSON, D. SMITH & J. MORLEY. 1990. Antigen challenge induces pulmonary airway eosinophil accumulation and airway hyperreactivity in sensitized guinea-pigs: The effects of anti-asthma drugs. Br. J. Pharmacol. **99:** 679–686.

23. BENTLEY, A. M., *et al.* 1992. Identification of T lymphocytes, macrophages, and activated eosinophils in the bronchial mucosa in intrinsic asthma. Am. Rev. Respir. Dis. **146:** 500–506.

24. GUNDEL, R. H., *et al.* 1990. Relationship between bronchoalveolar lavage (BAL) eosinophil-derived proteins and the onset and recovery of airway hyperresponsiveness. J. Allergy Clin. Immunol. **85:** 282.

25. GUNDEL, R. H., M. E. GERRITSEN, G. J. GLEICH & C. D. WEGNER. 1990. Repeated antigen inhalation results in a prolonged airway eosinophilia and airway hyperresponsiveness in primates. J. Appl. Physiol. **68:** 779–786.

26. LELLOUCH-TUBIANA, A., J. LEFORT, M. T. SIMON, A. PFISTER & B. B. VARGAFTIG. 1988. Eosinophil recruitment into guinea-pig lungs after PAF-acether and allergen administration. Modulation by prostacyclin, platelet depletion and selective antagonists. Am. Rev. Respir. Dis. **137:** 948–954.

27. PRETOLANI, M., *et al.* 1993. Role of eosinophil activation in bronchial reactivity of allergic guinea-pigs. Am. Rev. Respir. Dis. In press.

28. HUNT, T. C., *et al.* 1993. Monoclonal antibodies specific for guinea-pig major basic protein: Their use in an ELISA, immunocytochemistry and flow cytometry. Clin. Exp. Allergy **23:** 425–434.

29. AZZAWI, M., *et al.* 1990. Identification of activated T lymphocytes and eosinophils in bronchial biopsies in stable atopic asthmatics. Am. Rev. Respir. Dis. **142:** 1407–1413.

30. ROBINSON, D. S., *et al.* 1992. Predominant TH2-like bronchoalveolar T-lymphocyte population in atopic asthma. New Eng. J. Med. **326:** 298–304.

31. FREW, A. J., *et al.* 1990. Lymphocytes and eosinophils in allergen-induced late-phase asthmatic reactions in the guinea-pig. Am. Rev. Respir. Dis. **141:** 407–413.

32. LAPA E SILVA, J. R., *et al.* 1993. Immunopathological alterations in the bronchi of immunized guinea-pigs. Am. J. Respir. Cell. Mol. Biol. **9:** 44–53.

33. PRETOLANI, M., J. LEFORT & B. B. VARGAFTIG. 1988. Active immunization induces lung hyperresponsiveness in the guinea-pig: Pharmacological modulation and triggering role of the booster injection. Am. Rev. Respir. Dis. **138:** 1572–1578.

34. CURTIS, J. L. & H. B. KALTREIDER. 1989. Characterization of bronchoalveolar lymphocytes during a specific antibody-forming cell response in the lungs of mice. Am. Rev. Respir. Dis. **139:** 393–400.

35. GARSSEN, J., F. P. NIJKAMP, H. VAN DER VLIET & H. VAN LOVEREN. 1991. T-cell-mediated induction of airway hyperreactivity in mice. Am. Rev. Respir. Dis. **144:** 931–938.

36. SANDERSON, C. J. 1992. Interleukin-5, eosinophils, and disease. Blood **79:** 3101–3109.

37. BISCHOFF, S. C., T. BRUNNER, A. L. DE WECK & C. A. DAHINDEN. 1990. Interleukin-5 modifies histamine release and leukotriene generation by human basophils in response to diverse agonists. J. Exp. Med. **172:** 1577–1582.

38. COËFFIER, E., D. JOSEPH & B. B. VARGAFTIG. 1991. Activation by human recombinant IL-5 of guinea-pig eosinophils. Selective priming to PAF and interference of its antagonists. J. Immunol. **147:** 2595–2602.

39. NAKAMURA, M., *et al.* 1991. Molecular cloning and expression of platelet-activating factor receptor from human leukocytes. J. Biol. Chem. **266:** 20400–20405.

40. PRETOLANI, M., J. LEFORT, D. LEDUC & B. B. VARGAFTIG. 1992. Effect of human recombinant interleukin-5 on in vitro lung responsiveness to PAF in actively sensitised guinea-pigs. Br. J. Pharmacol. **106:** 677–684.

41. PRETOLANI, M., *et al.* 1990. Protection by nedocromil sodium of active immunization-induced bronchopulmonary alterations in the guinea-pigs. Am. Rev. Respir. Dis. **141:** 1259–1265.

42. WANG, J. M., *et al.* 1989. Recombinant human interleukin 5 is a selective eosinophil chemoattractant. Eur. J. Immunol. **19:** 701–705.

43. TRIGGIANI, M., W. C. HUBBARD & F. H. CHILTON. 1990. Synthesis of 1 acyl-2-acetyl-

sn-glycero-3-phosphocholine by an enriched preparation of the human lung mast cell. J. Immunol. **144:** 4773–4780.

44. PLAUT, M., *et al.* 1989. Mast cell lines produce lymphokines in response to cross-linkage of FcεRI or to calcium ionophores. Nature **339:** 64–67.
45. PRETOLANI, M., J. LEFORT & B. B. VARGAFTIG. 1993. Inhibition by nedocromil sodium of recombinant human interleukin-5 (rhIL-5)-induced lung hyper-responsiveness to platelet-activating factor in actively sensitized guinea-pigs. J. Allergy Clin. Immunol. **91:** 809–816.
46. RESLER, B., J. B. SEDGWICK & W. W. BUSSE. 1992. Inhibition of interleukin-5 (IL-5) effects on human eosinophils (eos) by nedocromil sodium (ned). J. Allergy Clin. Immunol. **89:** A362.
47. COËFFIER, E., D. JOSEPH & B. B. VARGAFTIG. 1992. Airway eosinophils from antigen-stimulated guinea-pigs exhibit enhanced migration. Allergy **47:** 231.
48. SEDWICK, J. B., *et al.* 1991. Immediate and late airway response of allergic rhinitis patients to segmental antigen challenge. Characterization of eosinophil and mast cell mediators. Am. Rev. Respir. Dis. **144:** 1274–1281.
49. CORRIGAN, C. J., *et al.* 1993. CD4 T-lymphocyte activation in asthma is accompanied by increased serum concentration of interleukin-5. Effect of glucocorticoid therapy. Am. Rev. Respir. Dis. **147:** 540–547.
50. SANJAR, S., P. McCABE & L. REYNOLDS. 1991. Recombinant human IL-5 (rhIL-5) induces a rapid and selective blood eosinophilia in the guinea-pig. Am. Rev. Respir. Dis. **143:** A14.
51. IWAMA, T., H. NAGAI, N. TSURUOKA & A. KODA. 1993. Effect of murine recombinant interleukin-5 on bronchial reactivity in guinea-pigs. Clin. Exp. Allergy **23:** 32–38.
52. IWAMA, T., H. NAGAI, H. SUDA, N. TSURUOKA & A. KODA. 1992. Effect of murine recombinant interleukin-5 on the cell population in guinea-pig airways. Br. J. Pharmacol. **105:** 19–22.
53. CHAND, N., *et al.* 1992. Anti-IL-5 monoclonal antibody inhibits allergic late phase bronchial eosinophilia in guinea-pigs: A therapeutical approach. Eur. J. Pharmacol. **211:** 121–123.
54. GULBENKIAN, A. R., *et al.* 1992. Interleukin-5 modulates eosinophil accumulation in allergic guinea-pig lung. Am. Rev. Respir. Dis. **146:** 263–265.
55. VAN OOSTERHOUT, A. J. M., *et al.* 1993. Effect of anti-IL-5 and IL-5 on airway hyperreactivity and eosinophils in the guinea-pigs. Am. Rev. Respir. Dis. **147:** 548–552.
56. RENZI, P. M., S. SAPIENZA, T. DU, N. S. WANG & J. G. MARTIN. 1991. Lymphokine-induced airway hyperresponsiveness in the rat. Am. Rev. Respir. Dis. **143:** 375–379.
57. RENZI, P. M., T. DU, S. SAPIENZA, N. S. WANG & J. G. MARTIN. 1991. Acute effects of interleukin-2 on lung mechanics and airway responsiveness in rats. Am. Rev. Respir. Dis. **143:** 380–385.
58. JAMES, A. L., P. D. PARE & J. C. HOGG. 1989. The mechanics of airway narrowing in asthma. Am. Rev. Respir. Dis. **139:** 242–246.
59. YAMAGUCHI, Y., *et al.* 1990. Role of IL-5 in IL-2-induced eosinophilia. *In vivo* and *in vitro* expression of IL-5 mRNA by IL-2. J. Immunol. **145:** 873–877.
60. KIPS, J. C., J. TAVERNIER & R. A. PAUWELS. 1992. Tumor necrosis factor causes bronchial hyperresponsiveness in rats. Am. Rev. Respir. Dis. **145:** 332–336.
61. PAUWELS, R. A., J. C. KIPS, R. A. PALEMAN & M. E. VAN DER STRAETEN. 1990. The effect of endotoxin inhalation on airway responsiveness and cellular influx in rats. Am. Rev. Respir. Dis. **141:** 540–545.
62. VINCENT, D., *et al.* 1993. Intratracheal *E. coli* lipopolysaccharide induces platelet-dependent bronchial hyperreactivity. J. Appl. Physiol. **74:** 1027–1038.
63. WATSON, M. L., D. SMITH, A. D. BOURNE, R. C. THOMPSON & J. WESTWICK. 1993. Cytokines contribute to airway dysfunction in antigen-challenged guinea-pigs: Inhibition of airway hyperreactivity, pulmonary eosinophil accumulation, and tumor necrosis factor generation by pretreatment with an interleukin-1 receptor antagonist. Am. J. Respir. Cell Mol. Biol. **8:** 365–369.
64. McCASKILL, A. C., C. S. HOSKING & D. J. HILL. 1984. Anaphylaxis following intranasal challenge of mice sensitized with ovalbumin. Immunology **51:** 669–677.

65. LEVITT, R. C. & W. MITZNE. 1988. Expression of airway hyperreactivity to acetylcholine as a simple autosomal recessive trait in mice. FASEB J. **2:** 2605–2608.
66. OHTA, K., et al. 1993. Expression of airway hyperreactivity in mice is mediated by M3 muscarinic receptors. Am. Rev. Respir. Dis. **147:** A571.
67. HARADA, M., R. MISAKI, H. FUKUSHIMA, M. NAGATA & S. MAKINO. 1989. Strain difference and mode of inheritance of the susceptibility to passive cutaneous anaphylaxis mediated by allogeneic IgE antibody in the mouse. Immunol. Invest. **18:** 723–735.
68. SOUZA, C. M., L. C. S. MAIA & N. M. VAZ. 1974. Susceptibility to cutaneous anaphylaxis in inbred strains of mice. J. Immunol. **112:** 1369–1372.
69. EWART, S. L., W. MITZNER & M. WILLS-KARP. 1993. T lymphocyte suppression attenuates airway reactivity in mice with genetically hyperreactive airways. Am. Rev. Respir. Dis. **147:** A571.
70. VIANNA, R. M. J., et al. 1993. Eosinophil recruitment into the mice airways is not sufficient to induce bronchopulmonary hyperresponsiveness. Am. Rev. Respir. Dis. **147:** A571.
71. LINDSAY, A., M. STRATH, A. L. MELLOR & C. J. SANDERSON. 1990. Eosinophilia in transgenic mice expressing interleukin 5. J. Exp. Med. **172:** 1425–1431.
72. NOGAMI, M., et al. 1990. Experimental pulmonary eosinophilia in mice by *Ascaris suum* extract. Am. Rev. Respir. Dis. **141:** 1289–1295.
73. NAKAJIMA, H., et al. 1992. CD4+ T-lymphocytes and Interleukin-5 mediate antigen-induced blood eosinophil infiltration into the mouse trachea. Am. Rev. Respir. Dis. **146:** 374–377.
74. METWALI, A., E. ELLIOT, R. MATHEW, A. BLUM & J. V. WEINSTOCK. 1993. IL-2 contributes to the IL-5 response in granulomas from mice infected with *Schistosoma mansoni*. J. Immunol. **150:** 536–542.

Eosinophil Tissue Mobilization in Allergic Disorders

P. L. B. BRUIJNZEEL

Department of Pharmacology
MBL/TNO
Rijswijk, The Netherlands

INTRODUCTION

Asthma and atopic dermatitis (=eczema) are both considered atopic disorders. It has become clear that different etiologic mechanisms are involved in the induction and maintenance of the disease. Therefore one distinguishes allergic (extrinsic) and nonallergic (intrinsic) asthma.[1,2] Whereas allergen interaction with specific IgE is a prerequisite for allergic asthma,[2,3] the etiology of nonallergic asthma is more difficult to demonstrate.[3,4] Postulated pathogenetic mechanisms include viral infections,[5] receptor imbalance,[6] and antigen–antibody reaction.[7] Although such a clear separation has not yet been made for atopic dermatitis, this patient group can also be divided into a group of patients with elevated and normal IgE antibody levels.[8] Also in the latter group the etiology is unclear. Therefore one may also distinguish extrinsic and intrinsic atopic dermatitis. Notwithstanding this etiologic diversification, both forms of asthma and atopic dermatitis do share some pathogenetic characteristics.

Both asthma and atopic dermatitis are inflammatory disorders in which T-cells and eosinophils are predominantly involved. Remarkably, other inflammatory cell types seem of less importance. Activated lymphocytes may be observed both in the circulation and in the tissue.[9–12] T-cell activation is reflected by increased expression of IL-2R and HLA-DR. Although there are differences in the activation pattern of T-lymphocytes from allergic and nonallergic asthma and/or atopic dermatitis patients, their activation state indicates that they actively release factors acting on other cells, for example, eosinophils. In this respect particularly cytokines are relevant. In the various body compartments (circulation, tissue, and alveolar space) activated T-lymphocytes and cytokine production and secretion by those cells have been demonstrated.[13–15] Interleukin-1 (IL-1), tumor necrosis factor-α (TNF-α), IL-3, IL-4, IL-5, granulocyte macrophage colony-stimulating factor (GM–CSF), IL-8, and RANTES are of importance with respect to eosinophil tissue mobilization.

Another feature of asthma and atopic dermatitis is the presence of increased levels of eosinophilic granulocytes in the circulation and more particularly in the tissue (and bronchoalveolar lavage fluid in asthma).[10,12,15–19] Tissue damage in both asthma and atopic dermatitis is due to release of granule-derived and membrane-derived mediators from eosinophil origin.[20] Tissue deposits of the following granule-derived mediators of the eosinophil have been demonstrated in the tissue of asthma and atopic dermatitis patients: eosinophil major basic protein (MBP), eosinophil cationic protein (ECP), and eosinophil peroxidase (EPO). The degree of eosinophilia and the tissue damage seem to correlate with the degree of the severity of the disease.[16,19,21–23] The formation of eosinophils in the bone marrow is mainly under the control of the cytokines IL-3 and GM–CSF,[24] whereas eosinophil

259

differentiation is under the control of IL-5.[24] Moreover, these cytokines have been shown to act as modulators of eosinophil activation and tissue infiltration.[25-31]

THE TISSUE RECRUITMENT OF INFLAMMATORY CELLS

Both lymphocytes and eosinophilic granulocytes are recruited at the site of inflammation in asthma and atopic dermatitis. In the past few years we have been able to show that activated T-lymphocytes from the circulation of both asthma and atopic dermatitis patients spontaneously secrete factors that prolong eosinophil survival *in vitro*.[10,12,24] Identification of these factors revealed that IL-3, IL-5, and GM–CSF were secreted by activated CD4+ T-cells from these patients and not by the same cell types from normal individuals. Furthermore, these cytokines could also be demonstrated in the sera of those patients.[10] This finding has stimulated us to further investigate in particular the role of these cytokines in modulating eosinophil infiltration in allergically inflamed tissue. Eosinophil tissue infiltration from the circulation is governed by the following processes:

1. The adherence to endothelium
2. The transmigration across endothelium
3. The chemotaxis within the tissue

This is schematically outlined in FIGURE 1.

THE ADHESION TO AND TRANSMIGRATION ACROSS ENDOTHELIAL CELL MONOLAYERS BY EOSINOPHILS

Although the eosinophil–endothelial cell interactions are extensively discussed by Moser *et al.*,[26,29] a brief summary of the most important findings is also given here. Eosinophils from the circulation of normal individuals have the capacity to adhere to IL-1 or TNF-α-activated endothelial cell monolayers, but they can hardly transmigrate this layer. In contrast, eosinophils from asthma or atopic dermatitis patients do show a slightly increased capacity to adhere to IL-1- or TNF-α-activated endothelium. These eosinophils also spontaneously transmigrate the endothelial layer.[26] This transmigration capacity can be induced by pretreatment of eosinophils from normal individuals with picomolar concentrations of IL-3, IL-5, or GM–CSF.[26] All cytokines proved to be equally potent in this respect. Obviously *in vitro* or *in vivo* priming of eosinophils is necessary to enable tissue infiltration. This transmigration capacity proved to be dependent on CD11b/CD18 expression on the eosinophil and intercellular adhesion molecule-1 (ICAM-1) expression on the endothelium, as demonstrated by blocking antibodies with specificity for these structures. These studies indicated that although similar structures are involved in adherence and transmigration, adherence does not automatically mean transmigration. Furthermore, transendothelial migration of eosinophils based on CD11b/CD18–ICAM-1 interaction cannot explain selective eosinophil tissue infiltration observed in allergic inflammation, since transendothelial migration of neutrophils is also determined by these structures.[32] To find an explanation for this selective eosinophil tissue, bilayer constructs were made consisting of endothelial cell monolayers on an extracellular matrix of fibroblasts. When these constructs were stimulated with IL-4, selective eosinophil infiltration of eosinophils

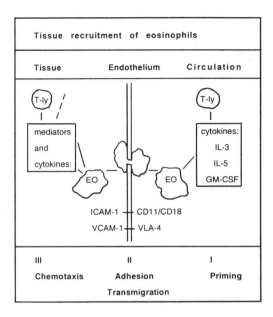

FIGURE 1. Selective recruitment of eosinophils in allergic inflammation is determined by the following three processes: **(I)** Priming of eosinophils in the circulation by the cytokines IL-3, IL-5, and GM–CSF. **(II)** Adhesion to and transmigration across endothelial cell layers. In this process the most important structures on the eosinophil are CD11/CD18 and VLA-4, on the endothelium ICAM-1 and VCAM-1. **(III)** Chemotaxis (and chemokinesis) of eosinophils by factors present in the circulation and the tissue. The chemotaxins may be divided into mediators and cytokines, which can originate from a variety of cell types. (Abbreviations used: T-ly: T-lymphocytes; EO: eosinophilic granulocyte.)

from the circulation of asthma or atopic dermatitis patients took place.[29] Hardly any infiltration of neutrophils occurred. Again eosinophils from normal individuals had to be primed *in vitro* with picomolar concentrations of IL-3, IL-5, and GM–CSF to allow tissue infiltration. This selective eosinophil infiltration proved to be dependent on the expression of very late antigen-4 (VLA-4) on the eosinophil and vascular adhesion molecule-1 (VCAM-1) on the endothelium. In this system IL-4 proved to be responsible for the induction of VCAM-1 on the endothelial cells. However, Moser *et al.* also pointed out that CD11b/CD18 structures on the eosinophil and ICAM-1 structures on the endothelium were involved.[29] Remarkably, IL-1 activation of those bilayer constructs did not induce eosinophil transmigration, whereas in the monolayer constructs it did (see the contribution of Moser in this issue for more details). Also the data with IL-4 indicated that eosinophils from allergic individuals were primed *in vivo*, whereas eosinophils from normal individuals were not. Pretreatment of eosinophils from normal individuals with the cytokines IL-3, IL-5, and GM–CSF seemed a prerequisite to allow transmigration of eosinophils across endothelium cell bilayer constructs just as it was for endothelial cell monolayers.[26,29] In addition the endothelial cell layer has to be stimulated in a specific way (e.g., IL-4) to allow selective eosinophil tissue infiltration without neutrophil tissue infiltration. Thus, priming of eosinophils in the circulation by IL-3, IL-5, and GM–CSF gives the eosinophils an increased capacity to extravasate.

CHEMOTAXIS OF EOSINOPHILS

Mediators as Chemotaxins

The response of eosinophils to certain chemoattractants may be an important pathophysiologic mechanism leading to specific eosinophil accumulation. However, most *in vitro* chemotaxis systems have used chemotaxis chambers in which the migration was measured through filter systems. In these systems the importance of the adherence to and the transmigration across the endothelial cell layer is ignored. As previously outlined, this process forms an essential part of the eosinophil extravasation. For this reason the relevance of *in vitro* chemotaxis studies for the *in vivo* situation should always be considered with some caution unless eosinophil mobilization has been demonstrated by the chemoattractant *in vivo* as well (e.g., after intracutaneous application). Therefore the *in vitro* chemotaxis data presented here should only be considered valid for cells being in the same body compartment [e.g., the circulation or the tissue (see FIG. 1)].

Many chemoattractants for eosinophils have been evaluated so far.[25,27,28,30,31,33] In TABLE 1 we have listed a number of eosinophil chemotaxins we have evaluated on their chemotactic potency for eosinophils from normal individuals. Some of the listed chemotaxins are potent chemotaxins, whereas others are not or are no chemoattractant at all [e.g., N-formyl-methionyl-leucyl-phenylalanine (FMLP), platelet factor 4 (PF4), and IL-8 (see TABLE 2)]. In addition, most of these chemoattractants have not been identified as being eosinophil selective, that is, they also act as chemotaxins on other cell types (e.g., neutrophils).[34] With respect to the selective eosinophil infiltration observed in allergic inflammation, these chemotaxins may therefore be of limited importance. In particular since most of these chemotaxins have a much greater chemoattractant potency toward neutro-

TABLE 1. Chemotaxis of Eosinophils: Mediators

Chemotaxin	Optimal Chemotactic Concentration	Cells per 10 hpf (Mean Values $\pm$ SEM)		
		Normals	Asthma	Eczema
PAF	0.1 μM	98 $\pm$ 15 (8)	102 $\pm$ 7 (6)	105 $\pm$ 10 (10)
	0.1 nM*	24 $\pm$ 5 (8)	101 $\pm$ 12 (6)	56 $\pm$ 7 (8)
C5a	10 nM	109 $\pm$ 27 (9)	135 $\pm$ 21 (8)	126 $\pm$ 20 (8)
LTB4	0.1 μM	47 $\pm$ 7 (8)	71 $\pm$ 7 (8)f	n.d.
20-OH-LTB4	0.1 μM	47 $\pm$ 7 (8)	65 $\pm$ 7 (8)f	n.d.
FMLP	10 nM	21 $\pm$ 4 (7)	67 $\pm$ 15 (8)	55 $\pm$ 8 (9)
PF4	1 nM	21 $\pm$ 4 (8)	105 $\pm$ 15 (8)	92 $\pm$ 15 (8)
Buffer	—	24 $\pm$ 5 (12)	26 $\pm$ 5 (8)	24 $\pm$ 5 (8)

Note: In parentheses: number of experiments.

Key: n.d.: not done; *: optimal chemotactic concentration for eosinophils from asthmatic patients; f: valid for intrinsic asthma patients; hpf: high-power field.

TABLE 2. Chemotaxis of Eosinophils: Cytokines

Chemotaxin	Optimal Chemotactic Concentration	Cells per 10 hpf (Mean Values ± SEM)		
		Normals	Asthma	Eczema
IL-3	10 nM	50 ± 8 (8)	42 ± 7 (8)	90 ± 15 (8)
IL-5	10 nM	70 ± 15 (8)	50 ± 5 (8)	90 ± 10 (8)
GM–CSF	10 nM	80 ± 11 (8)	35 ± 7 (8)	60 ± 9 (8)
	1 nM*	50 ± 10 (8)	n.d.	100 ± 9 (8)
IL-8	10 nM	21 ± 4 (8)	50 ± 7 (8)	71 ± 15 (8)
TNF-alpha	10 nM	35 ± 7 (8)	n.d.	35 ± 7 (8)
Buffer	—	24 ± 5 (12)	26 ± 5 (8)	24 ± 5 (8)

Note: In parentheses: number of experiments.
Key: n.d.: not done; *: optimal chemotactic concentration for eosinophils from eczema patients; hpf: high-power field.

phils than toward eosinophils.[33,34] This also holds for platelet activating factor (PAF), which was originally described to possess greater chemotactic potency for eosinophils than for neutrophils.[35]

When the migratory responsiveness of eosinophils from asthma and atopic dermatitis patients toward optimal chemotactic concentrations of some chemoattractants is compared to those of normal individuals, then a different response pattern to some of those chemoattractants is observed (see TABLE 1). In the case of complement factor 5a (C5a) and TNF-α no difference is observed. In contrast, the chemotactic response of eosinophils from the patients to PAF and to a lesser extent to leukotriene B4 (LTB4) is increased. Even more interesting, the migratory responsiveness of patient eosinophils to some chemoattractants turned out not to be chemotactic for eosinophils from normal individuals (i.e., FMLP, PF4, and IL-8). The latter finding indicates that certain factors present in the circulation of those patients must have influenced those responses. Indeed, we have been able to demonstrate that *in vitro* pretreatment of eosinophils from the circulation of normal individuals with picomolar concentrations of the cytokines IL-3, IL-5, and GM–CSF gives those cells the capacity to show an increased responsiveness to those chemotaxins. In this respect they all show an equal potency.[25,27,28,30,31] In addition these cytokines were able to induce a chemotactic responsiveness toward FMLP, PF4, and IL-8. These effects could be blocked by the addition of specific monoclonal antibodies against the priming cytokines.

These findings indicate that picomolar (or even lower) levels of the cytokines IL-3, IL-5, and GM–CSF, which may be present in the circulation or the tissue of asthma and atopic dermatitis patients, have the capacity to modulate the migratory responsiveness to a number of chemoattractants. To some chemoattractants the responsiveness will not be influenced, whereas in other cases there will be an increase or even an induction of the migratory responsiveness. Taking this latter finding into account it seems logical to assume that there are still eosinophil chemotaxins that have to be identified.

Cytokines as Chemotaxins

Of the cytokines that may be relevant to allergic inflammation IL-2, IL-3, IL-4, IL-5, IL-8, RANTES, and GM–CSF have been shown to possess the capacity to induce eosinophil migratory responses.[34] IL-8 and IL-4 show chemotactic activity for *in vivo* or *in vitro* primed eosinophils only (see the paper by Dubois & Bruijnzeel in this issue). Of particular interest are the chemotactic responses of eosinophils to the cytokines IL-3, IL-5, and GM–CSF. Eosinophils from the circulation of normal individuals do show a migratory response to IL-3, IL-5, and GM–CSF. In general this response is optimal at a concentration of 10 nM. Dose range studies for those chemokines performed with eosinophils from the circulation of asthma and atopic dermatitis patients has resulted in some interesting data, which are shown in TABLE 2. Eosinophils from the circulation of allergic asthma patients showed significantly decreased chemotactic responses ($p < 0.05$; paired Student's t-test), whereas eosinophils from atopic dermatitis patients showed significantly increased chemotactic responses ($p < 0.05$; paired Student's t-test). These responses could be fully blocked by specific monoclonal antibodies.

Thus, IL-3, IL-5, and GM–CSF seem to act as primers at picomolar or even lower concentrations and as chemoattractants at nanomolar concentrations. Although the chemotactic responsiveness of eosinophils from the circulation of asthma and atopic dermatitis patients toward various mediators is similar, the migratory response pattern to these cytokines is completely different.

CYTOKINE-INDUCED MIGRATION: CHEMOKINESIS OR CHEMOTAXIS ?

Taking into account that the cytokines IL-3, IL-5, and GM–CSF all prolong *in vivo* survival of eosinophils and induce an increased activation state of the eosinophil, as is reflected by our chemotaxis data, then the question arises whether eosinophils primed by these cytokines do show an increased chemokinetic responsiveness, and as a consequence a reduced chemotactic responsiveness toward the same cytokines. Indeed, when eosinophils from the circulation of normal individuals are preincubated with increasing concentrations of cytokines (exemplified for GM–CSF in FIG. 2), the blank value of migration (being the chemokinetic response) increases considerably with increasing concentration of the priming cytokine. How does this affect the net chemotactic response? In case of PAF, for example, the net chemotactic response will still be increased, particularly at PAF concentrations of around 10 pM and a cytokine priming concentration of 10 pM. When higher priming concentrations (around 1 nM) are being used, however, then chemokinesis will strongly affect the net chemotactic response. This also holds for the induction of the chemotactic response from normal individuals toward FMLP, PF4, IL-4, and IL-8 *in vitro* in eosinophils.[25,27,28,30,31] Nevertheless, the chemotactic responsiveness of eosinophils from asthma and atopic dermatitis patients toward these mediators is significantly increased, whereas the chemokinetic response is not. Therefore, further investigations into this matter have indicated that the problem of increased chemokinesis of eosinophils from normal individuals can be partly overcome by pretreatment of those cells with picomolar concentrations of the cytokines over a period of 24 to 48 hours *in vitro* at 37°C. Therefore most of the aforementioned is still valid. In the case of chemotaxis toward the cytokines IL-3, IL-5, and GM–CSF themselves, priming of the eosinophils should result in decreased chemotactic responsiveness toward the homologous cytokine. This is shown in FIGURE 2(A), and is also observed in eosinophils from asthma patients (see TABLE 2). Obviously the cytokine receptor is desensitized, leading to decreased responsiveness to the cytokine. Also, 3 hours after

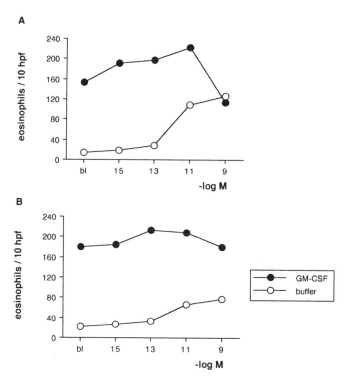

FIGURE 2. (A) Eosinophils from the circulation of a normal individual were exposed *in vitro* to increasing concentrations of GM–CSF for 30 minutes at 37°C. After washing the cells with buffer, the spontaneous migration (= chemokinesis) (○) and the chemotaxis (●) to 1-nM GM–CSF were determined. The net chemotactic response is the difference between these two lines. An illustrative example of $n = 3$ is shown. **(B)** See FIGURE 2(A). Here, eosinophils from the circulation of an atopic dermatitis patient were used. An illustrative example of $n = 3$ is also shown.

allergen provocation of allergic asthma patients this desensitization seems to take place already, possibly being the result of the release of cytokines in the circulation.[10,12] Although this explanation may seem logical, why do eosinophils from atopic dermatitis patients show an increased migratory responsiveness to the cytokines IL-3, IL-5, and GM–CSF? As shown in FIGURE 2(B), these eosinophils are less sensitive for desensitization by GM–CSF than eosinophils from normal individuals, even at nanomolar concentrations of GM–CSF. As a consequence the chemokinetic response is less and the net chemotactic response remains almost intact. Therefore these results indicate that eosinophils from atopic dermatitis patients do have either an altered receptor sensitivity for GM–CSF or an increased receptor number for GM–CSF. This is further supported by the fact that eosinophils from the circulation of atopic dermatitis patients can be further primed with GM–CSF, leading to an increased PAF responsiveness, whereas this does not occur in eosinophils from asthma patients.[31] Obviously there are spare receptors available. Possibly, this also is valid for IL-3 and other unidentified chemotactic factors. This phenomenon should be taken into account when comparing the eosinophil mobilizing capacity toward various factors or when comparing the migratory responsiveness of eosinophils from different patient groups to one factor.

IN CONCLUSION

Eosinophils from the circulation of normal individuals and asthma and atopic dermatitis patients show different chemotactic responses to various mediators and cytokines. Evidence is provided that the cytokines IL-3, IL-5, and GM–CSF present in the circulation and the tissue of allergic individuals, modulate the transendothelial migration capacity as well as the chemotactic responsiveness to various mediators and cytokines. The mechanism by which they modulate these responses is unclear at the moment, although it seems very likely that they influence the cytoskeleton. Therefore a better understanding of the modulatory role of these cytokines could be of help in developing new therapeutic strategies for allergic disorders.

REFERENCES

1. RACKEMANN, F. M. 1947. Am. J. Med. 3: 601–606.
2. DANIELLE, R. P. 1988. In Immunology and Immunologic Diseases of the Lung, R. P. Danielle, Ed.: 503–516. Blackwell. Boston.
3. ISHIZAKA, T. 1981. J. Allergy Clin. Immunol. 67: 90–98.
4. NEWHOUSE, T. 1989. In Intrinsic Asthma. M. Schmitz-Schumann, G. Menz, U. Costabel, and C. P. Page, Eds.: 17–26. Birkhäuser Verlag. Basel.
5. LI, J. T. C. & E. J. O'CONNELL. 1987. Ann. Allergy 59: 321–327.
6. SZENTIVANYI, A. 1968. J. Allergy 42: 203–212.
7. TURNER-WARWICK, M. 1974. Prog. Immunol. 11: 283–294.
8. BRUIJNZEEL-KOOMEN, C. A. F. M. 1989. Thesis, University of Utrecht, Utrecht, The Netherlands.
9. CORRIGAN, C. J. & A. B. KAY. 1988. Lancet i: 1129–1132.
10. WALKER, C., J.-C. VIRCHOW, JR., P. L. B. BRUIJNZEEL & K. BLASER. 1991. J. Immunol. 146: 1829–1835.
11. WALKER, C., M. K. KAEGI, P. BRAUN & K. BLASER. 1991. J. Allergy Clin. Immunol. 88: 935–942.
12. WALKER, C., et al. 1993. Clin. Exp. Allergy 23: 145–153.
13. AZZAWI, M., et al. 1990. Am. Rev. Respir. Dis. 142: 1407–1413.
14. HAMID, Q., et al. 1991. J. Clin. Invest. 87: 1541–1546.
15. WALKER, C., et al. 1992. Am. Rev. Respir. Dis. 145: 109–115.
16. GLEICH, G. J. 1990. J. Allergy Clin. Immunol. 85: 423–436.
17. VIRCHOW, J.-C., JR., U. HÖLSCHER & C. VIRCHOW. 1992. Am. Rev. Respir. Dis. 145: 127–132.
18. KAPP, A., W. CZECH, J. KRUTMANN & E. SCHÖPF. 1991. J. Am. Acad. Dermatol. 24: 555–558.
19. CZECH, W., J. KRUTMANN, E. SCHÖPF & A. KAPP. 1992. Br. J. Dermatol. 126: 351–355.
20. BRUIJNZEEL, P. L. B. 1989. Int. Arch. Allergy Appl. Immunol. 90: 57–63.
21. BOUSQUET, J., et al. 1990. New Eng. J. Med. 323: 57–63.
22. LEIFERMAN, K., et al. 1985. New Eng. J. Med. 313: 47–56.
23. BRUIJNZEEL, P. L. B., et al. 1993. Clin. Exp. Allergy. 23: 97–109.
24. OWEN, W. F. 1991. ACI News. 3: 85–89.
25. WARRINGA, R. A. J., L. KOENDERMAN, P. T. M. KOK, J. KREUKNIET & P. L. B. BRUIJNZEEL. 1991. Blood 77: 2694–2700.

26. MOSER, R., J. FEHR, L. OLGIATI & P. L. B. BRUIJNZEEL. 1992. Blood **79:** 2937–2945.
27. WARRINGA, R. A. J., *et al.* 1991. Blood **79:** 1836–1841.
28. WARRINGA, R. A. J., *et al.* 1992. Am. J. Respir. Cell Mol. Biol. **7:** 631–637.
29. MOSER, R., J. FEHR & P. L. B. BRUIJNZEEL. 1992. J. Immunol. **149:** 1432–1438.
30. WARRINGA, R. A. J., H. J. J. MENGELERS, J. A. M. RAAIJMAKERS, P. L. B. BRUIJNZEEL & L. KOENDERMAN. 1993. J. Allergy Clin. Immunol. **91:** 1198–1205.
31. BRUIJNZEEL, P. L. B., *et al.* 1993. J. Invest. Dermatol. **100:** 137–142.
32. MOSER, R., B. SCHLEIFFENBAUM, P. GROSCURTH & J. FEHR. 1989. J. Clin. Invest. **83:** 444–455.
33. BRUIJNZEEL, P. L. B., R. A. J. WARRINGA, P. T. M. KOK & J. KREUKNIET. 1990. Br. J. Pharmacol. **99:** 798–802.
34. RESNICK, M. B. & P. F. WELLER. 1993. Am. J. Respir. Cell Mol. Biol. **8:** 349–355.
35. WARDLAW, A. J., R. MOQBEL, O. CROMWELL & A. B. KAY. 1986. J. Clin. Invest. **78:** 1701–1706.

IL-4-Induced Migration of Eosinophils in Allergic Inflammation

G. R. DUBOIS[a] AND P. L. B. BRUIJNZEEL[b]

[a]Department of Dermato-Allergology
University Hospital Utrecht
Heidelberglaan 100
NL 3584 CX Utrecht, The Netherlands

[b]Department of Pharmacology
MBL/TNO
Rijswijk, The Netherlands

INTRODUCTION

Allergical inflammation is characterized by a specific cellular infiltration. This cellular infiltration consists of T-lymphocytes and eosinophils. The T-cells appear in an activated state both in the circulation and in the tissue. This is reflected by the presence of activation markers such as IL-2R and HLA-DR. In allergic asthma, activated T-cells can be detected in the bronchial mucosa and in atopic dermatitis activated T-cells can be found in the lesional skin.[1,2] Further characterization of these T-cells showed that they are mainly CD4 +ve and generate the cytokines IL-3, IL-4, IL-5, and GM–CSF.[1] Increased numbers of eosinophils are present in the circulation and the tissue of allergic asthma patients. Increased numbers of circulating eosinophils are also found in atopic dermatitis patients. Although hardly any intact eosinophils are present in lesional atopic dermatitis skin deposits of granule-derived eosinophil, mediators can be observed.[3] Of the aforementioned cytokines, IL-3, IL-5, and GM–CSF are important growth and differentiation factors for eosinophils; they also prolong eosinophil survival *in vitro*.[4-6] They can potentiate functional responses of eosinophils such as antibody-dependent cytotoxicity, respiratory burst activation, and migratory responsiveness.[5-10] In contrast to other inflammatory cells, eosinophils and some B-cell subpopulations express IL-5 receptors.[11] Therefore many effects of IL-5 are considered eosinophil specific.

In addition to IL-3, IL-5, and GM–CSF, IL-4 is also secreted by CD4 +ve T-cells. IL-4 was originally described as a costimulant of B-cells.[12] Other effects on B-lymphocytes include induction of class II major histocompatibility antigens[13] and induction of $Fc_\varepsilon RII$.[14,15] IL-4 induces the proliferation of human thymocytes and primary mast cells.[16] IL-4 also enhances the IgE and IgG1 production[17] and influences tumor infiltrating lymphocytes and lymphokine-activated killer cells.[18]

In recent years we have investigated which processes modulate eosinophil tissue infiltration in allergic inflammation. So far, these investigations have indicated that eosinophils in the circulation from allergic asthma and atopic dermatitis patients are in a "primed" state.[10,19] This primed state is most likely due to previous contact with the cytokines IL-3, IL-5, and GM–CSF and renders the eosinophils an increased capacity to respond chemotactically to various chemotaxins, for example, PAF, NAF, LTB_4, FMLP.[9,19] These chemotaxins may be responsible for the migration of eosinophils within the tissue. However, it is difficult to imagine that they are responsible for the tissue infiltration from the circulation. In this respect IL-4 may be an important cytokine. IL-4 can induce the expression of vascular cell adhesion molecule-1 (VCAM-1) on endothelial cells.[20] The expression of VCAM-1 allows eosinophils to attach to and migrate through the endothelium.[21] Eosinophils, but not neutrophils, do express the counterpart structure of VCAM-1, that is, very late antigen-4 (VLA-4).[22] Since IL-4 may act as a chemotaxin on fibroblasts,[23] we have investigated whether IL-4 could also act as a chemoattractant on eosinophils.

Here we report that IL-4 acts as a chemotaxin on eosinophils in allergic asthma and atopic dermatitis patients, but not on eosinophils from normal individuals. IL-4 possesses almost the same chemotactic potency as other cytokines, for example, IL-3, IL-5 and GM–CSF. These findings therefore further extend the importance of IL-4 for the pathogenesis of allergic inflammation.

MATERIALS AND METHODS

Cell Isolation

Blood was obtained from healthy volunteers or from patients with atopic dermatitis (AD). Eosinophils from the blood of normal donors were isolated from the buffy coat of 500 ml of blood, and eosinophils from the patients were isolated from 50 ml of blood anticoagulated with 0.4% (wt/vol) trisodium citrate (pH 7.4) as described before.[19] In short, the mononuclear cells were removed via separation of blood over isotonic Ficoll Paque (1.077 g/ml, pH 7.4). After isotonic lysis of the erythrocytes in an ice-cold solution containing 155-mM NH_4Cl, 10-mM $KHCO_3$ and 0.1-mM EDTA (pH 7.2), the mixed granulocytes were washed and resuspended in RPMI medium supplemented with human serum albumin (1% wt/vol) and incubated 30 minutes at 37°C to restore initial densities of the cells. After this incubation period, the cells were washed and resuspended in a phosphate-buffered salt solution supplemented with human serum albumin (1% wt/vol) and trisodium citrate (0.4% wt/vol). One milliliter of cell suspension (containing 50.10^6 cells at the maximum) was layered on 4 ml of an isotonic Percoll solution (density: 1.082 g/ml). To prevent contamination of the cells with cell debris and the remaining erythrocytes, 1 ml of Percoll (density: 1.100 g/ml) was brought under the Percoll 1.082 g/ml. After centrifugation (20 min, 1000 gmax, room temperature), the eosinophil-rich fraction was collected from the interface. After washing with buffer the eosinophils were further purified from this eosinophil-rich fraction using the immunomagnetic bead method as described by Hansel et al.[24] In short, neutrophils present in the eosinophil-rich granulocyte preparation were coated with a monoclonal antibody against CD16 during 30 min at 0°C. Afterward the cells were washed twice and subsequently coincubated head over head with beads at a ratio of 1 : 2 (cells/beads) for 20 min at 4°C. The neutrophils were subsequently removed by a magnetic particle concentrator. The eosinophils were washed with buffer and suspended in the buffer solution to be used for the migration experiments. Eosinophil purity was always >95% and the viability was over 98%.

Migration Assay

Microchemotaxis Assay

Migration was measured with a modified Boyden chamber assay using a 48-well microchemotaxis chamber. Chemotaxins or HEPES (N-2-hydroxyethylpiperazine-N'-2-ethanesulphonic acid) buffer (30 μl) were placed in the lower compartments. Two filters (cellulose nitrate) were placed between the lower and the upper compartments. The lower filter had a pore width of 0.45 μm and the upper filter had a pore width of 8 μm. Before use, the filters were soaked in HEPES buffer. Purified eosinophils were placed in the upper compartment (25 μl of 5 $\times$ 10^6 cells/ml). The chemotaxis chambers were subsequently incubated for 2.5 hr at 37°C, unless otherwise stated. Afterward the upper filters were removed, fixed in butanol/ethanol (20%/80%, v/v) for 10 min, and stained with Weigert solution [1% haematoxylin (v/v) in 95% ethanol (v/v) and an acidic FeCl$_3$-solution (70 mM) mixed in a volume ratio of 1 : 1]. The filters were dehydrated with ethanol, made transparent with xylene, and fixed upside down. The number of cells per 10 high-power fields (hpf) was determined with light microscopy (magnification 400×). The number of cells that had passed the upper filter was determined in this way.

Statistical Analysis

All data are presented as mean $\pm$ SEM. The Student's t-test for paired or unpaired data was applied. P values < 0.05 were considered significant.

RESULTS

The Migratory Responsiveness of Eosinophils from the Circulation of Normal Individuals, Allergic Asthma Patients and Atopic Dermatitis Patients toward IL-4

We examined the ability of IL-4 to mobilize eosinophils using a modified Boyden chamber assay. As depicted in FIGURE 1, eosinophils from allergic asthma and atopic dermatitis patients showed a dose-dependent migratory response to-

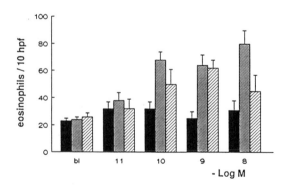

FIGURE 1. Migratory responses of eosinophils derived from the circulation of normal individuals (■), atopic dermatitis patients (▨), or allergic asthma patients (▨) toward dose ranges of IL-4. The results are expressed as the number of eosinophils/10 high-power fields (hpf). Mean values $\pm$ SEM are presented of n = 4–8 different experiments.

TABLE 1. Checkerboard Analysis of IL-4-Induced Migration of Eosinophils from the Circulation of Atopic Dermatitis Patients

[IL-4]	Lower Compartment		
	0	2.5 10^{-9}	10^{-8}
Upper Compartment 0	23 ± 8	63 ± 8	108 ± 8
2.5 10^{-9}	21 ± 4	25 ± 3	62 ± 10
10^{-8}	24 ± 4	28 ± 5	23 ± 3

Note: Mean values ± SEM are presented of four different experiments.

ward IL-4. Eosinophils from allergic individuals appeared to migrate significantly above [IL-4] = 0,1 nM. In contrast, eosinophils from normal individuals showed no significant migratory response toward IL-4.

Neutrophils from both patients and normal individuals did not respond to IL-4 (data not shown). Therefore the IL-4-induced migratory response is limited to eosinophils from allergic asthma and atopical dermatitis patients.

IL-4-Induced Chemotaxis

Checkerboard analysis was performed to investigate whether the IL-4-induced migration was due to chemokinesis or chemotaxis. TABLE 1 reveals that IL-4 acts as a chemotaxin on eosinophils from allergic patients and that the effect on the chemokinesis of eosinophils can be neglected.

The IL-4-induced chemotactic response of eosinophils from the circulation of atopic dermatitis patients could be completely inhibited by a specific monoclonal antibody against IL-4 (98 ± 3%, $n = 4$, mean ± SEM). The inhibition was cytokine specific since the antibody could not inhibit the chemotactic response toward other cytokines (data not shown). Desensitization with experiments with hu-IL-4 also showed a specific interaction between IL-4 and the eosinophils (data not shown).

Comparison of Chemotactic Potency of IL-4 with Other Chemotaxins

TABLE 2 shows a comparison of the chemotactic potency of IL-4 with other chemotaxins for eosinophils from the circulation of normal individuals, allergic asthma patients, and atopic dermatitis patients. As can be seen IL-4 possesses a similar chemotactic potency as IL-3, IL-5, IL-8, and GM–CSF for eosinophils from both allergic asthma and atopic dermatitis patients.

Induction of IL-4 Chemotactic Response in Eosinophils from Normal Individuals by GM–CSF

To find out whether the difference between the migratory response of eosinophils from normal individuals and allergic asthma and atopic dermatitis patients

TABLE 2. Comparison of IL-4-Induced Chemotaxis of Eosinophils from the Circulation of Normal Individuals, Allergic Asthma Patients, and Atopic Dermatitis Patients

	Chemotaxis of Eosinophils: Cytokines			
Chemotaxin	Optimal Chemotactic Concentration	Cells per 10 hpf (Mean Values ± SEM)		
		Normals	Asthma	Atopic Dermatitis
IL-3	10 nM	50 ± 8 (8)	42 ± 7 (8)	90 ± 15 (8)
IL-5	10 nM	70 ± 15 (8)	50 ± 5 (8)	90 ± 10 (8)
GM–CSF	10 nM	80 ± 11 (8)	35 ± 7 (8)	60 ± 9 (8)
	1 nM*	50 ± 10 (8)	n.d.	100 ± 9 (8)
IL-8	10 nM	21 ± 4 (8)	50 ± 7 (8)	71 ± 15 (8)
TNF-α	10 nM	35 ± 7 (8)	n.d.	35 ± 7 (8)
IL-4	10 nM	29 ± 6 (8)	45 ± 12 (4)	83 ± 10 (8)
	1 nM**	26 ± 3 (8)	62 ± 6 (4)	68 ± 16 (8)
Buffer	—	24 ± 5 (12)	26 ± 5 (8)	24 ± 5 (8)

Note: In parentheses: number of experiments.

Key: n.d.: not done; * optimal concentration for eosinophils from atopic dermatitis patients; ** optimal concentration for eosinophils from allergic asthma patients.

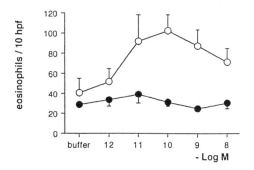

FIGURE 2. Migratory response of eosinophils derived from normal individuals toward dose-ranges of IL-4 before (–●–) and after (–○–) preincubation overnight with 10-pM GM–CSF. The results are expressed as the number of eosinophils/10 high-power fields (hpf). Mean values ± SEM are presented of $n = 6$ different experiments.

was due to previous *in vivo* contact of those cells with GM–CSF, experiments were performed with eosinophils from normal individuals that had been preincubated overnight with 10-pM GM–CSF. FIGURE 2 shows that the migratory response toward IL-4 increased significantly after pretreatment with GM–CSF and that the chemotactic response became similar to that of eosinophils from patients with allergic asthma or atopic dermatitis.

DISCUSSION

The eosinophil is recognized as an important effector cell capable of contributing to the pathogenesis of allergic inflammation. However, the function and recruitment of eosinophils is dependent on T-lymphocytes and their cytokine products.

Here we show that IL-4 is chemotactic for eosinophils from patients with allergic asthma and atopic dermatitis, but not for eosinophils from normal individuals. Recently we demonstrated that eosinophils from the circulation of patients with allergic asthma and atopic dermatitis exhibit a potentiated migratory response toward FMLP, NAF/IL-8, PAF, and PF4.[9,19] Other studies showed that the migratory response of eosinophils from normal individuals could be increased by pretreatment of those cells with IL-3, IL-5, or GM–CSF. Pretreatment with these cytokines resulted in the induction of a migratory response toward NAF/IL-8 and FMLP.[10] Here we show that GM–CSF is capable of inducing a migratory response of eosinophils toward IL-4 from normal individuals. Therefore these findings extend the evidence that eosinophils from the circulation of patients with allergic disorders are *in vivo* "primed," most likely due to previous contact with the cytokines IL-3, IL-5, or GM–CSF.

The presence of activated T-cells in the blood and the tissue of allergic asthma and atopic dermatitis patients, which according to their phenotype, will secrete IL-4 in addition to the priming cytokines, allows the suggestion that IL-4 may contribute to tissue recruitment of eosinophils, not only by inducing the expression of certain adhesion molecules but also by a direct action on eosinophils. Here we show that IL-4 is almost as potent a chemotaxin as other cytokines with documented chemotactic ability, most interestingly, only for eosinophils from patients with allergic disorders.

REFERENCES

1. WALKER, C., J. C. VIRCHOW, JR., P. L. B. BRUIJNZEEL & K. BLASER. 1991. J. Immunol. **146:** 1829–1836.
2. WALKER, C., *et al.* 1993. Clin. Exp. Allergy **23:** 145–153.
3. LEIFERMAN, K., *et al.* 1985. New Eng. J. Med. **313:** 47–56.
4. LOPEZ, A. F., D. J. WILLIAMSON, J. R. GAMBLE, C. G. BEGLEY & J. M. HARLAN. 1986. J. Clin. Invest. **78:** 1220–1226.
5. LOPEZ, A. F., *et al.* 1988. J. Exp. Med. **167:** 219–224.
6. ROTHENBERG, M. E., *et al.* 1988. J. Clin. Invest. **81:** 1986–1992.
7. SILBERSTEIN, D. S., *et al.* 1986. J. Immunol. **137:** 3290–3298.
8. YAMAGUCHI, Y., *et al.* 1988. J. Exp. Med. **167:** 1737–1743.
9. WARRINGA, R. A. J., L. KOENDERMAN, P. T. M. KOK, J. KREUKNIET & P. L. B. BRUIJNZEEL. 1991. Blood **77:** 2694–2700.
10. WARRINGA, R. A. J., *et al.* 1992. Blood **79:** 1836–1841.
11. CHIHARA, J., *et al.* 1990. J. Exp. Med. **172:** 1347–1351.
12. HOWARD, M., *et al.* 1982. J. Exp. Med. **155:** 914–923.
13. ROEHM, N. W., *et al.* 1984. J. Exp. Med. **160:** 679–694.
14. DEFRANCE, T., *et al.* 1987. J. Exp. Med. **165:** 1459–1467.
15. HUDAK, S. A., S. O. GOLLNICK, D. H. CONRAD & M. R. KEHLY. 1987. Proc. Natl. Acad. Sci. U.S.A. **84:** 4606–4610.
16. SPITS, H., *et al.* 1988. J. Immunol. **141:** 29–36.
17. SNAPPER, C. M., F. D. FINKELMAN & W. E. PAUL. 1988. J. Exp. Med. **167:** 183–196.
18. KAWAHAMI, Y., S. A. ROSENBERG & M. T. LOTZE. 1988. J. Exp. Med. **168:** 85–94.
19. BRUIJNZEEL, P. L. B., *et al.* 1993. J. Invest. Dermatol. **100:** 137–142.
20. THORNHILL, M. H., *et al.* 1991. J. Immunol. **146:** 592–598.
21. MOSER, R., J. FEHR & P. L. B. BRUIJNZEEL. 1992. J. Immunol. **149:** 1432–1438.
22. WALSH, G. M., J.-J. MERMOD, A. HARTNELL, A. B. KAY & A. J. WARDLAW. 1991. J. Immunol. **146:** 3419–3423.
23. POSTELETHWAITE, A. E. & J. M. SEYER. 1991. J. Clin. Invest. **87:** 2147–2152.
24. HANSEL, T. T., *et al.* 1989. J. Immunol. Methods **22:** 97–103.

Modulation of the Enhanced Migration of Eosinophils from the Airways of Sensitized Guinea Pigs: Role of IL-5

ELIANE COËFFIER, DANIELLE JOSEPH,
AND B. BORIS VARGAFTIG

Unité de Pharmacologie Cellulaire
Unité Associée Institut Pasteur/INSERM 285
25, Rue du Dr. Roux
75015, Paris, France

INTRODUCTION

An increased number of eosinophils in blood and bronchoalveolar lavage fluid (BALF) is frequently observed in patients with bronchial asthma,[1] as initially recognized by Hüber and Koessler,[2] but neither the mechanisms of eosinophil recruitment into tissues undergoing allergic reactions nor their pathophysiological role have been completely elucidated.[3,4] Platelet activating factor (PAF) and leukotriene (LT) B_4 are two recognized inflammatory mediators that share the ability to induce eosinophil chemoattraction *in vitro*[5-7] and *in vivo*.[8-11] T-cells also play an important role in the induction of eosinophilia, particularly via three well-characterized factors, interleukin-3 (IL-3),[12] granulocyte-macrophage colony-stimulating factor (GM–CSF),[13] and interleukin-5 (IL-5),[14-16] that are known to stimulate eosinophilopoiesis.

IL-5 can induce migration of guinea pig,[17] mouse,[18] and human[19] eosinophils. In addition, human recombinant (hr) IL-5 primes very intensively guinea pig eosinophils for an enhanced migration by PAF and LTB4,[17] as well as human eosinophils, to other chemoattractants.[20] This priming may be important for bronchopulmonary hyperresponsiveness. We hypothesized that eosinophil migration into antigen-challenged guinea-pig lungs is IL-5 dependent and that eosinophils might also be hyperresponsive and primed by IL-5 generated *in vivo* by lung lymphocytes. Experiments were thus performed with TRFK-5, a specific monoclonal antibody against IL-5.

MATERIALS AND METHODS

Materials and Buffers

Lipid-free bovine serum albumin (BSA), gamma globulin fraction II, calcium ionophore A23187, formyl-L-methionyl-L-leucyl-L-phenylalanine (FMLP), human recombinant C5a, calcium ionophore A23187, N-2-hydroxyethylpiperazine-N'-2-ethanesulphonic acid (HEPES), and metrizamide were from Sigma Chemical Co. (St. Louis, Missouri). Al(OH)3 was from Merck (Darmstadt, GFR). Synthetic PAF-acether (1-0-hexadecyl-2-acetyl-*sn*-glycero-3-phosphorylcholine) was from Bachem (Budendorf, Switzerland). Recombinant human Interleukin 5 (rhIL-5) was from Immugenex (Los Angeles, California). Chicken ovalbumin (OA) was from Miles (Naperville, Illinois). Sodium pentobarbitone was from Clin-Midy (Montpellier, France). Mepyramine maleate was from Rhône-Poulenc-Rorer (Vitry/seine, France). Nedocromil sodium, a generous gift of Dr. A. Norris (Fisons, UK) was dissolved in saline at the concentration of 10 mg/ml and further diluted in saline. In preliminary phases of this study, TRFK-5-derived rat anti-mouse IL-5 antibody and the GL-113-derived rat anti-*Escherichia coli*-β-galactosidase antibody were generous gifts from Dr. R. W. Egan of Schering-Plough Research (Bloomfield, New Jersey). Finally, the TRFK-5 was provided from Immugenex (Los Angeles, California).

Buffers were L-glutamine-free RPMI 1640, containing 2-g/l sodium bicarbonate from Eurobio, Paris, France, and Ca^{2+} and Mg^{2+}-free Hank's' balanced salt buffer (HBSS) from Gibco (Paisley, UK).

The 48-well microtaxis chambers and the cellulose nitrate filters (3-μm pore size) were purchased from Neuro Probe, Inc. (Cabin John, Maryland, USA).

Sensitization Procedure

Male Hartley guinea pigs (weighing 500 g) from the Saint-Antoine breeding (Pleudaniel, France) were sensitized s.c. with 0.5 ml of 0.15-M NaCl (saline) containing 10 μg of ovalbumin dispersed in 1-mg Al(OH)3. Nonsensitized animals received 0.5 ml of saline containing 1-mg Al(OH)3 alone. Fourteen days later, the guinea pigs were challenged by the intranasal instillation of ovalbumin (3 mg/ml in 0.15-M sterile saline, 1 mg per animal) or saline alone, under protection of mepyramine (1 mg/kg, i.p.), to prevent acute anaphylaxis. TRFK-5 was administrated i.p. at 30 μg/kg 2 hours before the intranasal challenge. This dose was shown to be effective in suppressing eosinophil infiltration by antigen in guinea-pig BALF.[21] Nedocromil sodium was administrated twice s.c. at 30 mg/kg, 10 minutes before and 9 hours after the intranasal challenge with ovalbumin. Control animals were treated with saline.

Harvest of Bronchoalveolar Cells

Airway eosinophils were obtained by bronchoalveolar lavage 24 hours after the intranasal challenge. Guinea pigs were anesthetized with sodium pentobarbitone (34 mg/kg, i.p.). Bronchoalveolar cells were collected in 10 successive lavages using 5-ml aliquots of 50 ml of sterile saline at room temperature through a polyethylene tracheal cannula. The 50-ml bronchoalveolar lavages were supplemented with 20-IU/ml heparin (Choay, Paris, France) and centrifuged (475 g, 10 minutes, 20°C). Cells were counted with a Malassez hemacytometer and the cell purity was analyzed after cytocentrifugation by a modified May–Grünwald–Giemsa staining (Diff-quick, American Scientific Products, McGaw Park, Illinois) and the viability was estimated with the Trypan Blue exclusion test.

Purification of Guinea-Pig Eosinophils from BAL

Eosinophils were isolated on a metrizamide gradient according to a modification[17] of the method of Vadas *et al.*[22] Gradients were prepared by placing the bronchoalveolar cell pellet in 3-ml metrizamide at 18 percent in a 15-ml plastic Falcon tube and underlaying this solution with a serie of 3-ml volumes of discontinuous metrizamide gradient (20–24 percent metrizamide). After two centrifugations (180 g, 11 minutes, 20°C, and 2200 g, 11 minutes, 20°C) the cells were collected from each density interface and washed once in HBSS. After counting with a Malassez hemacytometer, eosinophil numbers were adjusted to 4×10^6/ml in RPMI 1640 containing L-glutamine (2 mM), 0.4 percent BSA, and 27 mM HEPES. The cell purity was controlled after cytocentrifugation and a modified May–Grünwald–Giemsa staining (Diff-Quick, American Scientific Products, McGaw Park, Illinois), and the viability was estimated with the Trypan Blue exclusion test.

Migration Studies

Eosinophil migration was performed according to a modification of the Boyden chamber technique as already described,[17] using micropore filters with a 3-μm pore size.

Expression of Results

Results are expressed as the number of eosinophils migrating at 40 μm (mean ± SEM) through the cellulose nitrate filter in the presence of the agonist and of the solvent alone. The variability of the results was evaluated by the coefficient of variation among individual observations per test and among triplicate values. The statistical significance of differences between means of various groups were tested using analysis of variance with the Anova test, and $P < 0.05$ was considered significant. When individual groups were compared with only a single control condition, Student's t-test for paired samples was employed, $P < 0.05$ being considered significant.

RESULTS

Interference of Sensitization and of Provocation with Antigen with the Cell Numbers and Distribution

The sensitization procedure alone more than doubled the total number of cells recovered from the BALF, since animals treated with adjuvant alone had 10.9 ± 2.2 × 10^6 cells versus 44.5 ± 5.0 × 10^6 for sensitized animals 24 hours after the intranasal instillation of antigen (TABLE 1). However, the main differences in the cell composition of BALF from actively sensitized guinea pigs compared with that from nonimmunized animals were the number and proportion of eosinophils. Indeed, the eosinophil counts were further increased by antigen challenge (5.0 ± 0.8 × 10^6 eosinophils for immunized and challenged animals versus 0.6 ± 0.4 × 10^6 for nonimmunized guinea pigs). Finally, the proportion of eosinophils did not change in the unchallenged animals, being of 5–8 percent, but reached 12 percent after provocation. The number of macrophages was also increased after sensitization and challenge; no difference in the number of the other cell types, that is, polymorphonuclear neutrophils and lymphocytes, was detected (TABLE 1).

Eosinophil Purification

Two populations of eosinophils were separated from the BALF of control and sensitized animals upon the discontinuous metrizamide gradient, one of low density

TABLE 1. Cell Counts in BAL from Control and Sensitized Guinea Pigs

Treatment	Leukocytes Millions/BAL	Eosinophils %	Eosinophils Millions	Macrophages %	Macrophages Millions	Neutrophils %	Neutrophils Millions	Lymphocytes %	Lymphocytes Millions
Unsensitized (n = 6)									
Saline-challenged	21.2 ± 5.7	8 ± 3	2.3 ± 1.1	67 ± 11	12.9 ± 4.0	18 ± 11	5.2 ± 3.5	7 ± 4	0.8 ± 0.5
Ovalbumin-challenged	10.9 ± 2.2	5 ± 2	0.6 ± 0.4	66 ± 7	6.9 ± 1.1	29 ± 8	3.5 ± 1.5	3 ± 1	0.3 ± 0.1
Sensitized (n = 35)									
Saline-challenged	41.7 ± 3.5	7 ± 1	3.0 ± 0.7	80 ± 2	33.4 ± 3.0	7 ± 1	2.7 ± 0.5	5 ± 1	1.9 ± 0.3
Ovalbumin-challenged	44.5 ± 5.0	12 ± 2*	5.0 ± 0.8*	75 ± 3	32.8 ± 3.4	9 ± 2	5.0 ± 1.6	5 ± 1	1.6 ± 0.4

Note: Guinea pigs were sensitized s.c. with 0.5 ml of saline containing 10 μg of ovalbumin dispersed in 1-mg Al(OH)3. Nonsensitized animals received 0.5 ml of saline containing 1-mg Al(OH)3 alone. Guinea pigs were challenged 14 days later by the intranasal instillation of ovalbumin (3 mg/ml in saline, 1 mg per animal) or saline alone, under protection of mepyramine (1 mg/kg, i.p.). Airway eosinophils were obtained by bronchoalveolar lavage 24 hours after the intranasal challenge. Cells were counted and the cell purity was analyzed after cytocentrifugation.
* Represents statistical significance ($P < 0.05$) from both the unsensitized and sensitized, ovalbumin-challenged groups as tested by Anova test.

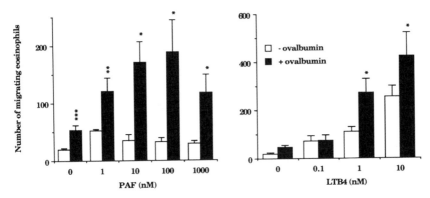

FIGURE 1. Increased migration of normodense eosinophil from BAL of guinea pig after challenge with ovalbumin. Airway eosinophils were obtained by bronchoalveolar lavage performed 24 hours after the challenge of sensitized guinea pigs with 1 mg of ovalbumin by the intranasal route. The eosinophils were isolated on a metrizamide gradient and migration was studied as described under "Methods." Spontaneous, PAF-, and LTB4-induced migration of eosinophils from sensitized and ovalbumin-challenged animals (*black column*) was evaluated, as compared to that of sensitized and saline-challenged (*white column*) animals. The results are expressed as the number of eosinophils migrating through the nitrocellulose filter (3-μm pore size) to 40 μm using an optical grid at 400× magnification (mean ± SEM of 4 to 16 experiments). (* $P < 0.05$; ** $P < 0.01$; *** $P < 0.001$; t test on the results from paired samples between sensitized, saline-challenged, and sensitized, ovalbumin-challenged guinea pigs.)

(at 20 and 22 percent of metrizamide, 20 ± 3 percent and 27 ± 4 percent of eosinophils for sensitized saline-challenged and ovalbumin-challenged guinea pigs, respectively; $n = 12$) and another of normal density (at 22 and 24 percent of metrizamide), of purity ranging between 67 and 96 percent (78 ± 3 percent and 82 ± 2 percent of eosinophils for sensitized saline-challenged, and ovalbumin-challenged guinea pigs, respectively; $n = 12$). Normodense eosinophils were used for further experiments.

Increased Migration of Normodense Eosinophil from the Guinea-Pig BALF after Challenge with Ovalbumin

As shown in FIGURE 1, eosinophils collected from ovalbumin-challenged animals migrated to a larger extent than controls to *in vitro* stimulation with PAF and LTB4. Spontaneous, PAF-, and LTB4-induced migration of eosinophils from sensitized and ovalbumin-challenged, was significantly augmented as compared to those of sensitized and saline-challenged, animals.

Modulation by TRFK-5, a Specific Monoclonal Antibody against IL-5, of the Accumulation and Migration of Normodense Eosinophils

TRFK-5 injected i.p. two hours before antigen challenge (30 μg/kg), inhibited eosinophil accumulation in BAL after ovalbumin provocation (FIG. 2). TRFK-5 also inhibited the enhancement of PAF- and LTB4-induced eosinophil migration, observed with eosinophils from sensitized and ovalbumin-challenged, as compared to sensitized and saline-challenged, animals (FIG. 3).

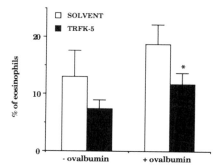

FIGURE 2. Interference of TRFK-5 with eosinophil recruitment into the BAL of guinea pigs challenged with intranasal ovalbumin. TRFK-5 was administrated i.p. at 30 μg/kg 2 hours before the intranasal challenge (*black column*). Control animals were treated with saline (*white column*). Airway eosinophils were obtained by bronchoalveolar lavage performed 24 hours after the challenge. Cells were counted with a Malassez hemacytometer and the cell purity was analyzed after cytocentrifugation and staining. The results are expressed as the total number of cells in the BAL (mean ± SEM of 4 to 10 experiments). (* $P < 0.05$; § $P < 0.05$; t test on the results from paired samples between sensitized, solvent-treated and ovalbumin-challenged animals, and sensitized, TRFK-5-treated and ovalbumin-challenged guinea pigs.)

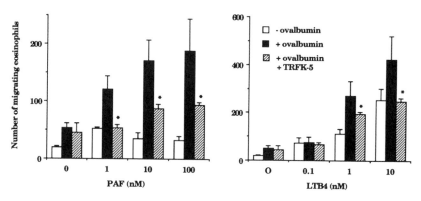

FIGURE 3. Modulation of the enhanced IL-5 responsiveness of airway eosinophils by anti-IL-5 antibody. TRFK-5 was administrated i.p. at 30 μg/kg 2 hours before the intranasal challenge, control animals being treated with saline. Airway eosinophils were obtained by bronchoalveolar lavage performed 24 hours after challenge. The eosinophils were isolated on a metrizamide gradient and migration was studied as described under "Methods." The results are expressed as in FIGURE 1 (mean ± SEM of 4 to 16 experiments). (* $P < 0.05$; t test on the results from paired samples between sensitized, solvent-treated and ovalbumin-challenged animals, and sensitized, TRFK-5-treated and ovalbumin-challenged guinea pigs.

DISCUSSION

The concept that inflammatory cells, particularly eosinophils, are involved with the development and/or expression of bronchopulmonary hyperresponsiveness is becoming increasingly popular. Airway and blood eosinophilia are associated with the allergen-induced, late-phase bronchoconstriction in asthmatic patients[1] and in animal models of allergic asthma.[9,23] Similarly, airway eosinophilia, associated with late-phase bronchoconstriction, is observed in antigen-challenged guinea pigs,[23,24] but little is known about the processes that control this infiltration of eosinophils *in vivo*.

The present study supports and extends those findings, since altogether the leukocyte numbers and the proportion of eosinophils in the BALF of ovalbumin-challenged guinea pigs increased markedly.

Eosinophils collected 24 hours after provocation migrated more intensively in response to PAF and LTB4 than those of paired sensitized unchallenged animals. Enhancement of eosinophil function, in response to antigen challenge, has been previously reported. Cerasoli *et al.*[24] demonstrated that eosinophils from the airways of actively sensitized guinea pigs release more superoxide anion in response to antigen challenge, and Moser *et al.*[25] showed that eosinophils from allergic patients show an increased adherence and transmigration capacity. On the other hand, Sedgwick *et al.*[26] compared the function of airway and blood eosinophil after *in vivo* antigen challenge and demonstrated that, after challenge, eosinophils from the BALF have an enhanced afflux of intracellular calcium, generate more anion superoxide, and express larger amounts of the integrin adherence receptor CR3 (CD 11b/CD 18).

Eosinophils from sensitized and challenged animals became hyperresponsive to PAF and LTB4. *In vitro,* IL-5 primes very intensively guinea pig eosinophils for an enhanced migration in response to PAF and LTB4,[17] and accordingly we hypothesized that eosinophils from sensitized and antigen-challenged animals might be primed *in vivo* by IL-5 generated by lung lymphocytes upon antigen challenge. This led us to study whether IL-5 accounts for the *in vivo* eosinophil recruitment to the lungs and for hyperresponsiveness of guinea-pig eosinophils using TRFK-5, a specific monoclonal antibody against IL-5. TRFK-5 indeed inhibited *in vitro* eosinophil migration by rhIL-5 and, administered *in vivo,* reduced eosinophil recruitment to the BALF of antigen-challenged animals, and decreased the enhanced responsiveness of eosoinophils collected from the challenged animals. The fact that TRFK-5 prevents lung and BAL eosinophilia has already been described for guinea pigs[21] and mice.[27]

Our findings suggest that IL-5 produced at the site of an antigen invasion may participate in the mechanism of the local accumulation of eosinophils, perhaps by both chemotactic activity and survival prolonging activity. Our results support the concept that IL-5 is essential for recruitment and priming of eosinophils from the guinea-pig BALF.

REFERENCES

1. DeMonchy, J. G. R., *et al.* 1985. Am. Rev. Respir. Dis. **131:** 373–376.
2. Huber, H. L. & K. K. Koessler. 1992. Arch. Intern. Med. **30:** 689–760.
3. Frigas, E. & G. J. Gleich. 1986. J. Allergy Clin. Immunol. **77**(4): 527–537.
4. Venge, P. 1990. Agents Actions. **29**(1/2): 122–126.
5. Czarnetzki, B. M. & R. Mertensmeier. 1985. Prostaglandins **30**(1): 5–10.

6. WARDLAW, A. J., R. MOQBEL, O. CROMWELL & A. B. KAY. 1986. J. Clin. Invest. **78:** 1701–1706.
7. COËFFIER, E., D. JOSEPH & B. B. VARGAFTIG. 1991. Intern. J. Immunopharmacol. **13**(2/3): 273–280.
8. SANJAR, S., *et al.* 1990. Br. J. Pharmacol. **99:** 267–272.
9. LELLOUCH-TUBIANA, A., J. LEFORT, M. T. SIMON, A. PFISTER & B. B. VARGAFTIG. 1988. Am. Rev. Respir. Dis. **137:** 948–954.
10. ARNOUX, B., *et al.* 1988. Am. Rev. Respir. Dis. **137**(4): 855–860.
11. SILBAUGH, S. A., *et al.* 1987. Am. Rev. Respir. Dis. **136:** 930–934.
12. LOPEZ, A. F., *et al.* 1987. Proc. Natl. Acad. Sci. U.S.A. **84:** 2761–2765.
13. THORNE, K. J. I., *et al.* 1986. Eur. J. Immunol. **16:** 1143–1149.
14. SANDERSON, C. J., D. J. WARREN & M. STRATH. 1985. J. Exp. Med. **162:** 60–74.
15. CAMPBELL, H. D., *et al.* 1987. Proc. Natl. Acad. Sci. U.S.A. **84:** 6629–6633.
16. YOKOTA, T., *et al.* 1987. Proc. Natl. Acad. Sci. U.S.A. **84:** 7388–7392.
17. COËFFIER, E., D. JOSEPH & B. B. VARGAFTIG. 1991. J. Immunol. **147:** 2595–2602.
18. YAMAGUCHI, Y., *et al.* 1988. J. Exp. Med. **167:** 1737–1742.
19. WANG, J. M., *et al.* 1989. Eur. J. Immunol. **19:** 701–705.
20. WARRINGA, R. A. J., *et al.* 1992. Am. J. Respir. Cell Mol. Biol. **7:** 631–636.
21. GULBENKIAN, A. R., *et al.* 1992. Am. Rev. Respir. Dis. **146**(1): 263–266.
22. VADAS, M. A., J. R. DAVID, A. BUTTERWORTH, N. T. PISANI & T. A. SIONGOK. 1979. J. Immunol. **122:** 1228–1238.
23. DUNN, C. J., G. A. ELLIOTT, J. A. OOSTVEEN & I. M. RICHARDS. 1988. Am. Rev. Respir. Dis. **137:** 541–547.
24. CERASOLI, F., J. TOCKER & W. M. SELIG. 1991. Am. J. Respir. Cell Mol. Biol. **4:** 355–363.
25. MOSER, R., J. FEHR, L. OLGIATI & P. L. B. BRUIJNZEEL. 1992. Blood **79**(11): 2937–2945.
26. SEDGWICK, J. B., *et al.* 1992. J. Immunol. **149**(11): 3710–3718.
27. OKUDAIRA, H., *et al.* 1991. Int. Arch. Allergy Appl. Immunol. **94**(1–4): 171–173.

Effects of Interleukin-5 Inhibition on Antigen-Induced Airway Hyperresponsiveness and Cell Accumulation in Guinea Pigs

A. A. Y. MILNE AND P. J. PIPER

Department of Pharmacology
The Royal College of Surgeons
London, WC2A 3PN
United Kingdom

INTRODUCTION

Chronic asthma is characterized by bronchial hyperresponsiveness to a variety of spasmogens including acetylcholine and histamine.[1] This state is also correlated with an increased number of eosinophils in bronchoalveolar lavage fluid (BALF) of asthmatic patients.[2] Eosinophil accumulation in the lung is dependent upon the presence of T-lymphocytes,[3] and may be mediated in part by cytokines released from these cells upon their activation.[4] Interleukin-5 (IL-5) is a cytokine that, unlike other interleukins, has many actions that are specific for eosinophils. Increased levels of IL-5 are found in the BALF[5] and serum[6] of asthmatic patients, and it has been suggested that inhibition of the actions of this cytokine could be a useful target for new therapies in asthma.

Previous work in a guinea-pig model has shown that blockade of IL-5 *in vivo* using a monoclonal antibody to IL-5, TRFK-5, leads to a reduction in the numbers of eosinophils recovered from BALF.[7,8] However, the effect on bronchial hyperresponsiveness was not studied. We have developed a model of antigen-induced airway inflammation in the guinea pig, which exhibits hyperresponsiveness and accumulation of leukocytes, especially eosinophils in BALF. Recently in our laboratory, using this model, we have shown that an antibody to the leukocyte CD18 integrin reduced eosinophil numbers in BALF by over 80 percent, but did not reduce bronchial hyperresponsiveness.[9] In the light of these results, it is of interest to examine the effects of TRFK-5 on bronchial hyperresponsiveness, to observe whether changes in the numbers of eosinophils would be paralleled by changes in airway responsiveness.

For this reason, we have studied the effects of the neutralizing monoclonal antibody to IL-5, TRFK-5, on antigen-induced bronchial hyperresponsiveness and cell accumulation in guinea pigs.

METHOD

Male Hartley guinea pigs (180–200 g) were sensitized to ovalbumin over a 2-week period. On day 0, the animals were injected intraperitoneally (i.p.) with 1-mg/ml ovalbumin/aluminium hydroxide mixture (1 ml) and B pertussis vaccine (0.25 ml). Then, on day 7, the guinea pigs were given a booster injection of ovalbumin/aluminium hydroxide (0.1 ml). On day 14, the animals sensitized in this way were exposed to an aerosol of ovalbumin (0.1 percent) for 1 hour, after receiving a protective dose of pyrilamine (10 mg/kg i.p., 1 hour before challenge). At 4, 24, or 48 hours following ovalbumin challenge, the guinea pigs were anesthetized and increases in resistance in response to acetylcholine (Ach) and histamine (Hist) (1–30 μg/kg i.v.) were measured using a computerized Pulmonary Monitoring System (Mumed). Following this, the guinea pigs were killed and their lungs lavaged with 40-ml buffer (bovine serum albumin in phosphate buffered saline, 0.25 percent). From this, total and differential counts were made of leukocytes in BALF.

The antibodies TRFK-5 or rat IgG, an isotype-matched control antibody, were administered intravenously to sensitized guinea pigs at a dose of 1 mg/kg, 1 hour prior to ovalbumin challenge ($n = 5$ guinea pigs in each group). Airway responsiveness to Ach and leukocytes in BALF were examined 24 hours post ovalbumin challenge.

RESULTS

Ovalbumin sensitization of guinea pigs alone did not alter the leukocyte populations in BALF. However, at 4 hours following ovalbumin challenge of sensitized guinea pigs, there was a significant increase in the number of neutrophils recovered from BALF (4-fold) (TABLE 1). In addition, there was a 5-fold increase in the eosinophil population, when compared to numbers in control guinea pigs. There was no significant change in the number of macrophages in BALF. At 24 hours post challenge, the number of neutrophils recovered from BALF was not different from that seen in control animals, while the eosinophil population of BALF had increased by 16-fold and the macrophages by 2-fold. At 48 hours post challenge, the number of eosinophils and macrophages remained elevated compared to control levels.

Measurement of increases in resistance to Ach and Hist (FIG. 1) showed that at 4 hours post ovalbumin challenge, there was no change in the responsiveness of the airways to either Ach or Hist, whereas at 24 hours post challenge, there was a bronchial hyperresponsiveness to both these agonists. At 48 hours post challenge, guinea pigs still showed a degree of hyperresponsiveness to Ach, but not to Hist.

Since at 24 hours post ovalbumin challenge of sensitized guinea pigs there appeared to be a maximal response of the airways to challenge, with both hyperresponsiveness and eosinophilia in BALF, this time point was chosen for the evaluation of test compounds on these parameters.

TABLE 1. Cellular Composition of BALF ($\times 10^6$) in Control Guinea Pigs or 4-, 24-, or 48-hours Post Ovalbumin Challenge of Sensitized Guinea Pigs

	Total	Macrophage	Neutrophil	Eosinophil
Control	9.2 ± 2.3	8.3 ± 2.3	0.0	0.5 ± 0.1
4 hours	20.5 ± 4.7	11.7 ± 1.7	4.7 ± 2.1*	2.9 ± 1.1*
24 hours	30.9 ± 3.1**	16.1 ± 1.2*	1.9 ± 0.9	10.9 ± 2.3**
48 hours	31.4 ± 9.5*	15.4 ± 4.3	0.1 ± 0.02*	13.1 ± 4.7*

Note: Ovalbumin sensitization alone had no effect on the composition of cells in the airways.

Key: * $p < 0.05$; ** $p < 0.01$; Student's t-test versus control.

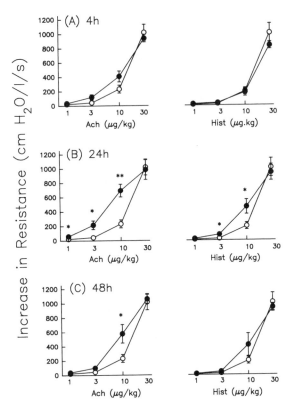

FIGURE 1. Effect of ovalbumin sensitization and challenge (●—●) on airway responsiveness to acetylcholine and histamine versus control (○—○). **(A)** Four hours post challenge. **(B)** Twenty-four hours post challenge. **(C)** Forty-eight hours post challenge.

Treatment of sensitized guinea pigs with TRFK-5, 1 hour before ovalbumin challenge, resulted in a significant reduction in both the total number of cells and the number of eosinophils recovered from BALF (FIG. 2). In addition, TRFK-5 significantly reduced the degree of bronchial hyperresponsiveness to Ach. Treatment with rat IgG had no effect on these parameters.

DISCUSSION

Ovalbumin sensitization and challenge of guinea pigs results in a bronchial hyperresponsiveness to Ach and Hist and an accumulation of eosinophils in the BALF, 24 hours later. These parameters are two important features of asthma, and this provides a useful model to study the mechanisms involved in the recruitment of eosinophils to the airways, and their relationship with the development of bronchial hyperresponsiveness.

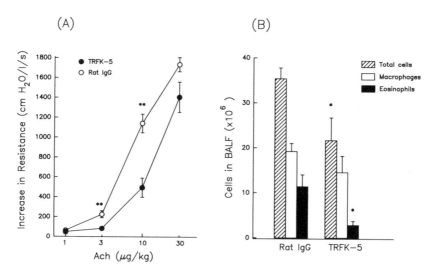

FIGURE 2. Effect of TRFK-5 or rat IgG on (**A**) bronchial hyperresponsiveness to acetyl-choline (●—●, TRFK-5; ○—○, rat IgG) and (**B**) cellular composition of BALF (× 10^6) (*hatched box:* total leukocytes, *open box:* macrophages, *filled box:* eosinophils).

The mechanisms for the selective recruitment of eosinophils to the lungs of asthmatics have not yet been fully elucidated, but there are a number of possibilities, including enhanced eosinophil–endothelial interactions[10] that are important for tissue emigration, and eosinophil-specific chemoattractants and activating factors.[11] Cytokines generally have many effects on leukocytes, for example, IL-2 exerts regulatory effects on virtually all cell types participating in the immune response.[12] However, IL-5 appears at present to exhibit many actions that are specific to eosinophils. It causes hyperadherence of eosinophils *in vitro via* a leukocyte integrin (CD11/18)-dependent mechanism.[10] It is a chemotactic agent for human and guinea pig eosinophils *in vitro*,[13,14] as well as a priming agent for chemotaxis in response to other agents, for example, IL-8,[15] PAF, and LTB$_4$.[16] IL-5 also promotes release of eosinophil granule proteins and prolongs survival *in vitro*.[17] In addition, it is a growth and differentiation factor for eosinophils.[18]

Our results are consistent with the findings of Gulbenkian *et al.*[7] and Chand *et al.*[8] showing that TRFK-5 reduces eosinophil accumulation in BALF in a guinea pig model of airway inflammation. As such, the evidence for involvement of IL-5 in the eosinophilia has been strengthened. However, the eosinophilia was not completely prevented—in fact, there was still a 4-fold increase, about 25 percent of the usual increase. This was also the case in the study by Chand *et al.*,[8] who found that a similar proportion of eosinophilia remained after treatment with anti-IL-5 or dexamethasone. These findings suggest that there may be a component of the eosinophilia that is mediated by a mechanism independent of IL-5, for example, IL-3 or GM–CSF, which may be released from T-lymphocytes.

Iwama *et al.*[19] demonstrated that in guinea pigs, intratracheal injection of murine recombinant (mr) IL-5 leads to an increase in the eosinophil number in BALF. It is interesting that the level of BALF eosinophils in response to mrIL-5 was similar to that seen in our animals after treatment with TRFK-5. Van Oosterhout *et al.*[20] administered mrIL-5 to guinea pigs by injecting IL-5-secreting cells intraperitoneally. This did not result in increased numbers of eosinophils in BALF. It is possible that giving IL-5 over a longer period of time resulted in a desensitization of eosinophils to this cytokine. Giving IL-5 to naive animals, in which the cell population is in a low state of activation, may not give large changes in cell numbers in the lung, since one of the actions of IL-5 is to enhance the chemoattractant properties of other mediators. It would be of interest to determine the effects of mrIL-5 given to ovalbumin-sensitized guinea pigs.

In addition to inhibition of eosinophil accumulation in BALF, our study shows that treatment of sensitized guinea pigs with TRFK-5 before ovalbumin challenge inhibits the development of bronchial hyperresponsiveness to Ach in this model. These results are in accordance with previous work in this laboratory using the antibody R15.7 to the leukocyte CD18 integrin.[9] In this study, treatment of guinea pigs with this antibody resulted in a significant reduction in bronchial hyperresponsiveness to Ach, as well as a reduction in the number of eosinophils recovered from BALF. In the same study, however, a different antibody to CD18, 6.5E, had no effect on bronchial hyperresponsiveness, but reduced the number of eosinophils in BALF. Iwama *et al.*[21] showed that treatment of guinea pigs with mrIL-5 resulted in an increase in the bronchial hyperresponsiveness to Ach. This was a dose of mrIL-5 that produced a modest increase in BALF eosinophilia.[19] In addition, Van Oosterhout *et al.*[20] administered mrIL-5 to guinea pigs, resulting in increased responsiveness of tracheal rings to agonists, but no change in the number of eosinophils recovered from BALF.

These results taken together suggest that IL-5 is involved in both the recruitment of eosinophils to the airways and the development of bronchial hyperresponsiveness, although these two parameters do not necessarily go hand in hand.

REFERENCES

1. BOUSHEY, H. A., M. J. HOLTZMAN, J. R. SHELLER & J. A. NADEL. 1980. Bronchial hyperreactivity. Am. Rev. Respir. Dis. **121:** 389–412.
2. WARDLAW, A. J., S. DUNNETTE, G. J. GLEICH, J. V. COLLINS & A. B. KAY. 1988. Eosinophils and mast cells in bronchoalveolar lavage in subjects with mild asthma. Relationship to bronchial hyperreactivity. Am. Rev. Respir. Dis. **137:** 62–69.
3. BASTEN, A. & P. B. BEESON. 1970. Mechanisms of eosinophilia. II. Role of the lymphocyte. J. Exp. Med. **131:** 1288–1294.
4. KAY, A. B. 1991. Asthma and inflammation. J. Allergy Clin. Immunol. **87:** 893–910.
5. WALKER, C., *et al.* 1992. Allergic and nonallergic asthmatics have distinct patterns of T-cell activation and cytokine production in peripheral blood and bronchoalveolar lavage. Am. Rev. Respir. Dis. **146:** 109–115.
6. CORRIGAN, C. J., *et al.* 1993. CD4 T-lymphocyte activation in asthma is accompanied by increased serum concentrations of interleukin-5. Effect of glucocorticoid therapy. Am. Rev. Respir. Dis. **147:** 540–547.
7. GULBENKIAN, A. R., *et al.* 1992. Interleukin-5 modulates eosinophil accumulation in allergic guinea pig lung. Am. Rev. Respir. Dis. **146:** 263–265.
8. CHAND, N., *et al.* 1992. Anti-IL-5 monoclonal antibody inhibits allergic late phase bronchial eosinophilia in guinea pigs: A therapeutic approach. Eur. J. Pharmacol. **211:** 121–123.
9. MILNE, A. A. Y. & P. J. PIPER. 1993. Different effects of two anti-CD18 antibodies

on antigen-induced airway hyperresponsiveness and cell accumulation in guinea pigs. Br. J. Pharmacol. **109:** 16 pp.

10. WALSH, G. M., *et al.* 1990. IL-5 enhances the in vitro adhesion of human eosinophils, but not neutrophils, in a leucocyte integrin (CD11/18)-dependent manner. Immunology **71:** 258–265.

11. RESNICK, M. B. & P. F. WELLER. 1993. Mechanisms of eosinophil recruitment. Am. J. Respir. Cell Mol. Biol. **8:** 349–355.

12. ANDERSON, T. D. 1992. Structure and function of interleukin-2. *In* Cytokines in Health and Disease, S. L. Kunkel and D. G. Remick, Eds.: 27–59. Dekker. New York.

13. WANG, J. M., *et al.* 1989. Recombinant human interleukin 5 is a selective eosinophil chemoattractant. Eur. J. Immunol. **19:** 701–705.

14. COËFFIER, E., D. JOSEPH & B. B. VARGAFTIG. 1991. Activation of guinea pig eosinophils by human recombinant IL-5. Selective priming to platelet-activating factor-acether and interference of its antagonists. J. Immunol. **147:** 2595–2602.

15. WARRINGA, R. A. J., *et al.* 1992. Modulation of eosinophil chemotaxis by interleukin-5. Am. J. Respir. Cell Mol. Biol. **7:** 631–636.

16. SEHMI, R., *et al.* 1992. Interleukin-5 selectively enhances the chemotactic response of eosinophils obtained from normal but not eosinophilic subjects. Blood **79:** 2952–2959.

17. KITA, H., D. A. WEILER, R. ABU-GHAZALEH, C. J. SANDERSON & G. J. GLEICH. 1992. Release of granule proteins from eosinophils cultured with IL-5. J. Immunol. **149:** 629–635.

18. SANDERSON, C. J., D. J. WARREN & M. STRATH. 1985. Identification of a lymphokine that stimulates eosinophil differentiation in vitro: Its relationship to interleukin-3 and functional properties of eosinophils produced in cultures. J. Exp. Med. **162:** 60–74.

19. IWAMA, T., H. NAGAI, N. TSURUOKA & A. KODA. 1992. Effect of murine recombinant interleukin-5 on the cell population in guinea pig airways. Br. J. Pharmacol. **105:** 19–22.

20. VAN OOSTERHOUT, A. J. M., *et al.* 1993. Effect of anti-IL-5 and IL-5 on airway hyperreactivity and eosinophils in guinea pigs. Am. Rev. Respir. Dis. **147:** 548–552.

21. IWAMA, T., H. NAGAI, N. TSURUOKA & A. KODA. 1993. Effect of murine recombinant interleukin-5 on bronchial reactivity in guinea pigs. Clin. Exp. Allergy **23:** 32–38.

Effects of Inhaled Steroids on Blood Eosinophils in Moderate Asthma[a]

MICHEL LAVIOLETTE, CLAUDINE FERLAND,
LUCE TRÉPANIER, HÉLÈNE ROCHELEAU,
AZZEDINE DAKHAMA, AND LOUIS-PHILIPPE BOULET

Unité de Recherche
Centre de Pneumologie de l'Hôpital Laval
Université Laval
Sainte-Foy, Québec, Canada

and

Réseau Canadien de Centres d'Excellence en Santé Respiratoire

INTRODUCTION

Asthma is a bronchial inflammatory disease characterized by a leukocyte mucosal infiltration, predominantly eosinophils.[1,2] These cells are recruited from blood marrow to the bronchial wall through a series of processes. Following inhalations of asthmogens such as allergen in sensitized subjects, cytokines and chemotactic factors are released by resident bronchial cells, probably mast cells and lymphocytes.[3,4] These mediators increase the eosinopoiesis, activate the eosinophil metabolism, increase their chemotaxis, the expression of adherence molecules by bronchial endothelial cells, and lead to increased expression of their ligands by eosinophils.[5,6] In the bronchial mucosa, eosinophils are believed to be activated and release mediators and cytokines that amplify the inflammatory process and increase bronchial responsiveness and asthma symptoms.[7,8] We and others showed that eosinophils of asthmatics have an increased capacity to produce the leukotriene (LT) C_4.[9,10]

Inhaled steroids are powerful anti-inflammatory drugs that are very effective in controlling asthma symptoms and are now considered to be the mainstay of asthma treatment.[11,12] However, the basic mechanisms through which they decrease airway inflammation and improve asthma control are not completely understood. At doses under the equivalent of 1500 mg of beclomethasone, the inhaled steroids have minimal or no systemic effects and their anti-inflammatory effects are very likely to be local.[13,14] Inhaled steroids could improve asthma by inhibiting the bronchial release of chemotactic factors and cytokines and, consequently, the recruitment and the activation of eosinophils. This study looked at the *in vivo* effects of inhaled steroids on blood eosinophils in mild and moderate asthma and showed that they decreased the eosinophil activation.

[a] This study was supported by the "Association pulmonaire du Québec," Montréal, Canada, and by Glaxo Canada, Inc., "Bureau d'affaires du Québec," Dorval, Canada.

MATERIALS AND METHODS

Subjects

Thirteen subjects with mild to moderate asthma were recruited in the study. All met the American Thoracic Society criteria for the diagnosis of asthma.[15] Subjects should have a $FEV_1 \geq 85\%$ predicted and require at least two inhalations of β_2 agonist twice a day, or a $FEV_1 < 85\%$ predicted with irregular use of β_2 agonist. The inclusion criteria were stable asthma symptoms for more than 3 months, no need for oral steroids during the 6 months preceding the study, no inhaled steroid use during the 2 months preceding the study, no history of other allergic symptoms but asthma, no medication use other than β_2 agonist, and no other disease than asthma. All had allergy skin prick tests with a battery of common airborne allergens to evaluate their degree of atopy. The subjects gave their informed consent to the study, which was approved by our local Ethics Committee.

Protocol

This is a double-blind crossover study with subjects taking beclomethasone dipropionate 200 μg dry powder administered via the Diskhaler delivery system (Beclodisk®) or placebo two inhalations twice daily for 6 weeks. They were randomly divided into two groups: group 1, placebo followed by beclomethasone; group 2, beclomethasone followed by placebo. Spirometry, measures of nonallergic airway responsiveness, and blood sampling were obtained at the first visit, and at the end of each treatment period (placebo or beclomethasone), during weeks 6 and 12. During the study, the subjects scored daily their symptoms, cough, dyspnea, wheezing, chest tightness, on a scale of 0 to 5 (0, no; 1, very light; 2, light; 3, moderate; 4, severe; 5 very severe symptom), β_2 agonist needs, and peak expiratory flows (PEF) on a diary card. They also visited the study supervisor at weeks 3 and 9 to verify the compliance to the medication and the procedures.

Forced expiratory flows were measured on a Vitalograph spirometer PFT II in the morning after withholding β_2 agonist for at least 8 hours and expressed as percent of Knudson predicted values. Nonspecific airway response to methacholine was measured according to the method described by Juniper *et al.*[16] and expressed as the dose provoking a fall of 20% in FEV_1. PEF were measured with a Mini-Wright peak flow meter, the subjects recording the better of three assays.

Blood-Cell Processing

Venous blood (120 ml) was collected early in the morning in EDTA tubes. The cell counts and differentials were obtained on a Cell Coulter STKS (Coulter Electronics Ltd., Florida). The blood was centrifuged to remove the plasma and the cell pellet was sedimented on Dextran (Sigma, St-Louis, Missouri). Leukocytes were centrifuged on Ficoll-Paque for 20 min at 700 g. The cell pellet containing the granulocytes was resuspended and red cells lysed with distilled water. Eosinophils were isolated using the technique described by Koenderman *et al.*[17] and modified in our laboratory.[18] Briefly, the granulocytes (75×10^6 cells in one ml of Ca^{++}/Mg^{++}-free Hank's balanced salt buffer (HBSS) supplemented with 5 percent fetal bovine serum, Gibco) were incubated with 10^{-8} M *N*-formyl-methionyl-phenylalanine (Sigma) for 10 minutes at 37°C. The cells were then suspended in HBSS and overlayed on a Percoll gradient with densities of 1.078 and 1.100 g/ml. After centrifugation, cells at the interfaces were recovered, washed, and counted. Cell counts were determined on a hemacytometer, cell viability by trypan blue exclusion, and cell differentials on Diff-Quik stained preparations. Eosinophil recovery was expressed as the percentage of eosinophils present at the interface 1.078–1.100 g/ml on Percoll gradient over the total number of eosinophils present at all interfaces and in the cell pellet.

Leukotriene C_4 Measurement

Eosinophils isolated at the interface 1.078–1.100 g/ml on Percoll gradients were suspended in RPMI with $MgCl_2$ (0.5 mM), $CaCl_2$ (2 mM), fetal bovine serum 10%, and 1% penicilline-streptomycine, and incubated with and without granulocyte-macrophage colony stimulating factor (GM–CSF) (100 U/ml) for 30 minutes. The cells were then stimulated for 15 minutes with 2 μM calcium ionophore A23187 in Eppendorf tubes. Control cell preparations were incubated with DMSO (Sigma) used to dissolve the ionophore. The cell suspensions were centrifuged and the supernatants kept at -70°C for LTC_4 determination. LTC_4 was measured using enzyme immunoassay kits (Cayman Chemical Co., Ann Arbor, Michigan).

Statistical Analysis

Results are expressed as mean ± SEM. The double-blind crossover design improves the sensitivity by eliminating the individual patient effect. To avoid a carryover effect of a treatment on the other, a crossover design was used to analyze the data.

RESULTS

Subjects

One subject of group 1 was withdrawn at the beginning of the study because of an asthma exacerbation following antigenic exposure (cat). No data are provided on this subject. Following randomization and excluding this withdrawal, group 1 included five subjects and group 2 included seven. All subjects tolerated the inhaled steroids well. Eleven subjects presented at least one positive reaction to allergy skin prick tests. No subject had allergic symptoms other than asthma during the study. One subject of group 2 required the use of inhaled steroids at the end of placebo treatment. The subjects' characteristics are presented in TABLE 1. Groups 1 and 2 were similar for the measured parameters, with a mean FEV_1 slightly under normal and a mean PC_{20} in the moderate asthma range.

Clinical and Physiological Parameters

FEV_1 remained stable during the study period and did not change significantly. Morning peak flows measured before β_2 agonist use showed a significant improve-

TABLE 1. Characteristics of Subjects

	Group 1	Group 2
Number	5	7
Sex (F/M)	3/2	3/4
Age (years)	27 ± 2.9*	26 ± 2.4
FEV_1 (l/sec)	2.65 ± 0.23*	2.88 ± 0.27
(% of predicted)	79 ± 5.7*	79 ± 6.1
PC_{20} (mg/ml)	0.2 ± 1.9†	0.38 ± 1.9
Blood eosinophil count (10^9/l)	0.40 ± 0.09*	0.34 ± 0.04

* Mean ± SEM.
† Geometric mean ± SEM.

ment during the beclomethasone period, increasing from 391 ± 30 to 472 ± 41 l/min (FIG. 1, $p = 0.007$). Inhaled steroids also decreased coughing ($p = 0.02$). Bronchodilator needs decreased from 3.1 ± 0.9 to 0.72 ± 0.5 inhalation(s)/day during beclomethasone period (FIG. 2, $p = 0.007$). Inhaled steroids increased the PC_{20} methacholine from 0.38 to 1.9 mg/ml (geometric mean) (FIG. 3, $p = 0.02$).

Eosinophil Count and LTC₄ Production

At the end of cell isolation procedures, eosinophil viability was always greater than 95 percent. With inhaled beclomethasone, blood eosinophil counts decreased from 0.35 ± 0.06 to 0.26 ± 0.04 cells × 10^9/l (FIG. 4, $p = 0.084$). The eosinophil recovery and purity on Percoll gradients at each visit were similar (FIG. 5). The purity was always higher than 90 percent and the recovery higher than 74 percent.

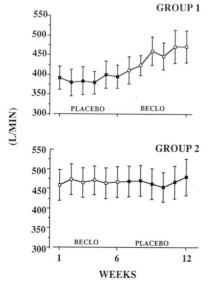

FIGURE 1. Morning PEF recorded during the study. Inhaled beclomethasone increased morning PEF ($p = 0.007$).

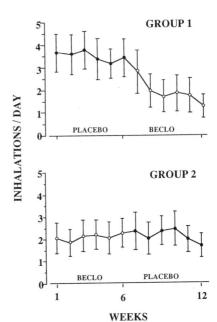

FIGURE 2. β_2 agonist need during the study. Inhaled beclomethasone decreased the use of β_2 agonist ($p = 0.007$).

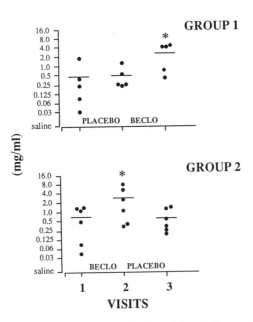

FIGURE 3. Methacholine PC_{20} measured at the first visit and after each treatment. Inhaled beclomethasone increased PC_{20} methacholine ($p = 0.02$).

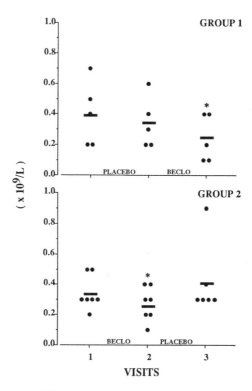

FIGURE 4. Blood eosinophil counts measured at the first visit and after each treatment. Inhaled beclomethasone decreased blood eosinophil counts ($p = 0.084$).

In the absence of ionophore A23187, eosinophils released no detectable LTC_4, even in the presence of GM–CSF. However, stimulation with ionophore induced the production of large amounts of LTC_4 by the eosinophils (FIG. 6), and the preincubation with GM–CSF enhanced the ionophore A27183-induced LTC_4 release (1.8-fold) ($p = 0.001$). Inhaled beclomethasone decreased the eosinophil A23187-induced LTC_4 release from 5571 ± 899 to 3129 ± 462 pg/250,000 eosinophils ($p = 0.04$), and the GM–CSF-enhanced LTC_4 production from $11,177 \pm 1597$ to 5950 ± 531 pg/250,000 eosinophils (FIG. 6, $p = 0.003$).

Correlation between Clinical and Cellular Parameters

Since inhaled beclomethasone improved both clinical and cellular parameters, we looked at correlations between these parameters. No significant correlation was found between the improvement in PC_{20} and the decrease in blood eosinophil counts with inhaled steroids. However, there was a significant correlation between the improvment in PC_{20} and the decrease in the GM–CSF-enhanced ionophore A27183-induced LTC_4 production with inhaled beclomethasone, $r = -0.57$ ($p = 0.02$) (FIG. 7).

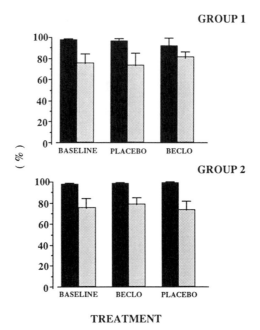

FIGURE 5. Eosinophil purity and recovery on Percoll gradients. Eosinophil purity (*closed bar*) and recovery (*open bar*) were similar at each visit.

DISCUSSION

This study shows that the clinical improvement induced by inhaled beclomethasone is accompanied by a decrease in blood eosinophil count and LTC_4 eosinophil production. Improvement of clinical and physiological parameters with inhaled steroids has been repeatedly reported.[19-21] However, this study shows a correlation between clinical improvement and a decrease in blood eosinophil LTC_4 production.

The technique used to isolate the eosinophils allows recovery of an eosinophil population, including normodense and hypodense cells, representative of the blood eosinophils rather than a specific eosinophil subpopulation.[18] Using this technique, we previously showed that eosinophils of moderate asthmatics release more LTC_4 than cells of normal or mild asthmatics.[9] Moreover we also showed that eosinophils isolated by this technique release similar amount of LTC_4 to eosinophils isolated by immunomagnetic selection using anti-CD16 monoclonal antibodies.[18] Therefore we do not believe that selection of different eosinophil subpopulations or an effect of the isolation procedure explains the differences obtained following treatment with inhaled beclomethasone.

The dose of inhaled steroids chosen in this study was 800 μg of beclomethasone dry powder daily in order to avoid any significant systemic effect of steroids. Indeed, with such a dose, the changes in blood eosinophil count and LTC_4 production are most likely to be due to the local effect of inhaled beclomethasone on the bronchial inflammatory processes. Some systemic absorption and effects can occur, but are likely to be minimal.[13,14]

The decrease in eosinophil counts and in ionophore A27183-induced and GM–CSF-enhanced LTC_4 productions probably indicate a decrease in blood eosinophil activation and recruitment to the bronchial mucosa. Since blood eosinophil activation and recruitment could be induced by other diseases than asthma and that these phenomena can mask the effect of the inhaled steroids on bronchial mucosa, we took care to avoid diseases such as allergic rhinitis, drug allergy, allergic dermatitis, or parasitic infestations. Therefore, we believe that the changes seen in blood eosinophil counts and LTC_4 productions are due to the bronchial effects of the inhaled steroids.

The improvement in asthma symptoms and in airway responsiveness are likely to reflect a decrease in bronchial inflammation. The association between the decrease in nonspecific airway responsiveness and in blood eosinophil LTC_4 production capacity support this hypothesis. Therefore we assume that the inhaled steroids decrease the release of chemotactic factors and cytokines by the cells present in the bronchial wall, and consequently decreased the recruitment and the activation of the blood eosinophils. Eosinophils are mostly tissue cells and the degree of blood eosinophil activation probably reflects the intensity of the inflammation going on in the tissue.

In conclusion, this study demonstrated that 800 μg/day of inhaled beclomethasone improves asthma symptoms and nonspecific airway responsiveness, and that

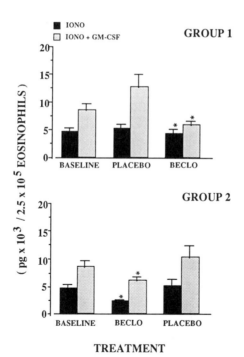

FIGURE 6. Eosinophil LTC_4 production. Inhaled beclomethasone decreased the ionophore A23187-induced and GM–CSF-enhanced LTC_4 productions ($p = 0.04$ and $p = 0.003$, respectively). $n = 4$ or 5 in group 1, and $n = 6$ or 7 in group 2.

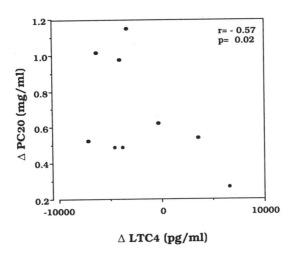

FIGURE 7. Correlations between beclomethasone-induced PC_{20} and GM–CSF-enhanced LTC_4 production changes. PC_{20} or LTC_4 production values were missing in three subjects at visit 2 or 3; therefore, ΔPC_{20} and ΔLTC_4 were available in 9 subjects.

these improvements are associated with a decrease in blood eosinophil count and activation.

ACKNOWLEDGMENTS

The authors thank M. S. Simard for assistance in statistical analysis.

REFERENCES

1. DJUKANOVIC, R., et al. 1990. Mucosal inflammation in asthma. Am. Rev. Respir. Dis.
    142: 434–457.
2. BOUSQUET, J., et al. 1990. Eosinophilic inflammation in asthma. New Eng. J. Med.
    323: 1033–1039.
3. KAY, A. B. 1991. Lymphocytes in asthma. Respir. Med. **85:** 87–90.
4. BARNES, P. J. 1989. New concepts in the pathogenesis of bronchial asthma. J. Allergy
    Clin. Immunol. **83:** 1013–1017.
5. SILBERSTEIN, D. S. & J. R. DAVID. 1987. The regulation of human eosinophil function
    by cytokines. Immunol. Today **8:** 380–385.
6. RESNICK, M. B. & P. F. WELLER. 1993. Mechanisms of eosinophil recruitment. Am.
    J. Respir. Cell Mol. Biol. **8:** 349–355.
7. GLEICH, G. J. 1990. The eosinophil and bronchial asthma: Current understanding. J.
    Allergy Clin. Immunol. **85:** 422–436.
8. SMITH, H. 1992. Asthma, inflammation, eosinophils and bronchial hyperresponsive-
    ness. Clin. Exp. Allergy. **22:** 187–197.
9. LAVIOLETTE, M., C. FERLAND, M. BOSSÉ, J.-F. COMTOIS & L.-P. BOULET. 1993.
    Eosinophil activation and asthma severity. J. Allergy Clin. Immunol. **91** (no. 1,
    part 2): 348.

10. KAJITA, T., *et al.* 1985. Release of leukotriene C4 from human eosinophils and its relation of the cell density. Int. Arch Allergy Appl. Immunol. **78:** 406–410.
11. INTERNATIONAL CONSENSUS REPORT ON DIAGNOSIS AND TREATMENT OF ASTHMA. 1990. Clin. Exp. Allergy **Suppl. 1:** 1–72.
12. WEBB, D. R. 1981. Steroids in allergy diseases. Med. Clin. North Am. **65:** 1073–1081.
13. JENNINGS, B. H., K. E. ANDERSSON & S. A. JOHANSSON. 1991. The assessment of the systemic effects of inhaled glucocorticosteroids. The effects of inhaled vs. oral prednisolone on calcium metabolism. Eur. J. Clin. Pharmacol. **41:** 11–16.
14. TOOGOOD, J. H. 1987. Corticosteroids. *In* Drug Therapy for Asthma. Research and Clinical Practice, J. W. Jenne and S. Murphy, Eds. Vol. 31: 719–761.
15. AMERICAN THORACIC SOCIETY. 1987. Standards for the diagnosis and care of patients with chronic obstructive pulmonary disease (COPD) and asthma. Am. Rev. Respir. Dis. **136:** 225–424.
16. JUNIPER, E. F., D. W. COCKCROFT & F. E. HARGREAVE. 1991. Histamine and methacholine inhalation tests: Tidal breathing method. Canadian Thoracic Society, A. B. Draco, Ed.
17. KOENDERMAN, L., P. T. M. KOK, M. L. HAMELINK, A. J. VERHOEVEN & P. L. B. BRUIJNZEEL. 1988. An improved method for the isolation of eosinophilic granulocytes from peripheral blood of normal individuals. J. Leukocyte Biol. **44:** 79–86.
18. LAVIOLETTE, M., M. BOSSÉ, H. ROCHELEU, S. LAVIGNE & C. FERLAND. 1993. Comparison of two modified techniques for purifying blood eosinophils. J. Immunol. Methods **165:** 253–261.
19. JUNIPER, E. F., *et al.* 1990. Effect of long-term treatment with inhaled corticosteroids on airway hyperresponsiveness and clinical asthma in nonsteroid-dependent asthmatics. Am. Rev. Respir. Dis. **142:** 832–836.
20. BEL, E. H., M. C. TIMMERS, J. HERMANS, J. H. DIJKMAN & P. J. STERK. 1990. The long-term effects of nedocromil sodium and beclomethasone dipropionate on bronchial responsiveness to methacholine in nonatopic asthmatic subjects. Am. Rev. Respir. Dis. **141:** 21–28.
21. KERREBIJN, K. F., E. E. M. VAN ESSEN-ZANDVLIET & H. J. NEIJENS. 1987. Effects of long-term treatment with inhaled corticosteroids and beta-agonists on the bronchial responsiveness in children with asthma. J. Allergy Clin. Immunol. **79:** 653–659.

Modulation of Macrophage Maturation by Cytokines and Lipid Mediators: A Potential Role in Resolution of Pulmonary Inflammation[a]

PETER M. HENSON AND DAVID W. H. RICHES

Department of Pediatrics
National Jewish Center for Immunology and
Respiratory Medicine
1400 Jackson Street
Denver, Colorado 80206

Macrophages are recognized to be pluripotential and their known properties span a wide array of cellular functions from migration and phagocytosis to key roles in the immune system and in protection against neoplasia. However, it is also becoming apparent that mononuclear phagocytes do not perform all these different functions at the same time. Rather they exhibit selective adaptation to the local environment (i.e., the pattern of signals impinging on their receptors) by exhibiting specific groups of coordinated activities analogous to distinct phenotypes. Developing in the bone marrow and circulating as relatively nondifferentiated monocytes, the cells are attracted to a tissue site, migrate through the vessel wall into the tissue, and there develop into mature macrophages. We have recently suggested that there are a number of distinct pathways for this maturation process that are dictated by both exogenous and endogenous regulatory factors,[1] and that the end product, the functional macrophage that is produced, may play quite different roles in the tissue depending on the maturation pathway that is engaged.

Shown in FIGURE 1 is an outline of three pathways of macrophage maturation that we have been studying *in vitro*. Each is defined by markers that are used as endpoints and each represents a distinct and mutually exclusive maturation process. The starting point in these experiments is bone-marrow-derived progenitor cells that are cultured in the presence of M-CSF for 5 to 7 days, and progress through monoblast, promonocyte, and monocyte stages to yield adherent monolayers of uncommitted macrophages that express many of the traits that are characteristic of monocyte-derived macrophages. They can then be induced by stimuli, such as those indicated in FIGURE 1, to further differentiate in different directions. The uncommitted cells are suggested to be similar to newly emigrated mononuclear phagocytes in the lung. While it is tempting to attribute specific *in vivo* functions to the cells deriving from the three maturational pathways, and even to dignify them with the term phenotypes, we believe that this designation is premature. The different cell types have not been formally demonstrated *in vivo*, their full characterization is not complete, and preliminary examination suggests that main-

[a] These studies were carried out in part in the F. L. Bryant, Jr. Laboratory for the Study of the Mechanisms of Lung Disease, and were supported by National Institutes of Health Grants GM48211 and HL27353.

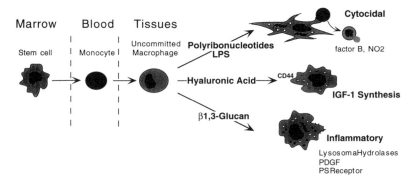

FIGURE 1. Three possible pathways of murine macrophage maturation.

tenance of the matured properties is dependent on the continued presence of the stimulus-induced cytokines.[1-3] Thus, the permanence of these changes has still to be determined, especially in the tissues themselves. Nevertheless, the demonstration of distinct and exclusive pathways for macrophage maturation, and determination of their regulatory mechanisms, clearly provides an hypothesis to account for macrophage heterogeneity and a potential explanation for its multiple postulated roles. It suggests an intriguing level of complexity to this cell type that will probably only begin to be resolved when distinct cell surface markers for the different pathways have been developed and can be used for single-cell analysis *in vitro* and *in vivo*. We would also suggest that there are many more pathways for macrophage maturation than those outlined here, but that analysis of these too will show similar combinations of external and endogenous regulatory mechanisms.

Most widely studied has been the controlled maturation of macrophages to a cytocidal state, capable of recognizing and killing transformed cells and thought to be important in tumor rejection.[4-6] Known to involve at least two major steps—priming and triggering[5,6]—the process represents a fascinating example of coordinated regulation of cell function by production of endogenous cytokines (even though when the process occurs *in vivo*, cytokines from external sources are also likely to be important). Our studies have focused on two markers for this pathway, synthesis of the complement protein factor B and production of reactive nitrogen intermediates derived from L-arginine, such as nitrite [an indication of the upregulation and action of inducible nitric oxide synthase (iNOS)]. This state can be induced by exposure of the uncommitted cells to polyribonucleotides or LPS[7,8] and requires the action of interferons and TNFα,[9-11] each of which can be produced by the macrophages themselves.

A second pathway is exemplified by the increased synthesis of insulinlike growth factor-1 (IGF-1) and is initiated, for example, by ligation of CD44 with hyaluronate.[12] IGF-1 is of potential interest to roles thought to be played by macrophages in wound healing and fibrosis, for example, in interstitial lung disease. To our surprise, TNFα seemed to be required for this path, too, even though polyribonucleotides were a poor stimulus for IGF-1 synthesis and hyaluronate did not induce the cytocidal cell.[13] The explanation of this paradox seems to lie in the role of interferon. When it is present, the cytocidal cell is induced by TNFα;

when it is not, the cell proceeds along the pathway to IGF-1 synthesis. Shown in
FIGURE 2 is the effect of exogenous IFNγ on induction of the two pathways by
TNFα. Once again the interferon (in this case IFNβ) could be endogenously
produced or could be supplied from surrounding cells. Thus, polyribonucleotides
stimulated the uncommitted macrophages to synthesize IFNβ and TNFα, whereas
hyaluronic acid induced only TNFα.[13] In this system, then, the action of interferon
can be thought of as a switch, allowing cells otherwise similarly stimulated to
mature to the cytocidal state rather than to synthesis of the fibroblast growth
factor IGF-1.

The third pathway depicted in FIGURE 1 is different yet again. The maturation
process is accompanied by increased synthesis (and secretion) of lysosomal hydrolases, and for largely historical reasons we have tentatively termed this an inflammatory macrophage (although this is certainly too general a term since it would
be expected that many different maturation pathways would be involved in creating
the different macrophage types seen in various types of inflammatory lesions).
Nevertheless, the cell that is induced by exposure to β-1, 3-glucan (the major
constituent of yeast cell walls) resembles in many ways the predominant macrophage found during chronic inflammation in the peritoneum or alveolus.[14,15] Uncommitted macrophages exposed to poly [I:C] (cytocidal pathway) do not develop
increased synthesis of lysosomal enzymes and, as shown in FIGURE 3, poly [I:C]
inhibits the ability of phagocytosable particles such as β-1,3-glucan to induce these
markers of the inflammatory pathway. In like manner, uptake of the particles does
not induce markers of the cytocidal cell and in fact prevents the ability of poly
[I:C] to induce this response.[1] In other words, the two pathways are mutually
exclusive. In more mechanistic terms, interferons and TNFα are inhibitory to the
inflammatory pathway, which seems to require the action of transforming growth
factor β (TGFβ) for induction.[3] In turn, TGFβ has been shown to be inhibitory
to induction of the cytocidal cell and thus might be considered the relevant
"switch" for the inflammatory pathway (FIG. 4).

The regulatory mechanisms for maturation of uncommitted cells to an "inflammatory" macrophage are proving of considerable complexity. Before developing this subject further, however, we will first digress into a brief consideration
of one aspect of resolution of pulmonary inflammation. In an acute alveolitis
there is first a massive emigration of granulocytes, then of monocytes which,

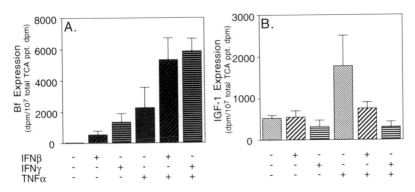

FIGURE 2. Interferons enhance the production of factor B (cytocidal pathway), but inhibit
upregulation of IGF-1 synthesis.

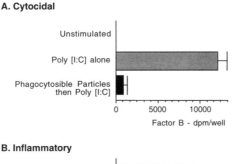

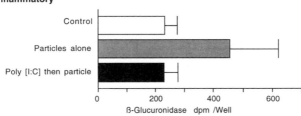

A. Cytocidal

B. Inflammatory

FIGURE 3. Maturation pathways induced by polyribonucleotides and digestible particles are mutually exclusive.

as previously indicated, mature into macrophages.[16-19] In self-limiting, resolving inflammation, the neutrophils are then removed. We have suggested (following the hundred-year-old lead of Elie Metchnikov) that the neutrophils are ingested by the mature macrophages[20] and that the recognition of neutrophils by the macrophages requires the former to undergo programmed cell death—apoptosis.[21] Apoptosis is a currently popular investigative area, first described and named by Andrew

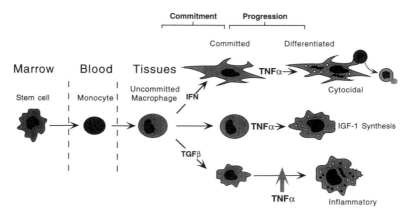

FIGURE 4. Endogenous or exogenous cytokines act as switches for the different maturation pathways.

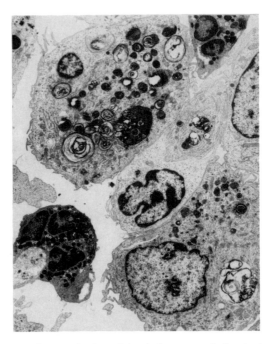

FIGURE 5. Electron micrograph of resolving inflammatory lesion in the rabbit lung. The remains of a neutrophil can be seen within a macrophage phagosome.

Wyllie,[22] that depicts a variety of processes in different cells, culminating in a nonnecrotic cell death that is active in nature, is accompanied by characteristic morphologic changes and intranucleosomal cleavage of the DNA, and usually results in rapid removal of the cells by surrounding mesenchymal cells and/or macrophages ([reference 23] and see FIG. 5). The process is of general interest in greatly disparate examples of tissue remodeling, is seen throughout the animal kingdom, and has received a further boost from its involvement in the complicated selection processes of the immune system.[24] Here we are interested in the removal process and, in particular, the mechanisms by which the macrophage recognizes the apoptotic neutrophil in the inflammatory lesion as a particle destined for engulfment. Its importance lies not only in the removal of inflammatory cells during the process of resolution, but also in the observation that the removal itself seems to be remarkably noninflammatory, that is, uptake of apoptotic cells is quite inefficient in stimulating the macrophage to produce further inflammatory mediators or proteins[25] (also Rose and Henson, unpublished). Presumably the net effect is to remove cells from tissues *in situ* without further damage and without (in ideal circumstances) perpetuating the inflammation.

To date at least three recognition mechanisms for apoptotic cells have been described:[23] (1) a lectin; (2) a complicated interaction involving thrombospondin and the vitronectin receptor (a $\beta 3$ integrin); and (3) a stereospecific recognition

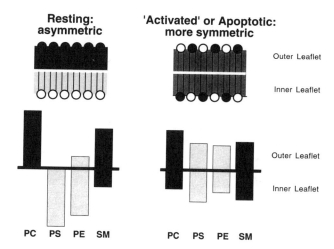

FIGURE 6. Expression of phosphatidylserine on the outer leaflet of cells.

of phosphatidylserine that is expressed on the surface of the apoptotic cell. Cells such as neutrophils and platelets normally exhibit significant asymmetry in the distribution of their membrane phospholipids with phosphatidylcholine (PC) on the outside and phosphatidylserine (PS) on the inside (FIG. 6). Activation of the cell leads to transient loss of this asymmetry, and thus expression of PS on the outside.[26] This is most easily seen in the platelet, where the PS expression after activation is critically involved in blood coagulation. In the activated neutrophil, the loss of asymmetry seems associated with the enhanced uptake and secretion of lipid mediators.[27] We have shown, however, that the apoptotic neutrophils or lymphocytes have also lost their membrane phospholipid asymmetry, here apparently in a permanent way. Thus these cells exhibit PS on the surface that is available for recognition by a putative receptor on the mature macrophage.[28] The recognition is stereospecific and can be inhibited by phosphatidylserine, glycerophosphoserine or L-phosphoserine, but not by other anionic phospholipids or D-phosphoserine.[28] Inflammatory macrophages from the mouse peritoneum or lung recognize and engulf apoptotic cells by this PS-dependent mechanism, but human monocyte-derived macrophages use the integrin and not the PS receptor. Resident alveolar macrophages were unable to take up effete neutrophils (i.e., apoptotic cells) at all,[20] suggesting, in a teleologic sense, the importance of allowing the newly incoming neutrophils to perform their normal function without risk of removal by resident cells. Only as part of the inflammatory process itself do the incoming macrophages appear to develop this ability. Since removal of neutrophils is expected to be critical to resolution of the inflammation, any abnormality of this removal process—for example, an inefficient influx of monocytes or an inappropriate maturation—might lead to more neutrophil-mediated damage.

Interestingly, the uncommitted mouse bone-marrow-derived macrophage also employs the vitronectin receptor and does not appear to express the PS receptor. By contrast, macrophages matured along the "inflammatory" pathway by exposure to β-1,3-glucan, now take up apoptotic cells by a PS-inhibitable process and no longer appear to use the vitronectin receptor.[29] Induction of the new receptor function requires new protein synthesis and appears to represent a legitimate marker of the inflammatory maturation pathway. While we are attempting to isolate and clone this receptor, its presence has been determined on macrophages by means of a simple rosetting assay. Erythrocytes that have been induced to express PS on their surface by treatment with diamide, or erythrocyte ghosts made in the presence of calcium so as to lose their membrane asymmetry, bind to macrophages that express the PS receptor in a PS-inhibitable fashion, and this binding is quantitated visually.[30] As shown in FIGURE 7, exposure of uncommitted macrophages to β-1,3-glucan induces new expression of this rosetting ability as well as enhanced synthesis of lysosomal hydrolases. Importantly, phagocytosis of latex beads, unlike glucan, was without effect, that is, the process of phagocytosis itself is not the stimulus for expression of the PS receptor or of maturation to the "inflammatory macrophage."

Initiation of the maturation pathway that leads to expression of this PS receptor function (i.e., the inflammatory pathway) could therefore be a consequence of engagement of specific receptors for β-1,3-glucan. However, we have long been intrigued by observations made by Axline and Cohn in the late 1960s that macrophages are able to distinguish between digestible and nondigestible particles, and respond to the former by increased synthesis of lysosomal hydrolases.[31] Using their approach, therefore, the requirement for digestibility was examined for induction of this maturation pathway.[1] Particles composed of L- or D-amino acids were assembled and compared as stimuli since only the former can be digested by macrophage enzymes. In the face of similar uptake, only the L-amino acid particles were able to stimulate expression of the PS receptor (FIG. 8). Importantly, the digestibility requirement could be overcome by prior treatment of the macrophages with TGFβ, showing that it came early in the induction pathway and presumably was a requirement for the synthesis and expression of the TGFβ, that is, of the cytokine "switch" for this pathway. Thus TGFβ-primed cells were able to respond to latex, glucan, or D-amino acid particles by rosetting with PS-expressing erythrocytes.

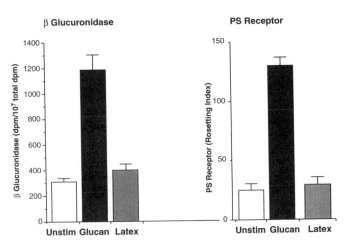

FIGURE 7. Stimulation of PS-receptor expression in uncommitted macrophages by β-1,3-glucan.

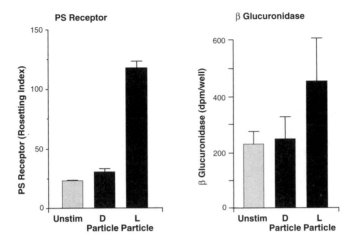

FIGURE 8. Only digestible particles (composed of L- rather than D-amino acids) are able to stimulate the uncommitted macrophage to develop markers of the "inflammatory state."

Questions then arise as to the mechanism by which macrophages discriminate between digestible or indigestible particles, as well as to the possible significance of this process. FIGURE 9 depicts some hypothetical mechanisms for this discrimination. One set of possibilities relates to the smaller products of digestion that escape the phagolysosome and might act as stimuli to the cell. Another focuses around condensation of the phagolysosome. Phagosome–lysosome fusion leads to the development of a phagolysosome that in the macrophage then condenses down over time into a secondary lysosome or residual body. For physical reasons relating the need to maintain a surrounding membrane, this condensation can be

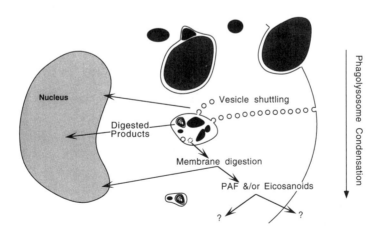

FIGURE 9. Some possible mechanisms by which particle digestibility might provide maturation signals.

presumed not to occur if the ingested particle is indigestible. Perhaps then the signals for inducing cell maturation derive from this condensation process. We have further reasoned that condensation must involve the removal of membrane and that this removal process might provide some of the signals, particularly if it is affected by the action of phospholipases. Secretory phospholipase A_2 in the phagolysosome, acting on membrane phosphatidylcholine could generate precursors of the eicosanoids and of PAF. Preliminary experiments indeed suggest that crude inhibitors of PLA_2 as well as an antagonist of PAF do inhibit the glucan-induced maturation process. We have also shown in the past, however, that sulphidopeptide leukotrienes can induce new synthesis of lysosomal hydrolases.[32] Thus at least two different products of phospholipase digestion and metabolism might contribute to the maturation pathway and might therefore represent the mechanism by which macrophages recognize the difference between digestible and indigestible particles. Here again, however, PAF or leukotrienes that have derived from other cells in the inflammatory environment would also contribute to this maturation process, so that both endogenous and exogenous signals can lead to the same endpoint.

Removal of granulocytes from inflammatory sites would be expected to be a critical step in the resolution of inflammation. The mechanisms described earlier achieve this step prior to granulocyte lysis (the apoptotic cell is still intact), and thus minimize the nonspecific release of toxic constituents. Because the uptake of apoptotic cells into macrophages seems to be itself inefficient at stimulating the macrophage to produce more inflammatory mediators[25] (also Rose and Henson, unpublished), this too would help maximize the resolution process. It is also noteworthy that any cells that were lysed in a lesion would be expected to expose their inner membrane leaflet PS and so be recognized by the mature macrophage and removed. The redundancy seen in the inflammatory cell removal mechanisms also argues for its importance. Enhancing these removal mechanisms would then seem to be a reasonable objective for limiting inflammatory reactions and preventing their progression to a more chronic state. By contrast it is intriguing to question whether low-grade inflammatory processes, such as those induced by tobacco smoke, might be inefficient at initiating the appropriate monocyte emigration or maturation, and thus might not provide the cells for neutrophil removal. The long-term consequences could then be elastolytic damage to the lung structure.

REFERENCES

1. LASZLO, D. J., et al. 1992. Development of functional diversity in mouse macrophages. Mutual exclusion of two phenotypic states. Am. J. Pathol. **143:** 587–597.
2. RICHES, D. W. H. & G. A. UNDERWOOD. 1991. Expression of IFNβ during the triggering phase of macrophage cytocidal activation. Evidence for an autocrine/paracrine role in the regulation of this state. J. Biol. Chem. **226:** 24785–24792.
3. NOBLE, P. W., et al. 1993. Transforming growth factor-β primes macrophages to express inflammatory gene products in response to particulate stimuli by an autocrine/paracrine mechanism. J. Immunol. **151:** 979–989.
4. HIBBS, J. B. J., R. R. TAINTOR, H. A. J. CHAPMAN & J. B. WEINBERG. 1977. Macrophage tumor killing: Influence of the local environment. Science **197:** 279–82.
5. RUSSELL, S. W., W. F. DOE & A. T. MCINTOSH. 1977. Functional characterization of a stable, noncytolytic stage of macrophage activation in tumors. J. Exp. Med. **146:** 1511–1520.
6. RUCO, L. P. & M. S. MELTZER. 1978. Macrophage activation for tumor cytotoxicity:

Development of macrophage cytotoxic activity requires completion of a sequence of short-lived intermediary reactions. J. Immunol. **121:** 2035–2042.

7. TORRES, B. A. & H. M. JOHNSON. 1985. Lipopolysaccharide and polyribonucleotide activation of macrophages: Implications for a natural triggering signal in tumor cell killing. Biochem. Biophys. Res. Commun. **131:** 395–401.

8. RICHES, D. W. H., P. M. HENSON, L. K. REMIGIO, J. F. CATTERALL & R. C. STRUNK. 1988. Differential regulation of gene expression during macrophage activation with a polyribonucleotide. The role of endogenously derived IFN. J. Immunol. **141:** 180–188.

9. MACE, K. F., M. J. EHRKE, K. HORI, D. L. MACCUBBIN & E. MIHICH. 1988. Role of tumor necrosis factor in macrophage activation and tumoricidal activity. Cancer Res. **48:** 5427–5432.

10. REMELS, L., L. FRANSEN, K. HUYGEN & B. P. DE. 1990. Poly I:C activated macrophages are tumoricidal for TNF-alpha-resistant 3LL tumor cells. J. Immunol. **144:** 4477–4486.

11. RICHES, D. W. H. & G. A. UNDERWOOD. 1991. Expression of IFNβ during the triggering phase of macrophage cytocidal activation. Evidence for an autocrine/paracrine role in the regulation of this state. J. Biol. Chem. **266:** 24785–24792.

12. NOBLE, P. W., F. R. LAKE, P. M. HENSON & D. W. H. RICHES. 1993. Hyaluronate activation of CD44 induces insulin-like growth factor-1 expression by a tumor necrosis factor-α-dependent mechanism in murine macrophages. J. Clin. Invest. **91:** 2368–2377.

13. LAKE, F. R., P. W. NOBLE, P. M. HENSON & D. W. H. RICHES. 1993. Functional switching of macrophage responses to TNFα by interferons. Implications for the pleiotropic activities of TNFα. J. Clin. Invest. In press.

14. SUGIMOTO, M., et al. 1978. Extracellular hydrolytic enzymes of rabbit dermal tuberculous lesions and tuberculin reactions collected in skin chambers. Am. J. Pathol. **90:** 583–606.

15. SUGA, M., A. M. DANNENBERG, JR. & S. HIGUCHI. 1980. Macrophage heterogeneity in vivo. Macrolocal and microlocal macrophage activation, identified by double-staining tissue sections of BCG granulomas for pairs of enzymes. Am. J. Pathol. **99:** 305–315.

16. HENSON, P., et al. 1979. Complement fragments, alveolar macrophages, and alveolitis. Am. J. Pathol. **97:** 93–110.

17. SHAW, J., P. HENSON, J. HENSON & R. WEBSTER. 1980. Lung inflammation induced by complement-derived chemotactic fragments in the alveolus. Lab. Invest. **42:** 547–558.

18. HENSON, P., et al. 1984. Resolution of pulmonary inflammation. Fed. Proc. **43:** 2799–2806.

19. DOHERTY, D., G. DOWNEY, G. WORTHEN, C. HASLETT & P. HENSON. 1988. Monocyte retention and migration in pulmonary inflammation. Requirement for neutrophils. Lab. Invest. **59:** 200–213.

20. NEWMAN, S., J. HENSON & P. HENSON. 1982. Phagocytosis of senescent neutrophils by human monocyte-derived macrophages and rabbit inflammatory macrophages. J. Exp. Med. **156:** 430–442.

21. SAVILL, J., et al. 1989. Macrophage phagocytosis of aging neutrophils in inflammation. Programmed cell death in the neutrophil leads to its recognition by macrophages. J. Clin. Invest. **83:** 865–875.

22. KERR, J. F. R., A. H. WYLLIE & A. R. CURRIE. 1972. Apoptosis: A basic biological phenomenon with wide-ranging implications in tissue kinetics. Br. J. Cancer **26:** 239–257.

23. SAVILL, J., V. FADOK, P. M. HENSON & C. HASLETT. 1993. Phagocyte recognition of cells undergoing apoptosis. Immunol. Today (Rev.) **14:** 131–136.

24. COHEN, J. J. 1991. Programmed cell death in the immune system. Adv. Immunol. **50:** 55–85.

25. MEAGHER, L. C., J. S. SAVILL, A. BAKER, R. W. FULLER & C. HASLETT. 1992. Phagocytosis of apoptotic neutrophils does not induce macrophage release of thromboxane B2. J. Leuk. Biol. **52:** 269–273.

26. BRATTON, D., J. KAILEY, K. CLAY & P. M. HENSON. 1991. A model for the extracellular release of PAF: The influence of plasma membrane phospholipid asymmetry. Biochem. Biophys. Acta **1062:** 24–34.

27. BRATTON, D., *et al.* 1992. The mechanism of internalization of PAF in activated human neutrophils: Enhanced transbilayer movement across the plasma membrane. J. Immunol. **148:** 514–523.

28. FADOK, V., *et al.* 1992. Exposure of phosphatidylserine on the surface of apoptotic lymphocytes triggers specific recognition and removal by macrophages. J. Immunol. **148:** 2207–2216.

29. FADOK, V., *et al.* 1992. Different populations of macrophages use either the vitronectin receptors or the phosphatidylserine receptor to recognize and remove apoptotic cells. J. Immunol. **149:** 4029–4035.

30. FADOK, V. A., *et al.* 1993. Particle digestibility is required for induction of the phosphatidylserine recognition mechanism used by murine macrophages to phagocytose apoptotic cells. J. Immunol. **151:** 4274–4285.

31. AXLINE, S. G. & Z. A. COHN. 1970. In vitro induction of lysosomal enzymes by phagocytosis. J. Exp. Med. **131:** 1239–1260.

32. LEW, D., C. LESLIE, P. HENSON & D. RICHES. 1991. The role of endogenously-derived leukotrienes in the regulation of lysosomal enzyme expression in macrophages exposed to β-1,3-glucan. J. Leuk. Biol. **49:** 266–276.

Proteinases and Cytokines in Neutrophil and Platelet Interactions *In Vitro*. Possible Relevance to the Adult Respiratory Distress Syndrome

MICHEL CHIGNARD AND PATRICIA RENESTO

Unité de Pharmacologie Cellulaire
Unité associée IP/INSERM 285
Institut Pasteur
25 rue du Dr Roux
75015 Paris, France

INTRODUCTION

While polymorphonuclear neutrophils are endowed with potent mechanisms for phagocytosis and the killing of microbes, and thus contribute to a host defense against microbicidal infections, they have also long been recognized as important effectors of inflammation. Indeed, when their migration in tissues is not regulated, their excessive accumulation could contribute to host tissue injury following release of two essential groups of toxic products: granular substances and toxic species of reduced oxygen.[1] Lungs are particularly exposed to such insults and constitute a primary site of damage caused by host defense mechanisms. Indeed, if only a few neutrophils are normally present in the lung interstitium and alveolar spaces, these cells are susceptible to respond to chemotactic stimuli and accumulate in the lung. Thus, neutrophils have been specifically implicated in the adult respiratory distress syndrome (ARDS) and emphysema.[2]

After several years, the concept that neutrophils contribute to inflammation not only alone but also through interactions with platelets, has emerged. For example, a neutrophil-dependent platelet deposition was observed in different experimental models such as dermal inflammation,[3] occlusion-reperfusion myocardial injury,[4] or subendothelial immune complex glomerulonephritis.[5] In a model of ARDS, it has been shown that not only neutrophils but also platelets contributed to lung injury.[6] In this pathology, characterized by a loss of integrity of the alveolar–capillary wall, platelets have been described as potential contributors.[7]

In vitro studies have revealed that such a cell-to-cell interaction was effective and was of extreme complexity. Different biochemical and biological pathways have thus been depicted: generation of oxygen derivatives, synthesis of arachidonate metabolites and platelet-activating factor (PAF), contact through the expression of P-selectin (GMP-140 or CD62), formation of neutrophil-activating peptide 2 (NAP-2), and participation of proteinases.[8,9]

We have focused our interest on one of these mechanisms, that is, the neutrophil-induced platelet activation mediated by proteinases and modulated by cytokines. This is one of the most apt to intervene in ARDS. The different reasons in support of this assertion are presented throughout the present review.

ACTIVATION OF PLATELETS BY STIMULATED NEUTROPHILS: ROLE OF PROTEINASES

As illustrated in the FIGURE 1, a strong platelet activation occurs when N-formyl-Met-Leu-Phe, a specific agonist of neutrophils, is added to a mixed cell suspension of neutrophils and platelets. The observation that cell-free supernatants of activated neutrophils also stimulated platelets, supported the involvement of a soluble mediator. The possible participation of PAF, arachidonic acid metabolites, and oxygen reactive species was quickly discarded. By contrast, the susceptibility of the activity to $PhMeSO_2F$ (PMSF) led us to conclude that neutrophil-induced platelet activation was due to a serine proteinase called neutrophilin, which is thought to be related to cathepsin G,[10] the only serine proteinase from neutrophils described so far as a potential platelet agonist.[11] These first works were followed by the effective identification of cathepsin G in supernatants of N-formyl-Met-Leu-Phe-activated neutrophils.[12] The participation of this proteinase in the neutrophil-mediated platelet activation was finally demonstrated by our group[13,14] and confirmed by another,[15,16] using specific antiproteinases. At the same time, it was shown that such a phenomenon

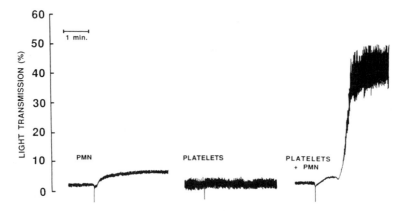

FIGURE 1. Platelet aggregation induced by addition of a neutrophil-specific agonist. Neutrophils (PMN) and platelets were purified from human blood and used alone or mixed together at a physiological concentration, that is, 5×10^6/ml and 2×10^8/ml, respectively. Cell suspensions were preincubated for 5 minutes at 37°C in the presence of 5-μg/ml cytochalasin B and 0.7-mg/ml fibrinogen prior to addition of 0.5-μM f-Met-Leu-Phe. Aggregations were recorded as the percentage of changes in light transmission as a function of time. Tracings from one experiment representative of a large number of others. Addition of f-Met-Leu-Phe to neutrophils or platelets alone was without marked effect, while its addition to mixed-cell suspensions induced a full aggregation.

was not restricted to N-formyl-Met-Leu-Phe, but was also observed with C5a,[13] leukotriene B4, or PAF[15] as neutrophil agonists. The addition of purified cathepsin G to platelets leads to intracellular calcium movement,[12] proteinase kinase C translocation,[17] thromboxane B2 synthesis,[14] release of the content of dense[12] and α granules,[18] and to aggregation.[12] This is supposedly mediated through a rapid, saturable, reversible binding characteristic of a specific receptor.[19] In fact, cathepsin G exhibits strong similarity with thrombin in its ability to activate platelets. Nonetheless, different indirect arguments led Selak[20] to postulate that the platelet receptors for these two agonists may be functionally, and possibly physically, different.

At this stage, the possible involvement of elastase, another serine proteinase released from activated neutrophils concomitantly with cathepsin G, was discarded since it failed to activate platelets by itself.[11,14,21,22] In fact, reported effects of elastase on these cells concerned the inhibition of platelet activation induced by thrombin,[11,21,23] collagen,[24] or von Willebrand factor,[23] and were the consequence of membrane glycoprotein cleavage. All these observations were obtained following 30- or 60-minute preincubation periods. Only one study performed with a 1-minute preincubation interval showed an effect on the glycoprotein Ib with the subsequent inhibition of thrombin-induced platelet aggregation.[21] It was only recently that a different effect of elastase was observed using a different experimental approach. Indeed, while it failed to directly activate platelets, elastase enhanced their reactivity to cathepsin G when added for time intervals of 10–60 seconds before cathepsin G,[20] or even simultaneously.[18] This led us to look for its participation to the neutrophil-mediated platelet activation. We first determined by spectrophotometric assays the amounts of cathepsin G and elastase secreted when neutrophils were stimulated by 0.5-μM N-formyl-Met-Leu-Phe, and susceptible to encounter nearby platelets. These concentrations of proteinases, estimated to be in the range of 240 nM for cathepsin G and 380 nM for elastase, were then tested either separately or together on a mixed neutrophils–platelets suspension. In these conditions, and as previously mentioned, elastase failed to activate platelets by itself in terms of aggregation, secretion, or thromboxane B2 synthesis. As shown in the FIGURE 2, the concentration of cathepsin G released from activated neutrophils induced a platelet activation that was of a lesser extent than that observed upon N-formyl-Met-Leu-Phe stimulation (maximal activation = 100 percent). By contrast, with the combination of both proteinases, the observed responses were comparable to those obtained with N-formyl-Met-Leu-Phe as agonist. Using elafin, which is endowed with a specific inhibitory effect toward elastase compared to cathepsin G,[25,26] it was proved that elastase effectively played a role.[18] Thus, when neutrophil degranulation leads to the activation of surrounding platelets, this effect is mediated by the synergistic effect of at least two serine proteinases, namely cathepsin G and elastase. It is of note that there are discrepancies between the specificity of this activity of elastase vis-a-vis cathepsin G. Thus, elastase potentiates platelet activation initiated by other platelet agonists according to us,[18] but not according to Selak.[20]

Proteinase 3 is the third serine proteinase stored in the azurophilic granules with enzymatic properties close to elastase, and which produces emphysema in hamsters.[27] We observed that purified proteinase 3, like elastase, although unable to directly trigger platelet activation, potentiated the platelet effect of cathepsin G (Renesto et al., J. Immunol., in press). Under our experimental conditions, the active concentrations were similar to those of elastase. Since proteinase 3 is at least as abundant in neutrophils as elastase,[28] it can be

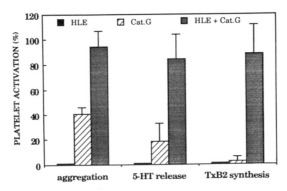

FIGURE 2. Platelet activation induced by cathepsin G, elastase, or both proteinases added together. Neutrophils and platelets were incubated together under conditions depicted in FIGURE 1, and challenged with 380-nM elastase (HLE), 240-nM cathepsin G (Cat. G), or both proteinases added simultaneously. Three minutes later, aggregation, serotonin (5-HT) release, and thromboxane B2 (TxB2) formation were evaluated. For each parameter, values were expressed as the percentage of responses obtained following addition of 0.5-μM f-Met-Leu-Phe. Each histogram is the mean $\pm$ SD of 3 to 5 distinct experiments. Elastase and cathepsin G alone were unable to mimic platelet responses obtained with f-Met-Leu-Phe. Only the concomitant addition of both proteinases was able to do so.

speculated that proteinase 3 also most probably participates to the neutrophil-mediated platelet activation process. This has to be proved, but a specific inhibitor has to be found.

These results called for the possible participation of a cell-to-cell interaction like that in ARDS. On the one hand, the formation of the activated fifth component of complement (C5a), an inducer of the PMN-mediated platelet activation,[13] is frequently associated with this disease.[29,30] On the other hand, one of the main mediators of this cooperative effect, namely elastase, was recovered in bronchoalveolar lavage fluids of patients with this pulmonary disease.[31,32] Up to now, the presence of cathepsin G has not been reported, but it can be conceived that its release occurs just as elastase does. It should be mentioned that McGuire *et al.*[32] failed to demonstrate the presence of cathepsin G in the bronchoalveolar lavage fluids of patients, but they hypothesized a possible binding of this proteinase to tissues at the site of injury and they raised the problem of the sensitivity of the test used.

Crossed immunoelectrophoresis studies of the sera of patients with ARDS have shown that, if the levels of most proteins were extremely low, this was not the case for acute-phase proteins, among which are α1-antitrypsin (or α1-proteinase inhibitor) and α1-antichymotrypsin, whose concentrations were increased.[33] Since the preservation of the functional integrity of tissues requires a delicate balance between proteinases and antiproteinases, it is not surprising to observe such an increased concentration of these antiproteinases under pathological conditions in which elastase and most probably cathepsin G levels are higher than in normal conditions. However, while antiproteinase concentrations were increased, it is of potential importance to note that the proteolytic activity of elastase can remain effective *in vivo*.[31,32] In fact, α1-antitrypsin in bronchoalveolar lavage fluids of patients with ARDS is largely inactivated, essentially by oxydation.[34] Failure of antiproteinases to inactivate their targets may have dramatic consequences. As an example, it is well known that individuals genetically deficient in α1-antitrypsin are predisposed to the development of pulmonary emphysema, a disease in which a progressive destruction of pulmonary parenchyma by elastase was observed.[35]

MODULATION OF NEUTROPHIL-MEDIATED PLATELET ACTIVATION BY TNFα

The intensity of the platelet response reflects the degree of neutrophil degranulation.[13] Consequently, substances promoting or inhibiting the stimulation of neutrophil can modulate this cell-to-cell interaction. A potential involvement of cytokines was thus envisaged in this context. Tumor necrosis factor alpha (TNFα) was the first one to be tested. The rationale for using this cytokine was that TNFα affects a broad range of neutrophil functions *in vitro*, either by a direct stimulatory activity[36,37] or by enhancing their response to secondary stimuli, referred to as the priming effect.[38,39,40] Moreover, not only *in vivo* experiments were in favor of a potential role for TNFα in pulmonary damage,[41] but this cytokine was identified in the pulmonary secretions of patients with ARDS as opposed to healthy individuals.[42,43] We thus performed experiments with this cytokine to investigate a possible modulation of neutrophil-mediated platelet activation. As expected, pretreatment of mixed-cell suspensions with TNFα, inactive by itself, resulted in strong platelet activation in response to a weak concentration of *N*-formyl-Met-Leu-Phe when compared with untreated controls (FIG. 3). This potentiating effect was the consequence of the enhanced release of proteinases from neutrophils and was unrelated to a nonspecific effect on platelets.[44] Thus, pretreatment of neutrophils with this cytokine enhanced β-glucuronidase release (chosen as an index of neutrophil

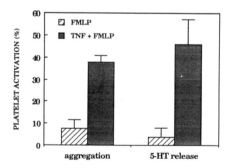

FIGURE 3. Enhancement by TNFα of platelet activation induced by f-Met-Leu-Phe-stimulated neutrophils. Neutrophils and platelets were preincubated together under conditions depicted in FIGURE 1 and in the presence or not of 10-ng/ml TNFα. Five minutes later, cells were challenged by a subthreshold concentration of f-Met-Leu-Phe (12.5 nM). Aggregation (expressed as the percentage of changes in light transmission) and serotonin (5-HT) release (expressed as the percentage of the total content of platelets) were measured. Each histogram is the mean ± SD of 5 distinct experiments. Preincubation of mixed-cell suspensions with TNFα resulted in a significant enhancement ($P < 0.05$) of platelet responses to a challenge by f-Met-Leu-Phe.

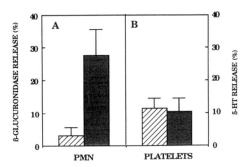

FIGURE 4. Effect of TNFα on neutrophil and platelet responses. Neutrophils and platelets were used separately and strictly under the same conditions as those depicted in FIGURE 3. Following preincubation (*stippled columns*) or not (*hatched columns*) with 10-ng/ml TNFα for 5 minutes, neutrophils (PMN) and platelets were challenged with 12.5-nM f-Met-Leu-Phe and 100-nM cathepsin G, respectively. Activation of both cell populations was evaluated by measuring β-glucuronidase release from neutrophils (**A**) and serotonin (5-HT) release from platelets (**B**). Values for both parameters are expressed as the percentage of the total content of cells. Each histogram is the mean ± SD of 3 distinct experiments. Preincubation with TNFα enhanced neutrophil activation induced by f-Met-Leu-Phe, but failed to affect platelet activation induced by cathepsin G.

degranulation), but failed to affect platelet activation induced by cathepsin G (FIG. 4(A) and (B), respectively). It should be noted that such an effect by TNFα was concentration-dependent and operative within 5 minutes of preincubation. This is not a common observation, since the usually described priming effect is obtained for longer preincubation times. Nonetheless, in a recent study Brandt et al.[45] also observed an enhancement of N-formyl-Met-Leu-Phe-induced degranulation with elastase release, upon a preincubation time of 5-minutes. This is an important point since TNFα is rapidly cleared from the circulation in human, having a half-life of 14 to 18 minutes.[46]

A potential regulatory mechanism concerning the interaction between TNFα and the neutrophil-derived proteinases should be mentioned at this stage. On the one hand, cathepsin G and elastase are able to inactivate TNFα. Scuderi et al.[47] have shown by Western blot analysis that cathepsin G and elastase degrade this cytokine into 11- and 7.6-kDa biologically inactive products. On the other hand, elastase releases a ligand-binding fragment from TNFα receptors. In fact, the proteinase affects only one type of receptor (the 75-kDa type), reducing by 85 to 96 percent the binding and releasing a soluble fragment that binds TNFα.[48] The overall consequence of these two biological properties, if happening *in vivo*, could be a negative feedback control of the inflammatory cascade.

EFFECTS OF INTERLEUKIN-1 ON NEUTROPHIL–PLATELET INTERACTION

Interleukin-1 (IL-1), which is close to TNFα in terms of biological effects,[49] presents a potentially important role in the development of ARDS. Indeed, it was shown that the IL-1β level was significantly higher in bronchoalveolar lavage fluids in severe ARDS than in patients at risk or before ARDS.[50] These results are consistent with the *in vitro* study of Jacobs *et al.*,[51] who reported that alveolar macrophages obtained from patients with ARDS released greater amounts of IL-1β than those obtained from individuals with pneumonia or from control subjects. However, when tested on the neutrophil-mediated platelet activation system within a wide range of concentrations and preincubation times, it was impossible to observe a potentiation by recombinant IL-1 of the response triggered by *N*-formyl-Met-Leu-Phe (unpublished data). This could be explained by the fact that although neutrophils are sensitive to natural IL-1, recombinant preparations in most laboratories have no direct effects on neutrophils.[52] Interestingly, the mature form of IL-1β is released along with a precursor inactive form. It has been shown that elastase and cathepsin G can process the precursor into a form similar in size and specific activity to the mature IL-1β.[53]

If neutrophil-mediated platelet activation can be modulated by cytokines that preferentially act on neutrophils, a possible effect on platelets has to be considered. Thus, Todoroki *et al.*[54] have shown that IL-1β and IFNγ increased the serotonin release from thrombin-treated platelets and their adhesion to monocytic leukemia cells (U937). Since the adhesion was observed using glutaraldehyde-fixed U937 cells, it was deduced that these cytokines were acting on platelets rather than on leukocytes. This is consistent with the fact that platelets bear a specific receptor for IFNγ.[55]

POTENTIAL ROLE OF NAP-1/INTERLEUKIN 8

NAP-1, also known as interleukin-8 (IL-8), is a neutrophil chemoattractant member of a new family of cytokines named chemokines. IL-8 stimulates various neutrophil functions, including degranulation.[56,57] Brandt *et al.*[45] have recently shown that elastase release induced by IL-8 is potentiated upon preincubation of the cells with TNFα. Using the neutrophil-mediated platelet activation system, we observed that IL-8 was a weak inducer of this cell-to-cell interaction. Nonetheless, the preincubation of the mixed cell suspension with mice recombinant TNFα, strongly modified the platelet response to an IL-8 challenge, and leads to a full platelet aggregation (Si Tahar *et al.*, to be published).

These data, with a synergism between TNFα and IL-8, are also in favor of the participation of the neutrophil–platelet interaction in ARDS, since IL-8 has been recovered in the airspace of these patients.[58,59] It has recently been shown that neutrophils synthesize IL-8[60,61] with an increase in the gene expression by LPS, TNFα, and IL-1β.[62] It is believed that such production by neutrophils themselves would constitute a positive feedback mechanism *in vivo*, that is, neutrophils at the inflammatory site would attract more neutrophils through the formation of IL-8.

POTENTIAL ROLE OF NAP-2

NAP-2 is another neutrophil-activating chemokine belonging to the C-X-C subfamily. Although its structure is homologous (46 percent) to IL-8, its biosynthesis is far from different. Unlike IL-8, which is secreted by monocytes and other cell types, NAP-2 appears to be generated extracellularly by proteolytic cleavage of platelet-derived products. It was first observed that NAP-2 corresponds to part of the sequence of the platelet basic protein, the connective tissue-activating peptide III and β-thromboglobulin, and is structurally homologous to platelet factor 4, these four proteins being contained in the α-granules of platelets.[63–65] In fact, platelet basic protein cleavage at bond 9 residue from the amino terminus creates the connective tissue-activating peptide III, and at bond 13 residues forms β-thromboglobulin.[66] These different molecules, released upon platelet activation, are susceptible to cleavage by proteinases to form NAP-2.[65] It was first reported that cathepsin G was likely to be involved in this process.[67] From several neutrophil-derived proteinases tested, only cathepsin G has the capacity to form NAP-2 with a high specificity and in a relatively short time period.[68,69] Thus, in pathological situations involving platelet activation, such as in ARDS, the following scenario can be envisaged in pulmonary capillaries. Activated neutrophils release cathepsin G, which first activates nearby platelets. As a consequence, the release of NAP-2 precursors from platelet granules occurs in the extracellular medium. Cathepsin G works again and cleaves the precursors to form NAP-2. The latter activates more neutrophils with more cathepsin G released. This possibly vicious circle is most probably restrained by plasma antiproteinases, but also by elastase. Indeed, elastase also cleaves NAP-2 precursors, but at a different point as compared to cathepsin G, thus preventing the formation of NAP-2.[69] A recent study[70] gives support to this speculative pathway. First, the authors, analyzing pulmonary edema fluids, found higher concentrations of NAP-2 in patients with ARDS than in control subjects. More interestingly, patients with ARDS had a higher concentration of β-thromboglobulin-like antigen (an assay measuring β-thromboglobulin, connective tissue-activating peptide III, and recombinant NAP-2) in their plasma than normal subjects, suggesting that platelets have degranulated into the plasma of these patients.[70]

IMPORTANCE OF A THIRD CELL POPULATION: ENDOTHELIAL CELLS

When considering ARDS, one has to keep in mind the involvement of endothelial cells. The effect of cytokines on the endothelium in relationships with neutrophil adhesion has been and is still widely studied.[71,72] Neutrophil proteinases have also been shown to affect endothelial cells. Thus, activated neutrophils trigger endothelial cell detachment,[73–75] and lysis,[76,77] an effect counteracted by inhibitors of proteinases. Addition of purified neutrophil elastase to cultured endothelial cells led to different observations, that is, a cell detachment but no lysis[75,78] or a cell detachment with lysis.[76,77] In our hands, elastase triggers detachment and lysis, with as a consequence, the release of von Willebrand factor,[79] a molecule considered to be a potential early predictor of acute lung injury.[80] This effect involved the enzymatic activity of elastase since the PMSF-treated proteinase was inactive. In view of the increased permeability observed in ARDS, it has also been observed that incubation of endothelial cells with elastase increased transendothelial albumin movement.[81] Nonetheless, this effect was apparently not related to the enzymatic activity of elastase, contrary to what was observed with detachment and lysis, but rather to its cationic charge.[81] Exactly the same results were obtained using cathepsin G.[82] Although, it has been shown that cathepsin G increases calcium efflux ($^{45}Ca^{2+}$ technic), we were unable to note movement of intracytoplasmic calcium (fura-2 technic) under our experimental conditions (unpublished data). In short, the reported effects of elastase and cathepsin G on endothelial cells seem to be more related to a cytotoxic effect than to a physiologic one.

CONCLUSION

The pathogenesis of ARDS is multifactorial, including neutrophils, platelets, endothelial cells, proteinases, cytokines, but also alveolar macrophages, epithelial cells, endotoxins, lipid mediators, complement, reactive oxygen species, and so forth.[83] This complexity has prevented any substantial progress in drug therapy. To better understand this complicated disease process, better laboratory animal

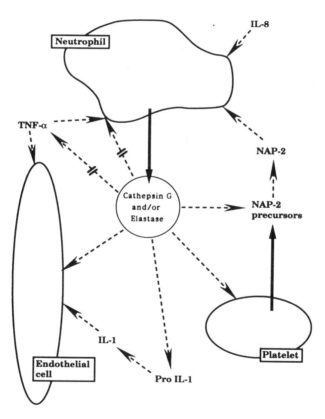

FIGURE 5. Simplified scheme illustrating some possible pathways involving cathepsin G and elastase interactions with blood and vascular cells and cytokines, and that are susceptible to intervene in ARDS. The different pathways represented are described in the present review.

models are needed.[84] As far as neutrophils and platelets are concerned, the rabbit is most probably not a good choice. Indeed, although the *in vitro* cooperation between neutrophils and platelets was also observed, the mediator involved is not a proteinase but PAF.[85,86] These results are consistent with the fact that cathepsin G was not found in rabbit neutrophils.[87] The guinea pig is probably not a good model either, since platelets respond poorly to a challenge by purified human cathepsin G (unpublished data). Rat and mice would be better species, since it has effectively been shown that cathepsin G is stored in the neutrophils of rat.[88] Mice constitute an attractive model because their neutrophils contain elastase and cathepsin G, while those of mutant, beige mice (Chediak-Higashi) are selectively deficient in these proteinases.[89] More precisely, the enzyme deficiency is just apparent and really due to the presence of an excess of inhibitors.[90] As an example, repeated intratracheal insults with endotoxin to normal mice result in the development of pulmonary emphysema, while beige mice do not incur a similar pathology.[91] Mice are also obviously an effective model due to the large array of murine recombinant cytokines that can be used without interspecies problems, and of antimurine cytokine specific antibodies.

Even if this review has not thoroughly focused on cytokines *per se,* it is our belief that nowadays they constitute one of the most attractive molecules to work with in order to successfully develop treatments for ARDS.[92]

In the neutrophil–platelet–endothelial cells network presented here, some other secondary loops are potentially operative. As an example, products released from activated platelets can affect surrounding cells, that is, serotonin by increasing endothelial cell permeability, or ATP by enhancing neutrophil response. A simplified picture can be drawn with cathepsin G and elastase at the center of a cross talk between the three cell populations (FIG. 5). This is obviously our bias, but our aim was to focus the attention of the reader on the possible importance of these two proteinases that could play a role at the crossroads of inflammation and thrombosis.

REFERENCES

1. WEISS, S. J. 1989. Tissue destruction by neutrophils. New Eng. J. Med. **320:** 365–376.
2. GADEK, J. E. 1992. Adverse effects of neutrophils on the lung. Am. J. Med. **92:** 27S–31S.
3. ISSEKUTZ, A. C., M. RIPLEY & J. R. JACKSON. 1983. Role of neutrophils in the deposition of platelets during acute inflammation. Lab. Invest. **49:** 716–724.
4. BEDNARD, M., B. SMITH, A. PINTO & K. M. MULLANE. 1985. Neutrophil depletion suppress 111In-labeled platelet accumulation in infarcted myocarde. J. Cardiovasc. Pharmacol. **7:** 906–912.
5. JOHNSON, R. J., *et al.* 1988. Platelets mediate neutrophil-dependent immune complex nephritis in the rat. J. Clin. Invest. **304:** 1225–1235.
6. TVEDTEN, H. W., G. O. TILL & P. A. WARD. 1985. Mediators of lung injury in mice following systemic activation of complement. Am. J. Pathol. **119:** 92–100.
7. HEFFNER, J. E., S. A. SAHN & J. E. REPINE. 1987. The role of platelets in the adult respiratory distress syndrome. Culprits or bystanders? Am. Rev. Respir. Dis. **135:** 482–492.
8. BAZZONI, G., E. DEJANA & A. DEL MASCHIO. 1991. Platelet-neutrophil interactions. Possible relevance in the pathogenesis of thrombosis and inflammation. Haematology **76:** 491–499.
9. CERLETTI, C., V. EVANGELISTA & G. DE GAETANO. 1992. Polymorphonuclear leucocyte-dependent modulation of platelet function: Relevance to the pathogenesis of thrombosis. Pharmacol. Res. **26:** 261–268.
10. CHIGNARD, M., M. A. SELAK & J. B. SMITH. 1986. Direct evidence for the existence

of a neutrophil-derived platelet activator (neutrophilin). Proc. Natl. Acad. Sci. U.S.A. **83:** 8609–8613.

11. BYKOWSKA, K., J. KACZANOWSKA, J. KARPOWICZ, J. STACHURSKA & M. KOPEC. 1983. Effect of neutral proteases from blood leukocytes on human platelets. Thromb. Haemostas. **50:** 768–772.

12. SELAK, M. A., M. CHIGNARD & J. B. SMITH. 1988. Cathepsin G is a strong platelet agonist released by neutrophils. Biochem. J. **251:** 293–299.

13. FERRER-LOPEZ, P., et al. 1990. Activation of human platelets by C5a-stimulated neutrophils: A role for cathepsin G. Am. J. Physiol. **258:** C1100–C1107.

14. RENESTO, P., P. FERRER-LOPEZ & M. CHIGNARD. 1990. Interference of recombinant eglin C, a proteinase inhibitor extracted from leeches, with neutrophil-mediated platelet activation. Lab. Invest. **62:** 409–416.

15. DEL MASCHIO, A., et al. 1990. Platelet activation by polymorphonuclear leukocytes exposed to chemotactic agents. Am. J. Physiol. **258:** H870–H879.

16. EVANGELISTA, V., G. RAJTAR, G. DE GAETANO, J. G. WHITE & C. CERLETTI. 1991. Platelet activation by fMLP-stimulated polymorphonuclear leukocytes: The activity of cathepsin G is not prevented by antiproteinases. Blood **77:** 2379–2388.

17. RENESTO, P., C. KADIRI & M. CHIGNARD. 1992. Combined activation of platelets by cathepsin G and platelet-activating factor, two neutrophil-derived agonists. Br. J. Haematol. **80:** 205–213.

18. RENESTO, P. & M. CHIGNARD. 1993. Enhancement of cathepsin G induced platelet activation by leukocyte elastase: Consequence for neutrophil-mediated platelet activation. Blood. **88:** 139–144.

19. SELAK, M. A. & J. B. SMITH. 1990. Cathepsin G binding to human platelets. Evidence for a specific receptor. Biochem. J. **266:** 55–62.

20. SELAK, M. A. 1992. Neutrophil elastase potentiates cathepsin G-induced platelet activation. Thromb. Haemostas. **68:** 570–576.

21. BROWER, M. S., R. I. LEVIN & K. GARRY. 1985. Human neutrophil elastase modulates platelet function by limited proteolysis of membrane glycoproteins. J. Clin. Invest. **75:** 657–666.

22. KORNECKI, E., et al. 1988. Granulocyte-platelet interactions and platelet fibrinogen receptor exposure. Am. J. Physiol. **255:** H651–H658.

23. WICKI, A. N. & K. J. CLEMETSON. 1985. Structure and function of platelet membrane glycoproteins Ib and V. Effects of leukocyte elastase and other proteases on platelets response to von Willebrand factor and thrombin. Eur. J. Biochem. **153:** 1–11.

24. BYKOWSKA, K., J. KACZANOWSKA, J. KARPOWICZ, S. LOPACIUK & M. KOPEC. 1985. Alterations of blood platelet function induced by neutral proteases from human leukocytes. Thromb. Res. **38:** 535–546.

25. WIEDOW, O., J.-M. SCHRÖDER, H. GREGORY, J. A. YOUNG & E. CHRISTOPHER. 1990. Elafin: An elastase-specific inhibitor of human skin. Purification, characterization, and complete amino acid sequence. J. Biol. Chem. **265:** 14791–14795.

26. SALLENAVE, J.-M., M. D. MARSDEN & A. P. RYLE. 1992. Isolation of elafin and elastase-specific inhibitor (ESI) from bronchial secretions: Evidence of sequence homology and immunological cross-reactivity. Biol. Chem. Hoppe-Seyler **373:** 27–33.

27. KAO, R. C., N. G. WEHNER, K. M. SKUBITZ, B. H. GRAY & J. R. HOIDAL. 1988. Proteinase 3. A distinct human polymorphonuclear leukocyte proteinase that produces emphysema in hamsters. J. Clin. Invest. **82:** 1963–1973.

28. CAMPENELLI, D., et al. 1990. Cloning of cDNA for proteinase 3: A serine protease, antibiotic, and autoantigen from human neutrophils. J. Exp. Med. **172:** 1709–1715.

29. HAMMERSCHMIDT, D. E., L. J. WEAVER, L. D. HUDSON, P. R. CRADDOCK & H. S. JACOB. 1980. Association of complement activation and elevated plasma-C5a with adult respiratory distress syndrome. Lancet **1:** 947–949.

30. ROBBINS, R. A., W. D. RUSS, J. K. RASMUSSEN & M. M. CLAYTON. 1987. Activation of the complement system in the adult respiratory distress syndrome. Am. Rev. Respir. Dis. **135:** 651–658.

31. LEE, C. T., et al. 1981. Elastolytic activity in pulmonary lavage fluid from patients with the adult respiratory distress syndrome. New Eng. J. Med. **304:** 192–196.

32. McGuire, W. W., R. G. Spragg, A. M. Cohen & C. G. Cochrane. 1982. Studies on the pathogenesis of the adult respiratory distress syndrome. J. Clin. Invest. **69:** 543–553.
33. Emmet, M., J. L. Miller & A. J. Crowle. 1987. Protein abnormalities in adult respiratory distress syndrome, tuberculosis and cystic fibrosis sera. Proc. Soc. Exp. Biol. Med. **184:** 74–82.
34. Cochrane, C. G., R. Spragg & S. D. Revak. 1983. Pathogenesis of the adult respiratory distress syndrome. Evidence of oxidant activity in brochoalveolar lavage fluid. J. Clin. Invest. **71:** 754–761.
35. Brantly, M., T. Nukiwa & R. G. Crystal. 1988. Molecular basis of alpha-1-antitrypsin deficiency. Am. J. Med. **84:** 13–31.
36. Klebanoff, S. J., et al. 1986. Stimulation of neutrophils by tumor necrosis factor. J. Immunol. **136:** 4220–4225.
37. Figari, S., N. A. Mori & M. A. Palladino, Jr. 1987. Regulation of neutrophil migration and superoxide production by recombinant tumor necrosis factor-α and -β: Comparison to a recombinant interferon-γ and interleukin-1α. Blood **70:** 979–984.
38. Berkow, R. L., D. Wang, J. W. Larrick, R. W. Dodson & T. H. Howard. 1987. Enhancement of the neutrophil superoxide production by preincubation with recombinant tumor necrosis factor. J. Immunol. **139:** 3783–3791.
39. Ferrante, A., M. Nandoskar, A. Waltz, D. H. B. Goh & I. C. Kowanko. 1988. Effects of tumor necrosis factor alpha and interleukin-1 alpha and beta on human neutrophil migration, respiratory burst and degranulation. Int. Arch Allergy Appl. Immunol. **86:** 82–91.
40. Atkinson, Y. H., W. A. Marasco, A. F. Lopez & M. A. Vadas. 1988. Recombinant human tumor necrosis factor-α. Regulation of N-formylmethionylleucylphenylalanine receptor affinity and function on human neutrophils. J. Clin. Invest. **81:** 759–765.
41. Ferrari-Baliviera, E., K. Mealy, R. J. Smith & D. W. Wilmore. 1989. Tumor necrosis factor induces adult respiratory distress syndrome in rats. Arch Surg. **124:** 1400–1405.
42. Millar, A. B., et al. 1989. Tumor necrosis factor in bronchopulmonary secretions of patients with adult respiratory distress syndrome. Lancet **2:** 712–714.
43. Roberts, D. J., et al. 1989. Tumor necrosis factor and adult respiratory distress syndrome. Am. Rev. Respir. Dis. **135:** 651–658.
44. Renesto, P. & M. Chignard. 1991. Tumor necrosis factor-α enhances platelet activation via cathepsin G released from neutrophils. J. Immunol. **146:** 2305–2309.
45. Brandt, E., F. Petersen & H.-D. Flad. 1992. Recombinant tumor necrosis factor-α potentiates neutrophil degranulation in response to host defense cytokines neutrophil-activating peptide 2 and IL-8 by modulating intracellular cyclic AMP levels. J. Immunol. **149:** 1356–1364.
46. Blick, M., S. A. Sherwin, M. Rosenblum & J. Gutterman. 1987. Phase I study of recombinant tumor necrosis factor in cancer patients. Cancer Res. **47:** 2986–2989.
47. Scuderi, P., P. A. Nez, M. L. Duerr, B. J. Wong & C. M. Vadez. 1991. Cathepsin-G and leukocyte elastase inactivate tumor necrosis factor and lymphotoxin. Cell. Immunol. **135:** 299–313.
48. Porteu, F., M. Brockhaus, D. Wallach, D. Engelmann & C. F. Nathan. 1991. Human neutrophil elastase releases a ligand-binding fragment from the 75-kDa tumor necrosis factor (TNF) receptor. Comparison with the proteolytic activity responsible for shedding of TNF receptors from stimulated neutrophils. J. Biol. Chem. **266:** 18846–18853.
49. Dinarello, C. A. 1992. Anti-cytokine strategies. Eur. Cytokine Network **31:** 7–17.
50. Suter, P. M., et al. 1992. High bronchoalveolar levels of tumor necrosis factor and its inhibitors, interleukin-1, interferon, and elastase, in patients with adult respiratory distress syndrome after trauma, shock, or sepsis. Am. Rev. Respir. Dis. **145:** 1016–1022.
51. Jacobs, R. F., D. R. Tabor, A. W. Burks & G. D. Campbell. 1989. Elevated interleukin-1 release by human alveolar macrophages during the adult respiratory distress syndrome. Am. Rev. Respir. Dis. **140:** 1686–1692.

52. CYBULSKY, M. I., H. Z. MOVAT & C. A. DINARELLO. 1987. Role of interleukin-1 and tumor necrosis factor-α in acute inflammation. Ann. Inst. Pasteur/Immunol. **138:** 505–516.

53. HAZUDA, D. J., J. STRICKLER, F. KUEPPERS, P. L. SIMON & P. R. YOUNG. 1990. Processing of precursor interleukin 1β and inflammatory disease. J. Biol. Chem. **265:** 6318–6322.

54. TODOROKI, N., et al. 1991. Enhancement by IL-1β and IFN-γ of platelet activation: Adhesion to leukocytes via GMP-140/PADGEM protein (CD 62). Biochem. Biophys. Res. Commun. **179:** 756–761.

55. MOLINAS, F. C., J. WIETZERBIN & E. FALCOFF. 1987. Human platelets possess receptors for a lymphokine: Demonstration of high specific receptors for HuIFN-γ. J. Immunol. **138:** 802–806.

56. SCHRÖDER, J.-M., U. MROWIETZ, E. MORITA & E. CHRISTOPHER. 1987. Purification and partial characterization of a human monocyte-derived, neutrophil-activating peptide that lacks interleukin 1 activity. J. Immunol. **139:** 3474–3483.

57. PEVERI, P., A. WALTZ, B. DEWALD & M. BAGGIOLINI. 1988. A novel neutrophil-activating factor produced by human mononuclear phagocytes. J. Exp. Med. **167:** 1547–1559.

58. MILLER, E. J., et al. 1992. Elevated levels of NAP-1/interleukin-8 are present in the airspace of patients with adult respiratory distress syndrome and are associated with increased mortality. Am. Rev. Respir. Dis. **146:** 427–432.

59. TORRE, D., et al. 1993. Levels of interleukin-8 in patients with adult respiratory distress syndrome. J. Infect. Dis. **167:** 505–506.

60. STRIETER, R. M., et al. 1990. Human neutrophils exhibit disparate chemotactic factor gene expression. Biochem. Biophys. Res. Commun. **173:** 725–730.

61. BAZZONI, F., et al. 1991. Phagocytosing neutrophils produce and release high amounts of neutrophil-activating peptide-1/interleukin 8. J. Exp. Med. **173:** 771–774.

62. FUJISHIMA, S., et al. 1993. Regulation of neutrophil interleukin 8 gene expression and protein secretion by LPS, TNF-α, and IL-1. J. Cell Physiol. **154:** 478–485.

63. WALTZ, A. & M. BAGGIOLINI. 1989. A novel cleavage product of β-thromboglobulin formed in cultures of stimulated mononuclear cells activates human neutrophils. Biochem. Biophys. Res. Commun. **159:** 969–975.

64. WALTZ, A., B. DEWALD, V. VON TSCHARNER & M. BAGGIOLINI. 1989. Effects of the neutrophil-activating peptide NAP-2, platelet basic protein, connective tissue-activating peptide III, and platelet factor 4 on human neutrophils. J. Exp. Med. **171:** 449–454.

65. WALTZ, A. & M. BAGGIOLINI. 1990. Generation of NAP-2 from platelet basic protein or connective tissue-activating peptide III through monocyte proteases. J. Exp. Med. **170:** 1745–1750.

66. WENGER, R. H., A. N. WICKI, A. WALTZ, N. KIEFFER & K. J. CLEMETSON. 1989. Cloning of cDNA for connective tissue activating peptide III from a human platelet-derived lambda gt11 expression library. Blood **73:** 1498–1503.

67. CAR, B. D., M. BAGGIOLINI & A. WALTZ. 1991. Formation of neutrophil-activating peptide 2 from platelet-derived connective tissue-activating peptide III by different tissue proteinases. Biochem. J. **275:** 581–584.

68. BRANDT, E., J. VAN DAMME & H.-D. FLAD. 1991. Neutrophils can generate their activator neutrophil-activating peptide 2 by proteolytic cleavage of platelet-derived connective tissue-activating peptide III. Cytokine **3:** 311–321.

69. COHEN, A. B., M. D. STEVENS, E. J. MILLER, M. A. ATKINSON & G. MULLENBACH. 1992. Generation of the neutrophil-activating peptide-2 by cathepsin G and cathepsin G-treated human platelets. Am. J. Physiol. **263:** L249–L256.

70. COHEN, A. B., et al. 1993. Neutrophil-activating peptide-2 in patients with pulmonary edema from congestive heart failure on ARDS. Am. J. Physiol. **264:** L490–L495.

71. MONTEFORT, S. & S. T. HOLGATE. 1991. Adhesion molecules and their role in inflammation. Respir. Med. **85:** 91–99.

72. WILLIAMS, T. J. & P. G. HELLEWELL. 1992. Adhesion molecules involved in the microvascular inflammatory response. Am. Rev. Respir. Dis. **146:** S45–S50.

73. HARLAN, J. M., P. D. KILLEN, A. HARKER, G. E. STRIKER, & D. G. WRIGHT. 1981. Neutrophil-mediated endothelial injury in vitro. Mechanism of cell detachment. J. Clin. Invest. **68:** 1394–1403.

74. VANDENBROUCKE-GRAULS, C. M. J. E., H. M. W. M. THIJSSEN, K. P. M. VAN KESSZEL, B. S. VAN ASBECK & J. VERHOEF. 1987. Injury to endothelial cells by phagocytosing polymorphonuclear leukocytes and modulatory role of lipoxygenase products. Infect. Immun. **55:** 1447–1454.

75. INAUEN, W., *et al.* 1990. Anoxia-reoxygenation-induced, neutrophil-mediated endothelial cell injury: Role of elastase. Am. J. Physiol. **259:** H925–H931.

76. SMEDLY, L. A., *et al.* 1986. Neutrophil-mediated injury to endothelial cells: Enhancement by endotoxin and essential role of neutrophil elastase. J. Clin. Invest. **77:** 1233–1243.

77. VARANI, J., *et al.* 1989. Endothelial cell killing by neutrophils. Synergistic interaction of oxygen products and proteases. Am. J. Pathol. **135:** 435–438.

78. HIEMSTRA, P. S., J. A. KRAMPS, T. M. DE VREEDE, F. C. BREEVELD & M. R. DAHA. 1991. Inhibition of polymorphonuclear leukocyte-mediated endothelial cell detachment by antileukoprotease: A comparison with other proteinase inhibitors. Immunobiology **182:** 117–126.

79. CHIGNARD, M., V. BALLOY & P. RENESTO. 1993. Leucocyte elastase-mediated release of von Willebrand factor from cultured endothelial cells. Eur. Respir. J. **6:** 791–796.

80. RUBIN, D. B., J. P. WIENER-KRONSNISH & J. F. MURRAY. 1990. Elevated von Willebrand antigen is an early plasma predictor of acute lung injury in nonpulmonary sepsis syndrome. J. Clin. Invest. **86:** 474–480.

81. PETERSON, M. W., P. STONE & D. M. SHASBY. 1987. Cationic neutrophil proteins increase transendothelial albumin movement. J. Appl. Physiol. **62:** 1521–1530.

82. PETERSON, M. W. 1989. Neutrophil cathepsin G increases transendothelial albumin flux. J. Lab. Clin. Med. **113:** 297–308.

83. REPINE, J. E. 1992. Scientific perspectives on adult respiratory distress syndrome. Lancet **339:** 466–469.

84. FLICK, M. R. 1986. Mechanism of acute lung injury: What have we learned from experimental animal models? Clin. Care Clin. **2:** 455–470.

85. ODA, M., K. SATOUCHI, K. YASUNAGA & K. SAITO. 1986. Polymorphonuclear leukocyte-platelet interactions: Acetylglyceryl ether phosphocholine-induced platelet activation under stimulation with chemotactic peptide. J. Biochem. **100:** 1117–1123.

86. COEFFIER, E., D. JOSEPH, M. C. PREVOST & B. B. VARGAFTIG. 1987. Platelet-leukocyte interaction: Activation of rabbit platelets by fMLP-stimulated neutrophils. Br. J. Pharmacol. **92:** 393–406.

87. OLSSON, I. & P. VENGE. 1980. The role of the human neutrophils in the inflammatory reaction. Allergy **35:** 1–13.

88. VIRCA, G. D., G. METZ & H. P. SCHNEBLI. 1984. Similarities between human and rat leukocyte elastase and cathepsin G. Eur. J. Biochem. **144:** 92–100.

89. TAKEUCHI, K., H. WOOD & R. T. SWANK. 1986. Lysosomal elastase and cathepsin G in beige mice. Neutrophils of beige (Chediak-Higashi) mice selectively lack lysosomal elastase and cathepsin G. J. Exp. Med. **163:** 665–677.

90. TAKEUCHI, K. & R. T. SWANK. 1989. Inhibitors of elastase and cathepsin G in Chediak-Higashi (Beige) neutrophils. J. Biol. Chem. **264:** 7431–7436.

91. STARCHER, B. & I. WILLIAMS. 1989. The beige mouse: Role of neutrophil elastase in the development of pulmonary emphysema. Exp. Lung Res. **15:** 785–800.

92. CHRISTIAN, J. W. 1992. Potential treatment of sepsis syndrome with cytokine-specific agents. Chest **102:** 613–617.

Modulation of IL-1 Receptor Antagonist and TNF-Soluble Receptors Produced by Alveolar Macrophages and Blood Monocytes

L. P. NICOD,[a] B. GALVE-DE-ROCHEMONTEIX,[b]
AND J. M. DAYER[b]

[a]Division of Respiratory Diseases
University Hospital
Geneva, Switzerland

[b]Division of Immunology and Allergy
University Hospital
Geneva, Switzerland

INTRODUCTION

Alveolar macrophages (AMs) can release inflammatory mediators such as interleukin-1α (IL-1α), β, or tumor necrosis factor-α (TNFα) in the alveoli and into the airways. AMs not only produce an IL-1 inhibitor that acts as a receptor antagonist,[1,2] they also release TNF inhibitors that are TNF-soluble receptors that inactivate the ligand, and thus up- or downregulating immune and inflammatory processes. The final biological result depends on the relative amount of proinflammatory cytokines and their respective inhibitors produced. The nature of these inhibitory substances and some aspects of the regulation of their production are reviewed in the following.

MODULATION OF IL-1RA, IL-1α, AND IL-1β

There are two biochemically distinct, but structurally related forms of interleukin-1: IL-1α and IL-1β. Both play an important role in inflammatory processes, cell growth, activation of immunocompetent cells, and both induce a wide range of hematologic and metabolic responses.[3] Cloning of cDNA of IL-1α and IL-1β[4,5] led to studies that have shed light on the mechanisms of gene expression.[3] The regulation of IL-1 activity is dependent on the presence of IL-1 receptors on target cells[6,7] and soluble inhibitors. Such an inhibitor was originally found in the urine of patients with monocytic leukemia, febrile patients, children with juvenile rheumatoid arthritis,[8,9] and *in vitro* in the supernatant of human monocytes stimulated with immune complexes.[10] By competing with IL-1 for its receptor,[11] the inhibitor counteracts recombinant human (rh) IL-1α and β in the lymphocyte-activating factor assay (IL-1/LAF), the mononuclear cell factor assay (IL-1/MCF) as assessed by the production of prostaglandin E_2 (PGE_2) and collagenase by synovial cells or dermal fibroblasts,[12] and it blocks the effect of rhIL-1 on Ca^{2+} release from fetal bone.[13] Since the IL-1 receptor antagonist (IL-1Ra) has been purified to homogeneity,[14] cloned,[15] and expressed, the understanding of regulation and functions has rapidly progressed.

IL-1Ra is a polypeptide of 17-kD and has 26 percent identity with IL-1β and 19 percent identity with IL-1α.[15,16] IL-1Ra apparently has no agonist activity, but inhibits the functions induced by both IL-1α and IL-1β. IL-1Ra produced in the supernatant of AMs after 48 hours in culture was analyzed by Western blot.[17] A single band around 20–22 kD was observed, slightly higher than the unglycosylated rhIL-1Ra that migrates around 17 kD. IgG-stimulated monocytes also produce an IL-1Ra of 22 kD. N-Glycanase digestion yields a molecule of 17 kD. This confirms that monocytes do produce glycosylated IL-1Ra as well as an unglycosylated form.[18] Northern blot performed on the RNA extract of six different preparations of AM within 1 hour after bronchoalveolar lavage did not reveal any basal expression of IL-1Ra mRNA.[17] However, when AMs were cultured on plastic dishes in a medium containing fetal calf serum, they became active and the presence of IL-1Ra mRNA was observed after 3 hours.[17] After 12 and 24 hours of culture, the steady-state level of IL-1 mRNA was decreased. The signal obtained after stimulation with phorbol myristate acetate (PMA) was much higher than with the medium alone. When AMs were simultaneously analyzed for the expression of IL-1α and IL-1β mRNA, both were detectable after as little as 15 minutes and both reached a peak at 3 hours. The level of IL-1α mRNA declined after 8 hours and was barely detectable after 24 hours. The kinetics of IL-1β mRNA expression were similar to those of IL-1α, but with weaker intensity. *In vitro,* the kinetics of production reveal that IL-1Ra, IL-1α, and IL-1β mRNA in the presence or absence of PMA are already expressed after 15 minutes, whereas the expression of IL-1Ra mRNA is slightly delayed and detected after 3 hours.[17] To induce IL-1Ra mRNA in peripheral blood monocytes after 4 hours of culture, medium conditions containing serum alone is not sufficient and a second signal is required, such as from IgG or IL-4.[18]

In studying the kinetics of secreted and cell-associated IL-1Ra protein, high concentrations of cell-associated IL-1Ra were found in freshly isolated AMs. Thus, when AMs of 14 subjects were analyzed for cell-associated IL-1Ra immediately after bronchoalveolar lavage (BAL); an average of 2.0 ± 0.5 ng/ml of IL-1Ra was found from 10^6 lysed AM/ml, whereas concentrations of cell-associated IL-1α and β were, respectively, 25- and 100-fold lower. In culture the amount of cell-associated IL-1Ra doubled after 8 hours and remained at this level for up to 24 hours.

IL-1Ra was released in traces in the supernatant after 3 hours, reaching 5 ng/ml after 8 hours and 12 ng/ml after 24 hours. Addition of LPS (10 μg/ml) did not markedly modify the amounts produced by AM in comparison with unstimulated conditions. After 8 hours the amount of secreted IL-1Ra was increased 2-fold, but it reached the same level as AM culture in the absence of lipopolysaccharide (LPS) after 24 hours. LPS did not modify significantly the amount of cell-associated IL-1Ra. The effect of LPS stimulation was most pronounced on IL-1β, with a 10-fold increase in production after 24 hours, whereas IL-1α release was enhanced 5-fold; ultimately, the total amounts of the two cytokines were similar. The concentration of IL-1α and β measured in the supernatants after LPS stimulation remained half of that of IL-1Ra measured after 24 hours with or without LPS.

Different cytokines were assessed as to their effect on the production of IL-1Ra by AMs. IL-4 induced a dose-dependent increase of IL-1Ra without affecting IL-1 production.[17,18] In order to demonstrate the specificity of this induction, IL-4-induced production of IL-1Ra was blocked by a specific antibody to IL-4. Regarding interferon-γ (IFN-γ) and granulocyte-macrophage colony stimulating factor

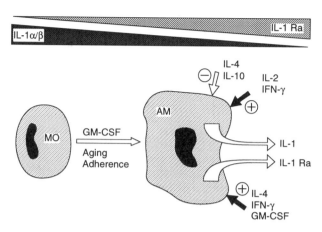

FIGURE 1. Effect of cytokines on the production of IL-1α, β, and IL-1Ra by MOs or AMs.

(GM–CSF), they enhanced the production of both IL-1Ra and IL-1α. Addition of IL-2 led to a significant increase of IL-1α production, but not of IL-1Ra. The effect of these cytokines on IL-1Ra mRNA expression was analyzed by Northern blot analysis. A slight increase of IL-1Ra mRNA (150 percent increase by optical density) was observed only in AM cultured with IL-4. This slight increase as compared to a tenfold increase in IL-1Ra, suggests that posttranscriptional factors may also be involved in the effect of IL-4 on AMs. The effect of cytokines on IL-1Ra and IL-1α or β is summarized in FIGURE 1.

AMs produce considerably less IL-1β than their precursors, the peripheral blood monocytes, and release less IL-1β in response to LPS.[19,20] But human AMs contain significant amounts of cell-associated IL-1Ra and produce it in much larger amounts than IL-1α and IL-1β.[17] Peripheral blood monocytes, on the contrary, produce little IL-1Ra before maturation induced by GM–CSF or specific stimuli such as IgG. Indeed, when monocytes mature into macrophages, IL-1β secretion is downregulated and IL-1Ra is favored due to a higher expression of its mRNA.[19] IL-1Ra production is increased by immune cells in the presence of IL-4 and to a smaller extent in that of IFN-γ and GM–CSF. AMs are the most important mononuclear population residing in the lung. Considering their ability to release preformed IL-1Ra or to produce it in large amounts after a certain delay, they are likely to play a crucial role in the homeostasis in the alveoli in that they neutralize locally the effects of IL-1. IL-1Ra has been measured in normal BAL fluid of four specimens with a range of 35 and 560 pg/ml.[18] In the event of endogenous or exogenous stimuli, however, AMs keep their capacity to trigger inflammatory processes by the rapid release of newly formed IL-1. While the anti-inflammatory role of IL-1Ra has been clearly demonstrated, we failed to find any evidence of antigen presentation or allogeneic reaction being affected by IL-1Ra.[21] This could be due to the fact that the occupancy of a few IL-1 receptors is sufficient to provide a second signal, or that molecules other than IL-1 can have the same effect.

EXPRESSION AND RELEASE OF TNF INHIBITORS

Tumor necrosis factor (TNF) was originally discovered as a serum protein with a necrotizing effect *in vivo* on certain transplantable mouse tumors[22] and with cytotoxic effects *in vitro* on some transformed cells.[23]

TNF is mainly produced by activated macrophages and lymphocytes, but also by mast cells and neutrophils.[23] It is now considered a pleiotropic cytokine/lymphokine with regulatory functions in immune and inflammatory reactions.[24] X-ray diffraction studies showed TNFα to be a tightly packed trimer.[25] TNFβ is 28 percent homologous with TNFα,[26] and competes with TNFα for cellular (TNF) binding sites.[27] Two types of TNF-R, type I (55 kD) and type II (75 kD), have been isolated in humans and their genes have been cloned.[28,29] Analysis of the extracellular domains of these receptors has revealed a pattern of cystein-rich repeats shared with the nerve growth factor. In contrast, the two TNF-R show no apparent similarity in their cytoplasmic portions, which suggests that they use different signaling mechanisms. Both types I and II TNF-R bind to TNFα and TNFβ with similar affinities,[30,31] but appear to mediate different functions. Human polymorphonuclear neutrophils (PMN), monocytes, and murine macrophages possess 500–2000 plasma membrane TNF binding sites per cell. The type I receptor is a 55-kD molecule that is expressed preferentially on T cells, fibroblasts, and cells of epithelial origin, whereas the 75-kD type II receptor is more abundant on B cells.[32,33]

Soluble TNF-binding proteins have been isolated from the urine of normal[34] and febrile individuals[35] and the sera of patients undergoing hemodialysis.[36] These soon proved to consist of TNF-R I and II, shed from blood white cells and probably other cells.[35,37] This notion was supported by the absence of transcript encoding for soluble forms of these receptors, suggesting that shedding of TNF-R results from proteolysis of their extracellular domains.

The balance between the production of TNFα and its inhibitors was studied on human AMs in the presence of PMA, LPS, or cytokines. Human AMs are capable of an enhanced production of TNFα contrary to blood monocytes.[38] The shedding of TNF-sR may be crucial in maintaining the alveoli free of deleterious inflammatory processes. The presence of TNF-inhibitor in the supernatant of AM

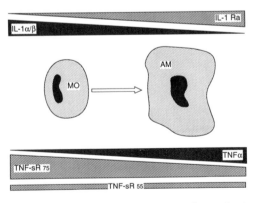

FIGURE 2. Effect of monocyte maturation into AMs on the production of IL-1Ra, TNF-soluble receptors (TNF-sR 55 and TNF-sR 75), and TNFα.

has been previously reported.[1] The link between this inhibitory activity and the shedding of TNF-R by AMs has been shown by using a specific immunoassay measuring the two soluble fragments of TNF-R (TNF-sR), as previously described.[39] After 48 hours in culture AMs each released similar amounts of each TNF-sR. In the presence of PMA or LPS the shedding of TNF-sR 55 was increased by 30 percent with the former and remained unchanged with the latter. TNF-sR 75 was more than doubled with PMA, but insignificantly increased with LPS.[40] The shedding of TNF-sR 75 from AMs and monocytes, respectively, was 4- and 5-fold higher than TNF-sR 55 after 48 hours of stimulation with PMA. TNF-sR 75 is released earlier from monocytes than from AMs, and in an amount that after 24 hours was twice as high as AMs. TNFα released from AMs was 2- to 3-fold more abundant than from monocytes (MOs). The relative proportion of TNFα and TNF-sR 75 or TNF-sR 55 produced by AMs versus MOs are schematized in FIGURE 2. In order to better understand the modulation of TNF-sR release, the expression of TNF-R mRNA was studied in AMs in the presence of LPS and PMA. LPS had no influence on TNF-R 55 or TNF-R 75 expression, whereas PMA increased both mRNAs. Thus, PMA increases both production and release of TNF-R mRNA. LPS has no influence on the expression of the TNF receptors, but in animal models it increases their internalization.[41] If this were to apply to human AMs or MOs, it would be easier to understand why the shedding of TNF receptors tends to be decreased or unchanged in the presence of LPS.

Of the cytokines analyzed, IFN-γ was the only one to increase the shedding of TNF-sR 55 (2-fold) and of TNF-sR 75 (3-fold) from both human MOs or AMs. Incubation of murine macrophages with 1 ng/ml of recombinant IFN-γ at 37°C for 18 hours led to a 2- to 3-fold increase in labeled TNFα binding.[23] If this observation can be extended to human monocytes or macrophages, IFN-γ would also increase the production as well as the shedding of TNF-Rs. The mechanisms controlling TNF-R shedding have not been elucidated. During the course of a study aimed at localizing the proteases involved in TNF-R shedding by activated PMN after a Percoll gradient, the activity was found in the azurophil granules. This activity was identified as elastase,[42] which acts on TNF-sR 75 but has no effect on TNF-sR 55. Thus, other enzymes are likely to be involved in the shedding of TNF-R.

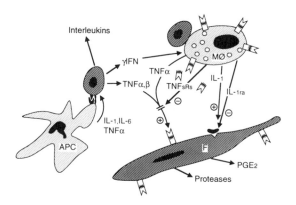

FIGURE 3. Immune and inflammatory cascade of events relative with IL-1 and TNFα and their respective inhibitors.

CONCLUSIONS

Overall, human MOs or AMs are a major source of IL-1α, IL-1β, and TNFα, although the differentiation of MOs into AMs changes their capacity to release them. At the same time MOs and AMs are capable of releasing inhibitors for these cytokines, the production of which is also influenced by the differentiation maturation process (FIG. 2). The balance or imbalance between these cytokines and their inhibitors can considerably affect the inflammatory cascade (FIG. 3). The precise regulatory processes remain to be explored in depth.

REFERENCES

1. GALVE-DE-ROCHEMONTEIX, B., A. F. JUNOD & J.-M. DAYER. 1990. Fibroblast-alveolar cell interactions in sarcoidosis and idiopathic pulmonary fibrosis: Evidence for stimulatory and inhibitory cytokine production by alveolar cells. Eur. Respir. J. **3:** 653–664.
2. GALVE-DE-ROCHEMONTEIX, B., L. P. NICOD, A. F. JUNOD & J.-M. DAYER. 1990. Characterization of a specific 20- to 25-kD interleukin-1 inhibitor from cultured human lung macrophages. Am. J. Respir. Cell Mol. Biol. **3:** 355–361.
3. DINARELLO, C. A. 1991. Interleukin-1 and Interleukin-1 antagonism. Blood **77:** 1627–1652.
4. AURON, P. E., et al. 1984. Nucleotide sequence of human monocyte interleukin-1 precursor cDNA. Proc. Natl. Acad. Sci. U.S.A. **81:** 7909–7911.
5. WINGFIELD, P., et al. 1986. Purification and characterization of human interleukin-1β expressed in recombinant Escherichia coli. Eur. J. Biochem. **160:** 491–497.
6. CHIZZONITE, R., et al. 1989. Two high-affinity interleukin 1 receptors represent separate gene products. Proc. Natl. Acad. Sci. U.S.A. **86:** 8029–8033.
7. BOMSZTYK, K., et al. 1989. Evidence for different interleukin 1 receptors in murine B- and T-cell lines. Proc. Natl. Acad. Sci. U.S.A. **86:** 8034–8038.
8. BALAVOINE, J.-F., et al. 1986. Prostaglandin E$_2$ and collagenase production by fibroblasts and synovial cells is regulated by urine-derived human interleukin 1 and inhibitor(s). J. Clin. Invest. **78:** 1120–1124.
9. PRIEUR, A. M., M. T. KAUFMANN, C. GRISCELLI & J.-M. DAYER. 1987. Specific interleukin-1 inhibitor in serum and urine of children with systemic juvenile chronic arthritis. Lancet **II:** 1240–1242.
10. AREND, W. P., F. J. JOSLIN & R. J. MASONI. 1985. Effects of immune complexes on production by human monocytes of interleukin 1 or interleukin 1 inhibitor. J. Immunol. **134:** 3868–3875.
11. SECKINGER, P., J. W. LOWENTHAL, K. WILLIAMSON, J.-M. DAYER & H. R. MACDONALD. 1987. A urine inhibitor of interleukin 1 activity that blocks ligand binding. J. Immunol. **139:** 1546–1549.
12. SECKINGER, P., et al. 1987. A urine inhibitor of interleukin 1 activity affects both interleukin 1α and 1β but not tumor necrosis factor. J. Immunol. **139:** 1541–1545.
13. SECKINGER, P., et al. 1990. Natural and recombinant human interleukin-1 receptor antagonists block the effects of interleukin-1 on bone resorption and prostaglandin production. J. Immunol. **45:** 4181–4184.
14. HANNUM, C. H., et al. 1990. Interleukin-1 receptor antagonist activity of a human interleukin-1 inhibitor. Nature (London) **343:** 336–340.
15. EISENBERG, S. P., et al. 1990. Primary structure and functional expression from complementary DNA of a human interleukin-1 receptor antagonist. Nature (London) **343:** 341–346.
16. CARTER, D. B., et al. 1990. Purification, cloning, expression and biological characterization of an interleukin-1 receptor antagonist protein. Nature (London) **344:** 633–638.
17. GALVE-DE-ROCHEMONTEIX, B., et al. 1993. Regulation of interleukin-1Ra, interleukin-1α, and interleukin-1β production by human alveolar macrophages with phorbol

myristate acetate, lipopolysaccharide, and interleukin-4. Am. J. Respir. Cell Mol. Biol. **8:** 160–168.

18. MOORE, S. A., *et al.* 1992. Expression and regulation of human alveolar macrophage-derived interleukin-1 receptor antagonist. Am. J. Respir. Cell Mol. Biol. **6:** 569–575.

19. ROUX-LOMBARD, P., C. MODOUX & J.-M. DAYER. 1989. Production of interleukin-1 (IL-1) and a specific IL-1 inhibitor during human monocyte-macrophage differentiation: Influence of GM-CSF. Cytokine **1:** 45–51.

20. WEWERS, M. D. & D. J. HERZYK. 1989. Alveolar macrophages differ from blood monocytes in human IL-1β release. J. Immunol. **143:** 1635–1641.

21. NICOD, L. P., F. EL HABRE & J.-M. DAYER. 1992. Natural and recombinant interleukin-1 receptor antagonist does not inhibit human T-cell proliferation induced by mitogens, soluble antigens or allogeneic determinants. Cytokine **4:** 29–35.

22. CARSWELL, E. A., *et al.* 1975. An endotoxin-induced serum factor that causes necrosis of tumors. Proc. Natl. Acad. Sci. U.S.A. **72:** 3666–3670.

23. DING, A. H. & F. PORTEU. 1992. Regulation of tumor necrosis factor receptors on phagocytes. Proc. Soc. Exp. Biol. Med. **200:** 458–465.

24. BEUTLER, B. & A. CERAMI. 1989. The biology of cachectin/TNF—A primary mediator of the host response. Ann. Rev. Immunol. **7:** 625–655.

25. JONES, E. Y., D. I. STUART & N. P. C. WALKER. 1989. Structure of tumour necrosis factor. Nature (London) **338:** 225–228.

26. PENNICA, D., *et al.* 1984. Human tumour necrosis factor: Precursor structure, expression and homology to lymphotoxin. Nature (London) **312:** 724–729.

27. STAUBER, G. B. & B. B. AGGARWAL. 1989. Characterization and affinity cross-linking of receptors for human recombinant lymphotoxin (tumor necrosis factor-β) on a human histiocytic lymphoma cell line, U-937. J. Biol. Chem. **264:** 3573–3576.

28. LOETSCHER, H., *et al.* 1990. Molecular cloning and expression of the human 55 kD tumor necrosis factor receptor. Cell **61:** 351–359.

29. SCHALL, T. J., *et al.* 1990. Molecular cloning and expression of a receptor for human tumor necrosis factor. Cell **61:** 361–370.

30. SMITH, C. A., *et al.* 1990. A receptor for tumor necrosis factor defines an unusual family of cellular and viral proteins. Science **248:** 1019–1023.

31. DEMBIE, Z., *et al.* 1990. Two human TNF receptors have similar extracellular, but distinct intracellular domain sequences. Cytokine **2:** 231–237.

32. ERIKSTEIN, B. K., *et al.* 1991. Independent regulation of 55-kDa and 75-kDa tumor necrosis factor receptors during activation of human peripheral blood B lymphocytes. Eur. J. Immunol. **21:** 1033–1037.

33. BROCKHAUS, M., *et al.* 1990. Identification of two types of tumor necrosis factor receptors on human cell lines by monoclonal antibodies. Proc. Natl. Acad. Sci. U.S.A. **87:** 3127–3131.

34. SECKINGER, PH., S. ISAAZ & J.-M. DAYER. 1988. A human inhibitor of tumor necrosis factor. J. Exp. Med. **167:** 1511–1516.

35. ENGELMANN, H., D. NOVICK & D. WALLACH. 1990. Two tumor necrosis factor-binding proteins purified from human urine: Evidence for immunological cross-reactivity with cell surface tumor necrosis factor receptors. J. Biol. Chem. **265:** 1531–1536.

36. PEETRE, C., H. THYSELL, A. GRUBB & I. OLSSON. 1988. A tumor necrosis factor binding protein is present in human biological fluids. Eur. J. Haematol. **41:** 414–419.

37. SECKINGER, PH., J. H. ZHANG, B. HAUPTMANN & J.-M. DAYER. 1990. Characterization of a tumor necrosis factor α (TNF-α) inhibitor: Evidence of immunological cross-reactivity with the TNF receptor. Proc. Natl. Acad. Sci. U.S.A. **87:** 5188–5192.

38. BACHWICH, P. R., J. P. LYNCH, J. LARRICK, M. SPENGLER & S. KUNKEL. 1986. Tumor necrosis factor production by human sarcoid alveolar macrophages. Am. J. Pathol. **125:** 421–425.

39. GIRARDIN, E., *et al.* 1992. Imbalance between tumor necrosis factor α and soluble TNF receptor concentrations in severe meningo-coccaemia. Immunology **76:** 20–23.

40. GALVE-DE-ROCHEMONTEIX, B., L. P. NICOD & J.-M. DAYER. Modulation of the expression and release of TNF-soluble receptors (TNF-sR) on human alveolar macrophages (AM) and monocytes (Mo). Eur. Respir. J. In press.

41. DING, A. H., E. SANCHEZ, S. SRIMAL & C. F. NATHAN. 1989. Macrophages rapidly internalize their tumor necrosis factor receptors in response to bacterial lipopolysaccharide. J. Biol. Chem. **264:** 3924–3929.
42. PORTEU, F., M. BROCKHAUS, D. WALLACH, H. ENGELMANN & C. F. NATHAN. 1991. Human neutrophil elastase releases a ligand-binding fragment from the 75-kDa tumor necrosis factor TNF receptor. Comparison with the proteolytic activity responsible for shedding of TNF receptor from stimulated neutrophils. J. Biol. Chem. **266:** 18846–18853.

Cells and Cytokines in Chronic Bronchial Infection

JORG ELLER,[a] JOSÉ R. LAPA E SILVA,[b]
LEONARD W. POULTER,[c] HARTMUT LODE,[a]
AND PETER J. COLE[d,e]

[a]Section of Infection and Immunology
Department of Pulmonology I
Krankenhaus Zehlendorf
Berlin, Germany

[b]Serviço de Pneumologia
Hospital Universitario Clementino Fraga Filmo
Federal University of Rio de Janeiro
Rio de Janeiro, Brazil

[c]Academic Department of Clinical Immunology
Royal Free Hospital School of Medicine
London, United Kingdom

[d]Host Defence Unit
Department of Thoracic Medicine
Royal Brompton National Heart & Lung Institute
Manresa Road
London SW3 6LR, United Kingdom

INTRODUCTION

Bronchiectasis is a chronic pulmonary disease with irreversible dilatation of one or more bronchi.[1] It is usually associated with chronic production of purulent infected sputum. Although a classic treatise on the histology of bronchiectasis was written 40 years ago,[2] it is only recently that the cellular immune response within the bronchial wall has been demonstrated.[3]

The pathogenesis of bronchiectasis is still not entirely clear. It has been proposed that initially a genetic and/or environmental impairment of mucus clearance[1,4,5] allows microorganisms to persist sufficiently long in the bronchial tree to establish themselves and produce exotoxins.[4,6,7] Their persistence in a normally sterile site stimulates an inflammatory response that fails to eliminate the bacteria but causes "innocent bystander" lung damage, leading to a "vicious circle" of events. Part of this inflammatory response is a considerable traffic of neutrophils to the lumen of the affected bronchial tree,[8] neutrophils rarely being found in healthy bronchial tissue or lumen. Because of their potential for damaging tissue,[9,10] these neutrophils may be the most significant component of the inflammatory response. The neutrophil influx is probably initiated by chemoattractant factors, which may be of bacterial[11] or host origin (e.g., complement components).[12]

---

[e] To whom correspondence should be addressed.

We have investigated the cellular immune component of the bronchial inflammatory response and the possibility that chemoattractant cytokines are produced during infective exacerbations of bronchiectasis. We have also determined the effect of antibiotic therapy on cytokine production.

METHODS

Investigation of the Cellular Component of the Chronic Inflammatory Infiltrate in Bronchiectasis

Patients

The aim of this study was to identify, by means of immunohistochemical techniques and a panel of monoclonal antibodies, the cells and their subsets present in the bronchial lesions of bronchiectasis and to determine whether the expression of activation markers can be demonstrated in the pathology of the disease. Twenty-two patients with bronchiectasis were included in this study. Bronchial specimens were obtained either from resected lobes/lungs of patients with localized bronchiectasis or by fiberoptic bronchoscopy of consecutive patients presenting with

TABLE 1. Clinical Details of Patients Included in the Investigation of the Bronchial Cellular Infiltration in Bronchiectasis

		Bronchiectasis ($n = 22$)	Controls ($n = 11$)
Age:		40.8 ± 14.7	57.0 ± 15.8
		%	%
Sex:	Male	27.3	45.5
	Female	72.7	54.5
Smoking:	Smokers	12.5	40
	Nonsmokers	75	40
	Exsmokers	12.5	20
Sampling:	Surgical	81.2	72.7
	Endoscopy	18.2	27.3
Area:	LLL	50	27.2
	RLL	13.3	36.4
	RUL	—	36.4
	Others	36.7	—
Aetiology:	Idiopathic	77.5	—
	Primary ciliary disk	4.5	—
	Cystic fibrosis	4.5	—
	ABPA[a]	9.0	—
	Foreign body	4.5	—
	Cancer	—	72.7
	Pneumonia	—	27.7
Imaging:	Cylindrical	63.6	—
	Saccular	18.2	—
	Mixed	18.2	—
Pathology:	Follicular	45.5	—
	Nonfollicular	55.5	—

[a] Allergic bronchopulmonary aspergillosis.

TABLE 2. Panel of Monoclonal Antibodies Employed in the Research

CD	Name	Specificity	Source	Reference
3	UCHT1	All T-cells	UCH	13
4	Leu3a	Helper/inducer T-cells	BD	14
8	RFT8	Suppressor/cytotoxic T-cells	RFH	15
7	RFT2	T-cell blasts	RFH	15
57	Leu7a	Natural killer cells	BD	16
22	RFBx	All B-cells	RFH	17
—	RFD6	Plasma cells	RFH	18
—	RFD1	Dendritic cells	RFH	19
—	RFD7	Mature macrophages	RFH	19
—	UCHM1	Monocytes	UCH	20
25	RFT5	Interleukin-2 receptor	RFH	21
—	RFDR2	MHC Class II	RFH	22
38	RFD10	Activated T/B-cells	RFH	23
45 RA	SN130	Virgin T-cells	RFH	24
45RO	UCHL1	Primed T-cells	UCH	25

Note: RFH = Royal Free Hospital, London, UK; UCH = University College Hospital, London, UK; BD = Becton Dickinson, Oxford, UK.

diffuse disease. Eleven control patients were also included. All patients gave informed written consent before the procedures and the study had the approval of the Ethics Committee of the Royal Brompton National Heart & Lung Hospital. The relevant clinical details are summarized in TABLE 1.

Handling of Samples

Resected lobes were dissected and macroscopically visible areas of bronchiectasis chosen. In the controls, most of them presenting with lung cancer, a bronchus away from the tumour was selected. Rings of bronchi of 0.5 cm were cut, placed in round cork disks, and covered with Tissue-Tek OCT (Miles, Illinois). A similar procedure was employed for endoscopic bronchial biopsies (at least five fragments). The cork disks were immersed in isopentane cooled by liquid nitrogen and stored at −70°C until use. Cryostat sections were placed on slides previously coated with poly-*l*-lysine (Sigma, St. Louis, Missouri), dried at room temperature, and fixed in chloroform-acetone. The slides were wrapped in cling film and stored at −20°C until use. Representative sections of each block were stained for conventional histology. Tonsil sections were used as positive controls for the immunohistochemical reactions.

Immunohistochemistry

Indirect immunoperoxidase was employed, using as first-step mouse antihuman monoclonal antibodies (TABLE 2),[13–25] followed by horseradish peroxidase conjugated to rabbit antimouse immunoglobulin (P161, Dakopatts, Copenhagen, Denmark) and by development with 3,3′-diaminobenzidine (Sigma) and hydrogen peroxide. Light haematoxylin counterstaining was performed and the sections dehydrated through graded alcohols, cleared with xylene, and mounted with DPX.

Indirect two-color immunofluorescence was used to study coexpression of different epitopes by a given cell. Monoclonal antibodies of different isotypes were employed, followed by a combination of goat antimouse IgM conjugated to TRITC and IgG-FITC (SBA, Alabama). The slides were examined under a Zeiss epifluorescence microscope equipped with filters for TRITC and FITC.

Quantitation and Statistics

The quantitation of the immunoperoxidase positive cells was performed in the bronchial lamina propria, between the epithelial basement membrane and the muscle coat, using an image analysis system (Seescan, Cambridge, UK). The results were expressed as number of positive cells per unit area (10^4 μ^2). The quantitation of immunofluorescence positive cells was performed by counting 150 cells and, by changing the filters, verifying which cells coexpressed the markers studied. The results were expressed as the percent of double-positive cells.

Results for each parameter analyzed were compared between bronchiectasis and controls, using the Mann-Whitney two-sample rank test. Results were considered statistically significant when $p < 0.05$.

Investigation of Cytokine Levels in Patients with Bronchiectasis

Patients

Twelve consecutive patients with acute infective exacerbations of radiologically proven bronchiectasis were recruited for this study. Seven were females, five males, and the age range was 21 to 64 years (mean $\pm$ SEM 47 $\pm$ 3.4). Ten patients were nonsmokers and two had stopped smoking 1 to 2 years previously. Spirometry was (% predicted $\pm$ SEM): FEV_1 63 $\pm$ 9%, FVC 79 $\pm$ 8%, FEV_1/ FVC 65 $\pm$ 7%, RV 113 $\pm$ 9%. Seven patients were admitted to hospital and five treated in the outpatient department. One patient had associated panhypogammaglobulinemia, one α1-antitrypsin deficiency, and one rheumatoid arthritis. Three patients had undergone previous surgical treatment for bronchiectasis and one had undergone decortication of an empyema. An acute infective exacerbation was defined by deterioration in symptoms (increase of sputum volume and sputum purulence). Seven patients received antibiotics intravenously for 10 days (four patients: piperacillin and gentamicin; two patients: imipenen and tobramycin; one patient: cefuroxime and gentamicin). Five patients received oral antibiotics for 4 to 6 weeks (two patients: amoxycillin/clavulanic acid; one patient: ciprofloxacin; one patient: cefuroxime axetil; one patient: cefaclor). Additional therapy on a continuous basis was as follows: all patients performed their own postural drainage, 10 patients received inhaled corticosteroids, 12 inhaled β1-sympathomimetics, two systemic corticosteroids, two prophylactic oral antibiotics, one prophylactic nebulized antibiotics and one theophylline.

The patients were divided into three groups: in Group I: interleukin-1α (IL-1α) and tumor necrosis factor-α (TNF-α), and in group II: IL-8 was measured before and at the end of antibiotic treatment. In Group III: IL-8 concentrations were determined at the end of and 2 weeks after antibiotic treatment.

Sputum

Sputum was obtained from each patient before, at the end of, and in six patients at least 2 weeks after antibiotic therapy. Sputum samples were collected during morning physiotherapy in sterile sputum pots. Sputum volume was measured and percentage sputum purulence was estimated. Sputum cell counts: after diluting with phosphate-buffered saline (PBS) and staining with crystal violet, cells were counted in a haemocytometer. Sol phase production: centrifugation at 20,000 rpm for 30 minutes produced sol phase, and this was diluted with 500 μmol of the proteinase inhibitor phenylmethylsulphonylfluoride (PMSF; Sigma)[26] aliquoted and stored at $-70°C$ until use. In addition, sputum sol phase was diluted $1:10$ and $1:300$ in PBS for measurements of IL-8.

Plasma

Ethylenediaminetetraacetic acid (EDTA) blood samples were obtained from each patient before and at the end of antibiotic treatment for a full blood count. In addition EDTA blood was taken from 6 healthy volunteers. Blood was centrifuged at 1000 rpm for 10 minutes, plasma aliquoted, and stored at $-70°C$ until use.

Determination of Cytokines

IL-1α, TNF-α, and IL-8 concentrations were measured in sputum sol phase and plasma using a quantitative "sandwich" enzyme-linked immunoabsorbent assay (ELISA) technique (Amersham International, Amersham, UK). Briefly, samples were added to a 96-well plate coated with one of the cytokines to be measured. After incubating for 2 hours at room temperatures the samples were removed and washed three times with buffer in order to remove all unbound protein. An enzyme-linked antibody specific for the cytokine was added to each well, which was again incubated for 2 hours at room temperature. Following a final wash to remove all unbound antibody, a substrate solution was added to each well that created a color in proportion to the amount of cytokine present in the sample. After incubating for 20 minutes, the reaction was stopped by adding a stop solution. The optical density was determined in a plate reader at 450 nm. For each ELISA a standard curve was created. By comparing the absorption of the samples with the standard, the concentration of the cytokine in the sample was determined. For each ELISA the influence of PMSF was tested by using one sample diluted in PMSF solution and one sample in distilled water. In the case of IL-8 the influence of PBS was tested in the same way. Forty samples could be measured in duplicate in each ELISA plate; therefore, each cytokine concentration was determined in plasma and sol phase of 8 patients.

Statistics

Changes in sputum volume and purulence, white cell count and cytokines were examined by Student's t-test for matched pairs. The results were considered statistically significant when $p < 0.05$.

RESULTS

Cellular Composition of the Chronic Inflammation in Bronchiectasis

All bronchiectasis samples showed intense mononuclear cell infiltration, compared to 9.1 percent of the controls. In 10 out of 22 bronchiectasis samples, the infiltrates showed a folliclelike arrangement. No control showed similar changes.

Phenotype of Immunocompetent Cells

The distribution and phenotype of the immunocompetent cell population in the bronchial lamina propria is presented in TABLE 3. The main finding was the large increment in the number of T-cells infiltrating the bronchial wall of all bronchiectasis samples. The difference between them and the controls was prominent ($p < 0.00005$). In about half the samples (those displaying follicular arrangements) large numbers of B-lymphocytes and plasma cells were seen in the follicles, but in the other half very few of these cells were found. The frequency of accessory cells was also greater in bronchiectasis. Mature macrophages were present in large numbers and many dendritic cells were also seen.

The ratios of CD4+ and CD8+ T-lymphocytes were evaluated by double immunofluorescence. An overall predominance of CD8+ cells was seen in 15 samples. In the others, all of them exhibiting folliclelike structures, the CD4+ subset was predominant, due to the large excess of this subset in the follicle.

Coexpression of Activation Markers and Other Molecules

Further analysis of the T-lymphocyte subsets was performed to determine coexpression of activation markers and other relevant molecules. The results for

TABLE 3. Phenotype of Immunocompetent Cells in the Bronchial Lamina Propria

	Bronchiectasis ($n = 22$)	Controls ($n = 11$)	p Value
CD3	7.4 ± 4.5	1.7 ± 0.7	<0.00005
CD57	0.6 ± 0.6	0.2 ± 0.2	<0.05
CD22	1.9 ± 3.7	0.01 ± 0.04	<0.05
RFD6	3.6 ± 4.0	1.0 ± 0.5	<0.05
UCHM1	2.3 ± 1.3	0.2 ± 0.2	<0.0001
RFD1	1.6 ± 0.9	0.7 ± 0.5	<0.05
RFD7	3.1 ± 1.6	0.8 ± 0.6	<0.00005

Note: Results presented as mean ± standard deviation of numbers of positively stained cells per 10^4 μ^2 of lamina propria.

TABLE 4. Expression of Functionally Relevant Molecules by CD8+ T-Cells in the Bronchial Lamina Propria

	Bronchiectasis ($n = 22$)	Controls ($n = 11$)	p Value
CD25	4.6 ± 3.9	0	<0.001
CD38	12.3 ± 8.9	0	<0.0005
CD7	72.2 ± 7.2	23.7 ± 21.7	<0.00005
HLA-DR	19.2 ± 7.3	2.8 ± 2.2	<0.00005
CD45RO	73.3 ± 8.9	46.0 ± 13.5	<0.001
CD45RA	18.6 ± 10.9	20.7 ± 4.5	NS

Note: Results presented as mean ± standard deviation of percents of double-labeled cells.

the CD8+ cells are presented in TABLE 4. Statistically significant differences between bronchiectasis and control samples were seen. The expression of the activation markers CD25 and MHC Class II was highly significant in bronchiectasis samples. Also, the expression of CD45RO was higher in bronchiectasis ($p < 0.0001$). The expression of the marker TIA-1, present in cells with cytolytic potential, was seen in 16 percent of the CD8+ cells.

In the case of the CD4+ T-cells, bronchiectasis samples were divided into two groups, according to the presence of follicular aggregates. The results are displayed in TABLE 5. In follicular bronchiectasis samples, a much larger and statistically significant proportion of CD4+ T cells coexpressing activation markers was found.

Determination of Cytokine Levels in Bronchiectasis

Cytokine Concentrations in Plasma

Cytokine concentrations of IL-1α, TNF-α, and IL-8 were below the lower limit of detection of the assays (including in the 6 volunteers). Limits of detection were: IL-1 α 3.9 pg/ml; TNF-α 15.7 pg/ml; IL-8 93.3 pg/ml.

Sputum Volume, Purulence, and Cell Count

In Group I, antibiotic treatment reduced sputum volume (mean ± SEM) from 38 ± 5 to 16 ± 6 ml ($p < 0.05$) and sputum purulence from 81 ± 5% to 40 ± 10%

TABLE 5. Expression of Functionally Relevant Molecules by CD4+ T-cells in the Bronchial Lamina Propria of Follicular and Nonfollicular Bronchiectasis

	Follicular ($n = 10$)	Nonfollicular ($n = 12$)	p Value
CD7	45.5 ± 14.5	7.9 ± 21.2	<0.005
CD25	2.6 ± 1.1	0.01 ± 0.01	<0.001
CD38	10.0 ± 4.3	2.2 ± 6.7	<0.05
RFDR	33.6 ± 26.4	10.0 ± 0.5	<0.05

Note: Results presented as mean ± standard deviation of percents of double-labeled cells.

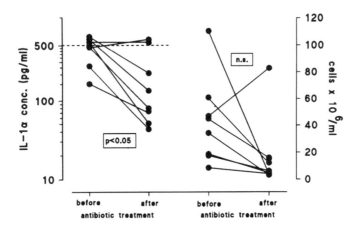

FIGURE 1. IL-1α concentration **(left side)** and sputum cell counts **(right side)** of patients in Group I before and immediately after antibiotic treatment.

($p < 0.005$). In Group II, it reduced sputum volume and purulence from 33 ± 6 ml to 14 ± 4 ml ($p < 0.02$) and from $75 \pm 8\%$ to $40 \pm 7\%$ ($p < 0.001$), respectively. In Group III, sputum volume and purulence remained unchanged from 15 ± 4 ml to 22 ± 7 ml (NS) and $35 \pm 9\%$ to $43 \pm 13\%$ (NS), respectively. The sputum cell count decreased from $43 \pm 12 \times 10^6$/ml to $18 \pm 10 \times 10^6$/ml (NS) after antibiotic treatment in Group I, from $44 \pm 15 \times 10^6$/ml to $11 \pm 6 \times 10^6$/ml ($p < 0.05$) in Group II, and from $13 \pm 7 \times 10^6$/ml at the end of antibiotic treatment to $14 \pm 5 \times 10^6$/ml (NS) 2 weeks later in Group III. In Group I, there was one patient who did not respond clinically to antibiotic treatment, and in this patient the sputum cell count increased after treatment.

Cytokine Concentrations in the Sputum

IL-1α (FIG. 1): Antibiotic treatment reduced sputum IL-1α concentrations in Group I from (mean $\pm$ SEM) 427 ± 46 pg/ml to 201 ± 69 pg/ml ($p < 0.01$). Sputum IL-1α concentrations decreased in 6/8 patients, remained above upper limit of detection in one patient and in the nonresponder. The nonresponder's sputum cell count and IL-1α increased after antibiotic treatment.

TNF-α (FIG. 2): Concentrations of TNF-α in Group I after therapy were decreased in 7/8 patients. In four patients the concentrations of the cytokine after therapy were below the lower limit of detection (31.4 pg/ml). Concentration decreased from 971 ± 281 pg/ml to 210 ± 147 pg/ml (NS). The nonresponder's sputum cell count and TNF-α increased after antibiotic treatment.

IL-8 (FIG. 3): In Group II there was no significant change in the concentration of the cytokine that remained elevated before (436 ± 144 pg/ml) and after (384 ± 193 pg/ml) antibiotic treatment, although the significant reduction ($p < 0.05$) in sputum cell count before ($44 \pm 15 \times 10^6$ cells/ml) and after ($11 \pm 6 \times 10^6$ cells/ml) associated with clinical improvement indicated effective antibiotic treatment.

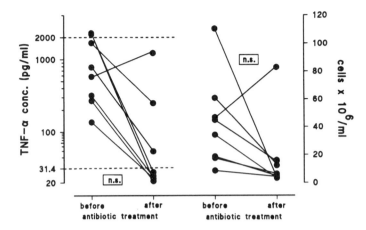

FIGURE 2. TNF-α concentrations **(left side)** and sputum cell counts **(right side)** of patients in Group I before and immediately after antibiotic treatment.

Because of this finding sputum samples were obtained from a further 6 patients 2 weeks after the end of antibiotic therapy (Group III). In comparison with the concentration at the end of antibiotic therapy (382 ± 128 pg/ml) again there was no significant change 2 weeks after antibiotic therapy (543 ± 259 pg/ml) (Fig. 4). The unchanged sputum cell count, however, suggested maintained remission, which was also clinically evident: $13 \pm 7 \times 10^6$ cells/ml; 2 weeks after antibiotic therapy: $14 \pm 5 \times 10^6$ cells/ml. Results are presented in TABLE 6.

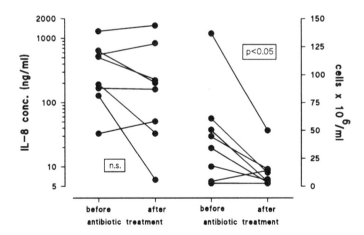

FIGURE 3. IL-8 concentrations **(left side)** and sputum cell counts **(right side)** of patients in Group II before and immediately after antibiotic treatment.

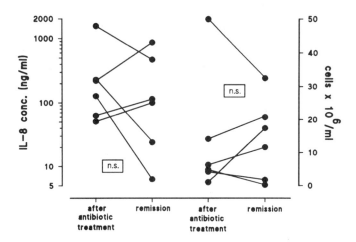

FIGURE 4. IL-8 concentrations **(left side)** and sputum cell counts **(right side)** of patients in Group III immediately after and 2 weeks after antibiotic treatment.

TABLE 6. Sputum Characteristics Before and Immediately after Antibiotic Treatment (above the Dotted Line; $n = 8$), and Immediately after and Two Weeks after Treatment (below the Dotted Line; $n = 6$)

	Percent of Purulence	Cell Counts $\times 10^6$/ml	IL-8 (pg/ml)
Pretreatment	75 ± 8	44 ± 15	438 ± 144
Immediately after treatment	40 ± 7^c	11 ± 6^b	384 ± 193^a
Immediately after treatment	35 ± 9	13 ± 7	328 ± 128
Two weeks after treatment	43 ± 12^a	14 ± 5^a	534 ± 259^a

Key: ^{a} NS; ^{b} $p < 0.05$; ^{c} $p < 0.001$.

DISCUSSION

Bronchiectasis is an understudied chronic respiratory disease,[27] particularly from the immunopathogenesis aspect. Here, the use of immunohistochemistry allowed characterization of the phenotypes of the immunocompetent cells that populate the affected bronchial wall in the disease. There was an increase in the numbers of all major types of immunocompetent cells in bronchiectasis samples. The most consistent finding was the increased number of T-lymphocytes. The infiltrating T-cells were loosely distributed in the bronchial wall of all samples with bronchiectasis, but in half of them folliclelike structures were present.

Important information is available about the role of T-cells, particularly of activated T-cells, in the development of chronic inflammatory diseases of the intestine. Trejdosiewics and colleagues[28] studied the phenotype of colonic mucosal T-lymphocytes in ulcerative colitis and found a large number of them exhibiting the activation marker CD7, in close association with increased expression of major histocompatibility complex (MHC) Class II molecules by colonic enterocytes during the inflammatory process. This was taken to suggest the existence of local immunostimulation of T cells. One of the consequences of this immunostimulation is the production of interferon-gamma, which leads to augmentation of nonconstitutive expression of MHC Class II antigens by colonic enterocytes and acquisition of antigen-presenting capacity by these cells. In those circumstances, HLA-DR positive epithelial cells might inappropriately present other antigens, exogenous, or autoantigens, and broaden the spectrum of local immune response, thus contributing to the perpetuation of the chronic inflammation. MacDonald[29] discussed the role of activated T-lymphocytes in intestinal disease, showing that these cells are capable of producing crypt gland proliferation, villous atrophy, and increased HLA-DR expression by enterocytes in different experimental systems. This picture is very similar to the one seen in coeliac disease, where a large number of cells is known to infiltrate the intestinal mucosa.[30]

In bronchiectasis, the major question is whether T-lymphocytes are implicated in the pathogenesis of the disease or are merely secondary consequences of the disease. The presence of excessive numbers of activated T-lymphocytes could contribute to the immunopathology of the condition. In these circumstances, production of cytokines would be a likely possibility, particularly of those with chemoattractant activity for neutrophils, a prominent cell in the pathogenesis of the condition.

Recently, some publications showed the association of obliterative bronchiolitis and bronchiectasis in patients undergoing heart-lung transplantation.[31] The involvement of an active immune process in the genesis of the complication was suggested by the apparent arrest of the process by augmented immunosuppression.[32] Griffith *et al.*[33] have proposed an immune-mediated basis for the process, beginning with epithelial injury induced by activated lymphocytes, resulting in epithelial necrosis with sloughing of cells into the lumen. Injury to the small airways causes them to dilate, due to the loss of smooth-muscle support, and results in cylindrical bronchiectasis with mucopurulent secretions retained within the airways. Glanville *et al.*[34] suggested that increased expression of Class II antigens by the bronchial epithelium during the rejection process made them a likely target for cytotoxic cells directed against alloantigens. Holland *et al.*[35] studied the composition of these lymphocyte infiltrates in posttransplant bronchiolitis and found a large preponderance of CD8+ cells, mainly in peribronchial areas.

In a recently developed model of experimental bronchiectasis,[36] the development of bronchial dilatation is paralleled by intense mononuclear cell infiltration in the bronchus and surrounding structures.[37] A large majority of these cells are activated T-lymphocytes and macrophages. Also, during the height of the bronchial inflammation, the bronchial epithelium expresses Class II molecules. This expression was measured by optic densitometry,[38] and a highly significant increase in the expression of these molecules was seen in bronchiectasis, as compared with controls, suggesting that in the development of experimental bronchiectasis, immune mechanisms may play a role.

Also, the pathogenesis of bronchiectasis has recently been shown, both in human disease[8,39] and in the animal model of experimental bronchiectasis,[40] to involve the traffic of neutrophil polymorphonuclear leukocytes from the circulation through the bronchial wall into the bronchial lumen where the chronically infecting microorganisms are situated. Such cell traffic can constitute nearly 50 percent of circulating neutrophils in severe bronchiectasis.[8] Although a degree of bronchial damage is probably due to bacterial exotoxins,[6,41-44] it is likely that the majority of bronchial damage is host-mediated via the release of proteinases[45] and oxidants[46] by neutrophils trafficking through the bronchial wall into the bronchial lumen. Progression of lung damage, which has been shown in a proportion of patients with bronchiectasis,[47] is likely to be due to continued infection with relentless recruitment of neutrophils to the site, resulting in continuous inflammatory damage.

Chemoattractants likely to provoke this cell traffic are of bacterial origin[11] and host origin.[12] Persistence of bacterial infection can induce IL-1 and TNF-α in many cells, and these cytokines stimulate expression of ICAM-1 and the CD11/CD18 integrin complex involved in a variety of cell adherence functions, including migration of neutrophils from endothelium into tissues.[48,49] They also induce the production of IL-8,[50] which itself is a powerful mediator of neutrophil transmigration[50,51] and activation.[52] IL-8 has been shown to be present systemically in sepsis[53] and is thought to play a role in the development of pulmonary disease.[54-56] The finding of IL-1 and TNF-α together with very high levels of IL-8 in the expectorated secretions of patients with infective exacerbations of bronchiectasis is consistent with the chemoattraction of considerable numbers of neutrophils to the bronchial lumen from which these secretions derive. Acute infective exacerbations in patients with bronchiectasis are usually associated with increased volume of expectoration, which has also increased purulence. This increase is due to polymorphonuclear leukocytes–eosinophils in allergic, asthmatic secretions and neutrophils in infected secretions. In the patients treated by antibiotics in this study there was a decrease in volume and purulence and in cell content, confirming clinical observations that the patients (with one exception) responded to treatment. In those patients IL-1 and TNF-α levels were also reduced by treatment, but IL-8 levels remained persistently high. Following patients for 2 weeks into remission after the conclusion of successful antibiotic treatment confirmed that the volume, purulence, and cell content of sputum remained low but that IL-8 remained high. While following patients for longer in remission might have revealed waning of IL-8 levels, the finding in this study might offer one explanation of the common clinical observation that patients frequently relapse with recurrence of purulent secretions soon after an antibiotic is withdrawn. This has been interpreted as due to reinfection, but from the results of this study, it could be due to local IL-8 levels remaining high and stimulating resumption of neutrophil recruitment to the bronchial tree. Nevertheless, the fact that sputum cell counts remained low in the face of high IL-8 levels after clinical response to antibiotic treatment suggests that for IL-8 to act as a chemoattractant in this situation, there might be an additional requirement. Alternatively, it is possible that the IL-8 might be inhibited in some way from acting in this manner.

The source of IL-8 has until recently been assumed to be mononuclear cells, and in bronchiectasis the high levels in secretions would be compatible with an origin from the florid cellular immune response within the bronchial wall described in this paper. Nevertheless, more recently bronchial epithelial cells have been demonstrated as a source of IL-8, and epithelial lining fluid from patients with cystic fibrosis (one cause of bronchiectasis) induces significant expression of mRNA for IL-8.[57] A third possible source is the neutrophil itself,[58] but the levels of IL-8 would be expected to fall with successful antibiotic treatment if the neutrophils were an important source.

The undetectable levels of IL-1, TNF-α, and IL-8 in the plasma of these patients, in contrast to, for example, TNF-α found in the plasma of patients with cystic fibrosis,[59] probably reflects the fact that bronchiectasis of non-cystic-fibrosis aetiology represents a more localized process, manifest clinically by lack of systemic features, for example, fever.

The results of the study of cells and cytokines in bronchiectasis suggest that cytokine-mediated neutrophil recruitment may underlie the majority of bronchial damage occurring in this condition—and that the cellular immune response within the bronchial wall may be associated with this.

REFERENCES

1. COLE, P. J. 1990. Bronchiectasis. In Respiratory Medicine, R. A. L. Brewis, G. J. Gibson, and D. M. Geddes, Eds.: 726–759. Baillière & Tindall. London.
2. WHITWELL, F. 1952. A study of the pathology and pathogenesis of bronchiectasis. Thorax 7: 213–239.
3. LAPA E SILVA, J. R., J. A. H. JONES, P. J. COLE & L. W. POULTER. 1989. The immunopathological component of the cellular inflammatory infiltrate in bronchiectasis. Thorax 44: 668–673.
4. COLE, P. J. & R. WILSON. 1989. Host-microbial interrelationship in respiratory infection. Chest 95: 217–221.
5. CURRIE, D. C., et al. 1987. Impaired tracheobronchial clearance in bronchiectasis. Thorax 42: 126–130.
6. WILSON, R., et al. 1987. Pyocyanin and 1-hydroxyphenazine produced by Pseudomonas aeruginosa inhibit the beating of human respiratory cilia in vitro. J. Clin. Invest. 79: 221–229.
7. MUNRO, N. C., et al. 1989. Effect of pyocyanin and 1-hydroxyphenazine on in vivo tracheal mucus velocity. J. Appl. Physiol. 67: 316–323.
8. CURRIE, D. C., et al. 1987. Indium-111-labelled granulocyte accumulation in the respiratory tract of patients with bronchiectasis. Lancet i: 1335–1339.
9. HOGG, J. C. 1991. Neutrophil traffic. In The Lung, Vol. 1, R. G. Crystal and J. B. West, Eds.: 565–579. Raven Press. New York.
10. PARKER, C. W. 1991. Neutrophil mechanisms. Am. Rev. Respir. Dis. 143: S59–S60.
11. RAS, G., R. WILSON, H. TODD, G. TAYLOR & P. J. COLE. 1990. Effect of bacterial products on neutrophil migration in vitro. Thorax 45: 276–280.
12. COLDITZ, I. & J. MORLEY. 1991. Mediators of inflammatory cell accumulation in the lung. In Mediators of Pulmonary Inflammation, M. A. Bray and W. H. Anderson, Eds.: 513–532. Dekker. New York.
13. BEVERLEY, P. C. L. & R. E. CALLARD. 1981. Distinctive functional characteristic of human T lymphocytes defined by E rosetting or a monoclonal anti-T-cell antibody. Eur. J. Immunol. 11: 329–334.
14. REINHERZ, E. L. & S. F. SCHLOSMAN. 1990. The differentiation and function of human T-lymphocytes. Cell 19: 821–827.
15. JANOSSY, G. & H. G. PRENTICE. T cell subpopulations, monoclonal antibodies and their therapeutic applications. Clin. Haematol. 11: 631–661.
16. ABO, T. & C. M. BALCH. 1981. A differentiation antigen of human NK and K cells identified by a monoclonal antibody (HNK-1). J. Immunol. 127: 1024–1029.
17. COLLINGS, L. A., L. W. POULTER & G. JANOSSY. 1984. The demonstration of cell surface antigens on T cells, B cells and accessory cells in paraffin-embedded human tissues. J. Immunol. Meth. 75: 227–239.
18. LING, N. R., I. C. M. MACLENNAN & D. Y. MASON. 1987. B-cell and plasma cell antigens: New and previously defined clusters. In Leukocyte Typing III, A. J. McMichael, Ed.: 302–336. Oxford Univ. Press. Oxford.
19. POULTER, L. W., D. A. CAMPBELL, C. MUNRO & J. JANOSSY. 1986. Discrimination of macrophages and dendritic cells of man using monoclonal antibodies. Scand. J. Immunol. 24: 351–357.
20. HOGG, N., S. MACDONALD, M. SLUSARENKO & P. C. L. BEVERLEY. 1984. Monoclonal

antibodies specific for human monocytes, granulocytes and endothelium. Immunology **53:** 753–767.

21. UCHIYAMA, T., S. BRODER & T. A. WALDMANN. 1981. A monoclonal antibody (anti-TAC) reactive with activated and functionally mature human T cells. J. Immunol. **126:** 7393–7397.

22. JANOSSY, G., et al. 1986. Separate ontogeny of two macrophage-like accessory cell populations in the human fetus. J. Immunol. **136:** 4354–4361.

23. JANOSSY, G., M. TIEDMAN, E. S. PAPAGEORGIOU, P. C. KUNG & G. GOLDSTEIN. 1981. Distribution of T-lymphocyte subsets in the human bone marrow and thymus—An analysis with monoclonal antibodies. J. Immunol. **126:** 1608–1613.

24. AKBAR, A. N., L. TERRY, A. TIMMS, P. C. L. BEVERLEY & G. JANOSSY. 1988. Loss of the CD45R and gain of UCHL1 reactivity is a feature of primed T cells. J. Immunol. **140:** 2171–2178.

25. SMITH, S. H., M. H. BROWN, D. ROWE, D. E. CALLARD & P. C. L. BEVERLEY. 1986. Functional subsets of helper-inducer cells defined by a new monoclonal antibody, UCHL1. Immunology **58:** 63–70.

26. JAMES, G. T. 1978. Inactivation of the protease inhibitor phenylmethylsulfonylfluoride in buffers. Ann. Biochem. **86:** 574–579.

27. BARKER, A. F. & E. J. BARDANA, JR. 1988. Bronchiectasis. Update of an orphan disease. Am. Rev. Respir. Dis. **137:** 969–978.

28. TREJDOSIEWICZ, L. B., et al. 1989. Colonic mucosal T lymphocytes in ulcerative colitis: Expression of CD7 antigen in relation to MHC Class II (HLA-DR) antigens. Dig. Dis. Sci. **34:** 1449–1456.

29. MACDONALD, T. 1990. The role of activated T lymphocytes in gastrointestinal disease. Clin. Exp. Allergy **20:** 247–252.

30. MACDONALD, T. T. & J. SPENCER. 1988. Evidence that activated mucosal T cells play a role in the pathogenesis of enteropathy in human small intestine. J. Exp. Med. **167:** 1341–1349.

31. BURKE, C. M., et al. 1984. Post-transplant obliterative bronchiolitis and other late lung sequelae in human heart-lung transplantation. Chest **86:** 824–829.

32. GLANVILLE, A. R., J. C. BALDWIN, C. M. BURKE, J. THEODORE & E. D. ROBIN. 1987. Obliterative bronchiectasis after heart-lung transplantation: Apparent arrest by augmented immunosuppression. Ann. Int. Med. **107:** 300–304.

33. GRIFFITH, B. P., et al. 1988. Immunologically mediated disease of the airways after pulmonary transplantation. Ann. Surg. **208:** 371–378.

34. GLANVILLE, A. R., et al. 1989. The distribution of MHC Class I and II antigens on bronchial epithelium. Am. Rev. Respir. Dis. **139:** 330–334.

35. HOLLAND, V. A., et al. 1990. Lymphocyte subset populations in bronchiolitis obliterans after heart-lung transplantation. Transplantation **50:** 955–959.

36. GUERREIRO, D., et al. 1990. Quantitation of experimental bronchiectasis. Eur. Respir. J. **3:** 296s.

37. LAPA E SILVA, J. R., et al. 1989. Immunopathology of experimental bronchiectasis. Am. J. Respir. Cell Mol. Biol. **1:** 297–304.

38. LAPA E SILVA, J. R., D. GUERREIRO, N. C. MUNRO, L. W. POULTER & P. J. COLE. 1993. Immunopathology of chronic bronchial inflammation: Contribution of animal models. In New Concepts in Asthma, J. Tarayre, B. Vargaftig, and J. Tisne-Versailles, Eds.: 266–279. Macmillan. London.

39. CURRIE, D. C., et al. 1990. Indium-111-labelled granulocyte scanning to detect inflammation in the lungs of patients with chronic sputum expectoration. Thorax **45:** 541–544.

40. GUERREIRO, D., et al. 1992. Bronchial wall neutrophils in experimental bronchiectasis. Am. Rev. Respir. Dis. **145:** A547.

41. WILSON, R. & P. J. COLE. 1988. The effect of bacterial products on ciliary function. Am. Rev. Respir. Dis. **138:** 549–553.

42. STEINFORT, C., et al. 1989. The effect of Streptococcus pneumoniae on human respiratory epithelium in vitro. Infect. Immun. **57:** 2006–2013.

43. FELDMAN, C., et al. 1990. The effect of Streptococcus pneumoniae pneumolysin on human respiratory epithelium in vitro. Microb. Path. **9:** 275–284.

44. WILSON, R., D. ROBERTS & P. J. COLE. 1985. Effect of bacterial products on human ciliary function in vitro. Thorax **40**: 125–131.

45. AMITANI, R., et al. 1985. Effects of human neutrophil elastase and bacterial proteinases on human respiratory epithelium. Am. J. Respir. Cell Mol. Biol. **4**: 26–32.

46. RAS, G. J., et al. 1990. Proinflammatory interactions of pyocyanin and 1-hydroxyphenazine with human neutrophils in vitro. J. Infect. Dis. **162**: 178–185.

47. MUNRO, N. C., L. Y. HAM, D. C. CURRIE, B. STRICKLAND & P. J. COLE. 1992. Radiological evidence of progression of bronchiectasis. Respir. Med. **86**: 317–401.

48. SCHUIMAAR, R. P., S. V. BENENATI, B. FRIEDMAN & B. S. BUCHNER. 1991. Do cytokines play a role in leukocyte recruitment and activation in the lung? Am. Rev. Respir. Dis. **143**: 1169–1174.

49. MANTOVANI, A., F. BUSSOLINI & E. DEJANA. Cytokine regulation of endothelial cell function. FASEB **6**: 2591–2599.

50. STRETER, R. M., et al. 1989. Endothelial cell gene expression of a neutrophil chemotactic factor for TNF-α, LPS and IL-1β. Science **243**: 1467–1469.

51. KUNKEL, S. L., T. STANDIFORD, K. KASAHARA & R. M. STRETER. 1991. Interleukin-8; The major neutrophil chemotactic factor in the lung. Exp. Lung Res. **17**: 17–23.

52. DJEU, J. Y., K. MATSUSHIMA, J. J. OPPENHEIM, K. SHIOTSUKI & D. K. BLANCHARD. 1990. Function activation of human neutrophils by recombinant monocyte-derived neutrophil chemotactic factor/IL-8. J. Immunology **144**: 2205–2210.

53. HACK, C. E., et al. 1992. Interleukin-8 in sepsis: Relation to shock and inflammatory mediators. Infect. Immun. **60**: 2835–2842.

54. DONELLY, S. C., et al. 1993. Interleukin-8 and the development of adult respiratory distress syndrome in at-risk patient groups. Lancet **341**: 643–647.

55. COURTNEY, B., et al. 1992. Interleukin-8 is a major neutrophilic chemotactic factor in pleural fluid of patients with empyema. Am. Rev. Respir. Dis. **146**: 825–830.

56. LYNCH, J. P., III, T. J. STANDIFORD, M. W. ROLFE, S. L. KUNKEL & R. M. STRETER. 1992. Neutrophilic alveolitis in idiopathic pulmonary fibrosis. Am. Rev. Respir. Dis. **145**: 1433–1439.

57. NAKAMURA, H., K. YOSHIMURA, N. G. MCELVANEY & R. G. CRYSTAL. 1992. Neutrophil elastase in respiratory epithelial lining fluid in individuals with cystic fibrosis induces interleukin-8 gene expression in a human epithelial cell line. J. Clin. Invest. **89**: 1478–1484.

58. CASSATELLA, M. A., et al. 1992. IL-8 production by human polymorphonuclear leukocyte. J. Immunol. **148**: 3216–3220.

59. SUTER, S., et al. 1989. Relation between tumor necrosis factor alpha and granulocyte elastase-α1-proteinase inhibitor complex in the plasma of patients with cystic fibrosis. Am. Rev. Respir. Dis. **140**: 1640–1644.

Cytokine Gene and Peptide Regulation in Lung Microvascular Injury: New Insights on the Development of Adult Respiratory Distress Syndrome

REUVEN RABINOVICI,[a] GIORA FEUERSTEIN,
AND LEWIS F. NEVILLE

Department of Surgery
Jefferson Medical College
Philadelphia, Pennsylvania 19107-5083

and

Department of Cardiovascular Pharmacology
SmithKline Beecham
King of Prussia, Pennsylvania 19406

INTRODUCTION

The incidence of the sepsis syndrome is on the rise in the United States, with at least 400,000 cases reported annually.[1] One of the more severe consequences of sepsis is microvascular lung injury [adult respiratory distress syndrome (ARDS)], which is the leading cause of death in these patients.[2]

Over the last 20 years, much progress has been made into the pathophysiology of septic lung injury with the identification and characterization of a variety of inflammatory mediators. These include cytokines [tumor necrosis factor α (TNFα), interleukin-1β (IL-1β)], phospholipids [platelet activating factor (PAF) prostaglandins, leukotrienes], adhesion molecules (ELAM-1, ICAM-1), proteases, complement and toxic oxygen radicals (for review, see reference 3).

The leading concept in the pathophysiology of septic lung injury is that processes leading to the production of proinflammatory mediators and ultimately to tissue injury are triggered by the release into the circulation of overwhelming amounts of lipopolysaccharide (LPS). Several considerations cast doubt on the validity of this hypothesis. First, the experimental basis of this postulate was provided by animal models of lung injury produced by the large doses of LPS or live bacteria that do not adequately mimic the settings of clinical sepsis-induced lung injury. Second, all clinical trials evaluating the efficacy of anti-LPS monoclonal antibodies in septic patients, which were developed as a direct consequence of these animal models, failed to abrogate the consequences of sepsis (for review, see reference 4).

---

[a] To whom correspondence should be addressed.

Based upon the preceding considerations, we hypothesized that septic lung injury might be initiated not by excessive amounts of circulating LPS, but rather by interactions among minuscule doses of LPS and rapidly induced inflammatory mediators. Such an interaction might induce the synthesis of additional inflammatory mediators that will further exacerbate the inflammatory response and tissue injury.

MINUSCULE LPS–PAF INTERACTIONS *IN VIVO:* A NEW MODEL OF SEPTIC LUNG INJURY AND ARDS

To evaluate our hypothesis, PAF was selected as the prototype inflammatory mediator since it is rapidly synthesized and previously has been implicated in the pathophysiology of septic lung injury.[5] Additionally, a number of *in vitro* studies have documented synergistic interactions between LPS and PAF in augmenting the production of TNFα,[6] a pivotal mediator of septic lung injury.[7]

When LPS was administered to rats as a bolus dose (0.1 μg/kg), followed immediately by PAF infusion for 60 minutes (60 pmol/kg), profound lung injury occurred 3 hours later as assessed by a variety of end points. For example, the LPS–PAF paradigm grossly elevated lung water content (FIG. 1), myeloperoxidase (MPO) activity, and protein and polymorphonuclear (PMN) accumulation in bronchoalveolar lavage (BAL) fluid.[8] In accord with increased MPO activity and PMN count in BAL fluid, electron micrographs of lung sections prepared from LPS–PAF-challenged rats realized pronounced neutrophil sequestration and adherence to endothelium (FIG. 2). None of these effects were observed from rats challenged with LPS or PAF alone.

The effects of PAF in this model were specific since they were ameliorated by the PAF receptor antagonist BN 50739,[9] and not induced by a combination of LPS and lyso-PAF, the inactive metabolite of PAF.[8] Furthermore, PAF appeared to prime for the effect of LPS and not vice versa since the paradigm of LPS given prior or after PAF infusion failed to elicit lung injury.[8]

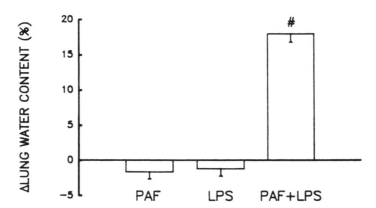

FIGURE 1. LPS (0.1 μg/kg) and PAF (1 pmol/kg/min over 60 min) synergize to elevate lung wet and wet–dry (lung water content) weight. □—change vs. control; # $P < 0.01$.

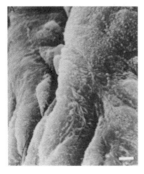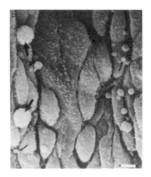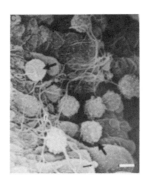

FIGURE 2. Scanning electron micrograph of the luminal surface of a pulmonary venule from rats given PAF **(A)**, LPS **(B)**, or PAF and LPS in combination **(C)**. Note that the endothelium in **(A)** is free of any adherent leukocytes or platelets, whereas a few platelets (*small arrows*) and leukocytes (*large arrows*), probably neutrophils, are adherent to the endothelium in **(B)**. In contrast, the endothelium in **(C)** is covered by adherent leukocytes (*large arrows*) and platelets (*small arrows*) embedded in branching fibrin (f) strands. The surface of the leukocytes in **(C)** is thrown into numerous blebs, evidence of activation. Final magnification = 799×. Bar equals 6 μm. These figures represent histopathological changes uniformly found in all lung areas.

APPARENT CENTRAL ROLE OF TNFα IN LPS–PAF-INDUCED SEPTIC LUNG INJURY

Based on numerous studies implicating TNFα in the pathogenesis of septic shock and septic lung injury, serum TNFα levels from LPS–PAF-challenged rats were evaluated. Whereas no elevation in serum TNFα was observed from rats challenged with either LPS or PAF alone, the combined LPS–PAF stimulus elicited a robust and monophasic increase in TNFα level (FIG. 3). The potential role of TNFα in mediating LPS–PAF-elicited lung injury was strengthened by the dose-dependent protective effect of anti-TNFα mAb.[10] Pretreatment of rats with anti-TNFα mAb (2.5 mg/kg–25 mg/kg) prior to LPS–PAF challenge was found to effectively attenuate the increased lung water, MPO (FIG. 4), protein, and neutrophil content of BAL as well as the histopathological aberrations associated with LPS–PAF-induced lung injury.

REPEATED LPS–PAF CHALLENGES FURTHER EXACERBATES PULMONARY DAMAGE TO PRODUCE "FULMINANT" ARDS-LIKE LUNG INJURY

Having established our LPS–PAF model, which induced lung injury highly reminiscent of the early stages of ARDS,[8] we further hypothesized that fulminant ARDS-like lung injury could be elicited by the more physiologic repeated exposure to minuscule LPS–PAF doses. Rats challenged with a second LPS–PAF insult, 4 hours after the primary one, exhibited severe lung injury comprising many pathophysiologic and histologic features of clinical ARDS.[11] This was exemplified by histopathological findings of severe pulmonary edema, proteinaceous exudates

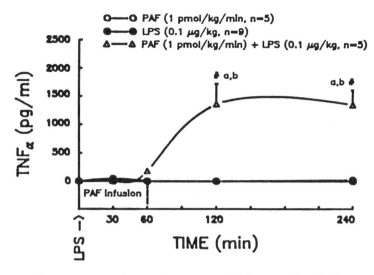

FIGURE 3. LPS and PAF synergize to elevate serum TNFα. **a**—vs. basal value; **b**—vs. all other groups. The sensitivity of the ELISA was 25 pg/ml.

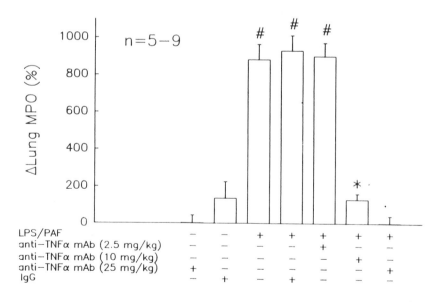

FIGURE 4. Effect of anti-TNFα mAb on LPS–PAF-induced MPO response. □—change vs. control (sham); anti-TNFα mAb—hamster antimurine TNFα monoclonal antibody; IgG—nonspecific hamster IgG at 25 mg/kg; anti-TNFα mAb doses are in mg/kg; #—vs. IgG alone, anti-TNFα mAb alone, anti-TNFα mAb (10 and 25 mg/kg)/LPS/PAF, and control (sham) groups; *—vs. anti-TNFα alone, LPS/PAF, IgG/LPS/PAF, anti-TNFα (2.5 and 25 mg/kg)/LPS/PAF, and control (sham) groups.

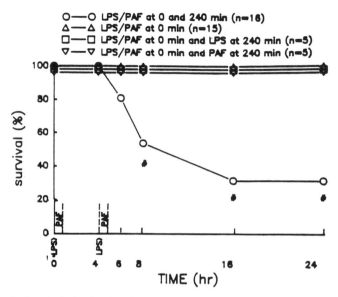

FIGURE 5. Survival of animals subjected to a double LPS–PAF stimulus. LPS–PAF was administered at 0 and 4 hours. LPS at 0.1 μg/kg and PAF at 0.1 pmol/kg/min over 60 minutes were used. #—vs. all other groups.

within alveoli indicative of interstitial pneumonia not observed in the single LPS–PAF paradigm. Two additional parameters also indicated the development of a fulminant ARDS-like lung injury: (1) The appearance of mortality associated with the second LPS–PAF insult (FIG. 5), and (2) the persistent presence of serum TNFα following the second LPS–PAF challenge (FIG. 6). The central role of TNFα in mediating LPS–PAF-induced lung injury and mortality was illustrated by the protective effect of anti-TNFα mAb.[11]

IS TNFα THE SOLE MEDIATOR OF LPS–PAF INDUCED LUNG INJURY?

As described earlier, *in vivo* observations have clearly showed a striking protective effect of anti-TNFα mAb against a single and repeated LPS–PAF insult. These data would therefore indicate a critical role for TNFα in mediating LPS–PAF lung injury.

Based on the multicytokine mediation of lung injury in other animal models, however, we investigated possible involvements of other cytokines in the LPS–PAF model. To that end, Northern blots were performed on total RNA isolated from lungs of rats challenged with the LPS–PAF paradigm. An increased hybridization signal (10-fold as compared to controls) for TNFα mRNA was ob-

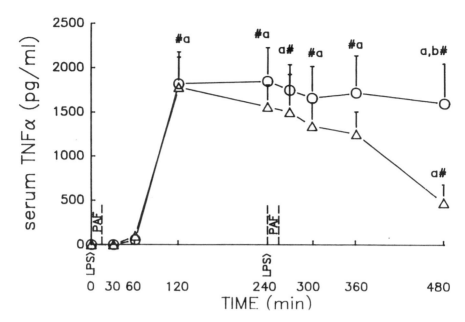

FIGURE 6. Serum TNFα response to a double LPS/PAF stimulus. **a**—vs. basal value; **b**—vs. all other groups. Please note the sustained elevation of TNFα in the serum of rats subjected to a double LPS–PAF challenge.

served (FIG. 7). Interestingly, we observed at least 100-fold enhancement in signal for IL-1β and IL-6 mRNA derived solely from LPS–PAF-treated rats (FIG. 7).

Lung histopathological findings of LPS–PAF-treated rats revealed adherence of neutrophils to the endothelium of pulmonary venules (FIG. 2). This phenomenon would indicate the likely involvement of a rat, IL-8-like chemotactic factor responsible for promoting neutrophil infiltration. To address this issue, stringent hybridization using a KC cDNA probe produced a striking hybridization signal to RNA extracted from lungs of LPS–PAF-treated rats (FIG. 7).

Furthermore, studies with the novel and highly selective complement inhibitor sCR1 supported a role of the complement in the LPS–PAF model of lung injury.[12] In these studies, pretreatment with sCR1 prevented lung edema and the increase in BAL fluid cell count and protein concentration. Also, sCR1 attenuated the deposition of C3 and C5b-9 to lung vessels. Interestingly, there was no effect on lung MPO activity and serum TNFα.

Therefore, in addition to the central role of TNFα in mediating LPS–PAF-induced lung injury, our data clearly support the involvement of a multimediator network that leads to tissue injury.

FUTURE GOALS AND DIRECTIONS

As described earlier, a multicytokine involvement would appear to prevail in the genesis of septic lung injury and ARDS. To further confirm this concept, the kinetics of appearance of IL-1β, IL-6, and IL-8 in the serum of LPS–PAF-treated

CYTOKINE mRNA INDUCTION IN ARDS-LIKE LUNG INJURY

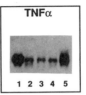

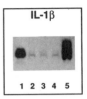

FIGURE 7. LPS–PAF administration to rats causes up-regulation in lung cytokine mRNA levels. Northern blots were performed on total RNA isolated from: 1. LPS (100 ng/ml)-stimulated peritoneal macrophages (positive control), and lungs from rats challenged with 2. LPS vehicle–PAF vehicle, 3. LPS vehicle–PAF, 4. LPS–PAF vehicle, and 5. LPS–PAF. RNA was hybridized to random-prime prepared [32P]-cDNA probes, washed, and taken for autoradiography. Note the pronounced and selective induction of TNFα, IL-1β, IL-6, and KC mRNA from LPS–PAF challenged rats (lane 5).

1. **LPS** - stimulated macrophages
2. **PAF vehicle - LPS vehicle**
3. **PAF** - LPS vehicle
4. **PAF vehicle** - **LPS**
5. **PAF** - **LPS**

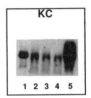

rats should be investigated. Establishing suitable bioassays for the interleukin members would facilitate such studies. Additionally, *in vitro* studies using alveolar macrophages will give insight into the mechanisms of LPS–PAF interactions. Such systems will provide data on possible synergistic relationships among the other cytokines involved in the pathogenesis of lung injury.

Our model described herein provides a new experimental paradigm to confirm our hypothesis that lung injury is elicited by interactions among minute doses of LPS and PAF. It should be noted that this paradigm may not imply the sole involvement or relative contribution of PAF in the genesis of septic lung injury. Instead, the model serves as an example that such interactions may indeed result in microvascular lung injury. Further investigations of interactions between rapidly induced inflammatory mediators and LPS should be ensued that could provide clues to the physiological triggering of ARDS. Insights into such interactions could provide new target sites for pharmacological intervention of septic lung injury.

REFERENCES

1. PARRILLO, J. E. 1993. Pathogenetic mechanisms of septic shock. New Eng. J. Med. **328:** 1471–1477.
2. DEMLING, R. H. 1990. Current concepts on the Adult Respiratory Distress Syndrome. Circ. Shock **30:** 297–310.
3. NEUGEBERGER, E. A. & J. W. HOLADAY, Eds. 1993. Handbook of Mediators in Septic Shock. CRC Press. Boca Raton, Fla.
4. BAUMGARTNER, J. D. 1992. Anti-endotoxin antibodies: A critical appraisal. *In* Mediators of Sepsis, M. Lamy and L. G. Thijs, Eds.: 315–328. Springer-Verlag. New York.
5. CHANG, S. W., C. O. FEDDERSEN, P. M. HENSEN & N. F. VOELKEL. 1987. Platelet-activating factor mediates hemodynamic changes and lung injury in endotoxin-treated rats. J. Clin. Invest. **79:** 1498–1509.

6. Dubois, C., E. Bissonnette & M. Rola-Pleszczynski. 1989. Platelet Activating Factor (PAF) enhances tumor necrosis factor production by alveolar macrophages: Prevention by PAF receptor antagonists and lipoxygenase inhibitors. J. Immunol. **143:** 964–970.

7. Mathison, J. C., E. Wolfson & R. J. Ulevitch. 1988. Participation of tumor necrosis factor in mediation of gram negative bacterial lipopolysaccharide-induced injury in rabbits. J. Clin. Invest. **81:** 1925–1937.

8. Rabinovici, R., *et al.* 1991. Priming by platelet activating factor of endotoxin-induced lung injury and cardiovascular shock. Circ. Res. **69:** 12–25.

9. Yue, T. L., R. Rabinovici, M. Farhat & G. Feuerstein. 1990. Pharmacologic profile of BN 50739, a new PAF antagonist in vitro and in vivo. Prostaglandins **39:** 469–480.

10. Rabinovici, R., *et al.* 1993. Tumor necrosis factor-α mediates endotoxin-induced lung injury in platelet activating factor-primed rats. J. Pharm. Exp. Ther. In press.

11. Rabinovici, R., *et al.* 1993. ARDS-like lung injury produced by endotoxin in platelet activating factor primed rats. J. Appl. Physiol. **74:** 1791–1802.

12. Rabinovici, R., *et al.* 1992. Role of complement in endotoxin/platelet-activating factor-induced lung injury. J. Immunol. **149:** 1744–1750.

Relationships between Polymorphonuclear Neutrophils and Cytokines in Patients with Adult Respiratory Distress Syndrome

S. CHOLLET-MARTIN, P. MONTRAVERS, C. GIBERT,
C. ELBIM, J. M. DESMONTS, J. Y. FAGON,
AND M. A. GOUGEROT-POCIDALO[a]

Service de Réanimation Médicale
Faculté Xavier Bichat
46, rue Henri Huchard
75877 Paris Cedex France

INTRODUCTION

Adult respiratory distress syndrome (ARDS) is a complex syndrome that results in increased permeability, pulmonary edema, severe hypoxemia, and mechanical abnormalities. Although the pathogenesis of ARDS is poorly understood, several observations point to an important role of polymorphonuclear neutrophils (PMN).[1,2] First, the vast majority of the cells recovered by bronchoalveolar lavage (BAL) in most patients with ARDS are PMN.[3] Second, there is considerable evidence linking neutrophil functions and the severity of ARDS, as assessed by circulating elastase and myeloperoxidase levels, and PMN oxidative burst measurement.[4-6] Moreover, it has been suggested that certain cytokines—interleukin-1β (IL-1β), tumor necrosis factor α (TNFα), interleukin-8 (IL-8), and interleukin-6 (IL-6)—play a critical role in the pathogenesis of ARDS, because of their powerful effects on PMN function and endothelial integrity. For example, high levels of TNFα have been found in bronchopulmonary secretions,[7] BAL fluid,[8,9] plasma[10,11] from patients with ARDS. A role of IL-8 in ARDS was further suggested by recent data showing elevated levels in the airspaces of patients with ARDS or at risk of ARDS.[12-14]

To gain further insight into the pathogenesis of ARDS, we studied the relationships between (1) hydrogen peroxide (H_2O_2) production by resting and *ex-vivo*-stimulated PMN, using a flow cytometric assay that permits the study of single cells and therefore the identification of subpopulations, and (2) plasma levels of TNFα, IL-1β, IL-8, and IL-6, together with their production by cultured monocytes and their BAL levels.

---

[a] To whom correspondence should be addressed.

MATERIALS AND METHODS

Patients and Controls

The 31 mechanically ventilated patients enrolled in this study were recruited from the medical and surgical intensive care units (ICU) of the Hôpital Bichat. Fifteen patients had ARDS, 8 without pneumonia, and 7 with pneumonia; 9 patients had pneumonia without ARDS; and 7 patients had neither ARDS nor pneumonia. Nine healthy volunteers served as control subjects. All the patients were studied within 3 days of the onset of ARDS or pneumonia. ARDS was defined using the lung injury score described by Murray *et al.*,[15] which includes the extent of roentgenographic densities, the severity of hypoxemia, and the level of positive-end-expiratory pressure (score > 2.5). The diagnosis of lung infection was based on clinical findings and the results of protected brush specimen cultures. The clinical severity of illness was assessed using two scoring systems, the simplified acute physiological score (SAPS)[16] and the number of abnormally functioning organs.[17]

Bronchoalveolar Lavage

BAL could be performed in 18 of the 31 patients and 6 healthy volunteers using a standard technique (5 × 20 ml of sterile saline aspirated via a hand-held syringe).[18] The recovered BAL fluid was rapidly filtered through sterile gauze and the cells were counted; cytospin preparations were made for differential cell counts and examination of intracellular microorganisms.[19] The supernatants were aliquoted and stored at −70°C for up to 15 days before assay.

Preparation of Blood Leucocytes

Blood was collected into sterile ethylenediaminetetraacetic acid (EDTA) treated vacuum tubes. Leucocytes were rapidly separated on a Dextran-Radioselectan gradient at +4°C to avoid PMN activation and adjusted to 10^6 PMN per milliliter in phosphate buffered saline (PBS).

Preparation of Monocyte Culture Supernatants

Monocytes were isolated from heparinized blood on a Ficoll-Isopaque gradient followed by an adherence step, as previously described.[20] Five × 10^5 monocytes were cultured for 24 hours with or without lipopolysaccharide (LPS, *E. coli* 055 = B5, Difco, 10 μg/ml). To determine extracellular cytokine production, cell-free supernatants were stored at −70°C.

Plasma Preparation

Blood was collected into sterile EDTA-treated vacuum tubes, transported on ice to the laboratory, and immediately centrifuged at 1500 g for 15 minutes at 4°C in order to avoid cytokine synthesis *in vitro*. Plasma samples were stored at −70°C.

Measurement of H_2O_2 Production by Blood PMN

Isolated PMN from the Patients

H_2O_2 production was measured using a flow cytometric assay of dichlorofluorescin (DCFH) oxidation as previously described.[21] Spontaneous and *ex vivo* phorbol myristate acetate (PMA)-stimulated DCFH oxidation were analyzed using a FACScan flow cytometer (Becton Dickinson, California), and a stimulation index (SI) was calculated.

Effect of the in vitro Preincubation with TNFα

After incubation with DCFH, blood from healthy donors was incubated with or without rh TNFα (0.1 to 1000 U/ml). *N*-Formyl-methionyl-leucyl-phenylalanine (FMLP) (10^{-6} M) was then added, the reaction was stopped on ice, and red cells were lysed. DCFH oxidation was then analyzed using a FACScan cytometer as previously described.[22]

Cytokine Assays

Cytokines were assayed using an immunoradiometric assay for TNFα (Medgenix, IRMA, Brussels, Belgium) and immunoenzymatic assays for IL-8, IL-6, and IL-1β (RD, Quantikine, Abingdon, UK and Medgenix, EASIA).

Statistical Analysis

All results are expressed as mean ±SEM. The significance of differences between groups was determined using the Mann-Whitney U test or analysis of variance and the Neuman-Keuls multiple range test, when appropriate. *P* values < 0.05 were considered significant. Correlations were tested for using the Spearman rank-correlation coefficient (ρ).

RESULTS

Clinical Results

Clinical characteristics of the 31 patients at the time of the assay are displayed in TABLE 1.

TNFα, IL-6, and IL-1β Plasma Levels

TNFα and IL-6 were detectable in the plasma of all 3 patient groups (FIG. 1) and the levels were significantly higher in both subgroups with ARDS than in those with other disorders ($p < 0.01$). In addition, plasma TNFα levels were significantly higher ($p < 0.01$) in the ARDS patients with pneumonia than in the

TABLE 1. Clinical Characteristics of the Patients

Parameters	ARDS without Pneumonia ($n = 8$)	ARDS with Pneumonia ($n = 7$)	Pneumonia without ARDS ($n = 9$)	Other Ventilated ($n = 7$)
Age (yr)	54 ± 6	62 ± 5	63 ± 5	64 ± 5
SAPS[a]	19 ± 3	19 ± 2	15 ± 1	12 ± 1
Organ dysfunction	3.8 ± 0.7	3.7 ± 0.6	2.8 ± 0.5	1.1 ± 0.1
Lung injury scoring	2.9 ± 0.1	2.8 ± 0.1	1 ± 0.1	0.7 ± 0.2
PaO_2/FiO_2 (mmHg)	100 ± 11	104 ± 12	237 ± 34	239 ± 37
Bacteremia[b]	3	3	4	—
Delay bacteremia/assay (days)	1 ± 0.5	1.3 ± 0.8	2.5 ± 0.9	—
Shock[b]	5	3	3	—

Note: Results are expressed as mean ± SEM.
[a] Simplified acute physiological score.
[b] Number of patients.

other groups. Lastly, IL-6 levels were significantly higher in the pneumonia group than in the ventilated group. IL-1β was never detectable.

Production of TNFα, IL-6, and IL-1β by 24-hour-Cultured Monocytes

Both spontaneous and LPS-induced TNFα and IL-6 production were significantly higher in the two subgroups of ARDS patients than in the control subjects (TABLE 2). IL-6 production was also significantly higher in patients with pneumonia, than in the patients with neither ARDS nor pneumonia and the control subjects. IL-1β production was normal in all groups of patients.

BAL Cytology and Cytokine Levels

The BAL fluids from the three groups of patients contained significantly higher percentages of PMN relative to the healthy controls (76 ± 13%, 79 ± 11%, 74 ± 9%, and 2 ± 1%, respectively, in ARDS without pneumonia, ARDS with pneumonia, pneumonia without ARDS, and controls; mean ± SEM, $p < 0.005$).

In the subgroup of patients in whom BAL could be performed, we compared IL-8 and TNFα levels both in plasma and BAL fluid (FIG. 2). IL-8 and TNFα were elevated in the plasma of all three patient groups relative to the control subjects. IL-8 plasma levels were significantly higher in the patients with ARDS and pneumonia compared to the other groups ($p < 0.05$). In BAL fluid, IL-8 and TNFα were increased in the two subgroups of ARDS patients relative to the pneumonia group ($p < 0.05$) and undetectable in the healthy controls. IL-8 levels were always greater than those of TNFα in all the patient groups. In addition, the BAL fluid-to-plasma ratios of the two cytokines were significantly greater for IL-8 than for TNFα only in the two ARDS groups, possibly reflecting greater local production of IL-8 than TNFα in the lungs of the patients with ARDS (TABLE 3).

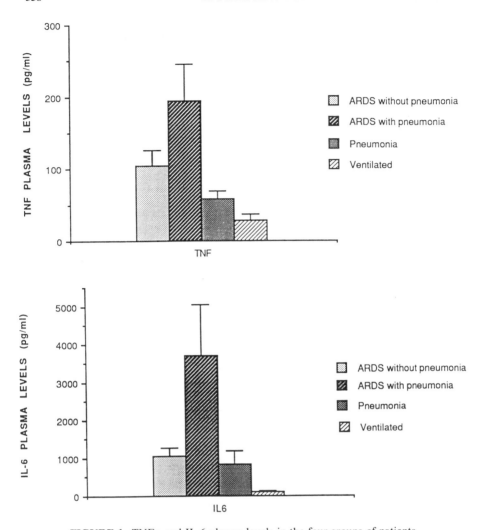

FIGURE 1. TNFα and IL-6 plasma levels in the four groups of patients.

H₂O₂ Production by Blood PMN

As shown in FIGURE 3, after stimulation with PMA, PMN from healthy subjects responded as a homogeneous population, with a median stimulation index (SI) of 4. In contrast, in the patients, PMN showed a bimodal response, with about half the PMN responding like cells from control subjects, and the other half showing a significantly increased SI. The significant largest increase in SI was observed in patients with ARDS.

In vitro addition of rhTNFα to whole blood from healthy controls induces various responses to FMLP, depending on the concentration of the rhTNFα. From

TABLE 2. Spontaneous and LPS-Induced Production of Cytokines by 24-hours-Culture Monocytes in the Different Groups of Patients and Control Subjects

	TNFα		IL-6		IL-1β	
	Spontaneous	LPS-Induced	Spontaneous	LPS-Induced	Spontaneous	LPS-Induced
Controls n = 9	248 ± 47	337 ± 57	415 ± 133	8135 ± 94	305 ± 15	5717 ± 802
ARDS without pneumonia n = 8	3995 ± 619[a]	30500 ± 8418[a]	5031 ± 1702[a]	14.522 ± 1382	1084 ± 433	5680 ± 1624
ARDS with pneumonia n = 7	3224 ± 1024[a]	19103 ± 5409[a]	3723 ± 1458[a]	32258 ± 12489[a]	353 ± 155	7177 ± 1689
Pneumonia n = 9	449 ± 91	3832 ± 598	2297 ± 807[a]	19603 ± 6046	747 ± 286	5456 ± 1281
Ventilated n = 7	217 ± 36	2779 ± 377	732 ± 256	4803 ± 1046	233 ± 116	7272 ± 2032

Note: Values are expressed in pg per 5–10^5 monocytes, as mean ± SEM.
[a] Significantly increased as compared to all other groups ($p < 0.05$). Not significantly together.

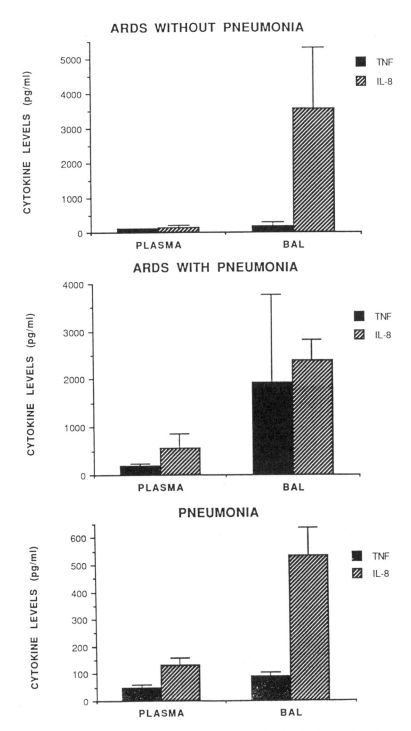

FIGURE 2. TNFα and IL-8 levels in plasma and bronchoalveolar lavage fluid in patients with ARDS and patients with pneumonia.

TABLE 3. BAL Fluid/Plasma Ratio of Cytokines

Patients	BAL Fluid/Plasma	
	IL-8	TNFα
ARDS without pneumonia ($n = 6$)	15.9 ± 9.2^a	5.8 ± 7.0
ARDS with pneumonia ($n = 6$)	12.8 ± 1.8^a	6.9 ± 3.1
Pneumonia ($n = 6$)	3.5 ± 1.2	1.6 ± 0.8

^{a} $p < 0.05$ vs. TNFα.

0.1 to 10 U/ml, a single PMN population was observed. As shown in FIGURE 4, from 10 to 750 U/ml, the SI of the more responsive population increased in a dose-dependent manner.

Correlations between Cytokine Levels and Biological Parameters

The SI of the second PMN subpopulation correlated with TNFα plasma levels ($\rho = 0.47$, $p < 0.01$), and both spontaneous ($\rho = 0.74$, $p < 0.001$) and LPS-induced TNFα production ($\rho = 0.74$, $p < 0.001$) in the overall patient population. There was no correlation between H_2O_2 production and IL-6 values, and this correlation was weak with IL-8 ($\rho = 0.4$, $p = 0.07$). There was no correlation between IL-8 levels and the percentage of PMN in BAL fluid in the overall population ($\rho = 0.22$, $p = 0.09$).

Correlations between Biological and Clinical Parameters

The lung injury score of individual patients but not the SAPS index correlated with the SI of their second PMN subpopulation in the DCFH assay ($\rho = 0.70$, $p = 0.001$) (FIG. 5). Moreover, the lung injury score correlated with TNFα plasma levels ($\rho = 0.63$, $p = 0.001$) (FIG. 5), and both spontaneous ($\rho = 0.81$, $p = 0.001$) and LPS-induced TNFα production ($\rho = 0.74$, $p = 0.001$) but not with SAPS index. On the contrary, IL-8 levels in BAL fluid correlated better with the SAPS value ($\rho = 0.05$, $p < 0.05$) than with the lung injury score. No correlations between lung injury and IL-1β parameters or IL-8 plasma levels were found. The patients who ultimately died or those with shock had significantly higher BAL IL-8 concentrations than the survivors or those normotensive (data not shown).

FIGURE 3. Distribution of fluorescence (DCF content) of PMN obtained from a normal control **(A)** and a patient with ARDS **(B)**, using flow cytometry to measure the H_2O_2 production. The *empty histograms* represent the production of H_2O_2 by resting PMN. The *solid histograms* show H_2O_2 produced by PMA-activated PMN, and show the appearance of a clearly hyperresponsive subpopulation of PMN in the ARDS patient.

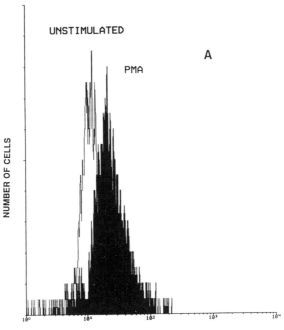

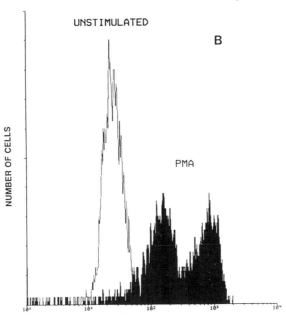

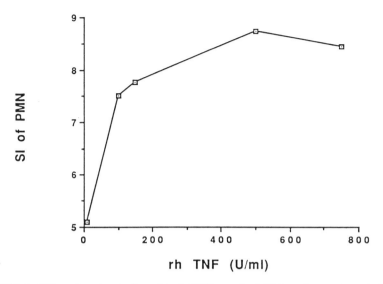

FIGURE 4. Effect of preincubation with rh TNFα on the PMN respiratory burst induced by FMLP in whole blood. The concentration of rh TNFα is related to the stimulation index (SI) of the hyperresponsive subpopulation. This curve represents a typical experiment.

DISCUSSION

Previous reports about the functional activities of circulating PMN in patients with ARDS differ in their findings. Using flow cytometric analysis, we found a bimodal response of H_2O_2 production by circulating PMN following PMA stimulation *ex vivo* in all the groups of patients, and a particularly hyperresponsive subpopulation in ARDS patients. We found that the PMN stimulation index correlated better with TNFα parameters than with IL-8 parameters in ARDS patients. This is consistent with *in vitro* studies showing that TNFα is a better priming agent than IL-8 for PMA-induced H_2O_2 production in the DCFH assay (unpublished personal data). These findings reinforce the recent work of De Forge,[23] who found, *in vitro,* that endogenously produced reactive oxygen metabolites directly induce the transcription and translation of IL-8.

We also investigated the levels of four cytokines, TNFα, IL-6, IL-8, and IL-1β, because these substances have been found to prime the PMN oxidative burst.[22] According to our results, TNFα emerged as the cytokine most closely related to diffuse lung injury, since levels in both plasma and supernatants of cultured monocytes were significantly higher in patients with ARDS than in the other groups of patients and controls. Our results are in accordance with the studies of Roberts *et al.*,[8] Hyers *et al.*,[9] and Marks *et al.*[10] who reported increased TNFα plasma levels in patients with ARDS. Tran Van Nhieu *et al.* recently described high levels of expression of TNFα gene in alveolar macrophages from patients with ARDS.[24] The correlations we found between the TNFα parameters studied and the PMN SI suggest that this cytokine may have a priming effect *in vivo,* thereby giving rise to a hyperresponsive PMN subpopulation. Our *in vitro* experiments can support this hypothesis since the addition of rhTNFα to normal whole blood, followed by *ex vivo* stimulation induced bimodal H_2O_2 production by PMN.[22] The existence of strong correlations between the lung injury score and

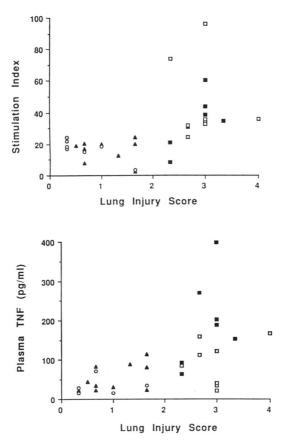

FIGURE 5. Correlations between lung injury score, SI of the hyperresponsive subpopulation of PMN, and TNFα plasma levels. Correlations were performed on the entire population: ARDS without pneumonia (□), ARDS with pneumonia (■), pneumonia (△), non-ARDS non-pneumonia (○).

both the PMN SI and TNFα parameters further supports the involvement of TNFα and PMN in the pathogenesis of ARDS as does the fact that the PMN SI and TNFα parameters correlated better with the lung injury score than with the general clinical indices (SAPS and number of organ dysfunctions). In contrast, levels of IL-8 in BAL correlated with an index of overall clinical severity (SAPS), but there was only a trend toward a correlation with the lung injury score. This correlation between SAPS values and BAL IL-8 levels is in accordance with the differences in IL-8 levels between the patients who died and those who survived and reinforces the relationship between IL-8 and overall clinical severity rather than lung injury.

IL-8 and TNFα were present in increased concentrations in the alveolar spaces of all the patients tested, and their levels were significantly higher in the two ARDS groups than in the pneumonia group and the controls. Similar results have been reported by Miller et al.,[14] Lynch et al.,[13] and Donnely et al.[12] in ARDS patients. Moreover, in our work, the BAL fluid-to-plasma ratio seems to indicate that more IL-8 than TNFα is produced in the lungs of patients with ARDS. Although alveolar macrophages appear to be the major cellular source of IL-8 in the lung,[12,25] cells that constitute the alveolar-capillary membrane have also been shown to produce IL-8, including endothelial cells, fibroblasts, type-II-like epithelial cells, and bronchial epithelial cells as well as neutrophils.

The presence of increased levels of IL-8 in the blood of patients with ARDS may play a role in the recruitment of neutrophils to the lung; indeed, it has been shown *in vitro* that IL-8 can increase the expression of L-selectin LAM-1[26] and can cause rapid and profound stimulation of F-actin polymerization of neutrophils.[27] The percentage of neutrophils found in the BAL fluid was not related to the corresponding IL-8 concentration in the overall patient group. These results are in accordance with those of Miller in ARDS[14] and of Lynch in idiopathic pulmonary fibrosis.[13] The fact that we failed to find a correlation suggests that IL-8 is not the only chemoattractant involved in transendothelial neutrophil migration in this setting.

As a conclusion, our results demonstrate the existence of a primed subpopulation of circulating PMN in patients with ARDS that is particularly hyperresponsive to subsequent stimulation *ex vivo*. The presence of significantly increased plasma TNFα levels in these patients, as well as the high capacity of their blood monocytes to produce TNFα *ex vivo,* both suggest a major role of this cytokine in the pathogenesis of ARDS; moreover, we show that high levels of IL-8 are potentially associated with neutrophil accumulation in the alveoli. In contrast, values of IL-6 show less and those of IL-1β show no involvement in this syndrome. The PMN and TNFα parameters that we measured correlated better with the lung injury score than with the general clinical severity scores, and reinforce the suggestion that the large amounts of TNFα in ARDS patients may prime blood PMN for subsequent activation; IL-8 and IL-6 may enhance this process. Therefore, ARDS-associated lung injury could be caused, at least in part, by an association of TNFα-induced pulmonary capillary endothelial cell damage and injury inflicted by TNFα-, IL-8-, and IL-6-primed PMN.

REFERENCES

1. SWANK, D. S. & S. B. MOORE. 1989. Roles of the neutrophil and other mediators in adult respiratory distress syndrome. Mayo Clin. Proc. **64:** 1118–1132.
2. SIBILLE, Y. & H. Y. REYNOLDS. 1990. Macrophages and polymorphonuclear neutrophils in lung defense and injury. Am. Rev. Respir. Dis. **141:** 471–501.
3. FOWLER, A. A., *et al.* 1987. The adult respiratory distress syndrome. Cell populations and soluble mediators in the air spaces of patients at high risk. Am. Rev. Respir. Dis. **136:** 1225–1231.
4. ZIMMERMAN, G. A., A. D. RENZETTI & H. R. HILL. 1983. Functional and metabolic activity of granulocytes from patients with adult respiratory distress syndrome. Evidence for activated neutrophils in the pulmonary circulation. Am. Rev. Respir. Dis. **127:** 290–300.
5. RIVKIND, A. I., *et al.* 1990. Neutrophil oxidative burst activation and the pattern of respiratory physiologic abnormalities in the fulminant post-traumatic adult respiratory distress syndrome. Circ. Shock **33:** 48–62.
6. MARTIN, T. R., B. P. PISTORESE, L. D. HUDSON & R. J. MAUNDER. 1991. The function of lung and blood neutrophils in patients with the adult respiratory distress syndrome. Implications for the pathogenesis of lung infections. Am. Rev. Respir. Dis. **114:** 254–262.

7. MILAR, A. B., *et al.* 1989. Tumor necrosis factor in bronchopulmonary secretions of patients with adult respiratory distress syndrome. Lancet **ii:** 712–714.

8. ROBERTS, D. J., J. M. DAVIES, C. C. EVANS, M. BELL & L. M. MOSTAFA. 1989. Tumor necrosis factor and adult respiratory distress syndrome. Lancet **ii:** 1043–1044.

9. HYERS, T. M., S. M. TRICOMI, P. A. DETTENMEIER & A. A. FOWLER. 1991. Tumor necrosis factor levels in serum and bronchoalveolar lavage fluid of patients with the adult respiratory distress syndrome. Am. Rev. Respir. Dis. **144:** 268–271.

10. MARKS, J. D., *et al.* 1990. Plasma tumor necrosis factor in patients with septic shock. Mortality rate, incidence of adult respiratory distress syndrome, and effects of methyl prednisolone administration. Am. Rev. Respir. Dis. **141:** 4–97.

11. ROTEN, R., *et al.* 1991. Plasma levels of tumor necrosis factor in the adult respiratory distress syndrome. Am. Rev. Respir. Dis. **143:** 590–592.

12. DONNELY, S. C., *et al.* 1993. Interleukin-8 and development of adult respiratory distress syndrome in at-risk patient groups. Lancet **341:** 643–647.

13. LYNCH, I. J. P., T. J. STANDIFORD, M. N. ROLFE, S. L. KUNKEL & R. M. STRIETER. 1992. Neutrophilic alveolitis in idiopathic pulmonary fibrosis. Am. Rev. Respir. Dis. **145:** 1433–1439.

14. MILLER, E. J., *et al.* 1992. Elevated levels of NAP-1/interleukin-8 are present in the airspaces of patients with the adult respiratory distress syndrome and are associated with increased mortality. Am. Rev. Respir. Dis. **146:** 427–432.

15. MURRAY, J. F., M. A. MATTHAY, J. M. LUCE & M. R. FLICK. 1988. An expanded definition of the adult respiratory distress syndrome. Am. Rev. Respir. Dis. **138:** 720–723.

16. LE GALL, J. R., P. LOIRAT & A. LPEROVITCH. 1983. Simplified acute physiological score for intensive care patients. Lancet **ii:** 741.

17. BIHARI, D., M. SMITHIES, A. GIMSON & J. TINKER. 1987. The effects of vasodilation with prostacyclin on oxygen delivery and uptake in critically ill patients. New Eng. J. Med. **317:** 397–403.

18. CHASTRE, J., *et al.* 1988. Diagnosis of nosocomial bacterial pneumonia in intubated patients undergoing ventilation: Comparison of the usefulness of bronchoalveolar lavage and the protected specimen brush. Am. J. Med. **85:** 499–506.

19. CHASTRE, J., *et al.* 1989. Quantification of BAL cells containing intracellular bacteria rapidly identifies ventilated patients with nosocomial pneumonia. Chest **95:** 190S–192S.

20. CHOLLET-MARTIN, S., G. STAMATAKIS, S. BAILLY, J. P. MERY & M. A. GOUGEROT-POCIDALO. 1991. Induction of tumor necrosis factor alpha during hemodialys. Influence of the membrane type. Clin. Exp. Immunol. **83:** 329–332.

21. CHOLLET-MARTIN, S., *et al.* 1992. Subpopulation of hyper-responsive polymorphonuclear neutrophils in patients with adult respiratory distress syndrome. Role of cytokine production. Am. Rev. Respir. Dis. **146:** 990–996.

22. ELBIM, C., S. CHOLLET-MARTIN, S. BAILLY, J. HAKIM & M. A. GOUGEROT-POCIDALO. 1993. Priming of polymorphonuclear neutrophils by tumor necrosis factor alpha in whole blood: Identification of two subpopulations in response to formyl-peptides. Blood. **82:** 633–640.

23. DE FORGE, L. A., J. C. FANTONE, J. S. KENNEY & D. G. REMICK. 1992. Oxygen radical scavengers selectively inhibit interleukin 8 production in human whole blood. J. Clin. Invest. **90:** 2123–2129.

24. TRAN VAN NHIEU, J., B. MISSET, F. LEBARGY, J. CARLET & J. F. BERNAUDIN. 1993. Expression of tumor necrosis factor alpha gene in alveolar macrophages from patients with the adult respiratory distress syndrome. Am. Rev. Respir. Dis. **147:** 1585–1589.

25. JORENS, P. G., *et al.* 1993. Interleukin-8 in the bronchoalveolar lavage fluid from patients with the adult respiratory distress syndrome and patients at risk for ARDS. Cytokine **4:** 592–597.

26. LUSCINSKAS, F. W., *et al.* 1992. In vitro inhibitory effect of IL-8 and other chemoattractants on neutrophil-endothelial adhesive interactions. J. Immunol. **149:** 2163–2171.

27. WESTLIN, W. F., J. M. KIELY & M. A. GIMBRONE. 1992. Interleukin-8 induces changes in human neutrophil actin conformation and distribution: Relationship to inhibition of adhesion to cytokine-activated endothelium. J. Leukoc. Biol. **52:** 43–51.

New Therapeutical Approaches in the Treatment of Asthma

PH. GODARD, P. CHANEZ, H. REDIER, J. BOUSQUET,
AND F. B. MICHEL

Clinique des Maladies Respiratoires
INSERM CJF 92 10
Hôpital Arnaud de Villeneuve
Avenue Doyen Girand
34059 Montpellier Cedex
France

INTRODUCTION

According to a recently proposed definition, bronchial asthma is a chronic inflammatory disorder of the airways.[1] It is a disabling condition, and all the epidemiologic data indicate an increase in its prevalence, morbidity, and mortality.[2] Despite the high efficiency of inhaled corticosteroids (ICS's), which to date remain one of the main treatments, there is a need for new therapeutical approaches. Indeed, first of all, ICS's do not cure asthma; within some weeks[3] or one year of cessation of the treatment, symptoms and other features of asthma (such as bronchial hyperreactivity, instability of PEFR) recur; secondly, side effects can be observed with the ICS's that are currently available;[4] thirdly, ICS's could prevent, but not totally abolish, the effect of various targeting factors.

Huge advances in knowledge over the past 10 years have made it possible to describe new therapeutical approaches; however, these new approaches are quite numerous. The aim of this paper is to go through some of them, keeping in mind that asthma is not a (unique) disease, but a rather complex disorder of the airways that combines inflammation and bronchospasm, and that is the consequence of several inherited and precipating factors, among which environmental factors (at large) take first place.

HISTORY

From a historic point of view it must be remembered that xanthins were introduced in the 1930s, corticosteroids in the 1950s, β agonists in the 1960s, and sodium cromoglycate in the 1970s. The last two decades have been characterized by the improvement of these drugs: xanthins once a day, ICS 250 mcg/puff, long-acting β2 agonists, Nedocromil sodium.

During the same period of time our knowledge has increased very rapidly, and it could be compared to the Big Bang that created the Universe. But we have not yet the new drugs to treat and cure asthmatic patients. In the 1970s, PGE2 analogs were thought to be helpful, but they failed; later on, platelet activating factor (PAF) antagonists were thought to be effective because PAF is quite a potent mediator that can imitate and induce all the findings that are observed in asthmatics, but, to date, no PAF antagonist has been successful in the treatment of chronic asthma. Inhibitors of 5-lipoxygenase and specific leukotriene antagonists are still in the pipeline, and some are promising. Any therapeutic impact at the cytokine or adhesion molecule level should also be carefully investigated, even if the design of such new drugs appears to be quite complex.

PATHOPHYSIOLOGY AND OBJECTIVES

In order to develop new therapeutic approaches in the treatment of asthma, we need to have a clear view of its pathophysiology. Bronchoscopy and saline-induced sputum analysis allow us to have direct access to the bronchi and the inflammatory lesions. Bronchoscopy can be safely performed in asthmatics;[5] with this method, broncho-alveolar (BAL) fluid, bronchial biopsies, and brushings can be obtained in various clinical conditions, according to the severity, as well as the presence or absence of any precipitating factor. Hargreaves' group recently developed a new methodology to assess, sequentially but not invasively, the cellular events that occur in the lower airways:[6,7] sputum can be induced safely by the inhalation of saline; after adequate procedures this method allows the clinician to check the presence of inflammatory cells (eosinophils, neutrophils, metachromatic cells, macrophages, lymphocytes) and to quantify inflammatory mediators in the sputum fluid.

For a long period of time, inhalation challenges have been considered as the gold standard to test the efficacy of a new drug. It is indeed a unique tool to dissect the complexity of events that occur after inhalation of an allergen or a precipitating factor. In recent years, A. B. Tonnel was the first to perform local antigen challenges via the fiberoscope;[8] many studies have since been made that allow us to better understand the inflammatory cascade at the site of the reaction itself.[9]

It is now clearly established, however, that chronic asthma is quite different from the acute inflammation induced by allergen challenge. Some drugs that can prevent or reverse allergic reactions are not always active in asthmatic patients.[10]

Chronic asthma is clearly an inflammatory disorder of the airways. The cellular component is related to the severity of the disease,[11] but could be different according to the condition of exposure: as assessed by BAL, during an acute reaction, eosinophils could be recruited preferentially in the proximal airways,[12] while during chronic exposure, the airway inflammation could take place throughout the bronchial tree.[13] The vascular component of the disease could be linked to the activity; in other words, to the variability or instability of airway obstruction.

To date, it is clear that many cells and mediators are involved in the pathophysiology of bronchial asthma. Moreover various stimuli are well known as precipitating agents (FIG. 1). It can be hypothetized that a common abnormal cellular pathway is involved and might be the target for a new drug. But this remains to be proved.

PREVENT THE EARLY INFLAMMATORY EVENTS

The time course and cellular involvement of the inflammatory cascade are not well known. However, it may be that resident cells that are present throughout the bronchial tree are able to initiate it, either spontaneously or after specific or nonspecific targeting.

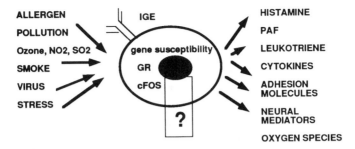

FIGURE 1. Is there any single abnormal cellular pathway of activation? The precipitating factors of asthma are numerous; cellular activation induces the synthesis and release of a lot of mediators that will injure the bronchi. It could be hypothesized that one single pathway is abnormal at the cellular level; it could be the target for a new drug.

1. Mast cells are present in normal airways. In bronchial asthma their number is increased;[14] as assessed by a high histamine, PGD_2 and tryptase content in BAL fluid, they appear to be activated.[15,16] After inhalation challenge, the number of metachromatic cells increases in sputum.[17] Recently S. Holgate demonstrated a substantial increase in mast cells, particularly outside the airway's smooth muscle, in patients who have died from asthma.[18] It is generally assumed that they act as the starter of the inflammatory cascade, especially after allergen challenge.

Cromones could act at this level,[19] but they have many more effects on different cells such as bronchial epithelial cells,[20] alveolar macrophages,[21] or bronchial receptors.

In 1991 C. Page proposed an interesting hypothesis suggesting that $\beta2$ agonists could decrease the release of inflammatory and also anti-inflammatory mediators from mast cells;[22] indeed heparin manifested antiasthmatic properties. J. G. Biet *et al.* demonstrated that low molecular mass heparin forms a tight complex with mucus proteinase inhibitor, the physiologic neutrophil elastase inhibitor of the upper respiratory tract.[23] Moreover it has been shown recently that a small dose of heparin (nebulized heparin, 20,000 units) inhibited the bronchospasm induced by the inhalation of house dust mite allergen in asthmatics.[24] However, additional data are required to confirm or not the "asthma paradox" that has been described by C. Page.

2. Bronchial epithelial cells (BECs) are present throughout the bronchial tree; they act as a barrier, indeed an active barrier. Van Houtte demonstrated that BECs released a bronchodilator agent, which has not yet been identified. Nitric oxide (NO) could be this bronchodilator agent, but this has not been proved. In bronchial asthma, BECs appear to be highly abnormal:

- Low viability,[25] which explains their increased number in BAL fluid, and the shedding of the epithelium[11,26] are abnormalities that have been linked to bronchial hyperreactivity[27] (unpublished personal results);
- As compared to normal subjects, they release higher quantities of inflamma-

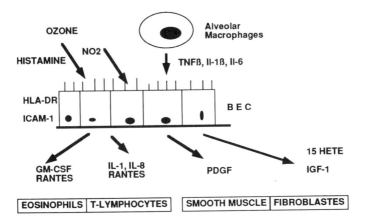

FIGURE 2. Activation and mediators release by BECs. BECs are present throughout the airways and can be activated by many aero contaminants and mediators; BECs have to be considered as an active barrier. Increasing evidence indicates their participation in the pathophysiology of asthma. BECs could be a good target for a new drug.

tory mediators such as 15 HETE;[28] BEC are also the potential source of many cytokines and growth factors, as assessed, at least, in animals (FIG. 2);
• They express abnormally high levels of HLA-DR[29] and intercellular adhesion molecule-1 (ICAM-1).[30] It has been shown in animals that anti-ICAM (2 mg/kg; daily; 10 days) was able to prevent eosinophil recruitment, eosinophil activation, and increased bronchial hyperreactivity.[31,32]

Because this kind of therapeutic approach [monoclonal antibody (MoAb)] could be responsible for the development of antibodies against MoAb, it might be best to modify the gene at the BEC level (cf. infra).

3. Alveolar macrophages (AM) can no longer be named "accessory" cells. They are present throughout the airways as assessed by segmental lavage[33] or analysis of the first recovery of BAL;[34] they are also present in the bronchial wall as assessed by biopsy, where they appear to be recruited from the blood monocytes;[35] moreover the DNA content in AMs and expression of Ki-67 by AMs do not support the theory that an important source of airway macrophages is due to local proliferation.[36] This could justify the modification of blood monocytes that appear highly abnormal in asthmatics.[37]

AM could be involved in the allergic- (and nonallergic-) induced mechanisms of asthma: antigen processing and IgE control, allergic-induced airway inflammation, and possibly repair after injury. Their suppressive activity on polyclonal-induced lymphocyte proliferation is decreased;[38] they express high quantities of HLA-DR and ICAM-1.[39] They appear to be activated in chronic asthma[40] and a high releasability, as assessed by reactive oxygen species release, has been shown to be correlated to the severity of asthma.[41] AMs are phagocytizing cells that make possible the development of specific targeting of drugs via liposomes. However, this possibility has not been evaluated to date.

Whether in the blood or in the airways, the cells appear to be activated even in stable asymptomatic asthmatic patients and in allergic patients with only rhinitis.

TABLE 1. Blood Monocytes cAMP Content

	Healthy Subjects	Asthmatics
Control	10.8 (21.8 − 0.0)	6.3 (11.3 − 1.7)
Isoproterenol	67.5 (27.8 − 64.6)[a]	6.6 (11.1 − 3.7)[b]
(10^{-7} mol/l)		

pmol/mg. prot.

Note: Results were obtained from 6 healthy subjects and 6 untreated allergic asthmatics, and expressed as median (range).

[a] $p < 0.001$ as compared to control.

[b] $p < 0.001$ as compared to healthy subjects.

This could be the consequence of a priming effect or of an intrinsic cellular defect: low intracellular cAMP (TABLE 1), high turnover of phosphoinositides,[42] translocation of the protein kinase C (PKC) (personal data, not shown). It might also be suggested that a high IgE binding to the cells can activate them, making it necessary to dampen the IgE synthesis. Another very interesting hypothesis has recently been highlighted by R. F. Herrscher *et al.*'s study: they demonstrated that physiological levels of serum cortisol can regulate IgE-dependent cutaneous inflammation by affecting the expression of cellular events at late-phase sites.[43] In an unpublished study, we have observed that, in asthmatics who develop an allergen-induced late-phase reaction, the cortisol levels in urine increase significantly less than those of asthmatics who develop only an early-phase reaction; this could suggest a deficit in cortisol response.

CURE AIRWAY INFLAMMATION

Bronchial asthma is really a chronic desquamative bronchitis with a high eosinophil and lymphocyte recruitment in the airways. Eosinophils are activated and release high quantities of various mediators such as LTC4, 15 HETE, ECP, and MBP; they are also the source of many cytokines.[44] T-cells express IL-2 receptor (CD25) and HLA-DR; they also express mRNA for IL-3, IL-4, IL-5, and granulocyte-macrophage colony stimulating factor (GM–CSF).[45] Many of these abnormalities have been correlated to the clinical severity of the asthma.[11] One of the main objectives of the treatment is to reverse clinical symptoms and to cure airway inflammation.

On an acute basis (from some days to some weeks), corticosteroids are able to reverse airway obstruction and bronchial hyperreactivity, and to clear inflammatory cells. To date, this class of drug is the best to rapidly (and completely in a majority of patients) improve an asthmatic patient. On a chronic basis, long-term treatment with ICS's has been shown to be very effective in maintaining the good results that have been obtained with oral corticosteroids[46] or to do the same thing as oral corticosteroids,[47] only in this case it takes weeks instead of days.

However, the efficacy of corticosteroids is not identical in all asthmatics. Many explanations have been proposed: heterogeneity of airway inflammation (involving mainly lymphocytes or neutrophils), different biodisponibilities of steroids, variable sensitivity of the glucocorticoid receptor.[48] There are corticoresistant asthmatic patients;[49] some authors have suggested the role of a specific cytokine, but additional data are required.

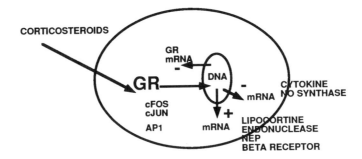

FIGURE 3. Glucocorticoid effects at the cellular and genomic levels. Glucocorticoid receptor (GR) is located in the cytosol; the AP1, which is formed by cFOS and cJUN could be a limiting step in the activation of GR by corticosteroids. Corticosteroids up-regulate the synthesis of many proteins that are involved in the pathophysiology of asthma, but also down-regulate some others. Corticosteroids down-regulate the expression of GR mRNA. (Personal results in collaboration with B. Terronane, I. Vachier, and J. C. Nicolas, INERM U58, Montpellier, France, unpublished.)

New therapeutic approaches could be as follows:

- Cyclosporine has been used with success and could act at the lymphocyte level;[50] the importance of side effects makes it indispensable to develop new drugs, with more specific activity;
- Methotrexate decreases the corticosteroid requirement,[51] but the mechanism of action is not clear; side effects could be severe;
- Other drugs, such as dapsone,[52] immunoglobulins, or gold salts,[53] have been successfully investigated in open studies.

These last findings are interesting because they open up new approaches in treatment with corticosteroids:

- Corticosteroids have to be used as starting drugs over a short period of time in order to reverse the inflammatory injury, preventive drugs being used afterwards;
- New drugs could be designed to increase corticosteroid sensitivity at the glucocorticosteroid receptor (GR) level (FIG. 3).

REPAIR THE AIRWAY INJURY

Bronchial asthma is a disease that remodels the airways.[54] In it at least two components seem to exist: a reversible one and an irreversible one that might be responsible for an aging of the airways. This last could be defined as a nonreversible impairment and disability, and could be expressed as a high FEV_1 decline over time.[55] From a pathological point of view, many abnormalities, such as pseudo-thickening of the base membrane, disruption of the elastic fibers, and hypertrophy of the bronchial smooth muscles, appear to be nonreversible.

Corticosteroids are able to restore a "normal" (at least from a morphological point of view) epithelial barrier,[56] but do not repair completely the airways. It seems very difficult to design new drugs that would be able to do that. This is an additional reason why preventive treatment has to be started early in the management of asthma.

It is interesting to observe that ICS's are not able to decrease the pseudo-thickening of the base membrane, but the removal from an occupational exposure is.

THE FUTURE

Bronchial asthma is a complex disorder, not just an inflammatory airway disease. Many components have to be taken into account.

Clinical Evaluation of Asthma

The various consensus reports and the quality-of-life questionnaires have made it necessary to report numerous clinical, physiological, and biological parameters. In order to better understand bronchial asthma, we have developed an expert system that takes into account all these parameters and proposes a management plan that has been validated by several academic experts in France. This kind of approach makes it possible to better classify the various asthmatic patients.[58]

In many textbooks, extrinsic asthma has been compared to intrinsic asthma; in fact, it appears more useful to check, in each patient, the presence and the responsibility of various precipitating factors and to give the name "intrinsic asthma" to cases where no precipitating factor has been identified.

The international guidelines indicate clearly that all precipitating factors have to be accounted for; the avoidance of allergen and desensitization have been proved to be very effective.[59]

In so-called intrinsic asthma, which appears to be more severe, an autoimmune mechanism could exist;[60] specific drugs could be used.

For the majority of patients, the up-to-date available drugs are effective and increase quality of life. However, compliance is very low and this makes it indispensable to explain, educate, and support the patients better.[61]

The Near Future

High-dose ICS therapy is a major clinical advance in the treatment of asthma. The ratio of efficacy/side effects is very high, and this needs to be improved. Biological abnormalities have also been observed, and clinical relevance of such observations has to be checked carefully. Fluticazone dipropionate (FP) has a higher receptor affinity than beclomethazone (BDP) and budesonide, and is transformed by a single metabolic pathway. FP and BDP have antiasthmatic equipotency in the dose ratio 1:2.

Many drugs are in the pipeline and could be on the market in the next few years.

- Zileuton is an orally active 5-lipoxygenase inhibitor (it is an iron ligand inhibitor, as compared to other compounds, which are redox or nonredox inhibitors) that has been shown to be active in rhinitis, and in mild to moderate asthma; in a recent randomized double-blind study, 139 asthmatics received either Zileuton (2.4 g/d or 1.6 g/d) or placebo for four weeks. FEV1 increased by 13.4 percent in the treated patients; mean urinary LTE4 decreased by 39 percent.[62] Zileuton was demonstrated to prevent the fall in FEV_1, and also the nasal–gastro intestinal and dermal symptoms that are observed after aspirin challenge in aspirin-sensitive patients. A new series of lipoxygenase inhibitors (ICI D2138, for example), which have neither iron liganding nor redox properties, are undergoing clinical evaluation and could provide improved clinical efficacy.[63]

- Several leukotriene antagonists (ICI 204219 and MK 571) are currently being evaluated, and they display antiasthmatic activities. The first one reduced the early-phase bronchconstriction by 80 percent and late-phase bronchoconstriction by about half, and attenuated the accompanying increase in bronchial hyperreactivity. They are undergoing clinical evaluation in chronic asthma.
- Specific phosphodiesterase (PDE) inhibitors are also being investigated; from a clinical point of view, these make it possible to decrease the side effects that are observed with theophylin. But more importantly, apart from a bronchodilatator effect, other actions have to be investigated: in rat HTC cells, Forskolin increased the glucocorticoid receptor (GR) mRNA expression; IBMX inhibited IL-4 and IL-5 mRNA expression in human PBMC. In guinea pigs, Rolipram (PDE IV inhibitor) reduced by 79 percent eosinophil infiltration evoked by leukotrienes B_4 and D_4 or by histamine in conjunctiva.[64] These new drugs could also have anti-inflammatory and antiallergic properties.[65]

Genes as Drugs

In the long term, within the next 10 years, it seems not unreasonable to hope that new therapeutic approaches will be available at the gene level. We can hope to correct, at least temporarily, the dysfunction of any particular cell that appears to be important in the pathophysiology of asthma.

From this point of view, epithelial cells could be considered as a good target for such gene therapy. The technology is available. Adenovirus DNA can accept exogenous DNA. The first treatment was administered to humans by R. Crystal in April 1993. Monocytes–macrophages and lymphocytes could also be good candidates.

Bronchial asthma is more a multifactorial syndrome than a single disease, and airway inflammation is a symptom of this disorder. Many mediators are involved in the pathophysiology and any improvement in the treatment must be compared to corticosteroids. All of the facets of this complex disorder (inflammation, bronchospasm, precipitating factors) must be taken into account in order to increase the quality of life for the patients.

REFERENCES

1. SHEFFER, A. L. 1992. International consensus report on diagnosis and treatment of asthma—International asthma management project. Clin. Exp. Allergy **22:** R7.
2. BURNEY, P. G. J. 1992. Epidemiology. Brit. Med. Bull. **48:** 10–22.
3. JUNIPER, E. F., et al. 1990. Effect of long-term treatment with an inhaled corticosteroid (budesonide) on airway hyperresponsiveness and clinical asthma in nonsteroid-dependent asthmatics. Am. Rev. Respir. Dis. **142:** 832–836.

4. ALI, N. J., S. CAPEWELL & M. J. WARD. 1991. Bone turnover during high dose inhaled corticosteroid treatment. Thorax **46:** 160–164.
5. VAN VYVE, T., *et al.* 1992. Safety of bronchoalveolar lavage and bronchial biopsies in patients with asthma of variable severity. Am. Rev. Respir. Dis. **146:** 116–121.
6. GIBSON, P. G., *et al.* 1989. Cellular characteristics of sputum from patients with asthma and chronic bronchitis. Thorax **44:** 693–699.
7. PIN, I., *et al.* 1992. Induced sputum cell characteristics in normal and asthmatic subjects. Thorax **47:** 25–29.
8. TONNEL, A. B., P. H. GOSSET & M. JOSEPH. 1983. Stimulation of alveolar macrophages in asthmatic patients after local provocation test. Lancet **1:** 1406–1408.
9. SEDGWICK, J. B., *et al.* 1991. Immediate and late airway response of allergic rhinitis patients to segmental antigen challenge—Characterization of eosinophil and mast cell mediators. Am. Rev. Respir. Dis. **144:** 1274–1281.
10. GODARD, PH., A. M. CLAUZEL, J. BOUSQUET & F. B. MICHEL 1991. Role of allergenic bronchial challenge in the evaluation of antiasthma drugs. Eur. Respir. Rev. **1:** 25–33.
11. BOUSQUET, J., *et al.* 1990. Eosinophilic inflammation in asthma. New Eng. J. Med. **323:** 1033–1039.
12. REDIER, H., *et al.* 1992. Inhibitory effect of cetirizine on the bronchial eosinophil recruitment induced by allergen inhalation challenge in allergic patients with asthma. J. Allergy Clin. Immunol. **90:** 215–224.
13. AALBERS, R., H. F. KAUFFMAN, B. VRUGT, G. H. KOETER & J. G. R. DEMONCHY. 1993. Allergen-induced recruitment of inflammatory cells in lavage three and 24 h after challenge in allergic asthmatic lungs. Chest **103:** 1178–1184.
14. TOMIOKA, M., S. IDA & Y. SHINDOH. 1984. Mast cells in bronchoalveolar lumen of patients with bronchial asthma. Am. Rev. Respir. Dis. **129:** 1000–1005.
15. CASALE, T. B., *et al.* 1987. Elevated bronchoalveolar lavage fluid histamine levels in allergic asthmatics are associated with metacholine bronchial hyperreactivity. J. Clin. Invest. **79:** 1197–1203.
16. DJUKANOVIC, R., *et al.* 1990. Mucosal inflammation in asthma. Am. Rev. Respir. Dis. **142:** 434–457.
17. PIN, I., *et al.* 1992. Changes in the cellular profile of induced sputum after allergen-induced asthmatic responses. Am. Rev. Respir. Dis. **145:** 1265–1269.
18. HOLGATE, S. T. 1993. Mediator and cytokine mechanisms in asthma. Thorax **48:** 103–109.
19. LEBEL, B., *et al.* 1988. Spontaneous and non specific releasibility of histamine and PGD2 by bronchoalveolar lavage cells from asthmatic and normal subjects effect of nedocromil sodium. Clin. Allergy **18:** 605–613.
20. MATTOLI, S., M. MEZZETTI, A. FASOLI, F. PATALANO & L. ALLEGRA. 1990. Nedocromil sodium prevents the release of 15-hydroxyeicosatetraenoic acid from human bronchial epithelial cells exposed to toluene diisocyanate invitro. Int. Arch Allergy Appl. Immunol. **92:** 16–22.
21. RADEAU, T., *et al.* 1993. Effect of nedocromil sodium on sulfidopeptide leukotriene-stimulated human alveolar macrophages in asthma. Pulm. Pharmacol. **6:** 27–31.
22. PAGE, C. P. 1991. One explanation of the asthma paradox—Inhibition of natural anti-inflammatory mechanism by beta2-agonists. Lancet **337:** 717–720.
23. FALLER, B., Y. MELY, D. GERARD & J. G. BIETH. 1992. Heparin-induced conformational change and activation of mucus protienase inhibitor. Biochemistry **31:** 8285–8290.
24. BOWLER, S. D., S. M. SMITH & P. S. LAVERCOMBE. 1993. Heparin inhibits the immediate response to antigen in the skin and lungs of allergic subjects. Am. Rev. Respir. Dis. **147:** 160–163.
25. CAMPBELL, A. M., *et al.* 1992. Viability of and mediator release from, bronchial epithelial cells from healthy subjects and asthmatics. Chest **131:** 25s–27s.
26. JEFFERY, P. K., A. J. WARDLAW, F. C. MELSON, J. V. COLLINS & A. B. KAY. 1989. Bronchial biopsies in asthma. An ultrastructure, quantitative study and correlation with hyperreactivity. Am. Rev. Respir. Dis. **140:** 1745–1753.
27. BEASLEY, R., W. R. ROCHE, J. A. ROBERTS & S. T. HOLGATE. 1989. Cellular events

in the bronchi in mild asthma and after bronchial provocation. Am. Rev. Respir. Dis. **139:** 806–817.

28. CAMPBELL, A. M., *et al.* 1993. Functional characteristics of bronchial epithelium obtained by brushing from asthmatic and normal subjects. Am. Rev. Respir. Dis. **147:** 529–534.

29. VACHIER, I., PH. GODARD, F. B. MICHEL, B. DESCOMPS & M. DAMON. 1990. Aberrant expression of antigen HLA-DR of class-II MHC in bronchial epithelial cells from asthmatic patients. C. R. Acad. Sci., Ser. III **311:** 341–346.

30. VIGNOLA, A. M., *et al.* 1993. HLA-DR and ICAM-1 expression on bronchial epithelial cells in asthma and chronic bronchitis. Am. Rev. Respir. Dis. In press.

31. WEGNER, C. D., *et al.* 1990. Intercellular adhesion molecule-1 (ICAM-1) in the pathogenesis of asthma. Science **247:** 456–459.

32. GUNDEL, R. H., C. D. WEGNER, C. A. TORCELLINI & L. G. LETTS. 1992. The role of intercellular adhesion molecule-1 in chronic airway inflammation. Clin. Exp. Allergy. **22:** 569–576.

33. RANKIN, J. A., *et al.* 1992. Human airway macrophages—A technique for their retrieval and a descriptive comparison with alveolar macrophages. Am. Rev. Respir. Dis. **133:** 928–933.

34. VAN VYVE, T. H., *et al.* 1992. Comparison between bronchial and alveolar samples of BAL fluid in asthma. Chest **102:** 356–361.

35. POSTON, R. N., *et al.* 1992. Immunohistochemical characterization of the cellular infiltration in asthmatic bronchi. Am. Rev. Respir. Dis. **145:** 918–921.

36. CHANEZ, P., *et al.* 1993. Proliferation of airway macrophages in asthmatics and normal subjects. J. Allergy Clin. Immunol. In press.

37. VACHIER, I., *et al.* 1992. Increased oxygen species generation in blood monocytes of asthmatic patients. Am. Rev. Respir. Dis. **133:** 1161–1166.

38. AUBAS, P., B. COSSO, PH. GODARD, F. B. MICHEL & J. CLOT. 1984. Decreased suppressor cell activity of alveolar macrophages in bronchial asthma. Am. Rev. Respir. Dis. **130:** 875–878.

39. CHANEZ, P., *et al.* 1993. ICAM-1 and LFA-1 expression on alveolar macrophages (AM) in asthma. Am. Rev. Respir. Dis. **147:** A520.

40. GODARD, PH., M. DAMON, P. CHANEZ & F. B. MICHEL. 1991. Releasability of airway macrophages in bronchial asthma. Int. Arch. Allergy Appl. Immunol. **95:** 97–101.

41. CLUZEL, M., *et al.* 1987. Enhanced alveolar cell luminol-dependent chemiluminescence in asthma. J. Allergy Clin. Immunol. **80:** 195–201.

42. DAMON, M., H. VIAL, A. CRASTES DE PAULET & PH. GODARD. 1988. Phosphoinositide breakdown and superoxide anion release in formyl-peptide-stimulated human alveolar macrophages. Comparison between quiescent and activated cells. FEBS Lett. **239:** 169–173.

43. HERRSCHER, R. F., C. KASPER & T. J. SULLIVAN. 1992. Endogenous cortisol regulates immunoglobulin E-dependent late phase reactions. J. Clin. Invest. **90:** 596–603.

44. CORRIGAN, C. J. & A. B. KAY. 1992. T-Cells and eosinophils in the pathogenesis of asthma. Immunol. Today **13:** 501–507.

45. BENTLEY, A. M., *et al.* 1993. Increases in activated T-lymphocytes, eosinophils, and cytokine messenger RNA expression for interleukin-5 and granulocyte/macrophage colony-stimulating factor in bronchial biopsies after allergen inhalation challenge in atopic asthmatics. Am. J. Respir. Cell Mol. Biol. **8:** 35–42.

46. SALMERON, S., *et al.* 1989. High doses of inhaled corticosteroids in unstable chronic asthma: A multicenter, double-blind, placebo-controlled study. Am. Rev. Respir. Dis. **140:** 167–171.

47. SZEFLER, S. J. 1991. Glucocorticoid therapy for asthma—Clinical pharmacology. J. Allergy Clin. Immunol. **88:** 147–165.

48. LANE, S. J. & T. H. LEE. 1991. Glucocorticoid receptor characteristics in monocytes of patients with corticosteroid-resistant bronchial asthma. Am. Rev. Respir. Dis. **143:** 1020–1024.

49. WOOLCOCK, A. J. 1993. Steroid resistant asthma: What is the clinical definition? Eur. Respir. J. **6:** 743–747.

50. CALDERON, E., R. F. LOCKEY, S. C. BUKANTZ, R. G. COFFEY & D. K. LEDFORD. 1992. Is there a role for cyclosporine in asthma? J. Allergy Clin. Immunol. **89:** 629–636.

51. MULLARKEY, M. F., J. K. LAMMERT & B. A. BLUMENSTEIN. 1991. Methotrexate for asthma. Ann. Intern. Med. **115:** 66–67.

52. BERLOW, B. A., M. I. LIEBHABER & Z. DYER. 1991. The effect of dapsone in steroid-dependent asthma. J. Allergy Clin. Immunol. **87:** 710–715.

53. BERNSTEIN, D. I., I. L. BERNSTEIN & S. BODENHEIMER. 1988. An open study of auranofin in the treatment of steroid-dependent asthma. J. Allergy Clin. Immunol. **81:** 6–10.

54. BOUSQUET. J. Asthma: A disease remodelling the airways. *In* Advances in Allergology and Clinical Immunology. Ph. Godard, J. Bousquet, and F. B. Michel, Eds. Parthenon.

55. PEAT, J. K., A. J. WOOLCOCK & K. CULLEN. 1987. Rate of decline of lung function in subjects with asthma. Eur. J. Respir. Dis. **70:** 171–179.

56. LAITINEN, L. A., A. LAITINEN & T. HAAHTELA. 1993. Airway mucosal inflammation even in patients with newly diagnosed asthma. Am. Rev. Respir. Dis. **147:** 697–704.

57. SAETTA, M., *et al.* 1992. Effect of cessation of exposure to toluene diisocyanate (TDI) on bronchial mucosa of subjects with TDI-induced asthma. Am. Rev. Respir. Dis. **145:** 169–174.

58. REDIER, H., J. P. DAURES, C. MICHEL, F. B. MICHEL & PH. GODARD. 1992. Validation of an expert system in asthmology. Eur. Respir. J. **4:** 326S.

59. BOUSQUET, J. & F. B. MICHEL. 1992. Advances in specific immunotherapy. Clin. Exp. Allergy **22:** 889–896.

60. LASSALLE, P., *et al.* 1993. T-cell and B-cell immune response to a 55-kDa endothelial cell-derived antigen in severe asthma. Eur. J. Immunol. **23:** 796–803.

61. FITZGERALD, J. M., D. SWAN & M. O. TURNER. 1992. The role of asthma education. Can. Med. Ass. J. Allergy Clin. Immunol. **147:** 855–856.

62. ISRAEL, E., P. RUBIN & J. KEMP. 1993. The effect of inhibition of 5-lipoxygenase by Zileuton in mild to moderate asthma. Ann. Intern. Med. In press.

63. MCMILLAN, R. M., K. E. SPRUCE, G. C. CRAWLEY, E. R. H. WALKER & S. J. FOSTER. 1992. Pre-clinical pharmacology of ICI-D2138, a potent orally-active non-redox inhibitor of 5-lipoxygenase. Br. J. Pharmacol. **107:** 1042–1047.

64. NEWSHOLME, S. J. & L. B. SCHWARTZ. 1993. cAMP-specific phosphodiesterase inhibitor, Rolipram, reduces eosinophil infiltration evoked by leukotrienes or by histamine in guinea pig conjunctiva. Inflammation **17:** 25–31.

65. ALABASTER, V. A. & B. A. MOORE. 1993. New perspectives on basic mechanisms in lung disease. 3. Drug intervention in asthma—Present and future. Thorax **48:** 176–182.

Index of Contributors